Third Edition

Deshpande's

Mechanical Ventilation

Clinical Application

Third Edition

Deshpande's Mechanical Ventilation

Clinical Application

Editor-in-Chief

R Vijai Kumar MD (Resp) DTCD
Senior Pulmonologist and Critical Care Specialist
Director, Hyderabad Chest Center
Hyderabad

Editor

Vijay Deshpande MS RRT FAARC
Emeritus Professor
Georgia State University
Atlanta, Georgia, USA

Visiting Faculty
School of Allied Health Sciences
Manipal, Karnataka (India)

Associate Editor

Srinivas Samavedam MD DNB FRCP FNB EDIC
Diploma in Health Care Quality Management
Diploma in Medical Law and Ethics MBA (Hosp Admin)
President, Elect ISCCM
Associate Editor, IJCCM

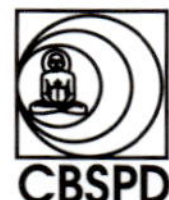

CBS Publishers & Distributors Pvt Ltd

New Delhi • Bengaluru • Chennai • Kochi • Kolkata • Lucknow • Mumbai
Hyderabad • Jharkhand • Nagpur • Patna • Pune • Uttarakhand

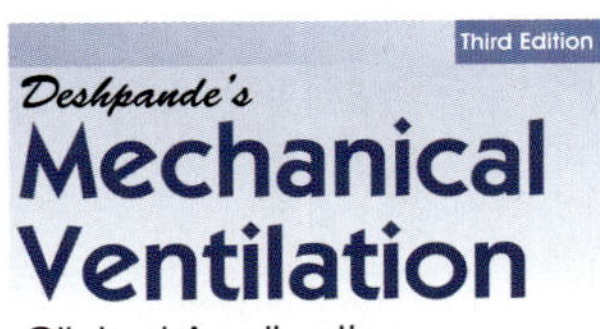

ISBN: 978-93-5466-765-7

Third Edition: 2025
First Edition: 2012
Second Edition: 2015
Reprint: 2017, 2018, 2020, 2022

Published by Satish Kumar Jain and produced by Varun Jain for

CBS Publishers and Distributors Pvt Ltd

4819/XI Prahlad Street, 24 Ansari Road, Daryaganj, New Delhi 110 002, India.
Ph: 011-23289259, 23266838 Website: www.cbspd.com
e-mail: delhi@cbspd.com;

Corporate Office: 204 FIE, Industrial Area, Patparganj, Delhi 110 092, India
Ph: 011-4934 4934 Fax: 011-4934 4935 e-mail: publishing@cbspd.com;
publicity@cbspd.com

Branches

- **Bengaluru:** Seema House 2975, 17th Cross, K.R. Road, Banasankari 2nd Stage, Bengaluru 560 070, Karnataka, India
  Ph: +91-80-26771678/79 Fax: +91-80-26771680 e-mail: bangalore@cbspd.com
- **Chennai:** 18/8B, Subbarayan Street, Shenoy Nagar, Chennai 600 030, Tamil Nadu, India.
  Ph: +91-44-42032115, 26681266 e-mail: chennai@cbspd.com
- **Kochi:** 42/1325, 36, Power House Road, Opposite KSEB, Kochi-682 018, Kerala, India.
  Ph: +91-484-4059061-67 Fax: +91-484-4059065 e-mail: kochi@cbspd.com
- **Kolkata:** 147, Hind Ceramics Compound, 1st Floor, Nilgunj Road, Belghoria, Kolkata-700 056, West Bengal, India
  Ph: +91-33-25633055–56 e-mail: kolkata@cbspd.com
- **Lucknow:** Basement, Khushnuma Complex, 7-Meerabai Marg (Behind Jawahar Bhawan), Lucknow-226 001, Uttar Pradesh, India.
  Ph: +91-522-4000032 e-mail:tiwari.lucknow@cbspd.com
- **Mumbai:** PWD Shed, Gala No. 25/26, Ramchandra Bhatt Marg, Next to JJ Hospital Gate No. 2, Opp Union Bank of India, Noorbaug, Mumbai-400009, Maharashtra, India
  Ph: +91-22-66661880, 66661889 e-mail: mumbai@cbspd.com

Representatives

- **Hyderabad** 0-9885175004
- **Jharkhand** 0-9811541605
- **Nagpur** 0-8692091830
- **Patna** 0-9334159340
- **Pune** 0-9664372571
- **Uttarakhand** 0-9716462459

Printed at: Magic International Pvt. Ltd., Greator Noida, UP, India

to

my patients and my students

Dr R Vijai Kumar

all my students and my grandchildren— Deven and Bodhi

Prof Vijay Deshpande

Contributors

Anand Vinaykumar Joshi
MBBS; DNB (Gen. Med), FRCP (Lon), FCICM (Aus and NZ), FNB (Critical Care-India), EDIC (UK), PGCC (Echo-Uni Melb.)
Intensivist and Physician
Gaman Hospital, Hyderabad, India.
Campbeltown Hospital, Sydney, NSW, Australia
Mater Private Hospital, Townsville, Queensland, Australia
St Vincent Hospital, Towoomba, Queensland, Australia

Anil Kumar Chillimuntha
BRT, MBA, MA, MPhil, PhD, PhD, CPQIH, FAGE
Executive Vice President
METAS Adventist Group of Colleges and Hospitals
Surat, India

Anitha Patil GK PG Diploma in Respiratory Therapy
Respiratory Therapist
CARE Hospital Hitech-City
Hyderabad, India

Anitha Shenoy MD, FRCA
Professor
Department of Anaesthesiology
Kasturba Medical College, Manipal
Karnataka, India

Ashfaq Hasan MD (Pulmonary Medicine)
Professor
Department of Pulmonary Medicine
Deccan College of Medical Sciences
Hyderabad, India

Balasubrahmanyam CH MD EDIC IDCCM FCCP
Senior Consultant, Critical Care Medicine
Citizens Specialty Hospital
Hyderabad, India

Chandresh Kumar Sudani
DNB (Anesthesia), IDCCM, PGDHHM
Consultant Intensivist
Department of Critical Care Medicine
Pulse Heart Super Specialty Hospital
Hyderabad, India

Chris Sara Mathew MSRT
Lecturer, Respiratory Care
Liwa College
Abu Dhabi, UAE

Dharani Narendra MD; FCCP
Assistant Professor and Director
Critical Care Fellowship Program,
Pulmonary Critical Care and Sleep Section
Baylor College of Medicine
Ben Taub General Hospital
Houston Texas, USA

Hari Prasad A MBBS, DNB, FNB
Consultant, Critical Care Medicine
Yashoda Hospitals,
Hyderabad, India

Hillary Vaughan MD
Fellow, Pulmonary, Critical Care and Sleep Medicine Section
Baylor College of Medicine
Ben Taub General Hospital
Houston Texas, USA

Jayaprakash Narayana Reddy
BSc BLSS & ACLS, PGDM, BMPH
Senior Respiratory Therapist
Respiratory Therapy Unit
Salmaniya Medical Complex
Manama, Kingdom of Bahrain

Jithin K Sreedharan
BSc RT, MSc RT, PhD, FiSQua, FIARC
Assistant Professor and Head
Department of Respiratory Therapy
College of Health Sciences
University of Doha for Science and Technology
Doha, Qatar

Kalpalatha K Guntupalli
MD, FCCM, Master FCCP, MACP
Frances K. Friedman and Oscar Friedman, MD '36
Endowed Professor for Pulmonary Disorders
Program Director, Critical Care Fellowship
Department of Medicine
Baylor College of Medicine
Houston, Texas, USA

K Hima Bindu MBBS, DNB
Pulmonologist, KPBH, Hyderabad

Krushna Chandra Misra MBBS, DNB, IDCCM, CPHCM
Head, Department of Critical Care
Yashoda Hospitals
Somajiguda, Hyderabad, India

Lisha PV MBBS, MD, DNB, DM
Assistant Professor Pulmonary Medicine
Amala Institute of Medical Sciences
Thrissur, Tamil Nadu, India

Madhuragauri Shevade MSc, RRT-NPS, FIARC
Manager (Training Programs)
Chest Research and Training Pvt Ltd
Pune, Maharashtra, India

Manjush Karthika PhD, PDF
Head
Department of Health and Medical Sciences
Associate Professor, Respiratory Care
Liwa College
Abu Dhabi, United Arab Emirates

Maneendra Singarapu MD,FNB,EDIC
Head Department of Critical Care Medicine
Gleneagles Global Hospitals
Hyderabad, India

Manimala S Rao MD, DA (Lond), FCCP, FICCM
Senior Consultant in Critical Care
Director, Medical Education (Academics)
Krishna Institute of Medical Sciences and Hospitals
Secunderabad, India

Monalisa Sahu MD, DM (AIIMS, New Delhi)
Consultant, Department of Infectious Diseases
Yashoda Hospitals, Hyderabad, India

Nagarjuna Maturu MD, DM, FCCP, (USA), FAPSR, FICS
Senior Consultant and Head
Department of Pulmonary Medicine
Yashoda Hospitals
Hyderabad, India

Nalini Nagalla MD, FSM (ISDA)Consultant Pulmonologist
Head, Sleep Disorders Center
Continental Hospital
Hyderabad, India

Narasimha Murthy T
PG Diploma in Respiratory Therapy
Senior Respiratory Therapist
Nizam Institute of Medical Sciences
Hyderabad, India

Palepu B Gopal MD, FRCA, FCCM
Senior Consultant, Critical Care Medicine
Citizens Specialty Hospital
Hyderabad, India

Pavan Gorukanti MD, (Pulmonary Critical Care)
Director, Yashoda Hospitals
Hyderabad, India

Pavan Kumar Reddy N
MD, FNB, EDIC, FICCM, MBA (HA)
Associate Clinical Director and Head
Department of Critical Care Medicine
Director, Sparsh Critical Care
Hyderabad, India

Rakesh Venuturumilli
MBBS, DA, DNB, IDCCM, FECMO, FIDM
Consultant and Head
Department of Critical Care and ECMO
GEM Care Poulomi Hospitals
Hyderabad, India

Raj Kumar Jupally MD, FNB
Consultant, Critical Care
Apollo Health City
Hyderabad, India

Ravi Krishna M
DNB (Pulmonary Medicine), DM (Critical Care), FECMO
Lead Consultant, Critical Care Medicine
ECMO Department, KIMS-ICON Hospital
Visakhapatnam, India

Rinoosha BR MD, FIP, FSM
Associate Consultant
Interventional Pulmonology
Yashoda Hospitals
Hyderabad, India

Ruben Restrepo MD, RRT, FAARC, FCCP
Coordinator of Research-Division of Respiratory Care
Distinguished Teaching Professor
UT Health SAN Antonio
SAN Antonio TX

R Vijai Kumar
MD (Resp), DTCD
International Fellow AARC (USA)
Governor's Community Service Award (ACCP, USA)
Director, Pulmonary Academics
Yashoda Hospitals
Consultant Pulmonologist
Hyderabad Chest Center
Vice Chairman, TB Alert (India)
Vice President, Indian Chest Society
Editorial Board of Indian Journal Respiratory Care
Editorial Board of Indian Journal Sleep Medicine
Hyderabad, India

Sagar Sunka MBBS, MD, FNB, EDIC
Consultant Intensivist
CARE Hospitals (Banjara), Hyderabad, India
sagarocean49@gmail.com

Sai Praveen Haranath MBBS, MPH, FCCP
American Board Certified in Internal Medicine
Pulmonary and Critical Care Medicine
Senior Consultant Pulmonologist and Critical Care Specialist
Medical Director
Apollo eACCESS Tele-ICU Service,
Clinic Director, Apollo LAM Clinic, part of the LAM Foundation International Clinic Network
Apollo Hospitals
Hyderabad, India

Sambit Sahu
Director, Medical Services, and
Head, Department of Critical Care
KIMS Hospitals
Hyderabad, India

Sanjay Sasikumar MSRT
Respiratory Therapist
Rashid Hospital
Dubai, UAE

Saumy Johnson
BSc RT, MSc RT, PhD, RPSGT, FNIV, FIARC
Associate Professor and In-charge of Respiratory Therapy
Department of Anesthesiology and Critical Care
Amrita Institute of Medical Sciences
Kochi, India

Saurabh Biswal MBBS, DA, DNB, IDCCM, IFCCM, EDIC
Consultant Intensivist
STAR Hospital, Hyderabad, India
biswal.saurabh@gmail.com

Shyamsunder Tipparaju MD, PDCC, FICCM
Director, Virinchi Hospital
Hyderabad, India

Shwethapriya R MD
Professor and Head
Department of Critical Care Medicine
Kasturba Medical College, Manipal
Karnataka, India

Shweta Ram Chandankhede
MBBS, MD, IDCCM, IFCCM
Consultant Intensivist
CARE Hospitals (Banjara), Hyderabad, India
shwets0106@gmail.com

Sricharan G MD, IDCCM
Consultant, Critical Care
Yashoda Hospitals
Hyderabad, India

Srinivas Samavedam
MD, DNB, FRCP, FNB, EDIC, FICCM, DMLE, MBA
Chief Intensivist, Ramdev Rao Hospital
Hyderabad, India

Srinivas Jakkinaboina MD, DM, EDIC
Head
Department of Critical Care Medicine, and
Medical Director
Amor Hospitals
Hyderabad, India

Subba Reddy K MD PDCC IDCCM IFCCM EDIC
Senior Consultant, Critical Care
Apollo Health City
Hyderabad, India

Sudipta Mukherjee MBBS, MD (Anaesthesiology), IDCCM, FNB (Critical Care Medicine), EDICM
Senior Consultant and Head
Department of Critical Care Medicine
Tata Medical Center, Kolkata, India

Sumita Agrawal MD; DM; MRCP (UK); FIP
Consultant and Head
Department of Pulmonary, Critical Care and Sleep Medicine
Medpulse Hospital Jodhpur, Rajasthan

Swarna Deepak
MD, MRCP, EDIC, IDCCM, IFCCM, FIDM
Senior Consultant, Critical Care Medicine
Apollo Health City, Hyderabad

TR Chandrashekar MD
Intensivist
Liver Transplantation
Department of SGE and LT
Bangalore Medical College and Research Institute
Superspeciality Hospital
Bangalore, India

Tisha Ann Skariah BSRT, MSRT
Neonatal and Paediatric Respiratory Care
Liwa College
Abu Dhabi, United Arab Emirates

Uthara Vijai Kumar MBBS, DNB (Resp.Med)
Consultant Pulmonologist
Sri Lakshmi Medical Centre and Hospital
Coimbatore, Tamil Nadu, India

Venkat Raman Kola
MD, DNB, IDCCM, EDIC, FICCM, HCM (ISB)
Clinical Director
Yashoda Hospitals
Hyderabad, India

Vajrapu Rajendra
MD, FNB, EDIC
Head, Department of Internal Medicine, and Critical Care
Gleneagles Aware Hospitals
Hyderabad, India

Vijay Deshpande MS RRT FAARC
Emeritus Professor
Georgia State University
Atlanta, Georgia, USA
Visiting Faculty
School of Allied Health Sciences
Manipal University
Manipal, Karnatak, India

Viswesvaran Balasubramanian
MD; DNB; DM (Pulmonary and Critical Care);
Consultant
Interventional Pulmonology and Sleep Medicine
Yashoda Hospitals
Hyderabad, India

Foreword

I am very pleased to write the Foreword to the book *Deshpande's Mechanical Ventilation: Clinical Application* edited by Dr Ratnavelu Vijai Kumar.

Having been a teacher and a practitioner of critical care for over 4 decades. I have been a witness to the evolution of sophisticated technology in mechanical ventilatory support. This is in response to the needs of the clinicians and the changing patient population.

The beginning of the specialty of respiratory care practitioners and the maturation of the scope of their practice also brought forth significant contributions to the art and science of providing mechanical ventilatory support. The integration of the intensivist, respiratory care practitioner, residents, fellows, and nurses into the ICU team requires that they all be familiar with the workings of the ventilator albeit at various levels of expertise. It also means there should be educational tools that are suitable for the entire team.

What do these various learners want from a book on mechanical ventilation?

A book that is written by authors who are reputable, scholarly and experts in the content matter.

Table of contents, that is comprehensive addressing different disease conditions.

Chapters cover historical perspectives to make the reading interesting and put it in today's perspective.

This book incorporates all of the above and more mechanical ventilation, being a life-supporting/life-sustaining intervention, necessarily is technically advanced, complicated, and sophisticated. While fulfilling the changing and varied nature of the patient, it should also have several modes to respond to the differing needs of the patient.

Being the life support device for a major organ system, ventilator also affects other organs systems, and all these nuances must be understood by the clinicians. This book addresses all these requirements.

Data from reputable journals/trials is reviewed and recommendations are based on high-grade peer-reviewed articles.

Contributors are respiratory care practitioners, intensivists, and pulmonologists from the global community, which makes it relevant to a larger audience.

A book that allows you to recognize the pros and cons of using different modalities and their use in varied conditions in an ICU.

This book on mechanical ventilation satisfies the needs of all levels of learners. It is comprehensive. Dr Vijai Kumar has built upon the first edition by Mr Vijay Deshpande incorporating the newer developments, and adding almost 10 new chapters. Chapters on communication, transport of patient on mechanical ventilator, ultrasound for a patient on ventilator, maintenance of ventilator after their use, etc. are welcome additions.

The many years of bedside experience of the chapter contributors are obvious and highlights the context of the recommendation as it relates to the local conditions.

It will be a "must have" and "must read" book on mechanical ventilation for intensivists, pulmonologists, respiratory therapists, nurses, and postgraduate students.

I congratulate Dr R Vijai Kumar for pulling this yeoman's task together and wish him the very best!

Kalpalatha K Guntupalli
MD, FCCM, Master FCCP, MACP
Frances K. Friedman and Oscar Friedman, MD'36
Endowed Professor for Pulmonary Disorders
Department of Medicine
Baylor College of Medicine
Houston, USA

Foreword

Mechanical ventilation stands as a beacon of modern medicine, illuminating the path toward life-saving interventions in critical care settings. As we embark on this journey through the intricate mechanisms of ventilatory support, it is with great honor that I introduce, *Deshpande's Mechanical Ventilation: Clinical Application* this profound and updated exploration into the realm of mechanical respiration. Ventilators, once deemed marvels of technology, have become indispensable allies in the fight against respiratory failure. From the early prototypes born out of necessity to the sophisticated computers adorning modern intensive care units, the evolution of mechanical ventilation mirrors the relentless pursuit of excellence in medical science. In this comprehensive, third edition, expert contributors delve into the fundamental principles underlying mechanical ventilation, unraveling the complexities of graphic waveforms that govern decisions with each breath. Some information on the modes of ventilation are meticulously orchestrated by the interplay of pressure, volume, and flow, describing the management of each possible disease or syndrome. Yet, beyond the realm of technical prowess of the practitioner lies the essence of patient care. Mechanical ventilation transcends mere mechanical support; it embodies the essence of empathy, dedication, and unwavering commitment to preserve life as the discussion on sedation and analgesics is used to combat asynchrony. Each breath delivered through the ventilator serves as a lifeline, as you learn of newer forms of ventilation, such as neurally adjusted assist and interplay the addition of extracorporeal membrane oxygenation bridging ventilation and oxygenation

Within these pages of *Deshpande's Mechanical Ventilation: Clinical Application*, clinicians and students will find a treasure trove of knowledge, ranging from the basic principles of respiratory physiology to the intricacies of ventilator management. Through explanations, illustrative diagrams, and clinical vignettes, the authors aim to demystify the enigma of mechanical ventilation, empowering learners to navigate its complexities with confidence and competence. As you embark on this odyssey through the realm of mechanical ventilation, let us remember the patients whose lives are entrusted to our care. May their resilience inspire us, their struggles humble us, and their triumphs fuel our relentless pursuit of excellence. I am so grateful to all the contributing authors for continuing this work and the dedication to my good friend and colleague, Prof Vijay Deshpande.

Douglas S Gardenhire
EdD, RRT, RRT-NPS, FAARC
Assistant Dean, International Initiatives
Lewis College of Nursing and Health Professions
Chair and Clinical Professor
Department of Respiratory Therapy
Georgia State University
Atlanta, Georgia, USA

Preface to the Third Edition

This textbook *Deshpande's Mechanical Ventilation: Clinical Application* is just out of the printing press, and is being served hot to all those who were eagerly waiting for a long time.

This book is packed in its 534 pages, very comprehensive, authentic, contemporary, knowledge on almost all aspects of mechanical ventilation.

The right place for this book, is on the study table of every doctor connected with the care of patient who needs mechanical ventilation. Of course, this textbook is not just a reference book but also a quick guide to questions arising in everyday critical care work in the hospital. Every intensive care unit (ICU) dealing with mechanical ventilation should have a copy in an easily accessible place.

This book is special, because it has 35 chapters covering almost every aspect of mechanical ventilation. Many of us desperately will be searching for answers to some issues, while engaged in care of patients on mechanical ventilation.

This book has 57 contributing authors, who are highly accomplished and are leaders in their field of expertise. Many of these authors have published their own books, contributed chapters to various textbooks, and have been authors of original research papers.

This book is special because almost all chapters from the previous edition have been rewritten by new authors, and 10 new chapters and revised old chapters will fill the void arising out of evolving critical care practice. These new chapters include the following topics:

1. How to perform suctioning
2. How to transport a patient who is on a ventilator
3. How to use an ultrasound bedside of a patient on ventilator
4. Neonatal ventilation
5. How to talk to the family of a patient on a ventilator
6. How to organize an ICU to provide MV
7. How do we maintain the MV support system
8. Role of ECMO and its relation to MV
9. How to perform bronchoscopy on a patient on MV
10. However, there is one new chapter which is very close to my heart, and that is

"Role of a Respiratory Therapist" in the management of MV.

As a result of rewriting, the existing chapters and adding new chapters, the book may look slightly bulkier but certainly provides interesting and immersive reading.

As Sir William Osler, an all-time great physician has said "that to study medicine without books is to sail an uncharted sea, but to study books alone, is not to go to sea at all." This book provides the much-needed down to earth practical knowledge.

R Vijai Kumar

Contents

CHAPTER 1

Indications for Mechanical Ventilation

❐ Krushna Chandra Misra ❐ Hari Prasad A

INTRODUCTION

The importance of positive pressure ventilation was well known since its use by Bjorn Ibsen in polio epidemics of 1950s. Since then there has been growing knowledge among the intensivists regarding patient–ventilator interactions which helped in reducing ventilator related complications.[1–4] With the advancement of computers and electronic technology ventilators have changed markedly in their appearances and minimising dyssynchrony. However, the fundamental principles of ventilator treatment of the critically ill patient remain unchanged, although there are several new nuances in their applications.[5–7]

Mechanical ventilation utilises positive pressure devices to provide O_2 and CO_2 transport between the pulmonary capillary bed and the environment. The goal of mechanical ventilation is to relieve the inspiratory muscles while maintaining sufficient levels of PO_2 and PCO_2 in arterial blood. The lungs and other organ systems should not be damaged during this operation, which should be carried out carefully.[8–10]

A mechanical ventilatory support system's essential elements are:

- An artificial airway that serves as the interface between the mechanical ventilator and the patient's airways (or, occasionally, a mask).
- A source of oxygen-enriched positive pressure breaths that are given either in reaction to a patient's effort or according to a predetermined timer.
- The ability to sustain a positive end expiratory pressure.

The following categories represent the main indications for invasive mechanical ventilation:

- Illness of the compromised airways.[11]
  - Airway protection in patients with dynamic airways or obtunded airways, such as those caused by trauma or oropharyngeal infections.
  - Angioedema, for example, causes proximal obstruction of the airways, while asthmatic bronchospasm and acute exacerbations of chronic obstructive pulmonary disease cause distal obstruction.
- Hypercapnic respiratory failure is caused by hypoventilation as a result of impaired drive, pump failure, or inability to exchange gases.

The following subcategories of the aetiology can be made:

- Central drive impairment, such as drug overdose[12]
- Muscular weakness in the respiratory muscles (including myositis and muscular dystrophy)[13]
- Defects of the peripheral nerve system, such as Guillain-Barré syndrome and myasthenic crises[14]
- Restrictive ventilatory problems (such as large pneumothorax, illness, or trauma to the chest wall)

✦ The inability to exchange oxygen or supply it to the peripheral tissues may be the cause of hypoxemic respiratory failure for one of the following reasons:
  - Acute respiratory distress syndrome (ARDS), pneumonia, and pulmonary edoema are a few examples of alveolar filling abnormalities.
  - Massive pulmonary embolism or air emboli caused by pulmonary vascular abnormalities that result in a mismatch between ventilation and perfusion (VQ)
  - Insufficiencies in diffusion (advanced pulmonary fibrosis)

✦ Increased ventilatory demand as a result of shock, acute metabolic acidosis, or severe sepsis.[15]

Controller Failure

The brain stem is the primary location of the ventilatory control system, which comprises an intrinsic ventilator pattern generator with three different types of inputs.[16] Afferent nerves from mechanoreceptors in the lung and chest wall make up one input. These detect irritants, ventilatory muscle loads, and respiratory system stretch. The central and peripheral chemoreceptors that sense pH, PCO_2, and PO_2 provide a second set of inputs. Cortical signals are a last input that alter the breathing rhythm during voluntary activities. The control system's goal is to maintain an appropriate degree of ventilation to facilitate CO_2 and O_2 transport while reducing the mechanical demands placed on the ventilatory muscles. This control system strategy results in the typical resting ventilatory pattern of 10–12 breaths/min, tidal volumes of 5–7 mL/kg, and inspiratory:expiratory timing of 1:2–1:3.[17]

Any central nervous system (CNS) injury, but particularly those that disrupt brain stem function, can weaken this system. General anaesthesia, a number of medications, particularly sedatives and opioid analgesics, and CNS damage can also impact its function. Respiratory arrest is the result of ventilatory controller failure at its worst. The controller's capacity to deliver sufficient inspiratory muscle stimulation will be compromised by damage to efferent neurons, particularly the phrenic nerve.

Although some CNS injuries might result in unwarranted hyperventilation, most diseases and medications that impact the ventilatory control system typically have as their side effect insufficient ventilation, which leads to a respiratory acidosis (hypercarbic respiratory failure). The clinical context determines the pH threshold from a respiratory acidosis that necessitates mechanical ventilatory support. Clinical investigations have demonstrated that pH levels as low as 7.15 (or maybe lower) do not hurt when there are no substantial cardiac dysrhythmias, pressor-dependent hypotension, or high intracranial pressure.[18] However, the decision to start mechanical ventilation is typically based on the clinical judgement that the ventilatory drive is unreliable for maintaining a safe level of ventilation for a protracted period of time in patients with hypoventilation and respiratory acidosis due to CNS reasons.

The mechanical ventilation strategy must ensure that an appropriate minute ventilation is given if mechanical ventilation is necessary for a ventilatory controller that is defective. In order to ensure proper tidal volumes, this frequently necessitates clinician-controlled ventilator breath rates as well as either set tidal volumes or pressure-targeted feedback devices. Correctly set alarm systems are essential.

Inappropriate flow demands and breath timing patterns may also result from abnormal ventilatory control systems. These can be particularly difficult for medical professionals who want to keep patients as awake as possible while also giving them assisted breaths that match their needs.[19]

Demand/Capability Imbalances

The airway resistance, compliance/elastance of the respiratory system, and minute ventilation demands are the main mechanical pressures on the ventilatory muscles.[9] The amount of minute ventilation wasted (dead space ventilation, or VD) and metabolic needs, such as oxygen intake (VO_2) and carbon dioxide generation (VCO_2), are what determine minute ventilation requirements. Both the patient's airway geometry and the characteristics of the artificial airway contribute to airway resistance. Both parenchymal lung abnormalities and abnormalities of the chest wall (such as tight surgical dressings, abdominal compartment syndrome, anasarca, ascites, and obesity) influence compliance/elastance qualities. Artificial airway resistance and patient ventilator dyssynchrony are examples of imposed stresses from the ventilator itself.[20] The amount of inspiratory muscle work necessary to begin breathing can increase when intrinsic positive end expiratory pressure (PEEP) is present.

The strength and endurance of the inspiratory muscle make up the ventilatory system's capacity in the patient. Metabolic disorders, systemic inflammation, dietary variables, electrolyte problems, and medications can all have an impact on these. Given that the diaphragm is the primary muscle used for inspiration, its resting position is extremely crucial. Inspiratory muscle power is severely reduced if the diaphragm is flattened due to lung hyperinflation, bullous illness, or intrinsic PEEP.

When the demands exceed the capacity, ventilational muscle failure and inadequate ventilation follow **(Fig. 1.1)**. Rapid, shallow breathing, which is a muscular "protective" reaction regulated by the ventilatory control centre, is frequently the first clinical sign of this.[21] As overworked muscles continue to contract, injury to the muscles, worsening hypoventilation, and a respiratory acidosis (hypercarbic respiratory failure) take place. Respiratory arrest is the result of ventilatory muscle failure at its worst.

Conceptual relationship between ventilatory muscle demands (left side of balance) and capabilities (right side of balance). As demands overwhelm capabilities, the balance shifts to the left and indications for mechanical ventilatory support increases.

The therapeutic decision to begin mechanical ventilatory support for demand/capability imbalances is best guided by mechanical assessments because gas exchange may be sufficient in the face of progressive ventilatory muscle overload for a protracted period of time. Importantly, this is done more through an assessment of muscle load tolerance than it is by an assessment of mechanical loads (such as work of breathing

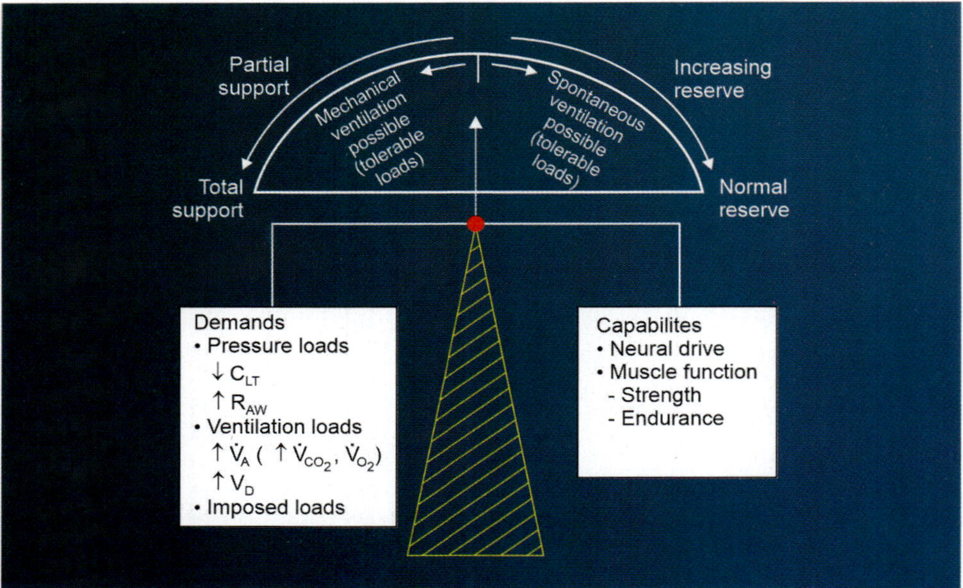

Fig. 1.1: Conceptual relationship between ventilatory muscle demands (left side of balance) and capabilities (right side of balance). As demands overwhelm capabilities, the balance shifts to the left and indications for mechanical ventilatory support increases. (*Courtesy:* MacIntyre NR, 'Respiratory factors in weaning from mechanical ventilatory support', Respiratory Care, 40, pp. 244–8, © The Journal Respiratory Care Company 1995.)

or pressure time product, which may be multiplied multiple times in patients needing mechanical ventilation). Conceptually, this can be stated by calculating a pressure time index (P_{TI}[22]) using a transdiaphragmatic pressure compared to muscular strength:

$$P_{TI} = (PD_{tidal}/PD_{max}) \times (T_i/T_{tot})$$

where PD_{tidal} is the transdiaphragmatic pressure change during inspiration, PD_{max} is the maximal voluntary transdiaphragmatic pressure, and T_i/T_{tot} is the fraction of the ventilator cycle spent in inspiration. A PTI value greater than 0.15 is associated with impending inspiratory muscle failure.

Clinically, tachycardia, abdominal paradox, auxiliary muscle usage, diaphoresis, and the difficulty to talk in short sentences are all signs of load intolerance.[21,23,24] In this situation, the decision to introduce mechanical ventilation is typically driven by clinical assessment that load intolerance is becoming lethal. Under these conditions, objective measurements or laboratory results may support the decision to start mechanical ventilation support, but they rarely offer conclusive data that would overturn the clinical evaluation.

When there is a demand/capability imbalance, mechanical ventilation techniques concentrate on increasing muscle capabilities and decreasing muscle loads. Positive pressure breaths are used to properly unload the ventilatory muscles in this process. However, support measures should not completely deplete the muscles used for breathing because this can lead to muscular atrophy.[25] This refers to a mechanical ventilation method that is centred on patient-triggered aided modes of breathing that are titrated to comfort. The ability to provide effective breath triggering (including the use of circuit PEEP in the setting of intrinsic PEEP), proper flow synchrony so that ventilator flow matches patient demand, and proper breath cycling to correspond with neural cycling are required for this.[18,20] To ensure appropriate lung emptying and reduce intrinsic PEEP, it also calls for the proper setting of the respiratory rate and I:E ratio. Importantly, this assistance does not necessarily necessitate the insertion of an endotracheal tube. Non-invasive (mask) ventilation may prevent endotracheal intubation in patients with load/capability mismatches but adequate airway protection abilities, especially in the COPD population experiencing an acute exacerbation.

Maintaining Alveolar Patency

Alveoli can flood or collapse as a result of numerous lung illnesses that affect the lung parenchyma. There are many factors that can be involved, including inhalation injuries, infections, systemic inflammation (such sepsis or pancreatitis), blunt chest trauma, aspiration, congestive heart failure, and fluid overload. Ventilation perfusion mismatching, which results in shunts and hypoxaemia (hypoxaemic respiratory failure), is the main clinical symptom of alveolar patency loss. The compliance/elastance loads that come from alveolar instability, if they are severe enough, can potentially lead to ventilatory muscle overload and hypercarbic respiratory failure.

Arterial PO_2 values above 55 mmHg are often sufficient to provide tissue oxygen supply, provided that other aspects of oxygen delivery (such as cardiac output and hemoglobin concentration) and tissue oxygen extraction are acceptable. Alterations in mental status, cardiac dysrhythmias, and other organ dysfunction are all clinical indicators that oxygen delivery is insufficient and that therapy is required. The emergence of a metabolic (lactic) acidosis is one piece of objective evidence supporting poor tissue oxygenation.

PEEP should be used carefully to stabilise alveoli while also providing more oxygen to individuals whose alveolar function is reduced.[26] Continuous positive airway pressure (CPAP), delivered using either a mask or an endotracheal tube, may be all that is necessary to achieve this if a tolerable load/capability balance exists (for instance, in patients with certain types of cardiogenic pulmonary edema). Concomitant ventilatory support is also frequently required, though. In these circumstances, it is critical to keep in mind that PEEP has two sides. The risk of over distention injury increases with the addition of the expiratory pressure to the total intrathoracic pressure, which is especially true when combined with an excessive tidal volume.[26–28] On the other hand, the expiratory pressure can help preserve alveolar patency during exhalation. It is obvious that balancing PEEP and FiO_2 to give adequate oxygenation in the case of alveolar injury is a significant therapeutic problem.

Support for an Artificial Airway

There are numerous diseases that can affect airway function.[29] Coughing and/or other airway defence reflexes may stop working as a result of CNS disorders (such as CNS damage, tumors, or medications). Aspiration of posterior pharyngeal debris and the inability to ventilate due to airway compromise are examples of clinical implications. Structure-related injuries to the pharynx, larynx, and main airways can potentially impair airway function.

Clinical signs of loss of airway patency include difficulty breathing, insufficient ventilation, and occasionally stridor. Weak or non-existent cough (particularly when being suctioned), the requirement for frequent suctioning (e.g. more frequently than every two hours), and clinical aspiration are signs of insufficient airway protection.[29]

The placement of an artificial airway (endotracheal tube or tracheostomy) is frequently necessary due to compromised airway function and/or the inability to protect the airway, even though a mask system with constant positive airway pressure can often alleviate airway compromise from some structural abnormalities (such as obstructive sleep apnea). 89% of patients with oral tracheal tubes, 4% with nasal tracheal tubes, and 4.9% with facial masks had them, according to a comprehensive survey of more than 5000 patients undergoing mechanical ventilation.[30] Two percent of the patients had a tracheostomy. Intriguingly, 22% of the 85 COPD patients who got non-invasive ventilation (NIV) in this sample afterwards needed tracheal intubation. 138 patients with different types of respiratory failure were given NIV, and 36.5% of them later needed tracheal intubation.

Many patients can tolerate an artificial airway (particularly a tracheostomy) for isolated airway difficulties quite well, barring the need for positive pressure breathing. Nevertheless, endotracheal tubes in particular can place a heavy resistive load on the inspiratory muscles, especially if they are small (i.e. less than 7 mm internal diameter) and/or partially obstructed by secretions.[31] In order to ensure tolerance, endotracheal tubes can potentially be painful and necessitate sedation and/or painkillers. In these circumstances, mechanical ventilation support could be required to help patients tolerate the artificial airway. This involves targeted ventilation at low pressure levels with possible back-up rates and PEEP (for example, inspiratory pressure support of 5 to 10 cmH_2O). Some gadgets come with an automatic tube or airway compensation feedback mechanism that gives inspiratory pressure support in a manner particularly intended to discharge the calculated resistance loads of the artificial airway. Although intriguing on paper, there is currently little evidence that this feedback capability enhances clinical results.

Conclusion

In ICUs all across the world, mechanical ventilation is a widespread method. The concept of mechanical ventilation is that it should be used when a patient's capacity to effect gas transport across the alveolar capillary interface and/or ventilate the lung is seriously damaged to the point of danger. In actuality, this entails dealing with one or more of the three basic pathophysiological processes—lack of adequate ventilatory control, imbalances in the demand-capability of the ventilatory muscle, and/or loss of alveolar patency. A patient who is unable to maintain a patent, protected airway requires positive pressure assistance as a fourth general indication in order to tolerate an artificial airway.

Despite the fact that there are some hard-and-fast thresholds for starting mechanical ventilation (such as respiratory arrest, refractory hypoxemia, severe acidosis from ventilatory muscle failure, and inability to protect the airway), the choice to start mechanical ventilation typically involves a comprehensive evaluation of the patient. This evaluation should cover the patient's mental state, capacity for protecting the airways, tolerance for ventilatory muscle strain, spontaneous ventilatory pattern, and any indications of organ dysfunction brought on by acidosis or hypoxemia. A great degree of clinical competence is required for this. Giving mechanical ventilatory support has the potential to save lives, but it has a high level of danger and should only be used when necessary.

References

1. Ibsen B. The anaesthetist's viewpoint on the treatment of respiratory complications in poliomyelitis during the epidemic in Copenhagen, 1952. Proc R Soc Med. 1954;47(1):72–74.
2. Gibney RTN, Wilson RS, Pontoppidan H (1982) Comparison of work of breathing on high gas flow and demand valve continuous positive airway pressure systems. Chest 82:692
3. Marini JJ, Capps JS, Culver BH (1985) The inspiratory work of breathing during assisted mechanical ventilation. Chest 87:613
4. Hubmayr, Rolf D. MD; Abel, Martin D. MD; Rehder, Kai MD. Physiologic approach to mechanical ventilation. Critical Care Medicine 18(1):p 103-113, January 1990.
5. Slutsky AS (1993) Mechanical ventilation. American College of Chest Physicians' Consensus Conference. Chest 104: 1833–1859
6. Kacmarek RM, Meklaus GJ. The new generation of mechanical ventilators. Crit Care Clin. 1990 Jul;6(3):551-78. PMID: 2198996.
7. Tobin MJ: Mechanical ventilation. N Engl J Med 1994:330:1056-60.
8. Gattinoni L, Protti A, Caironi P, and Carlesso E. (2010). Ventilator-induced lung injury: the anatomical and physiological framework. Critical Care Medicine, 38(10, Suppl.), S539–48.
9. Tejerina E, Frutos-Vivar F, Restrepo MI, et al. (2006). Incidence, risk factors, and outcome of ventilator-associated pneumonia. Journal of Critical Care, 21, 56–65.10.1016/j.jcrc.2005.08.005
10. Girard TD, Kress, JP, Fuchs BD, et al. (2008). Efficacy and safety of a paired sedation and ventilator weaning protocol for mechanically ventilated patients in intensive care (awakening and breathing controlled trial): a randomized controlled trial. Lancet, 371, 126–34.
11. Pham T, Brochard LJ, Slutsky AS. Mechanical Ventilation: State of the Art. Mayo Clin Proc. 2017 Sep;92(9):1382-1400.
12. Farkas A, Lynch MJ, Westover R, Giles J, Siripong N, Nalatwad A, Pizon AF, Martin-Gill C. Pulmonary Complications of Opioid Overdose Treated With Naloxone. Ann Emerg Med. 2020 Jan;75(1):39-48.
13. Jablonski R, Bhorade S, Strek ME, Dematte J. Recognition and Management of Myositis-Associated Rapidly Progressive Interstitial Lung Disease. Chest. 2020 Jul;158(1):252-263.
14. Neumann B, Angstwurm K, Mergenthaler P, Kohler S, Schönenberger S, Bösel J, Neumann U, Vidal A, Huttner HB, Gerner ST, Thieme A, Steinbrecher A, Dunkel J, Roth C, Schneider H, Schimmel E, Fuhrer H, Fahrendorf C, Alberty A, Zinke J, Meisel A, Dohmen C, Stetefeld HR., German Myasthenic Crisis Study Group. Myasthenic crisis demanding mechanical ventilation: A multicenter analysis of 250 cases. Neurology. 2020 Jan 21;94(3):e299-e313.
15. Jung B, Martinez M, Claessens YE, Darmon M, Klouche K, Lautrette A, Levraut J, Maury E, Oberlin M, Terzi N, Viglino D, Yordanov Y, Claret PG, Bigé N., Société de Réanimation de Langue Française (SRLF). Société Française de Médecine d'Urgence (SFMU). Diagnosis and management of metabolic acidosis: guidelines from a French expert panel. Ann Intensive Care. 2019 Aug 15;9(1):92.
16. Ramirez JM, Zuperku EJ, Alheid GF, et al. (2002). Respiratory rhythm generation: converging concepts from in vitro in vivo approaches? Respiratory Physiology and Neurobiology, 131, 43–56.10.1016/S1569-9048(02)00036-8

17. Otis AB, Fenn WO, and Rahn H. (1950). Mechanics of breathing in man. Journal of Applied Physiology, 2(11), 592–607.
18. Hickling KG, Walsh J, Henderson S, and Jackson R. (1994). Low mortality rate in adult respiratory distress syndrome using low-volume, pressure-limited ventilation with permissive hypercapnia: a prospective study. Critical Care Medicine, 22, 1568–78.
19. Tobin MJ, Jubran A, and Laghi F. (2001). Patient-ventilator interaction. American Journal of Respiratory and Critical Care Medicine, 163, 1059–63.10.1164/ajrccm.163.5.2005125
20. MacIntyre NR. McConnell R, and Cheng KC. (1997). Applied PEEP reduces the inspiratory load of intrinsic PEEP during pressure support. Chest, 1111, 188–93.10.1378/chest.111.1.188
21. Tobin MJ, Chadha TS, Jenouri G, et al. (1983). Breathing patterns 2: diseased subjects. Chest, 84, 286–94.
22. Bellemare, F and Grassino A. (1982). Effect of pressure and timing of contraction on human diaphragm fatigue. Journal of Applied Physiology, 53(5), 1190–5.
23. Pierson DJ. (2002). Indications for mechanical ventilation in adults with acute respiratory failure. Respiratory Care, 47, 249–62.
24. Hudson LD. (1983). Evaluation of the patient with acute respiratory failure. Respiratory Care, 28, 542–52.
25. Petrof BJ, Jaber S, and Matecki S. (2010). Ventilator-induced diaphragmatic dysfunction. Current Opinion in Critical Care, 16, 19–25.10.1097/MCC.0b013e328334b166.
26. MacIntyre NR. (2008). Is there a best way to set positive end expiratory pressure for mechanical ventilatory support in acute lung injury. Clinical Chest Medicine, 29, 233–40.
27. Gattinoni L, Carlesso E, and Cressoni M. (2011). Assessing gas exchange in acute lung injury/acute respiratory distress syndrome: diagnostic techniques and prognostic relevance. Current Opinion in Critical Care, 17, 18–23.10.1097/MCC.0b013e32834272d8.
28. Briel M, Meade M, Mercat A, et al. (2010). Higher vs lower positive end-expiratory pressure in patients with acute lung injury and acute respiratory distress syndrome: systematic review and meta-analysis. Journal of the American Medical Association, 303, 865–73.10.1001/jama.2010.218.
29. Shaker R. (1995). Airway protective mechanisms: current concepts. Dysphagia, 10, 216–27.10.1007/BF00431413.
30. Esteban A, Anzueto A, Frutos F, et al. (2002). Characteristics and outcomes in adult patients receiving mechanical ventilation. Journal of the American Medical Association, 287(3), 345–55.10.1001/jama.287.3.345.
31. Shapiro M, Wilson RK, Casar G, et al. (1986). Work of breathing through different sized endotracheal tubes. Critical Care Medicine, 14, 1028–31.10.1097/00003246-198612000-00007.

CHAPTER 2

Terms and Definitions Related to Mechanical Ventilation

❐ Vijay Deshpande ❐ TR Chandrashekar

In mechanical ventilation the delivery of air to the lungs is accomplished in two ways—by providing positive pressure at the airways or creating sub-atmospheric pressure at the chest wall. Secondly, these delivery methods can be given invasively or non-invasively (**Fig. 2.1**).

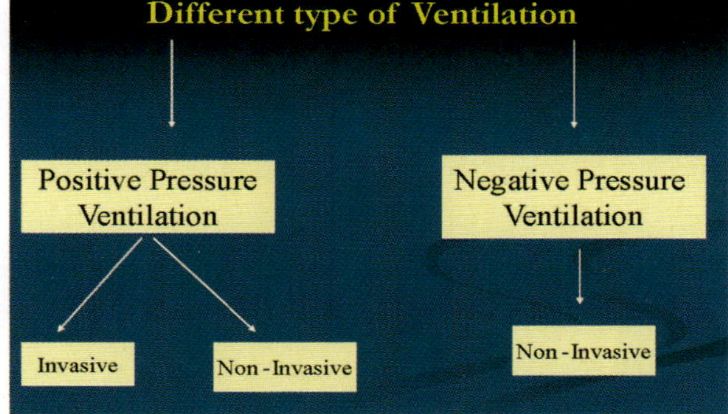

Fig. 2.1

Negative Pressure Ventilation

This type of ventilation, not requiring tracheal intubation, is also known as non-invasive ventilation (NIV). A negative extrathoracic pressure is applied to the chest wall.

This causes a rise in the chest wall resulting in decreased intra-thoracic pressure and creates a pressure gradient from the mouth to alveoli. Inspiration occurs (**Figs 2.2 and 2.3**).

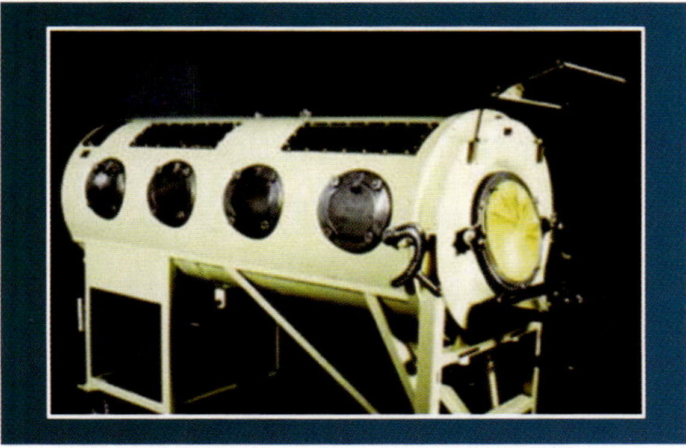

Fig. 2.2: Iron lung, an early developed negative pressure ventilator. The patient is placed in the cabinet with his head outside. A pump creates extrathoracic negative pressure increasing thoracic volume and thus, decreases intrathoracic pressure. Inspiration occurs. This type of ventilation is also non-invasive ventilation, since the patient does not require tracheal intubation

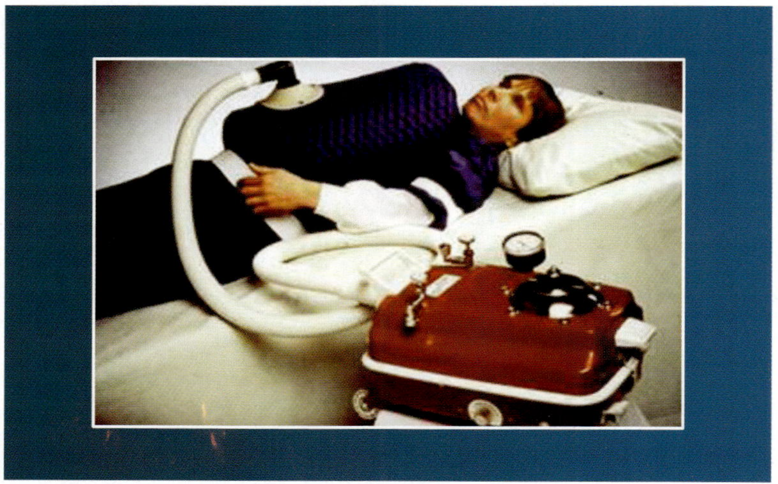

Fig. 2.3: Chest Curraise represents another negative pressure ventilator where a negative pressure is generated by a suction pump at the chest. Chest wall is lifted to create negative extrathoracic volume providing negative intrathoracic pressure to promote inspiration

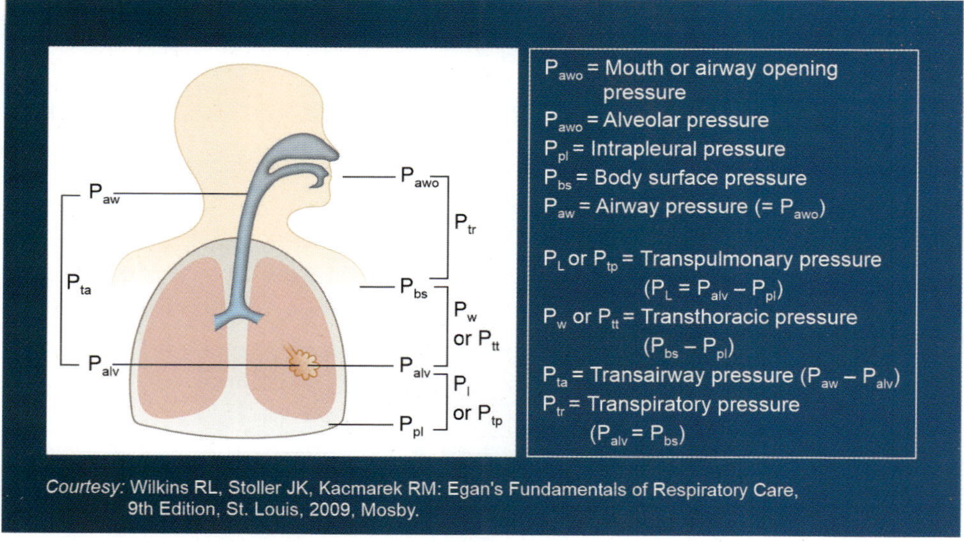

Fig. 2.4

Airway Opening Pressure (P_{awo})

Other terms: Mouth Pressure (P_m), Airway Pressure, Mask Pressure, Proximal Airway Pressure, Upper-airway Pressure. Since the baseline pressure is atmospheric, in pulmonary medicine P_{awo} is normally considered as Zero or Atmospheric. In situations such as positive pressure ventilation the P_{awo} is positive and during tracheal suction it is negative.

Body Surface Pressure (P_{bs}) is also zero or atmospheric in normal conditions. P_{bs} increases when a patient is placed in a Hyperbaric Chamber for treatment. During Negative Pressure Ventilation P_{bs} is negative.

Intrapleural Pressure (P_{pl}) is always less than atmospheric. It is the pressure in the potential space between the parietal and visceral pleura. It is difficult to reach this space to measure P_{pl}. A special balloon catheter is inserted in the esophagus to obtain Esophageal Pressure which is a close estimation of the pleural pressure. P_{pl} is approximately –5 cm H_2O at the end expiration during normal spontaneous breathing and becomes more negative (~ –10 cm H_2O) at the end of inspiration.

Alveolar Pressure (P_{alv}) or Intrapulmonary Pressure is directly dependent on the pleural pressure (P_{pl}). During normal spontaneous breathing, at the end expiration when P_{pl} is –5 cm H_2O, the alveolar pressure (P_{alv}) is the same as P_{awo} or mouth pressure with no gas flow. At the beginning of exhalation P_{alv} is greater than atmospheric (~ +3–4 cm H_2O) promoting exhalation. During mechanical ventilation P_{alv} is obtained from plateau pressure (Pp). This will be discussed in details in later chapters.

Transairway Pressure (P_{TA}) is the pressure gradient between P_{awo} and P_{alv}. PTA is the pressure gradient required to generate airflow against the frictional resistance. In situations of increased airway resistance (P_{RAW}) the transairway pressure needs to be increased to overcome airway resistance to ventilate the lung.

Transpulmonary pressure (P_L), the gradient between alveolar pressure and pleural pressure ($P_L = P_{alv} - P_{pl}$). During exhalation, the alveolar pressure decreases. However, PL at end exhalation does not allow alveoli to close, thus, it is also referred to as Alveolar Distending Pressure. P_L is essential to open alveoli during inspiration. In spontaneous breathing, contraction of the diaphragm increases the negative intrapleural pressure (more negative) resulting in increased P_L and expansion of the lung. In mechanical ventilation application of positive pressure at the airway opening increases P_{alv} and thus, increases P_L which results in lung expansion.

Positive Pressure Ventilation

A positive pressure (greater than atmospheric) is applied to the mouth (P_{awo}) providing a positive pressure gradient from mouth to alveoli (P_{TA}) resulting in inspiration. This can be applied with a mask (non-invasive) or with a tracheal tube (invasive). Current ICU ventilators are primarily positive pressure ventilators.

Volume Ventilation

Generally referred to as Volume Targeted Ventilation. Tidal volume, set by the clinician, is delivered by the ventilator during each mechanical breath. Ventilating pressure is variable, and depends on the lung characteristics such as airways resistance or lung compliance.

Pressure Ventilation

Also called Pressure Targeted Ventilation. Ventilator uses clinician set ventilating pressure as the target. It delivers this pressure to the patient's airways. Lung characteristics determine the volume delivered to the lung. In situations of increased airways resistance some of the delivered pressure is used up in overcoming the airways resistance. Thus, lesser pressure is available for lung expansion and lesser volume delivery. During pressure ventilation when lung compliance is decreased (stiffer lung), strong elastic forces allow lesser volume to be delivered at the set pressure. Thus, changes in lung characteristics affect volume delivery at the same applied pressure **(Table 2.1)**.

Table 2.1

	Tidal Volume (V_T)	Pressure
Volume Ventilation	Clinician Set	Varies as Resistance and Compliance change
Pressure Ventilation	Varies as Resistance and Compliance change	Clinician Set

Essential Parameters in Mechanical Ventilation

Triggering (Initiation of a Breath)

Triggering refers to initiation of a mechanical breath

1. **Patient Triggered or Assisted Ventilation** where a mechanical breath results from an inspiratory effort made by the patient.
2. **Time Triggered or Controlled Ventilation** is a term used when a mechanical breath is generated by a timer allowing delivery of breaths at fixed time intervals.
3. Triggering can be secondary to a negative pressure generated by the patient **(Pressure triggering)** or it results when patient removes a specific amount of flow from the circuit during inspiratory effort **(Flow triggering)**.
4. **Figure 2.5** demonstrates two mechanical breaths, an assist breath indicating a small negative deflection on the P/T scalar before the breath is traced, whereas, the time triggered control breath begins at the baseline.

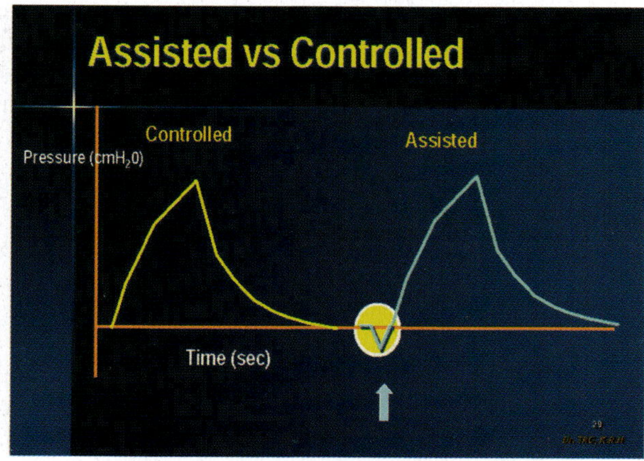

Fig. 2.5

Cycling (Termination of a Breath)

Termination of a mechanical breath is called "cycling". Cycling parameters are characteristics of different ventilator modes (**Figs 2.6A to C**).

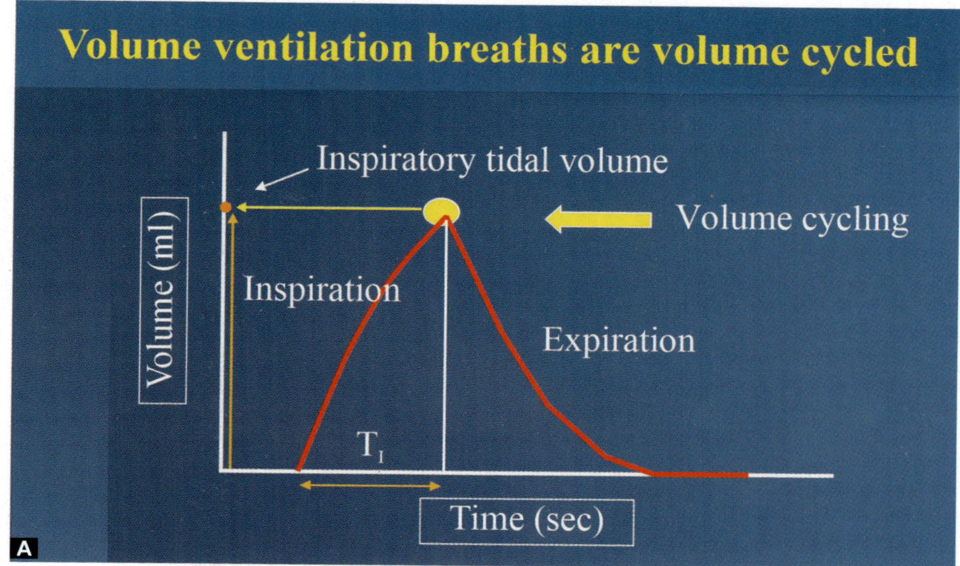

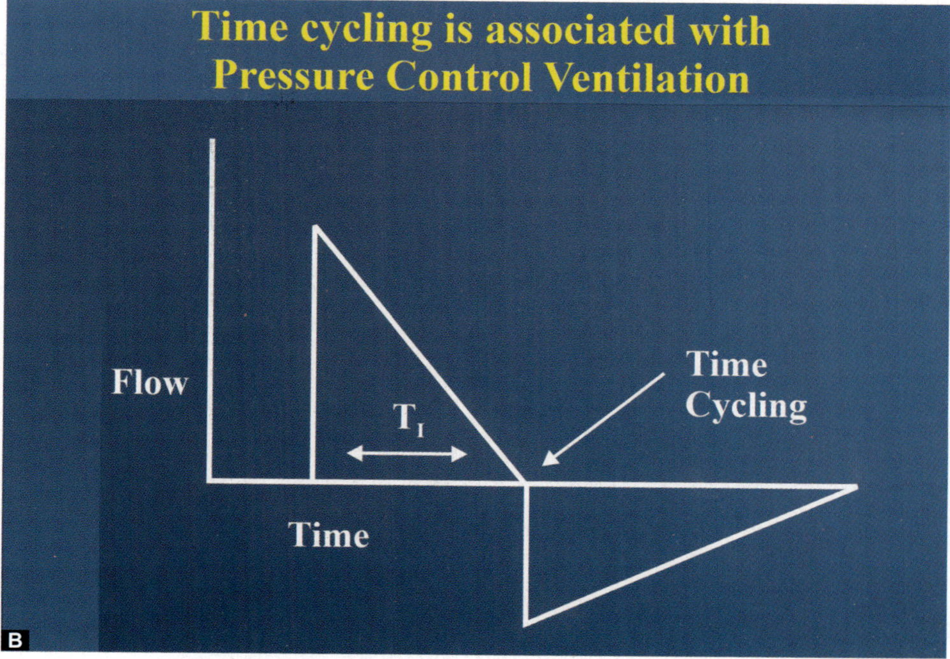

Fig. 2.6A and B

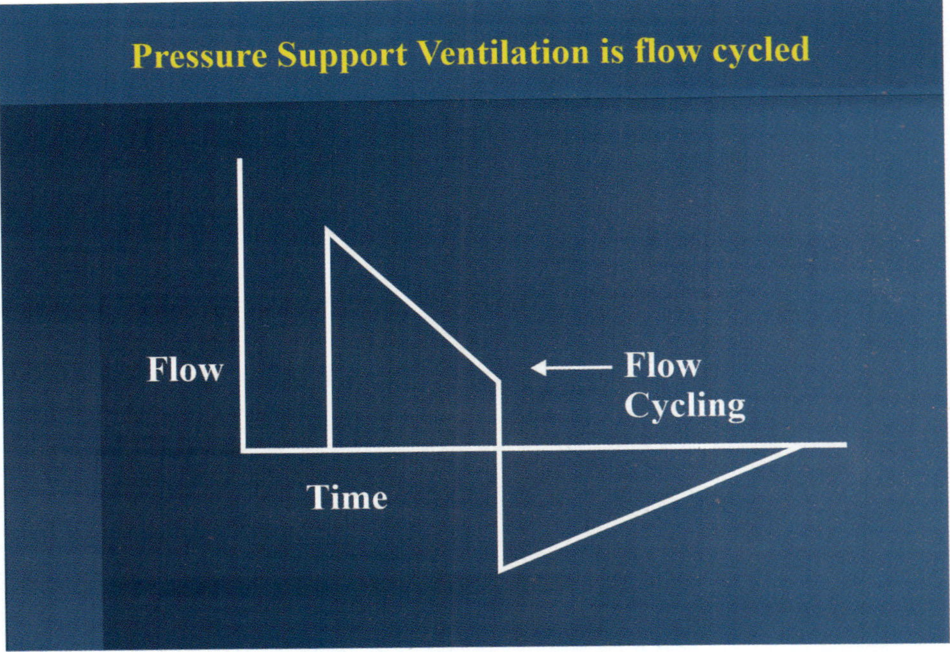

Fig. 2.6C

1. **Pressure-Cycled:** Inspiration is terminated when the preset pressure reaches.
2. **Volume-Cycled:** Inspiration is terminated when the preset volume is delivered by the ventilator.
3. **Time-Cycled:** When the preset inspiratory time elapses, inspiration is terminated.
4. **Flow-Cycled:** Inspiration is terminated when flow decreases to a system specific flow rate.

Interrelationship between Ventilator Parameters

Tidal Volume (V_T)

Volume delivered by the ventilator per breath. It is also the average volume inspired by a spontaneously breathing patient per minute (minute volume). Tidal volume can be calculated by dividing minute volume by the respiratory frequency. Measured in milliliters (ml) or liters (l).

Inspiratory flow rate ($\dot{V}$)

$\dot{V}$ = Inspiratory flow = $V_T \times f$

$V_T = \dot{V} \times T_I$

Respiratory Frequency (*f*)

Number of breaths taken spontaneously or delivered by the ventilator or in combination of spontaneous and mechanical breaths in one minute. Frequency is expressed in number of breaths per minute. f = breaths/min.

Minute Volume (V_E)

Volume delivered spontaneously or by the ventilator or in combination of spontaneous and mechanical breaths per minute. It is the volume delivered per breath (tidal volume) times the frequency $V_E = V_T \times f$.

Inspiratory Flow Rate ($\dot{V}$)

Inspiratory flow rate determines the rate of delivery of tidal volume. How fast or slow the volume is delivered.

$\dot{V}$ = Inspiratory flow = V_T/T_I

Inspiratory time and tidal volumes can be calculated,

$V = \dot{V} \times T_I$ and $T_I = V_T/\text{flow rate}$

Inspiratory Time (T_I)

This is the time required to deliver the set tidal volume at a given inspiratory flow rate $T_I = V_T/\text{flow rate}$

As the inspiratory flow rate is increased, the volume is delivered in shorter time. Conversely, for a fixed tidal volume slower flow rates will require longer inspiratory time to deliver the volume.

Cycle Time (T_C)

Respiratory rate or frequency (f) is expressed in cycles or breaths per minute. Thus, time needed to complete one cycle or breath is called cycle time (T_C).

$$T_C = 60 \text{ seconds/respiratory frequency}$$
$$= 60 \text{ sec}/f$$

Typical time parameters in mechanical ventilation are Inspiratory time, Expiratory time and Cycle time. They are interrelated.

$$T_C = T_I + T_E$$

Thus, $T_I = T_C - T_E$

and $T_E = T_C - T_I$

Expiratory Time (T_E)

This is the time used for expiration and is the remainder of the cycle time after the inspiration is completed.

$T_E = T_C - T_I$. For a given cycle time (60 sec/respiratory frequency) as inspiratory time is decreased (by increasing inspiratory flow rate), the expiratory time increases. Conversely, for a given Inspiratory Time and Expiratory Time, as the respiratory frequency is decreased the expiratory time increases.

Inspiratory Time %

This expresses the % of cycle time used for inspiration. If the cycle time is 4 seconds and the T_I% is set at 25%, the actual Inspiratory Time is 25% of 4 seconds or 1 second.

I–E ratio

An I–E ratio indicates the ratio of inspiratory time to expiratory time, i.e. $T_I{:}T_E$. It is conventionally expressed as a ratio with left side of the equation reduced to 1. If the inspiratory time is 2 seconds and expiratory time is 3 seconds, the actual I–E ratio is 2 : 3. However, conventionally it is written as, 1 : 1.5. Similarly if T_I is 3 seconds and T_E is 6 seconds the I–E ratio is 1 : 2 (3 seconds: 6 seconds).

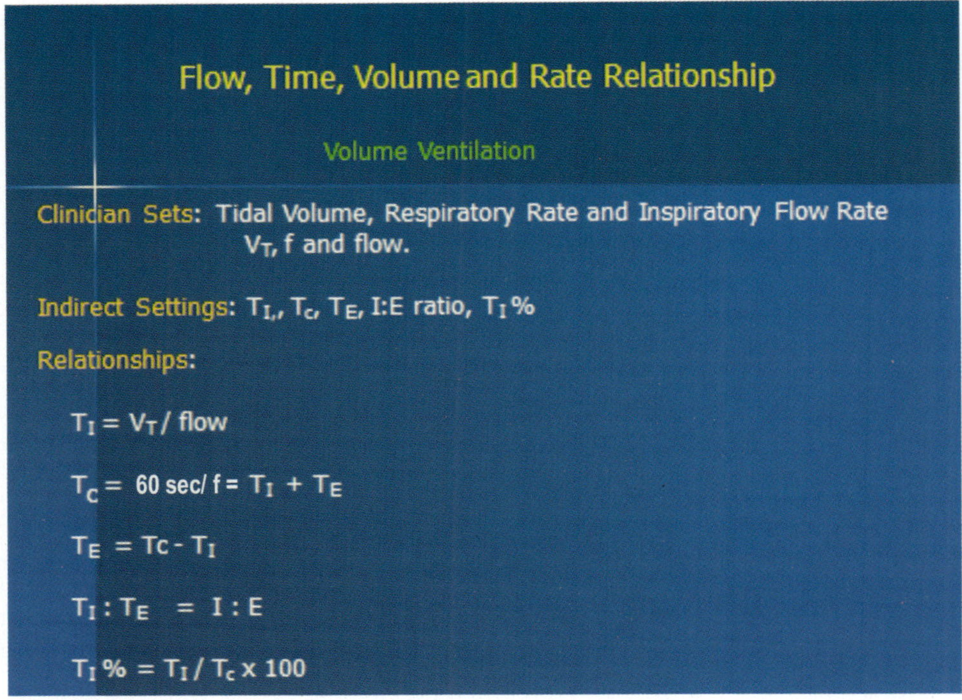

Fig. 2.7: Summarizes the interrelation ship between the above basic parameters. Based on clinical situation clinician is generally involved in making changes in one or more parameters. These changes may have an effect on other parameters. For example, when a clinician changes inspiratory time, it changes inspiratory flow rate and also change expiratory time

Some of the above material will be repeated in later chapters to re-emphasize the basic concepts.

CHAPTER 3

Initial Settings

❑ Madhuragauri Shevade ❑ Vijay Deshpande

INTRODUCTION

What we have seen so far in the previous chapters, is the foundation for mechanical ventilation. This forms the basis of ventilatory management for any disease or condition. However, it is pertinent for any clinician to first understand and then implement the correct strategies for mechanical ventilation using the appropriate settings. The fundamentals of the disease pathology and how it affects the functioning of the lung, followed by the outcome of the patient assessment, should be evaluated while making the decision. They must also understand the differences in the ventilator, and the similar as well as unique settings that each ventilator comes with. With that basic information, we will now look at the initial settings that a clinician must know and understand while initiating a patient on mechanical ventilation.

Initial Considerations

Before initiating any mode of mechanical ventilation, it is important to keep in mind some initial considerations. Firstly, we need to understand the reasons for the need and the goal for mechanical ventilation. Then, the diseases/conditions for which the patient requires ventilatory support should be considered as well. Finally, one must also understand why the patient is not able to support their own respiration and what is the status of the lungs. Once that is decided, then one can proceed with setting up of the ventilator.

Ventilator Parameters

When initiating mechanical ventilation, there are several points that one must consider and arrive at a decision to successfully ventilate a patient (**Fig. 3.1**). Although there is no set rank in which each setting needs to be selected, once it is determined that the patient needs ventilatory support, generally the selection of the mode and the control variable is done followed by the selection of values for the variables for the mode. Modes for invasive mechanical ventilation have more variables to be set as compared to noninvasive mechanical ventilation. **Table 3.1** enlists some of the basic parameters that are set when initiating mechanical ventilation.

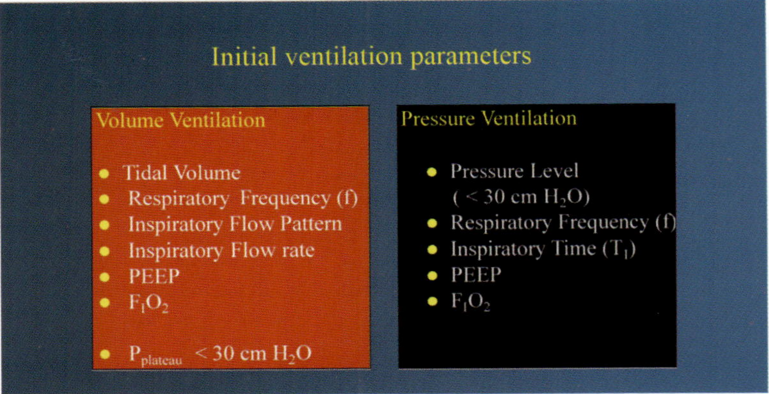

Fig. 3.1

Table 3.1: Ventilator parameters
✦ Mode
✦ Tidal volume
✦ Inspiratory pressure
✦ Frequency (rate)
✦ FiO_2
✦ Flow rate
✦ I:E ratio
✦ Sensitivity
✦ PEEP
✦ Alarms

Table 3.2: Modes of mechanical ventilation
✦ Control Mode Ventilation (CMV)
✦ Assist/Control (A/C)
✦ Synchronous Intermittent Mandatory Ventilation (SIMV)
✦ Pressure Support Ventilation (PSV)
✦ Continuous Positive Airway Pressure (CPAP)
✦ Bilevel Positive Airway Pressure (BIPAP)
✦ Volume Support (VS)
✦ Airway Pressure Release Ventilation (APRV)
✦ Mandatory Minute Ventilation (MMV)
✦ Inverse Ratio Ventilation (IRV)
✦ High-Frequency Oscillatory Ventilation (HFOV)

Mode

Primarily one can decide on whether the patient requires full ventilatory support or partial support for respiration. One can then select a mode of ventilation based on whether the patient needs a set volume or a set pressure. Based on these decisions the parameters are set as per the mode and the ventilator. **Table 3.2** enlists the various modes of mechanical ventilation. The modes of mechanical ventilation are discussed in more detail in the next chapter of this book.

Tidal Volume

The volume of air you inhale or exhale when at rest is known as the tidal volume V_T. The normal V_T is considered as 500 ml, however, it changes in various diseases.[1] On the mechanical ventilator it also changes depending on other settings such as the rate, mode, pressures, etc. When initiating the patient on volume ventilation mode on the mechanical ventilator, the V_T is calculated using the ideal body weight **(Figs 3.2 to 3.4)**.[2]

$$V_T = IBW \times ml$$

V_T is desired tidal volume, IBW is ideal body weight and ml is the volume of air

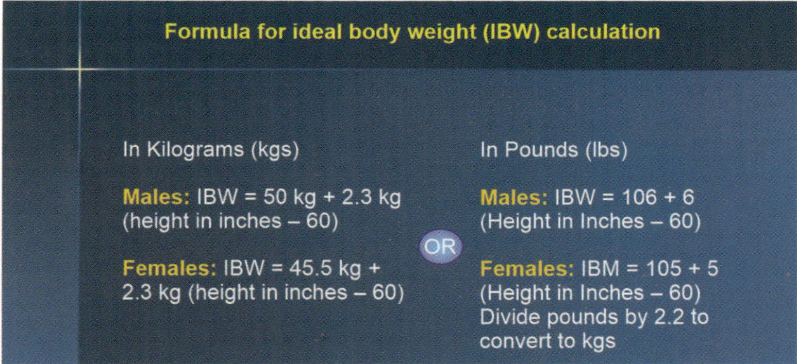

Fig. 3.2: Ideal body weight formulas for calculation in kilograms or pounds

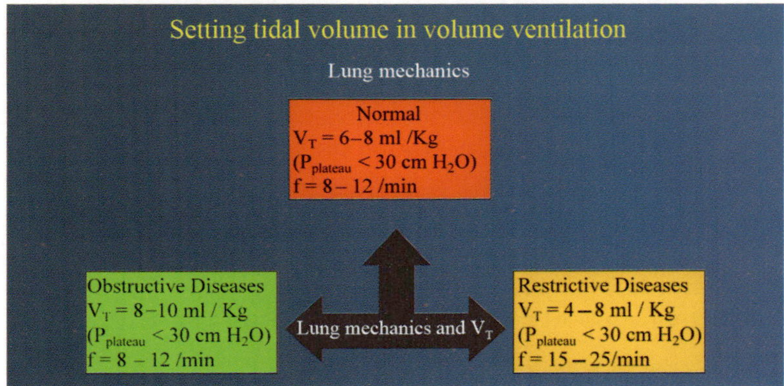

Fig. 3.3

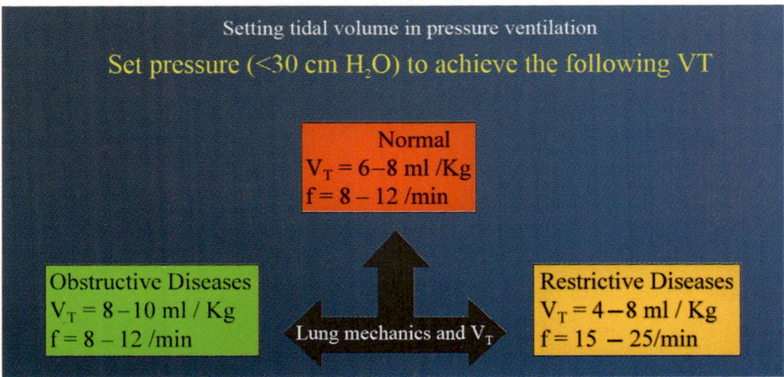

Fig. 3.4

Example 1: Calculate the IBW for a 5′ 7″ Male with actual weight 90 kg

IBW in kgs = 50 + 2.3 (67 – 60)
= 50 + 16.1
= 66.1 kgs

IBW in lbs = 106 + 6 (67″–60)
= 106 + 42
= 148 lbs

Example 2: Calculate the IBW for a 5′ 4″ Female with actual weight 80 kg

IBW in kgs = 50 + 2.3 (64–60)
= 50 + 9.2
= 59.2 kgs

IBW in lbs = 106 + 6 (64–60)
= 106 + 24
= 130 lbs

Fraction of Inspired Oxygen (FiO_2)

Patients who require ventilatory support often have oxygenation issues. For that we can provide them oxygen which is higher than the amount that is available in the atmosphere. This setting is called the fraction of inspired oxygen (FiO_2) measured in percentage. While initiating a patient on a ventilator, if the extent of hypoxia is unknown, or one suspects severe oxygenation issues, we often begin with 100% oxygen.[1,3] This amount is then titrated down to the value that is required for the patient to oxygenate the body tissues. If the patient was already being given supplemental oxygen, then the amount of oxygen that was being given can be set in the ventilator as well.

Peak Inspiratory Pressures (PIP)

Peak inspiratory pressure is the pressure that is delivered to above the set positive end expiratory pressure (PEEP). In pressure control modes, the inspiratory pressure is set and titrated to achieve the desired V_T and safeguard the lungs from barotrauma. Very high pressures, may lead to barotrauma and volutrauma the lungs whereas with too low a pressure the desired volume and pressures to oxygenate and ventilate the lungs may not be achieved. The oxygen saturation (SpO_2), V_T, and the airway pressures on the ventilator reflect the effect of the PIP that is set.

Other forms of pressure settings that are available on the ventilator commonly available in noninvasive ventilation are pressure support, continuous positive airway pressure (CPAP) and bilevel positive pressure ventilation (BiPAP). These variables provide pressures that support the spontaneous breath of the patient.

Frequency or Respiratory Rate (RR)

Frequency or respiratory rate (RR) is a parameter that is set on the ventilator in most of the modes of mechanical ventilation. It is an important parameter in controlled modes where most of the work is done by the ventilator thereby allowing the patient to recover. Respiratory rate is set at 14–20 breaths per minute and increased or decreased as per the need of the patient. A higher respiratory rate is effective in situations where reduction in carbondioxide (CO_2) levels is needed. This is used to normalize the pH values in patients who have respiratory acidosis. A higher RR is also used to reduce the intracranial pressures (ICP) in neurotrauma patients.[4]

A low RR can lead to hypercapnia and acidosis. The effects of RR can be seen on the oxygen saturation levels, the end tidal CO_2 levels, the arterial blood gases (ABG) and the ICP in neurotrauma patients.

RR is also set in modes that are partially controlled or just provide support to spontaneously breathing patients. Setting this assures minimum delivery of breaths in partially controlled modes. And can be set as a backup rate in case the spontaneously breathing patient is apneic.

Inspiratory : Expiratory Ratio (I:E ratio)

In some ventilators you can set an inspiratory expiratory ratio or commonly known as I:E ratio. The ratio of the amount of time needed for inspiration to the amount of time needed for expiration is set depending on the disease condition. Under normal circumstances, the I:E ratio is 1:2 which means the exhalation is twice the amount of time longer than the inhalation. In diseases or situations which does not involve the lungs, you can set the ratio to 1:2.[1,5] For example, patients of stroke or those who do not have a respiratory disease. For patients with respiratory diseases requiring prolonged exhalation time, you can set the ratio to 1:3 or 1:4. Chronic Obstructive Airways Diseases patients require a longer expiratory time to remove all the trapped air due to airway inflammation and obstruction.[6] If enough time is not given for exhaling the air in the lungs, air trapping or breath stacking occurs. This leads to hyperinflation of the lungs and an increase in the pressures in the lungs. I:E ratio is affected by the flow, inspiratory time, the respiratory rate that is set and minute ventilation. In most ventilators you have to calculate the desired ratio based on other settings.

Positive End Expiratory Pressure (PEEP)

Positive end expiratory pressure, as the name suggests is the baseline pressure that remains in the lungs at the end of expiration. The pressure that is set on the ventilator is done so to keep the small airways and the alveoli open with the objective of improving oxygenation and gas exchange. PEEP also helps prevent atelectatic trauma. Without PEEP, there are high chances of atelectasis due to the underlying pathology. Atelectasis is open and collapse of the airway due to sudden loss of pressure during exhalation.

A PEEP level of 5 cmH_2O is ideal to begin with and can be titrated based on the requirement of the patient.[5] PEEP levels can be set anywhere between 4 to 15 cmH_2O. Higher PEEP levels may be required when there is a severe oxygenation issue and no other parameter is providing the oxygenation as needed. A very high level of PEEP may lead to a raised intrathoracic pressure. This will impair the venous return to the heart and give rise to hypertension.

Titration of PEEP levels will affect the inspiratory pressures, the oxygen saturations, the blood pressures and airway pressures, which can be used to monitor the effects of PEEP.

Inspiratory Flow Rate

The inspiratory flow rate setting is set based on how fast the breath needs to be delivered. The higher the flow, the faster the volume is delivered. Flow rates are set on the patient's inspiratory requirements. If the flow is set too low, it will not meet the patient's demands and result in increased work of breathing and asynchrony between the patient and the ventilator. Higher values lead to increased airway pressures and decreased oxygenation. However, higher flows are used in certain disease conditions where there is air trapping and the requirement of a longer expiratory time. The normal inspiratory flow rate is set between 60 L/min and 120 L/min.[7]

Trigger Sensitivity

Sensitivity is a setting that can be set that allows the ventilator to "trigger" or begin the cycle of breath to the patient. It can be ventilator-initiated or patient-initiated breath. A ventilator-initiated or triggered breath is time-dependent. That means if you have set the respiratory rate to 20 breaths per minute, the ventilator will trigger a breath every 3 seconds for the patient. This happens when the mode is set to a "controlled" mode and the patient is not breathing on their own.

A patient-initiated breath is when the patient initiates the breath and the ventilator delivers the set volumes and flows to support or assist the patient's breathing. This type of sensitivity setting can be either a pressure trigger or flow trigger. In the pressure trigger, the ventilator detects the change in the pressure in the circuit and once it reaches the value that is set by the operator, it delivers the breath. Similarly, in flow trigger, it detects a change or drop in the flow within the circuit and delivers the breath. While initiating the ventilator, we can decide the type of trigger to be set. However, the most commonly set trigger variable is the flow trigger.

Normal pressure triggers are set between –1 to –2 cmH_2O or 1–2 L/min below the bias flow that is present in the ventilator circuit.[1,8] If the setting is too high, it can cause auto triggering and deliver higher than the set number of breaths. A low setting will result in difficulty for the patient to initiate a breath.

Alarms

Setting the alarms on the ventilator no matter what mode is set is one of the crucial steps while putting a patient on the ventilator. Alarms are a safeguard measure for all settings in case the set amount is not delivered to the patient. **Table 3.3** describes the different types of alarms, the settings and reasons for the alarms.[1] The alarm is an alert to the ventilator operator to check on the patient as well as on the device. A higher limit and a lower limit are set for pre-pressure, volumes, respiratory rate, etc. In spontaneous breath modes, you can also set an alarm for apnea spells in case the condition of the patient worsens and is unable to take a breath. Some ventilators also have a backup apnea mode that activates after a certain amount of apnea period or apneic spell. This is generally a control mode that takes over the patient's breathing

Table 3.3: Different ventilator alarms, the suggested settings and reasons for alarms

Alarms	Suggested settings	Reasons for the alarm
High pressure	Max 35 cmH_2O or 5–10 cmH_2O above the set PIP	✦ Decreased Lung Compliance ✦ Increased airway resistance ✦ Coughing ✦ Secretions ✦ Biting the endotracheal tube ✦ Kinking in the circuit or artificial airway ✦ Endotracheal tube pushing on the carina ✦ Herniation of the endotracheal tube cuff
Low pressure	2 cmH_2O below PEEP	✦ Leak in circuit or ETT ✦ Disconnection in the circuit ✦ Leak in the exhalation valve ✦ Loose connections ✦ Leak in the pilot balloon ✦ Dislocation of endotracheal tube ✦ Deflated endotracheal tube cuff ✦ Improvement in patient lung characteristics

Contd.

Table 3.3: Different ventilator alarms, the suggested settings and reasons for alarms

Alarms	Suggested settings	Reasons for the alarm
Low volume	200 ml from tidal volume	✦ Leak in circuit or ETT ✦ Disconnection in the circuit ✦ Leak in the exhalation valve ✦ Loose connections ✦ Leak in the pilot balloon ✦ Dislocation of endotracheal tube ✦ Deflated endotracheal tube cuff ✦ Improvement in patient lung characteristics
High frequency	30–35 breaths per minute	✦ Auto triggering due to incorrect trigger setting ✦ Patient dyspneic
Apnea	20 seconds	✦ Patient breathing below set rate. ✦ Leak or disconnection in the circuit ✦ Leak or disconnection in the artificial airway ✦ Alarm limit set incorrectly
High PEEP	3–5 cmH_2O above set PEEP	✦ Air trapping incorrect alarm setting
Low PEEP	2 cmH_2O below set PEEP	✦ Leak in circuit ✦ Leak from the airway
Low FiO_2	10–20% below the set value	✦ Leak in circuit or airway ✦ Sensor malfunction ✦ Malfunction with oxygen source

Figures 3.5 to 3.7 enlists the various parameters with its initial settings that can be used while starting a patient on mechanical ventilator.

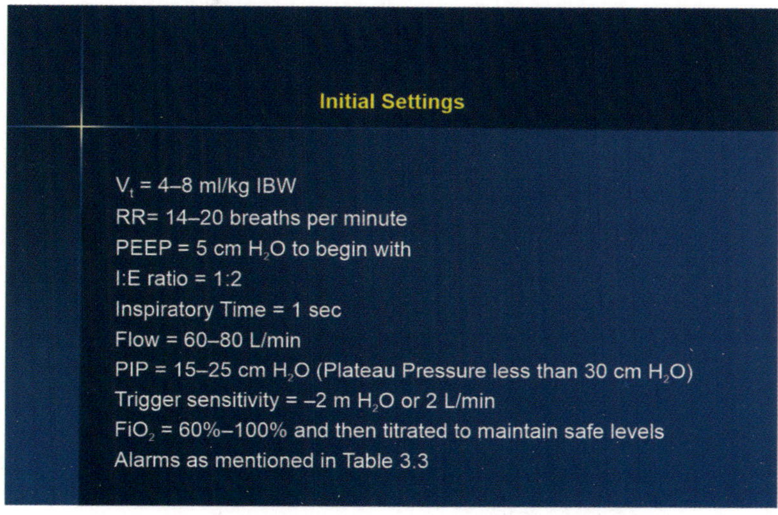

Fig. 3.5: Ventilator parameter and the initial settings

Inspiratory flow setting

- High flow rates result in:
  - Short T_I
  - High PIP
  - Poor gas distribution
- Slow flow rates result in:
  - Low PIP
  - Improved gas exchange
  - Increased T_I and I:E ratio
  - Increased mean airway pressure
  - Decreased T_E that may lead to air trapping

Fig. 3.6

Initial Flow Settings

- **Inspiratory flow rates**
  - Normal lungs: High flows are desirable
  - In ARDS: Slow T1 (3–4 time constant)
  - In COPD: Fast flow allows longer T_E
  - Set flow rate to achieve I: E of 1:2 or less (approx.50–80 L/min)

Fig. 3.7

Conclusion

As soon as the decision to mechanically ventilate the patient is made, the next step is to select the mode and the parameters based on the requirements. Typically, mode is selected followed by settings such as tidal volume, PEEP, FiO_2, respiratory rate, inspiratory time or inspiratory to expiratory ratio and so on. As technology advances and newer types and modes of mechanical ventilation are available, there may be slight variations in the ventilator parameters. This chapter described the basic parameters and the rationale behind these parameters while selecting initial settings of the mechanical ventilator. The subsequent chapters will describe in detail the various modes and the strategies to use each mode in different pulmonary related scenarios.

References

1. Kacmarek R, Stoller J, Heuer A. Egan's Fundamentals of Respiratory Care. 12th Edition. Vol. 12th edition. Mosby; 2019.
2. Peterson CM, Thomas DM, Blackburn GL, Heymsfield SB. Universal equation for estimating ideal body weight and body weight at any BMI. Vol. 103, American Journal of Clinical Nutrition. American Society for Nutrition; 2016. p. 1197–203.
3. Andres L. Mora Carpio, Jorge I. Mora. Ventilator Management [Internet]. StatPearls [Internet]. 2022 [cited 2022 Sep 20]. Available from: https://www.ncbi.nlm.nih.gov/books/NBK448186/
4. Miller JD, Ledingham IMcA. Reduction of Increased Intracranial Pressure: Comparison Between Hyperbaric Oxygen and Hyperventilation. Arch Neurol [Internet]. 1971 Mar 1;24(3):210–6. Available from: https://doi.org/10.1001/archneur.1971.00480330038003.
5. Kilickaya O, Gajic O. Initial ventilator settings for critically ill patients. Vol. 17, Critical Care. 2013.
6. Ahmed SM, Athar M. Mechanical ventilation in patients with chronic obstructive pulmonary disease and bronchial asthma. Vol. 59, Indian Journal of Anaesthesia. Indian Society of Anaesthetists; 2015. p. 589–98.
7. Warner M, Patel B. Mechanical Ventilation. In: Benumof and Hagberg's Airway Management (Third Edition). 2013. p. 981–97.
8. Hamahata NT, Sato R, Daoud EG. Go with the flow—Clinical importance of flow curves during mechanical ventilation: A narrative review. Canadian Journal of Respiratory Therapy. 2020;56:11–20.

CHAPTER 4

Indications of Mechanical Ventilation

❐ Vijay Deshpande ❐ TR Chandrashekar ❐ Srinivas Jakkinaboina

Initiation of Gas Flow

Once a patient is diagnosed with Acute Respiratory Failure (ARF) mechanical ventilation should be instituted. Physiological definition of ventilation describes it as movement of gas in and out of the lungs. To ventilate the lungs, gas must flow from the airway opening to the alveoli. This requires a pressure gradient, meaning gas always flows from high pressure to low pressure area. Without a pressure gradient (ΔP), gas flow cannot be generated. The pressure gradient required to deliver gas to alveoli is referred to as Transairway Pressure ($\Delta P = P_{airway\ opening} - P_{alveolar}$). During spontaneous breathing, at end-inspiration and at end-exhalation the pressures in the alveoli and at the airway opening are equal and thus, there is no pressure gradient and no gas flow. A mechanical ventilator must generate either a negative intra-alveolar pressure or a positive airway opening pressure. The negative pressure ventilators such as Iron Lung and Curraise apply sub-atmospheric pressure to the chest wall. Consequently, the chest wall rises creating a negative intra-thoracic pressure ($< P_{atm}$). A Pressure gradient from atmospheric, at the airway opening, and negative pressure in the alveoli is generated resulting in gas flow. The Positive pressure ventilators are designed to deliver greater than atmospheric ($>P_{atm}$) pressure to the airways resulting in increased transairway pressure. The pressure gradient between the airway opening and alveoli produces gas flow. Figures 4.1 and 4.2 show anatomy of

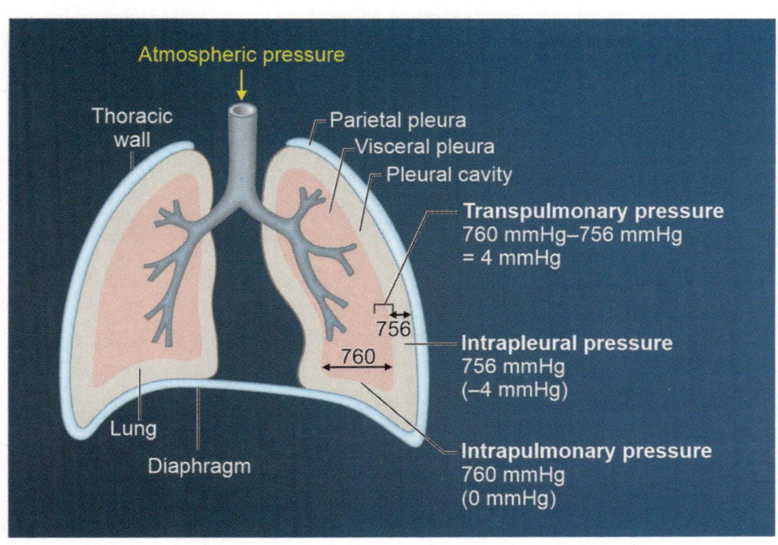

Fig. 4.1: Pressures at end exhalation

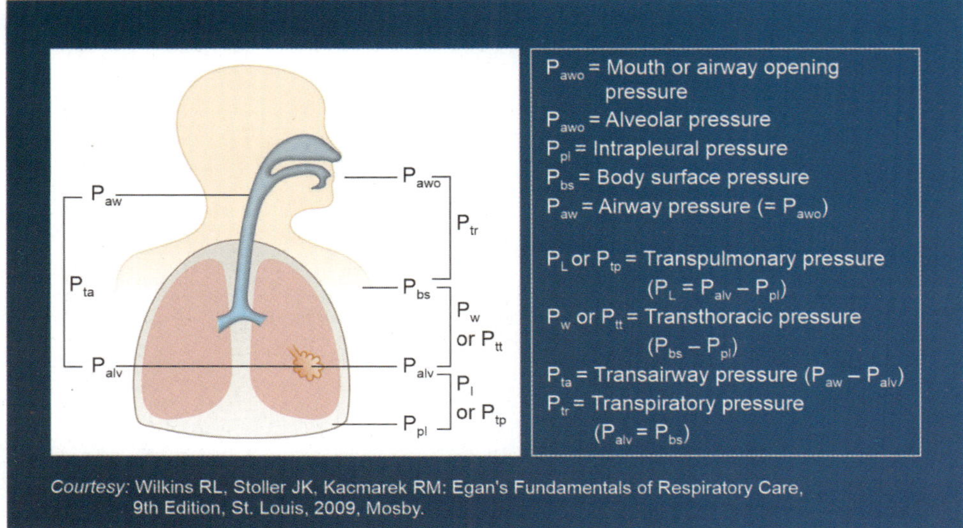

Courtesy: Wilkins RL, Stoller JK, Kacmarek RM: Egan's Fundamentals of Respiratory Care, 9th Edition, St. Louis, 2009, Mosby.

Fig. 4.2

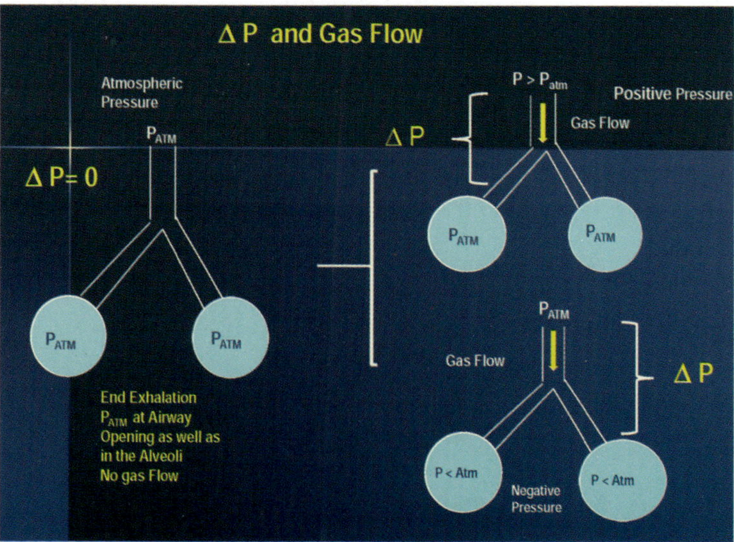

Fig. 4.3

thorax and lung pressures. **Figure 4.3** shows situation at end expiratory level with pressures at atmospheric (P_{atm}) with no gas flow, whereas, a delivery of positive pressure at the airway opening or generating a sub-atmospheric pressure in the alveoli results in a pressure gradient (ΔP) and gas flow to the alveoli.

Phases of Ventilation and the Four (4) Parameters

In clinical practice, the positive pressure ventilators are commonly used. From early mechanical ventilators with moving parts, advances in technology have progressed to the development of current microprocessor driven computerized ventilators. The positive pressure ventilators deliver pressure to the airway opening to ventilate the patient's lungs. Clinicians manipulate not only the pressure but also other parameters such as volume delivered, inspiratory flow rate and termination of ventilatory cycle. The entire cyclic operation of the positive pressure ventilation involves four phases, beginning of inspiration with closed exhalation valve, inspiration, end of inspiration and beginning of expiratory phase by opening exhalation valve and finally, exhalation. The cycle repeats itself at a set frequency or on patient demand (**Fig. 4.4**).

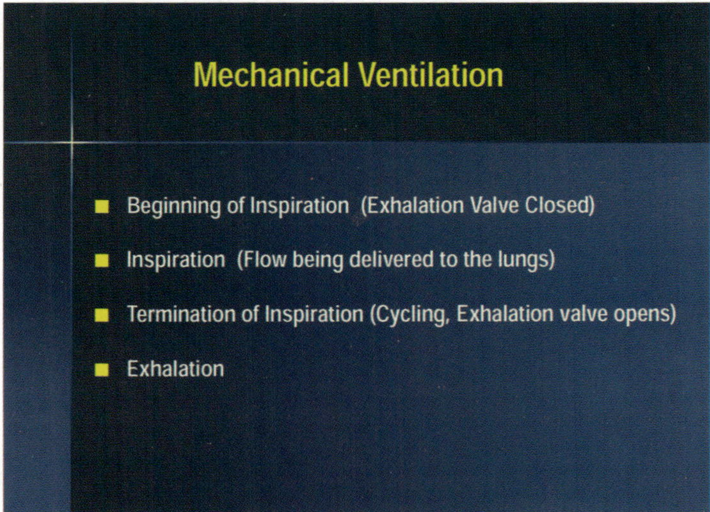

Fig. 4.4

Mechanically ventilated breaths incorporate four parameters; pressure, flow, volume and time. The ventilator at any given point of time can only control the volume (Flow × Time) or control the pressure levels, but both these parameters cannot be controlled simultaneously. Manipulation can be done in these parameters to deliver breaths most suitable for the patient's need based on clinical judgment. There are parameters that trigger the ventilator to begin inspiration (pressure, time and flow). Some parameters or variables are limited and do not exceed their maximum (preset) value during inspiratory phase. It should be noted that reaching the limiting value does not terminate inspiration. In different modes of ventilation, as will be demonstrated in later chapters, specific variables are limited indicating a square pattern for that parameter on the scalar waveform. A mechanical breath that has started must be terminated at some point. Cycle variables terminate the inspiratory phase (pressure cycled, volume cycled, flow cycled and time cycled). Ventilator classification system describes triggering, limiting and cycling variables (**Fig. 4.5**).

Triggering, Limiting and Cycling

Initiation of a mechanical breath (triggering) is provided when the patient makes an inspiratory effort, patient triggered, generally termed as "Assisted" breath or time triggered referred to as "Controlled" breath. The ventilator can be adjusted to provide

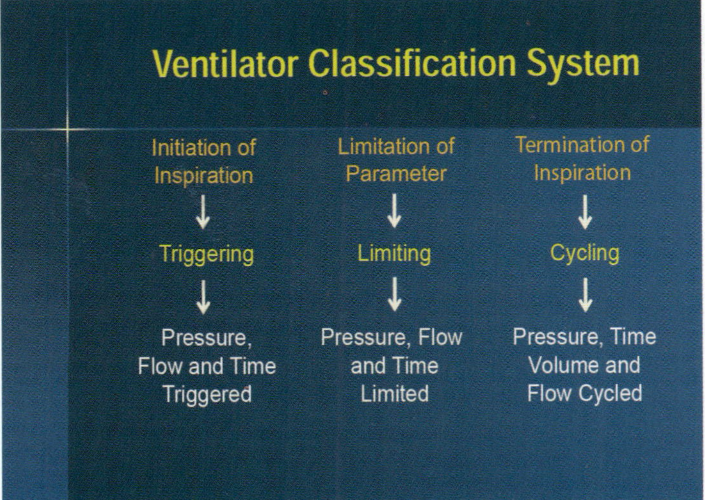

Fig. 4.5

triggering by any one of the two mechanisms, patient or time, whichever comes first (Assist/Control) – **Fig. 4.6**. Patient triggering requires generation of a negative pressure from the patient. A sensitivity control is set to recognize this patient effort and initiate mechanical breath. A more sensitive flow triggering is introduced in most new ventilators. On the pressure-time scalar, a patient triggered breath shows a small negative deflection just before the breath is delivered, whereas a time triggered breath begins at the baseline **(Fig. 4.7)**.

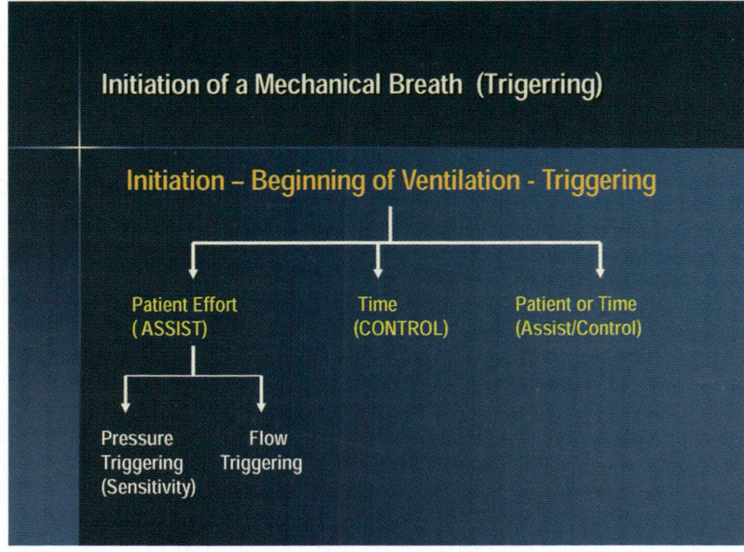

Fig. 4.6

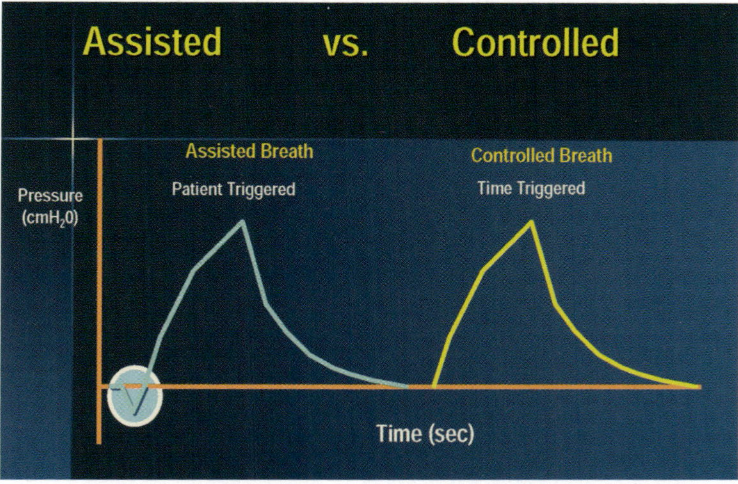

Fig. 4.7

Termination of inspiration and beginning of exhalation, termed as cycling, can be accomplished by all four parameters. **Figure 4.8** defines the cycling mechanisms by volume, time, flow and pressure parameters. As mentioned earlier in this chapter limiting a parameter does not allow it to exceed its preset value, even when the lung compliance and/or airway resistance deteriorate. **Figure 4.9** identifies examples of limited variables and **Fig. 4.10** graphically shows square patterns of the parameters that are limited. In Pressure Control Ventilation the pressure and inspiratory time parameters are preset by clinician. The pressure-time scalar illustrates pressure and time are limited. In volume control ventilation the flow parameter is limited as indicated by the square pattern.

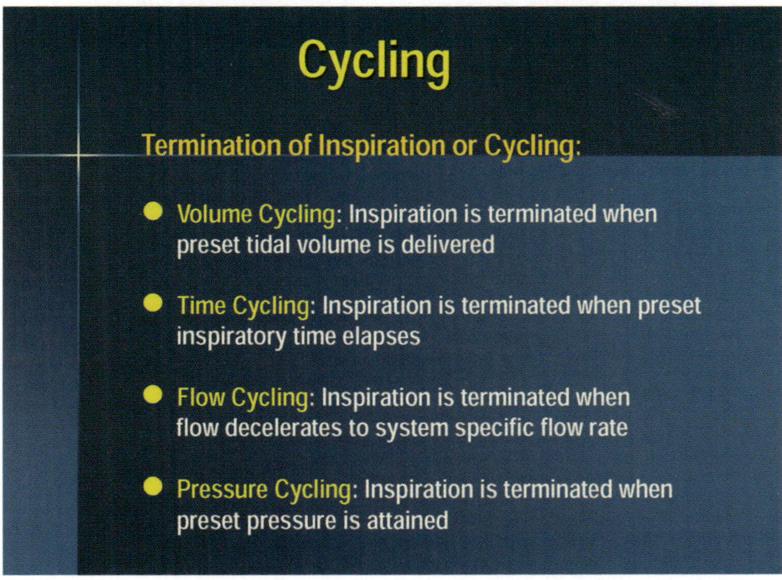

Fig. 4.8

Limiting

Limiting parameter is a preset level of the variable which does not exceed the set level irrespective of the lung characteristics (Compliance and Resistance). Examples:

- In Pressure Control Ventilation (PCV) the pressure level is preset and Limited.
- In PCV the inspiratory time (T_I) is also preset and limited. Any changes in compliance and/or resistance have no effect on T_I. In Volume Ventilation with constant flow the flow level is preset and limited.

Fig. 4.9

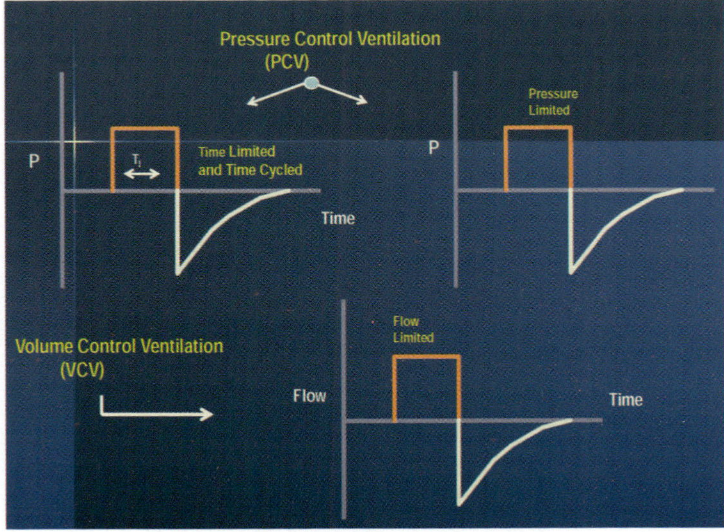

Fig. 4.10

Volume Targeted Ventilation

When a decision is taken to initiate mechanical ventilation the clinician has to select the type of ventilation from three options—Volume Targeted Ventilation, Pressure Targeted Ventilation or Dual Mode (**Fig. 4.11**).

Volume targeted ventilation is commonly used in clinical practice. Typical features of volume ventilation are listed in **Fig. 4.12**. Since the delivered tidal volume (V_T) is constant, it can be used to titrate $PaCO_2$ by adjusting V_T. It should be recognized that

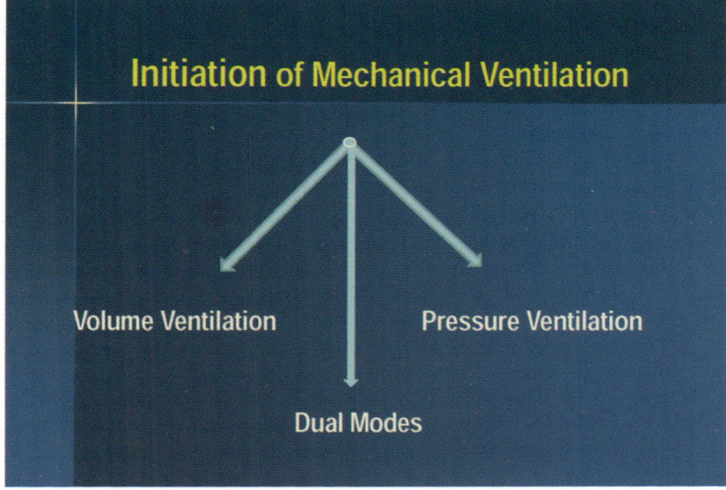

Fig. 4.11

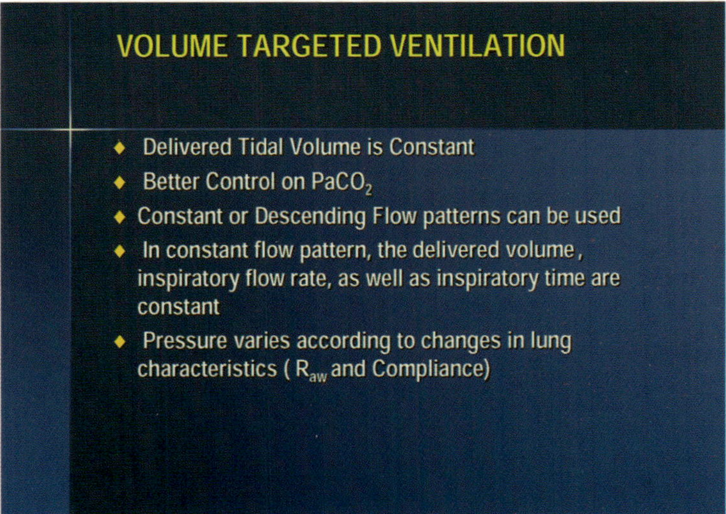

Fig. 4.12

in volume targeted ventilation or commonly referred to as Volume Control Ventilation (VCV) with constant flow setting, not only the volume but also, flow and inspiratory time are constant, as long as the driving force is high. Clinicians can use a descending flow setting to improve gas distribution during inspiration.

The only variable parameter in volume ventilation is pressure which is dependent on Airway Resistance (R_{aw}), Lung Compliance (C_L), inspiratory flow rate and the delivered tidal volume. In setting a volume ventilator the clinician sets desired tidal volume, respiratory frequency and inspiratory flow rate **(Fig. 4.13)**.

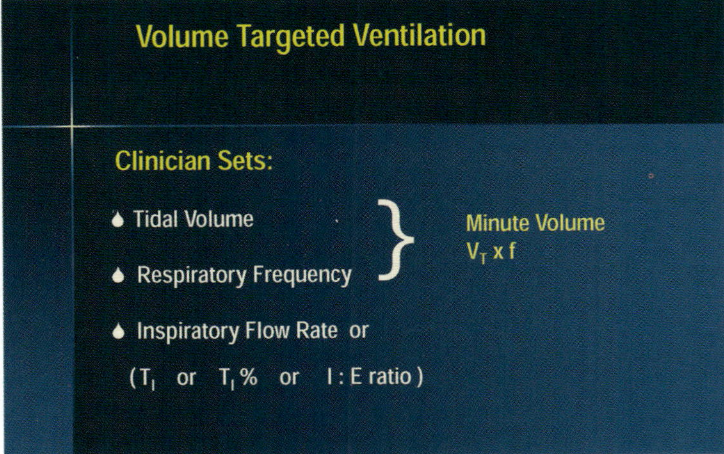

Fig. 4.13

Setting Inspiratory Flow

In many current ventilators inspiratory flow rate is set indirectly and thus, do not have a flow rate control on the panel. Interrelationships between the time parameters allow a clinician to set inspiratory flow rate indirectly. If the ventilator has a "Flow Rate" setting, then it can be set directly. Some ventilators have an "Inspiratory Time" setting. Since inspiratory Flow Rate = Tidal Volume/Inspiratory Time, by adjusting inspiratory time at the given set tidal volume, flow rate can be obtained (flow rate = V_T/ T_I) and adjusted as needed. Some ventilators adjust their inspiratory time by using T_I% control. T_I% is the percent (%) of cycle time (TCT) utilized for inspiration where the cycle time represents time required to complete one breathing cycle determined by the respiratory rate or frequency (f). Thus, TCT= 60 sec /F and T_I % = T_I/TCT × 100 (**Fig. 4.14**).

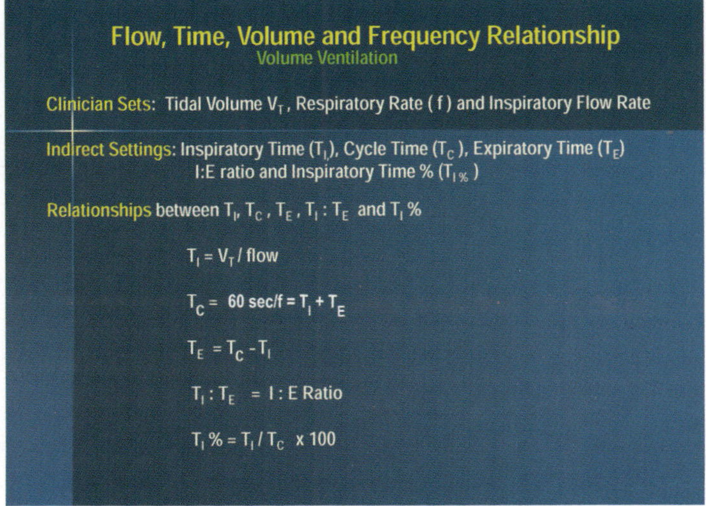

Fig. 4.14

Some ventilators use the $T_I - T_E$ ratio, commonly known as I–E ratio, and respiratory frequency to calculate inspiratory time to deliver preset tidal volume. An example is given in **Fig. 4.15**. Some ventilators have a T_I% setting to give the percent of T_I in relation to the total cycle time (TCT). The relationship between I:E ratio and T_I% is shown in **Fig. 4.16**. In summary, in Volume Ventilation, Inspiratory Flow Rate can be set with controls on a given ventilator. The flow rate can be set directly, or indirectly via T_I, or T_I% or I–E ratio depending on the ventilator.

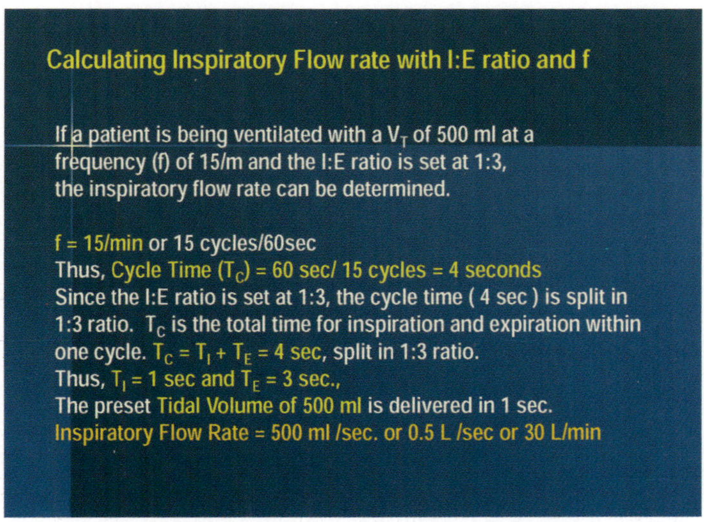

Fig. 4.15

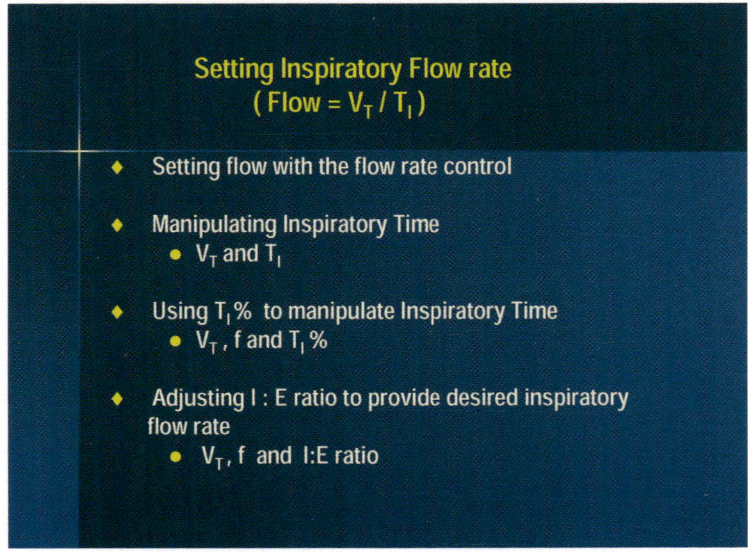

Fig. 4.16

Monitoring Pressures during Volume Ventilation

During volume targeted ventilation a clinician monitors pressures and lung characteristics **(Fig. 4.17)**. PIP represents Peak Inspiratory Pressure (PIP) or the maximum pressure attained during the mechanical breath. P_P refers to Plateau Pressure which is the same as Alveolar Pressure (P_A). This pressure (P_P) is obtained by activating Inspiratory Pause or Inflation Hold control on the ventilator. The difference between PIP and PP provides the Transairway Pressure (P_{TA}) or the pressure required to overcome airway resistance. From the measurement of Plateau Pressure (P_P) which is also termed as Static Pressure, we can determine Static Lung Compliance = V_T/P_P – PEEP. The value of PIP facilitates calculation of Dynamic Compliance = V_T/PIP–PEEP.

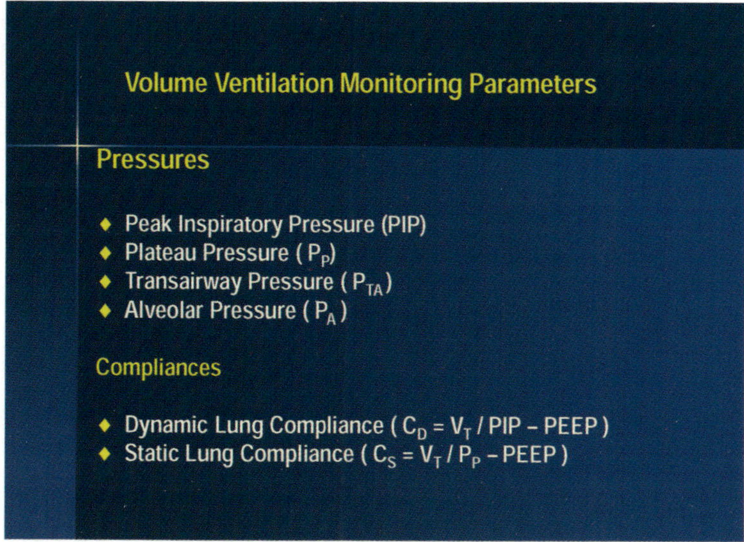

Fig. 4.17

Figure 4.18 represents a tracing of pressure as the lung is inflated during inspiratory phase in volume ventilation. Upon initiation of inspiratory flow, the gas molecules experience frictional resistance during their transit through the airways all the way to terminal bronchioles. This generates transairway pressure, P_{TA} **(Fig. 4.18)**. The tidal volume enters the alveolar zone against the recoiling force of the elastic fibers. Resulting pressure gradually increases until all the tidal volume is delivered. The pressure pattern depends on the compliance of the lung. At the end of tidal volume delivery the highest pressure, peak inspiratory pressure (PIP), is attained. The exhalation valve is supposed to open at this point to allow for exhalation. However, if the inspiratory hold control is activated, the exhalation valve remains closed. Now the tidal volume is trapped in the lungs indicating alveolar pressure or plateau pressure (P_P). Since there is no gas flow the transairway pressure resulting from inspiratory flow is eliminated. Thus, P_P is always less than PIP in volume ventilation.

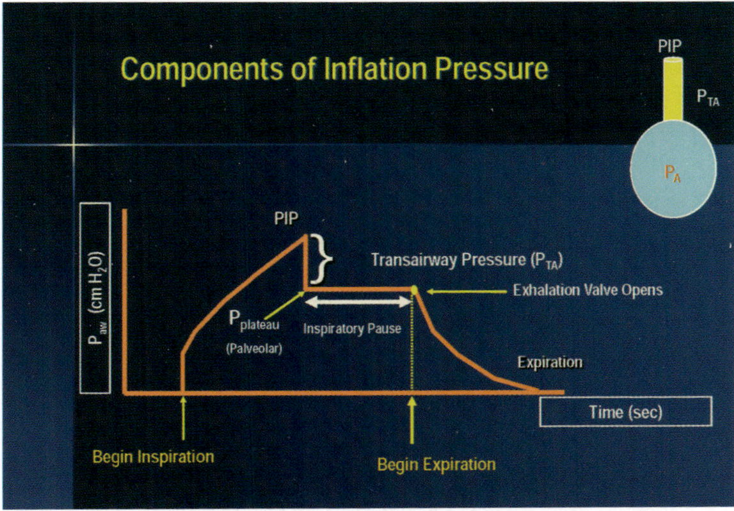

Fig. 4.18

The exhalation valve opens when the inspiratory pause time elapses. Patient exhales the inspired tidal volume. The difference between PIP and PP provides the pressure required to overcome airway resistance (P_{TA}). During every ventilator check, the clinician is expected to monitor and record the above pressures. It is imperative that alarms should be set appropriately. In volume ventilation the two essential alarms are the High Pressure Alarm, indicating that the pressure has reached the set high pressure limit and the Low Pressure or Low Volume Alarm signifying that a leak in the circuit is causing the loss of pressure (**Fig. 4.19**). As a rule of thumb, the high pressure alarm level is set at 5–10 cm H_2O higher than the ventilating pressure and the low pressure alarm level is set at 5–10 cm H_2O below the ventilating pressure (**Fig. 4.20**).

Volume Targeted Ventilation

Key Alarms	Significance
▪ High Pressure Alarm	↑ Airway Resistance ↓ Compliance
▪ Low Pressure Alarm	Leak in the system
▪ Low Volume Alarm	Leak in the system

Fig. 4.19

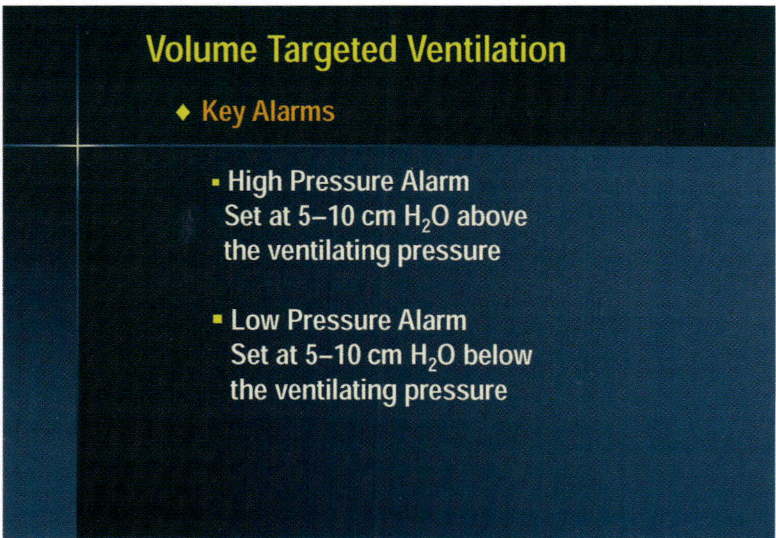

Fig. 4.20

In summary, during volume targeted ventilation the clinician sets V_T, respiratory rate (f) or minute volume ($V_E = V_T \times f$). Actually, some ventilators do not have a tidal volume setting, instead it is set indirectly from V_E and frequency ($V_T = V_E / f$) as shown in **Fig. 4.13**. The third parameter, Inspiratory Flow Rate, is derived from T_I or T_I % or I– E ratio.

Pressure Targeted Ventilation

Pressure Targeted Ventilation or Pressure Control Ventilation (PCV) provides preset pressure to the airways that does not exceed the set level irrespective of the changes in lung compliance and airway resistance (Pressure Limited). The volume delivered is dependent on Lung Compliance, R_{aw}, the Set Pressure and Patient effort during delivery of the pressure. Tidal volume is variable and so is $PaCO_2$ level **(Figs 4.21 and 4.22)**.

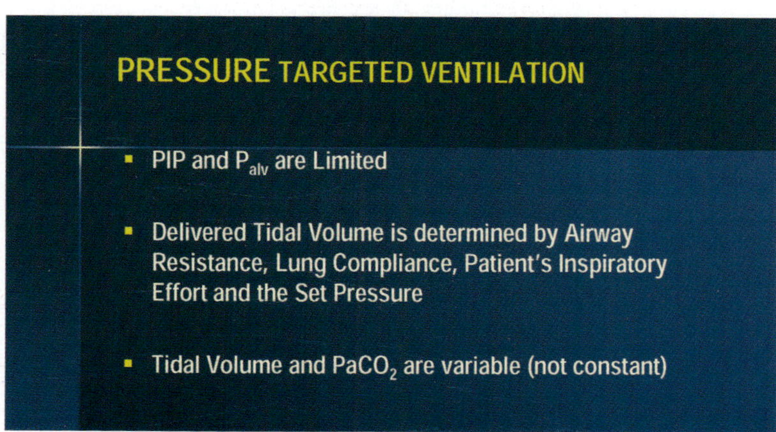

Fig. 4.21

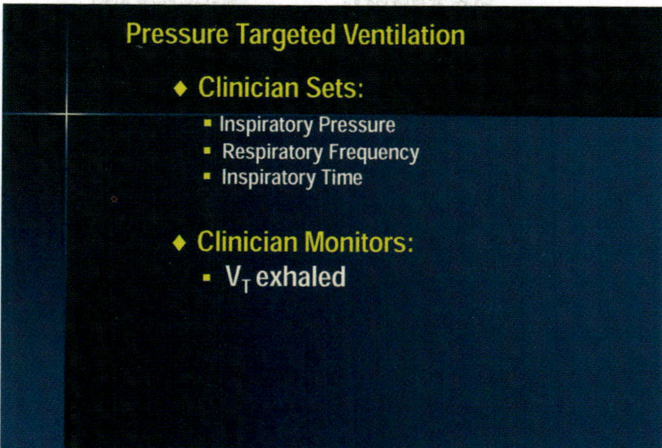

Fig. 4.22

To initiate Pressure Control Ventilation (PCV) the clinician sets the Pressure level, Respiratory Frequency (*f*) and Inspiratory Time (T_I). Since delivered tidal volume is variable, it is monitored and a low volume alarm (or Low Minute Volume alarm) is set appropriately **(Fig. 4.23)**.

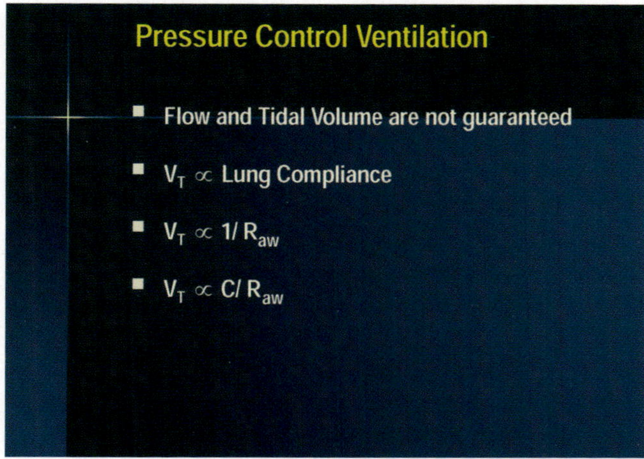

Fig. 4.23

It is important to recognize that, unlike in volume ventilation, activation of Low Volume Alarm is not associated with a circuit leak but it indicates increased R_{aw} or decreased CL. In PCV, the volume delivered is directly proportional to the lung compliance. Lower the lung compliance lower the tidal volume delivered at the preset pressure control level. However, changes in R_{aw} inversely affect the delivered volume. As R_{aw} increases the delivered volume decreases during PCV. Thus, the delivered volume is proportional to the ratio of C/R_{aw} **(Fig. 4.23)**. The low volume alarm in PCV is identical to high pressure alarm in VCV, both alert the clinician that the lung characteristics have deteriorated (Decreased Compliance or Increased Airway Resistance, **Figs 4.24 and 4.25**.

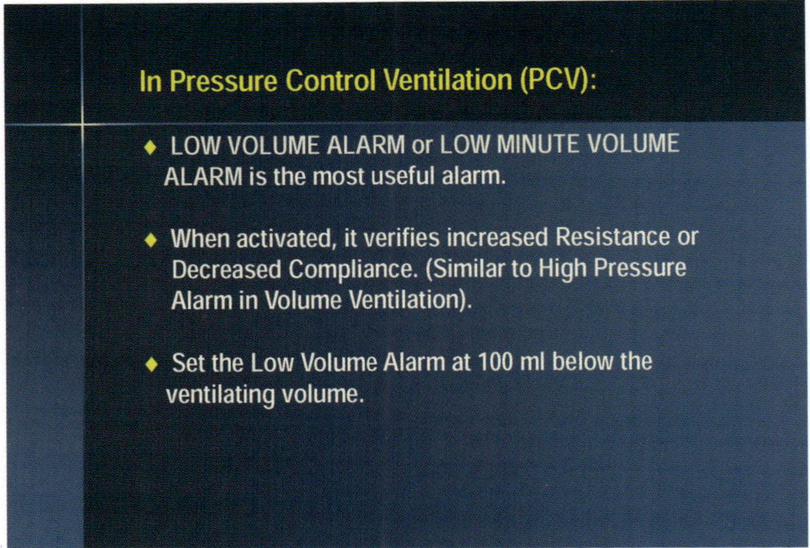

Fig. 4.24

Pressure Controlled Ventilation

Key Alarms	Significance
▪ Low Volume Alarm	↑ Airway Resistance ↓ Compliance
▪ Low Pressure Alarm	Leak in the system

Fig. 4.25

Figure 4.26 Summarizes the role of a clinician in initiating volume or pressure ventilation. Drawbacks in Volume and Pressure Ventilation

Drawbacks in Volume and Pressure Ventilation

The clinicians had a choice of selecting either volume targeted ventilation or pressure targeted ventilation. Researchers recognized the limitations of both the volume and

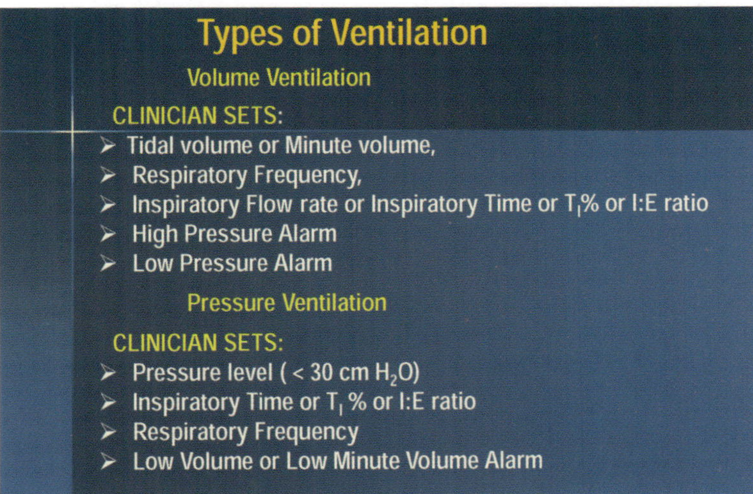

Fig. 4.26

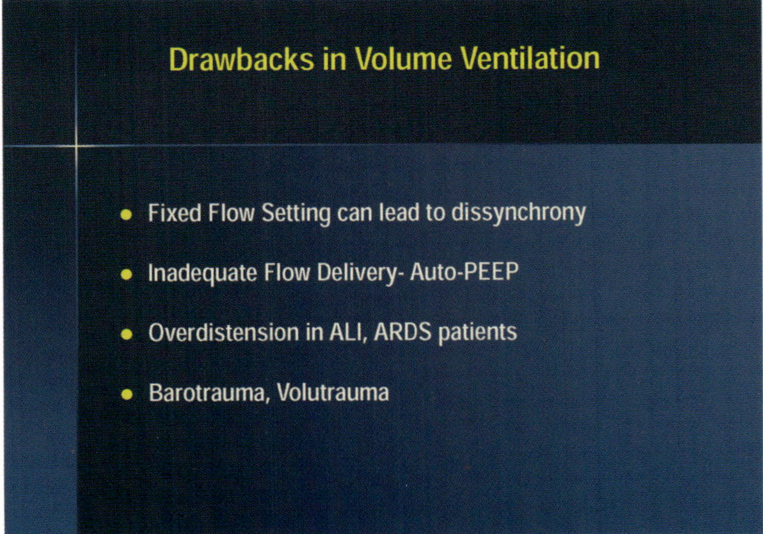

Fig. 4.27

pressure ventilation causing dissynchrony between the patient and ventilator. **Figure 4.27** identifies the drawbacks in Volume Ventilation.

Since the inspiratory flow rate (or T_I) is set by the clinician, the patient cannot set their own flow demand. Consequently, the patient attempts to breathe spontaneously during the delivery of the mechanical breath resulting in dissynchrony. If the set flow rate is slower than the patient's demand it may increase inspiratory time leaving shorter expiratory time. This can result, in some cases, in air trapping or auto-PEEP. The pressure during volume ventilation is dependent on the lung characteristics (R_{aw} and C_L). In stiff lungs or emphasematous regions, delivery of positive pressure can cause barotraumas–trauma resulting from high intrathoracic pressures. Barotrauma is recognized from pneumothorax, pneumomediastinum, subcutaneous air when a patient is receiving positive pressure ventilation. Moreover, in situations like Acute Lung Injury (ALI) or Acute Respiratory Distress Syndrome (ARDS), where the lungs have regions of non-homogenously spread partially and completely collapsed alveoli. The open alveoli receive most of the delivered tidal volume resulting in overdistention which promotes release of chemical mediators and further damages the lung. Thus the use of volume ventilation has limitations.

The positive aspects of pressure ventilation are the adequacy of flow since the demand valve opens during inspiration allowing the patient to receive as much flow as needed and the pressure can be set at a safe level (<30 cm H_2O). Pressure Ventilation has also, some disadvantages. The major problem with Pressure Ventilation is that the delivered pressure is fixed and the delivered volume depends on the set pressure, airway resistance, lung compliance and patient effort. If the lung characteristics deteriorate, the delivered volume decreases at the fixed set pressure. This can promote hypoventilation and hypercapnia (increased $PaCO_2$). If the set pressure is high it may lead to barotrauma (**Fig. 4.28**).

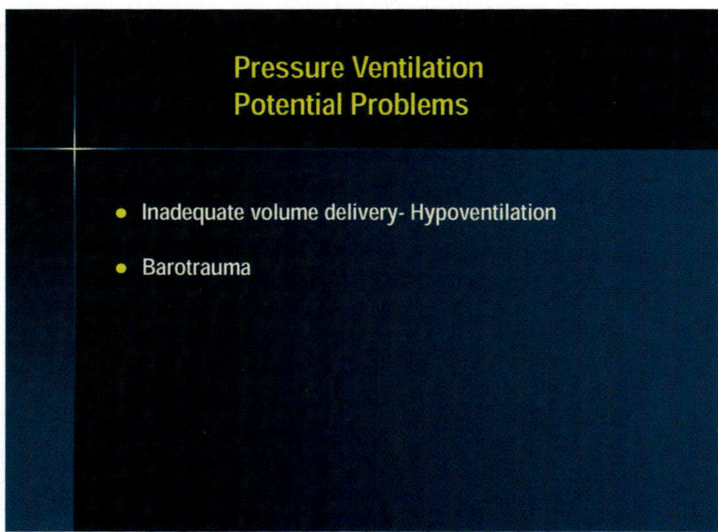

Fig. 4.28

Dual Modes of Ventilation

Recognizing the limitations of volume and pressure ventilation, manufacturers introduced dual ventilation system. Essentially, Dual Ventilation uses the beneficial aspects of both volume ventilation and pressure ventilation. In most cases, it delivers pressure ventilation with volume target. Thus the patient is protected from high pressure levels and yet, receives desired tidal volume. The ventilator adjusts pressure (<30 cm H_2O) based on calculated dynamic compliance and delivers desired volume (**Fig. 4.29**). Currently, different ventilators employ dual modes. **Figure 4.30** lists the names of commonly use Dual Modes. Subsequent chapters will discuss these modes in details.

Dual Modes of Ventilation

- Combine Pressure and Volume Ventilation in one mode
- Exploit beneficial effects of both Pressure and Volume Ventilation
- Improve Patient-ventilator Synchrony
- Prevent ventilator induced lung injury
  - Barotrauma
  - Volutrauma

Fig. 4.29

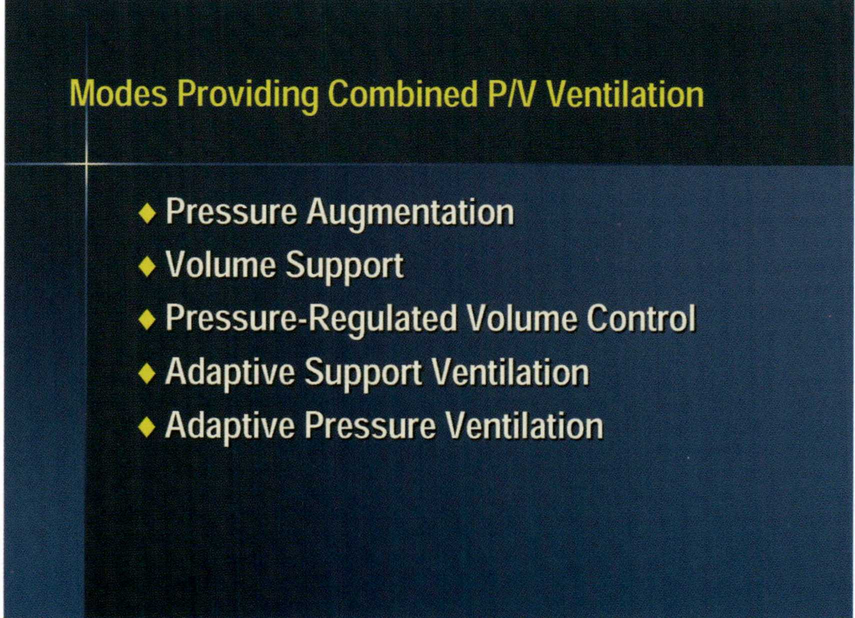

Fig. 4.30

After taking into consideration all aspects of the types of mechanical ventilation discussed in this chapter, the clinician should also consider the patient's underlying cause for respiratory failure before initiating mechanical ventilation.

CHAPTER 5

Basic Modes of Ventilation

❒ Shyamsunder Tipparaju ❒ Swarna Deepak ❒ K Hima Bindu ❒ Vijay Deshpande

INTRODUCTION

The ventilator delivers positive pressure breaths during ventilation. This mechanism is dependent upon the compliance and resistance of airways. This determines how much pressure should be generated by the ventilator to deliver the tidal volume required by the patient.

Clinicians can efficiently commence ventilation by utilizing appropriate ventilation strategies by having a clear understanding of the concepts of elastance and compliance (Fig. 5.1).

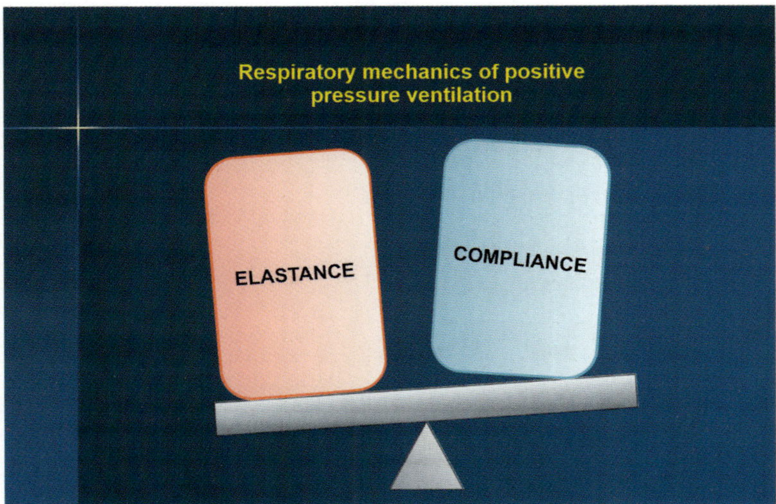

Fig. 5.1: Elastance and compliance determines the respiratory mechanics of positive pressure ventilation

ELASTANCE AND COMPLIANCE

Lung and chest wall movement depends upon the impedance of the respiratory system. This further depends upon elastic resistance to the tissue and non-elastic resistance to the gas flow. Elastic recoil of the lung depends upon surface tension forces and lung compliance. Surface tension forces within the alveoli create a tendency for the alveoli to collapse. The presence of surfactant reduces the surface tension and prevents alveolar collapse. Elastic recoil of the lung also depends upon compliance.

COMPLIANCE

Compliance is defined as the change in volume divided by a change in distending pressure. Compliance can be calculated individually for either the lung or chest wall or both. Compliance also depends upon whether there is no airflow (static compliance) or when there is flow of air in the lungs (dynamic compliance). **Figure 5.2** shows the formula for calculation of compliance and its normal values.[1]

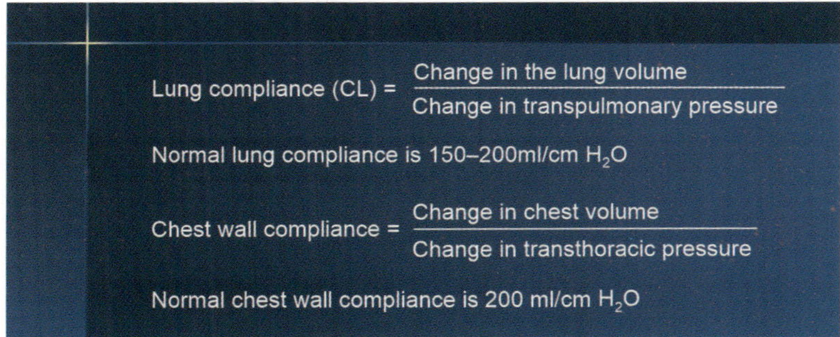

Fig. 5.2: Shows the formula for calculation of lung and chest wall compliance and its normal values

Total compliance of the system is the sum of both lung and chest wall compliance which is around 100 ml/cm H_2O. **Figure 5.3** shows the pressures at different levels of airway and lungs. This helps us to calculate the elastance and compliance. Transthoracic pressure is the difference between alveolar pressure and body surface pressure. Transpleural pressure is the difference between alveolar pressure and the pleural pressure.

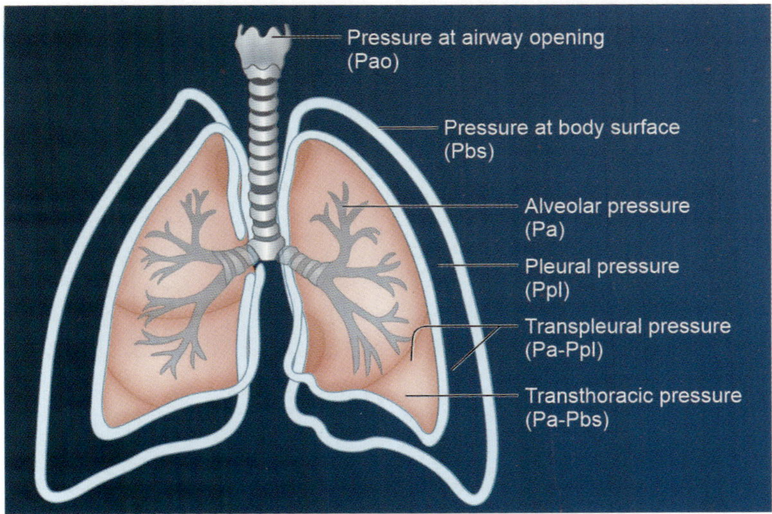

Fig. 5.3: Airway pressure (Pao), alveolar pressure (Pa), pleural pressure (Ppl), transthoracic (Pa-Pbs) and transpleural pressure (Pa-Ppl)[4]

ELASTANCE

Elastance or reciprocal of compliance (1/Compliance) represent the pressure required to overcome the recoiling force of the lungs against which the volume is being delivered. Elastance denotes how much pressure change occurs for change in the lung volume. It also denotes the work done to inflate the entire system. Half of it is used to expand the lungs and the other half is used to expand the chest.

Basic Mode of Mechanical Ventilation

A predetermined pattern of communication between the patient and the ventilator might be referred to as a mode of ventilation. Basic modes of mechanical ventilation were designed to deliver and meet basic ventilation needs of the patient.

Basic ventilatory modes are Controlled mode (VCV/PCV), Assist Control (AC-VC or AC-PC) mode, SIMV, PS mode, CPAP and BIPAP. The necessity for improved patient control of the ventilator, the potential of respiratory mechanics and respiratory drive monitoring in aided modes, and improved patient-ventilator synchrony led to the development of advanced modes of mechanical ventilation. Advanced modes of ventilation are Volume Assured Pressure Support (VAPS), Proportional Assist Ventilation (PAV), Neurally Adjusted Ventilatory Assist (NAVA), Adaptive Support Ventilation (ASV), and Intellivent-ASV.[1]

Basic mode initially designed was a control mode. Control variable could be either volume (volume controlled ventilation) or pressure (pressure controlled ventilation or both) (dual mode) (**Fig. 5.4**). Breath triggered by the patient is assisted breath and breath triggered by the machine is usually time triggered.

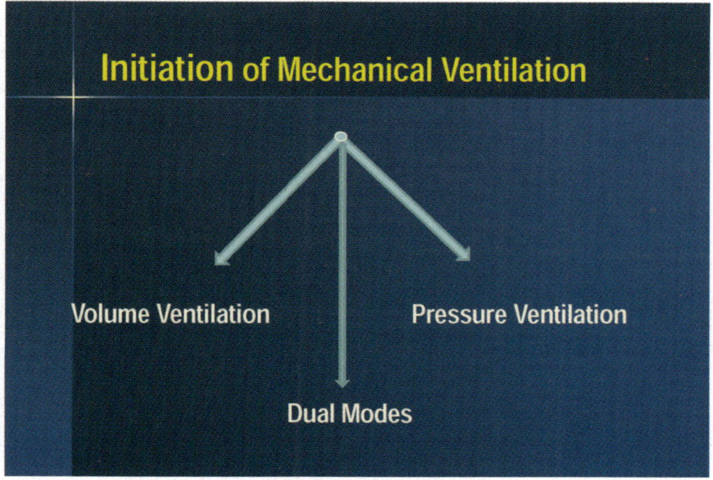

Fig. 5.4

There are 4 stages for initiation of mechanical ventilator breath:

1. Trigger
2. Inspiratory phase
3. Cycle
4. Expiratory phase

The phases of a mechanical breath are controlled by phase variables in mechanical ventilation. Trigger, limit, and cycle variables drive the phases of inspiration and expiration. **Figure 5.5** depicts the trigger, limit, and cycle variables.

Trigger

The variable that determines the initiation of inspiration. This can be either a flow trigger or time trigger or pressure trigger or volume trigger. Usually, time/pressure triggers are the common variables.

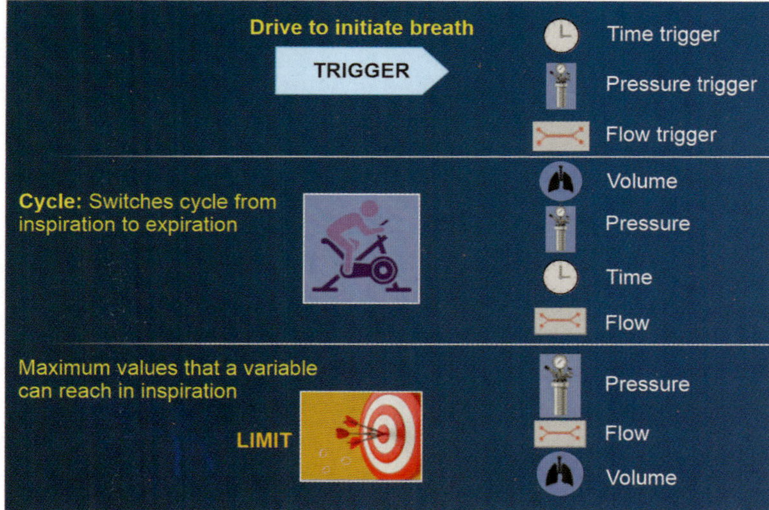

Fig. 5.5: Depicts trigger, cycle and limit variables[4]

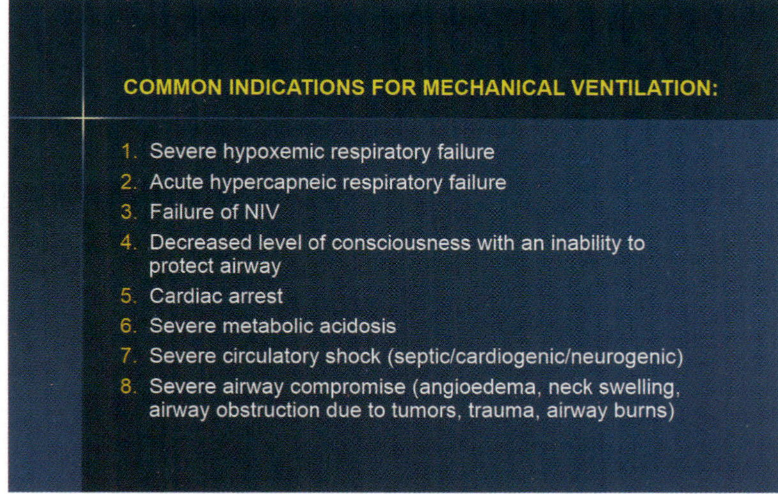

Fig. 5.6: Indications for mechanical ventilation

Cycle Variable

The variable that determines the end of inspiration and the beginning of expiration. The inspiratory phase ends and the expiratory phase begins when this pre-set variable is reached. The common cycle variables are either volume-cycled or time-cycled.

Limit Variable

This pre-set variable is fixed (pressure, volume, flow). It is not allowed to rise during the inspiratory phase. Inspiration does not end even when the variable reaches its pre-set value. Breath delivery continues even after pre-set value is reached.

CONTRAINDICATIONS FOR MECHANICAL VENTILATION

Except for the patient and their family's unwillingness to start mechanical ventilation, there are no absolute contraindications to mechanical ventilation.

Volume Control Ventilation (VCV)

In VCV, the preset variable tidal volume (TV) is fixed. The TV and minute ventilation (MV) remain constant irrespective of variations in respiratory mechanics (lung characteristics, elastance, and compliance). Hence there is a high risk of barotrauma. In volume-controlled ventilation, the clinician should set certain parameters for proper ventilation of the patient. The parameters are inspiratory flow rate, respiratory rate (*f*), and TV or MV. Each of the modes associated with mandatory breaths is described in Figs 5.7 to 5.9.

There are no absolute contraindications for control ventilation. A conscious and spontaneously breathing patient does not require a mandatory controlled ventilation.

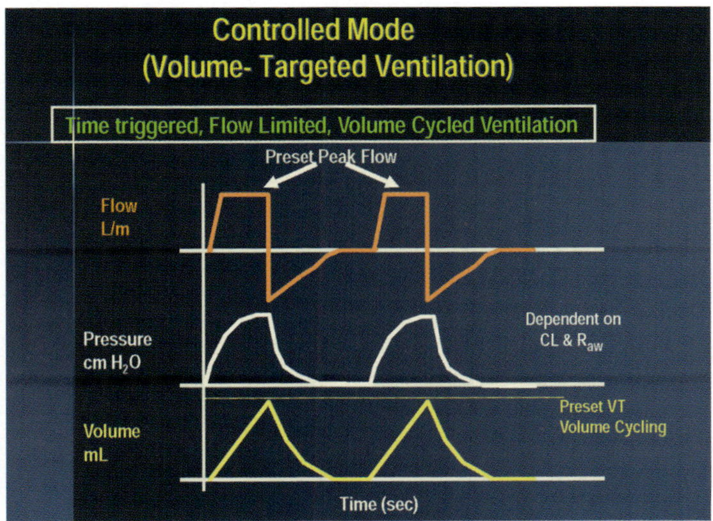

Fig. 5.7: Shows scalars-Flow/Time, Pressure/Time and Volume/Time-for Controlled Ventilation (Time Triggered, Flow Limited and Volume Cycled) in Volume Targeted or Volume Controlled or simply Volume Ventilation

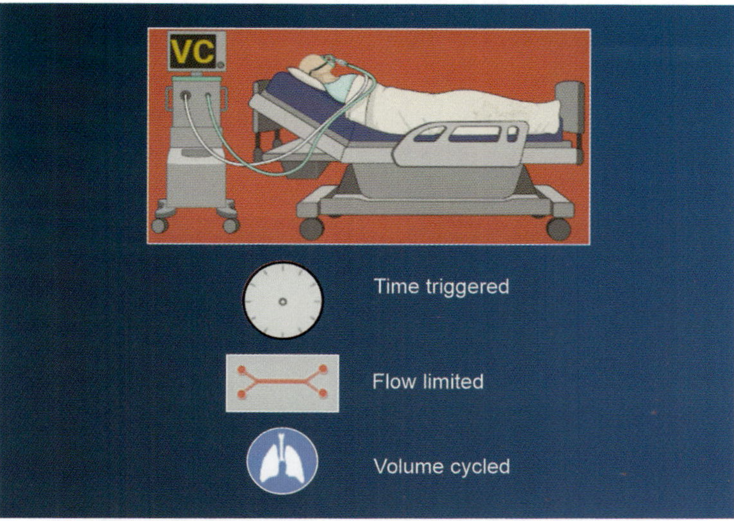

Fig. 5.8: Time triggered, flow limited and volume cycled in volume targeted or volume controlled ventilation[4]

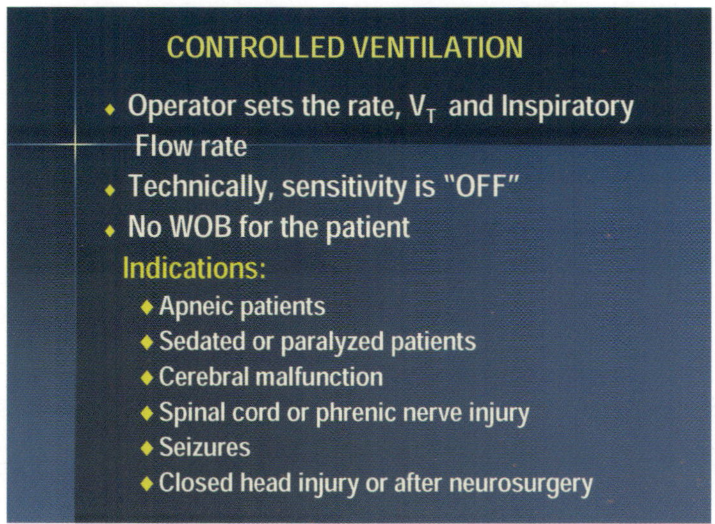

Fig. 5.9: Lists common medical conditions requiring controlled ventilation

The risks of controlled ventilation are clear. Since every breath is time-triggered, the ventilator will not permit the patient to take a spontaneous breath. As a result, the patient becomes anxious and loses synchrony with the ventilator. The patient is regarded as "fighting" the ventilator when the pressure alert sounds. Additionally, the patient must use the TV and flow that the clinician has specified, which may not be sufficient.

ASSIST CONTROL–VOLUME CONTROL

The most common initial mode used for a patient is volume-controlled ventilation. By changing the volume-controlled mode to assist mode we are encouraging the patient's spontaneous initiation of inspiration. This creates a negative deflection on the pressure-time scalar is shown in **Fig. 5.10**. In assist control mode, in addition to mandatory ventilator-delivered breaths, patient-triggered breaths are also delivered. Breaths are delivered at a pre-set TV for patient-triggered or time-triggered breaths.

Figure 5.10 shows scalars for assisted ventilation (Patient triggered, Flow limited, Volume cycled ventilation).

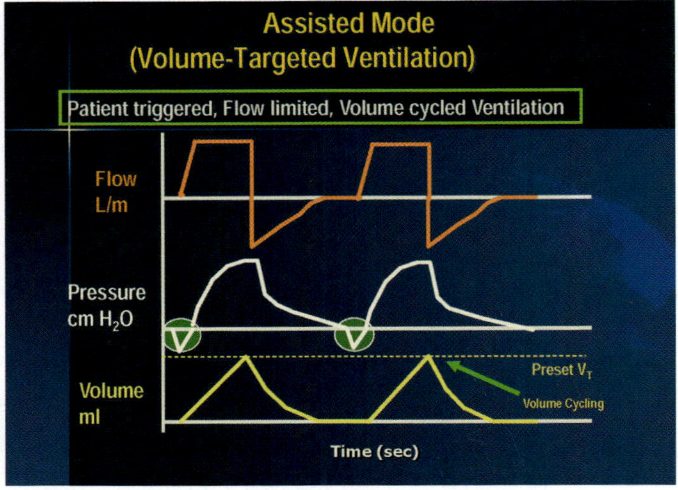

Fig. 5.10: Scalars for assisted ventilation

Pressure Control Ventilation (PCV)

In PCV, the pre-set variable of peak inspiratory pressure is fixed. TV and MV vary with changes in pulmonary compliance and airway resistance. In pressure control ventilation the clinician sets target pressure, respiratory rate, and inspiratory time. **Figure 5.11** shows variables for pressure control ventilation.

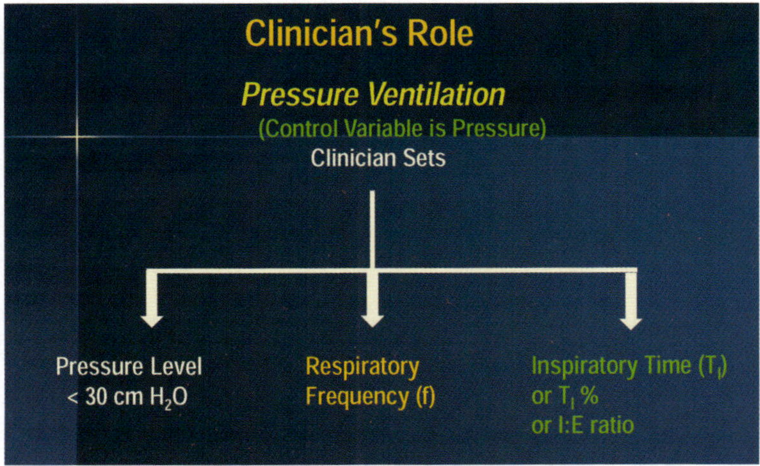

Fig. 5.11: Variables for pressure control ventilation

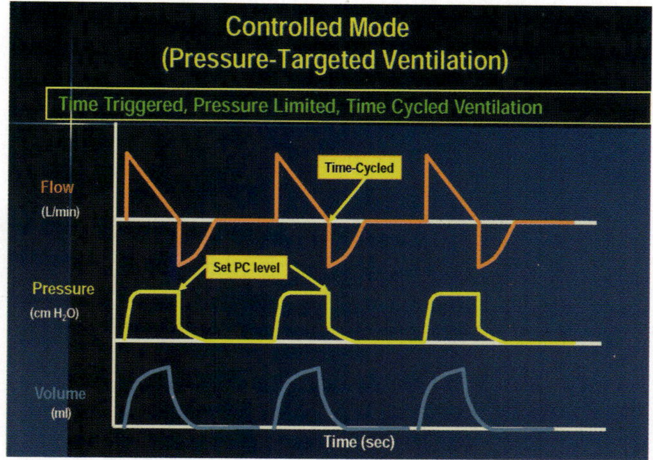

Fig. 5.12: Indicates the scalar for pressure control ventilation (time triggered, pressure limited, time cycled ventilation)

In the control modes, the patient will have no respiratory efforts generated and literally have no work of breathing. The patient should be adequately sedated with or without paralysis during the mode to ensure there is no bucking of the patient on the ventilator.

CONTROL MODE ALARMS

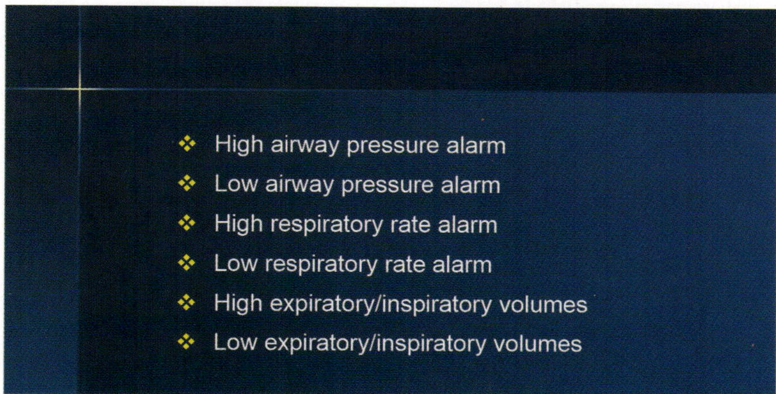

Fig. 5.13: Alarms in control mode

Complications of Control Ventilation

- Accidental disconnections from the ventilator causes hypoxia as the patient is completely dependent on the ventilator
- Patient-ventilator asynchrony
- Reduced diaphragm function/diaphragmatic muscle atrophy
- Low-pressure alarms

There are several technological advancements in the field of medicine over the past 40 years. One of the major development is in the evolution of different ventilator modes that help clinicians in managing various clinical scenarios.

Advances to the control mode include the development of assist modes of ventilation like SIMV, SIMV with pressure support and continuous positive airway pressure.

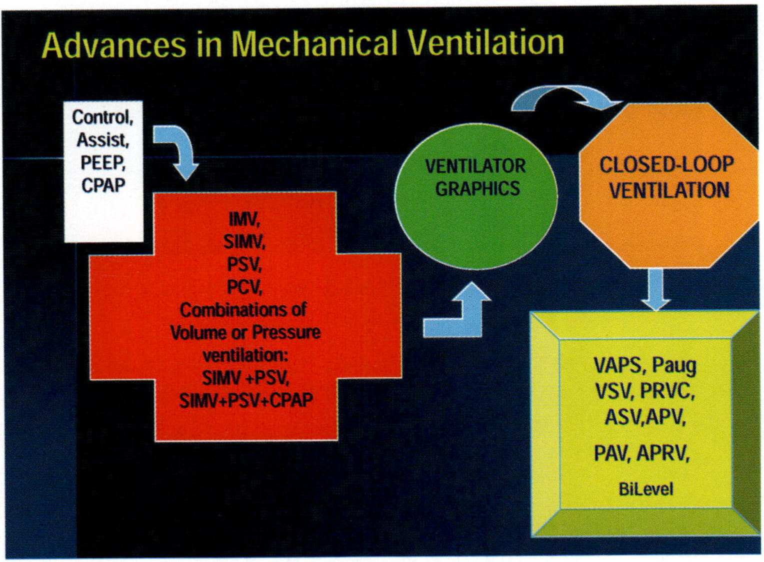

Fig. 5.14: Identifies technological advancement in modes of ventilation from assist/control to currently introduced closed loop ventilation

The following text describes the modes of ventilation with graphs and line diagrams.

COMMONLY USED VENTILATORY MODES

Synchronised Intermittent Mandatory Ventilation (SIMV)

The purpose of SIMV's initial development in the 1970s was to help patients wean themselves off of artificial ventilation. In a 1980s survey, 90.2% of hospitals preferred SIMV, making it the most popular and commonly utilized ventilator mode for weaning.

Because SIMV enables patients to attain normal alveolar ventilation with an intact ventilatory drive, it offers the benefit of preventing acute respiratory alkalosis.[2]

Indications for SIMV Mode

SIMV has two main indications since it may adaptably give ventilatory support at various levels: as a primary method of ventilatory support and as a tool for weaning.

The fact that utilizing SIMV may make breathing more difficult is one issue. By adding pressure support to the SIMV, one can combat this. In general, severe hypoxia and hypercapnic respiratory failure call for mechanical ventilation, frequently following a failed attempt at non-invasive ventilation. Trans airway pressure, also known as the pressure differential between PIP and Plateau pressure, is a measurement of the amount of pressure necessary to overcome the resistance provided by the tracheal tube (alveolar pressure). As a result, a doctor can add pressure support at a level equal to PIP-P_{plat} and then adjust it based on the patient's clinical status which is typically 5 cm.

In the SIMV mode, patient-triggered assisted breaths are delivered along with the time/machine-triggered mandatory breaths. In this mode, patient-triggered breaths are synchronized with the mandatory breaths to avoid breath stacking. It allows the patient's spontaneous breathing and hence maintains an intact ventilator drive.

If a patient makes a spontaneous inspiratory effort, just prior to the delivery of a time-triggered breath, then it will be assisted by the machine and mandatory breath will be delivered to the patient. In between the mandatory breaths in SIMV mode, the machine permits the patient to breathe spontaneously to any TV the patient wishes to.

SYNCHRONISATION WINDOW

To permit synchronization and avoid delivery of mandatory breath during spontaneous breathing, spontaneous breath can be delivered only during the synchronization window. If no spontaneous breathing is attempted during synchronization window, machine-triggered mandatory breaths can be delivered. Thus the TV and MV remain constant over time. Synchronization window duration is approximately 0.5 sec. Although it differs from manufacturer to manufacturer.

For example, if the SIMV mandatory frequency is 10/min, the ventilator should time trigger every 6 seconds. If the synchronisation window is 0.5 seconds, the ventilator automatically becomes sensitive to any spontaneous inspiratory effort at 5.5 seconds from the start of the previous mandatory breath, i.e. the synchronisation window becomes active. When the synchronisation window is active and the patient makes a spontaneous inspiratory effort, the ventilator is patient-triggered to deliver an assisted mandatory breath.

Given that SIMV comprises two different types of breaths, the doctor managing MV must be aware of both necessary and spontaneous breaths.

When SIMV was first developed, it was a widely used mechanical ventilation technique. Recent research suggests that it might not be the most efficient ventilation method. In comparison to pressure support ventilation with volume guarantee, a study of preterm infants reveals that SIMV has significantly worse mean airway pressure, length of time from the start of weaning to extubation, duration of nasal continuous positive airway pressure support after extubation, and extubation failure rate.[3] When compared to SIMV, adaptive support ventilation demonstrated statistically lower levels of atelectasis, the frequency of mechanical ventilator setting changes, the frequency of ventilator alarms, and hospital duration of stay in adult patients after coronary artery bypass grafting.

Scalars for SIMV in volume and pressure ventilation are shown in **Figs 5.15–5.17**.

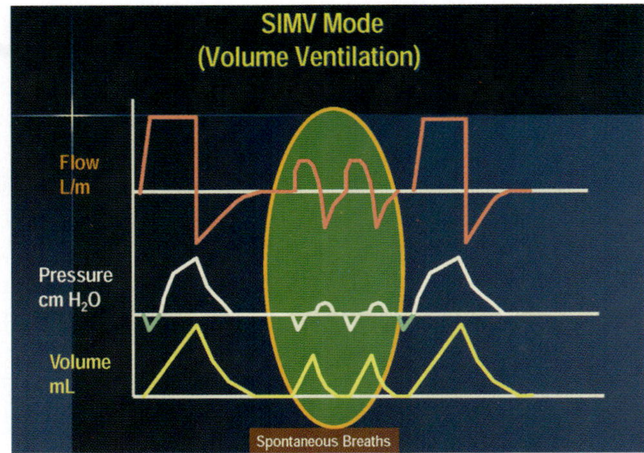

Fig. 5.15: Scalars for SIMV-volume control mode of ventilation

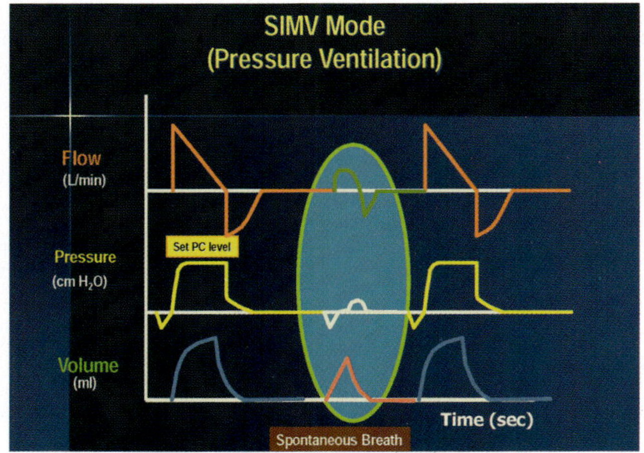

Fig. 5.16: Scalars for SIMV-pressure control mode of ventilation

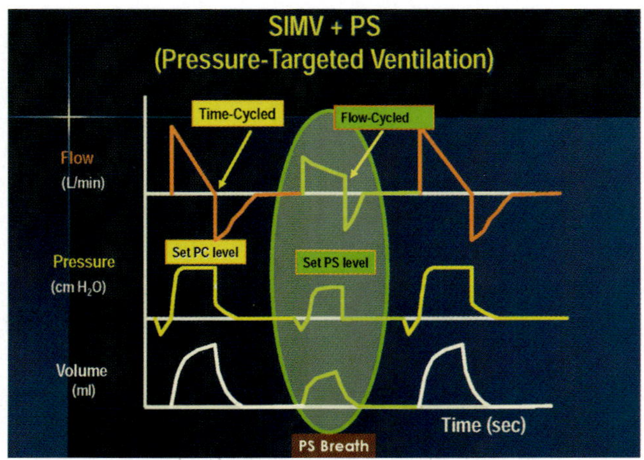

Fig. 5.17: Scalars for SIMV-volume control + pressure support mode of ventilation

PRESSURE SUPPORT VENTILATION

Pressure assistance will aid the patient's spontaneous breathing and increase the TV. PSV lessens the effort required for spontaneous breathing. For the length of spontaneous breathing, pressure support is provided to the patient's airway at the pre-set pressure plateau. Machine-triggered required breaths with predetermined inspiratory pressure are given if the frequency of spontaneous breathing is less than the preset backup frequency or if there is no spontaneous breathing. The flow pattern connected to this ventilation mode is typically downward. The delivery of TV and MV can both change with a change in lung mechanics. **Figure 5.18** depicts scalar for PSV.

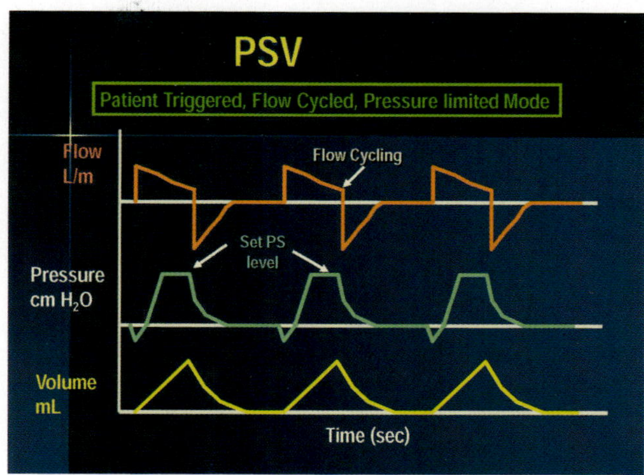

Fig. 5.18: Scalars for pressure support mode of ventilation

Indications of Spontaneous Mode

Mainly as a method of weaning spontaneous mode is used to liberate the patient from the ventilator.

Contraindications of Spontaneous Mode

1. There is no desire to breathe.
2. Very low oxygen status/high CO_2 levels necessitate complete control of breathing.
3. Unstable vitals necessitate advanced medical intervention—the patient should be sedated and controlled ventilated.

Continous Positive Airway Pressure (CPAP)

For those who are spontaneously breathing, continuous positive airway pressure (CPAP) is a type of positive airway pressure in which airflow is provided to maintain a constant pressure to keep the airways open. The pressure in the alveoli above atmospheric pressure at the conclusion of expiration is known as positive end-expiratory pressure (PEEP). PEEP can be administered with CPAP, which likewise keeps the target pressure constant during the entire breathing cycle, including both inspiration and expiration. Water pressure is measured in centimeters (cm H_2O). Bilevel positive airway pressure (BiPAP), in a contrast to CPAP, delivers a different amount of pressure depending on whether the patient is inhaling or exhaling. Expiratory positive airway pressure (EPAP) and inspiratory positive airway pressure (IPAP) are the names for these pressures. **Figure 5.19** shows the scalars for CPAP mode

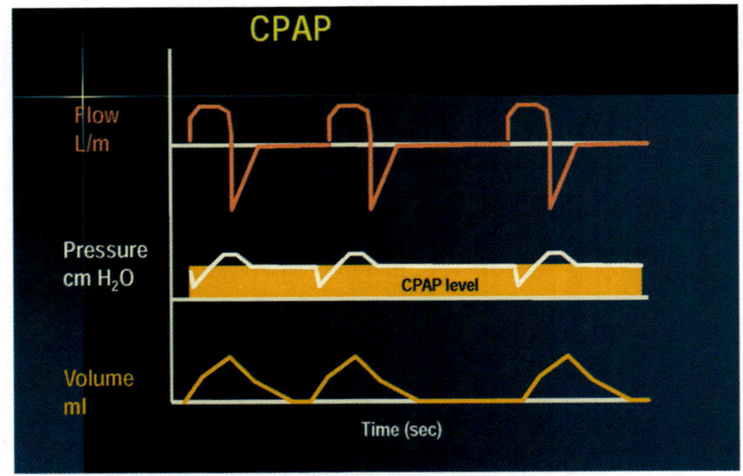

Fig. 5.19: Scalars for CPAP mode of ventilation

Common Complications of Mechanical Ventilation

1. VAP
2. Barotrauma
3. Atelecto trauma
4. Volutrauma
5. Biotrauma
6. Patient-ventilator asynchrony

Conclusion

Multiple modes of ventilation are available in the present day and each can be used based on the clinical scenario. Even though we have various advanced modes, many of them need to be yet incorporated into routine use as there is little evidence of their superiority over conventional modes. Finally, the decision of choosing the mode of ventilation remains with the astute bedside clinician.

References

1. Chang, D. (2014) Clinical Application of Mechanical Ventilation. 4th Edition, Delmar, New York.
2. Lazoff SA, Bird K. Synchronized Intermittent Mandatory Ventilation. [Updated 2022 Jul 4]. In: StatPearls [Internet]. Treasure Island (FL): StatPearls Publishing; 2022 Jan
3. Hideaki Imanaka, Masaji Nishimura, Hiroshi Miyano, Hideki Uemura, Toshikatsu Yagihara; Effect of Synchronized Intermittent Mandatory Ventilation on Respiratory Workload in Infants after Cardiac Surgery. *Anesthesiology* 2001; 95:881–88.
4. Images created with BioRender.com

CHAPTER 6

Interpretation of Arterial Blood Gases and Acid–Base Disorders

Ashfaq Hasan

INTRODUCTION

Arterial blood gas (ABG) analysis is now considered an indispensable test, both inside and outside of intensive care units. In current medical practice, ABG interpretation has become routine not only for ICU physicians but also for respiratory therapists and respiratory nurses. Yet, the processing of the data becomes second nature only after years of practice; for the novice, the analysis of blood gas can be frankly intimidating.

In this chapter, the essentials of ABG analysis are set out in a concise and easily assimilable form. Given the size limitations of the chapter, the emphasis has been primarily on a pragmatic approach to ABG interpretation. For this reason the chapter does not include discussion on the pathobiology of the various gas-exchange and acid–base derangements.

Seasoned healthcare professionals are of course familiar with the handful of 'step-wise' approaches to ABG analysis. In this chapter an analogous approach is described, further simplified, the "Alpha-Numeric (A-1) approach".[1]

In this algorithm, acid–base disorders are initially classified into one of two possible tracks. When an acid–base disorder is primarily metabolic in nature, the Metabolic Track, "(A)–(B)–(C)–(D)–(E)", is selected.

When an acid–base disorder is primarily respiratory in nature, the Respiratory Track "(O)—(.1)–(.2)–(.3)–(.4)–(.5)", is selected. In this track, the first two 'fractions' (0.1 and 0.2) are assigned to acute disorders and the last two to chronic disorders. For purposes of retention, acidosis has been dealt with before alkalosis in each instance.

Most biological fluids are alkaline: the 'narrow' pH range that is compatible with life 6.8–7.8 actually represents a very large range of the hydrogen ion concentration: from 16 nanomoles/L (pH 7.8) to 160 nanomoles/L (pH of 6.8). The concept of pH was introduced by Soren Peter Sorensen a Danish biochemist. A hydrogen ion concentration of 0.00000001 (10^{-7}) represents a pH of 7. To make it easier to handle a string of such numbers, Sorensen proposed the concept of pH which is essentially the negative logarithm of the H^+ ion concentration in moles per liter of solution. The pH has no units.

Among the disadvantages of the pH is that the scale for measuring the hydrogen ion concentration in the blood gets compressed at one end: thus, relatively small changes of pH are produced by the addition of a certain quantity of H^+ ions to the blood when it is very acidic than when to is less acidic. In other words changes in pH at the acidic end of the spectrum are liable to be misconstrued as small changes in the H^+ concentration, as compared to equivalent changes at the alkaline end of the spectrum.

A couple of basic questions will be addressed first:

Is the primary acid–base disturbance respiratory or metabolic:

Is the pH < 7.36?

If so, acidemia exists

Is the pH > 7.44?

If so, alkalemia exists

And, is the primary acid–base disturbance respiratory or metabolic?

Remember that:

In a primary metabolic acidosis the HCO_3^- is lower than normal
In a primary metabolic alkalosis the HCO_3^- is higher than normal
In a primary respiratory acidosis the CO_2 is higher than normal
In a primary respiratory alkalosis the CO_2 is lower than normal
Thus,

a. When the pH is acidemic (< 7.36), the relevant questions to ask are:
   - Is the bicarbonate low?
     - If so, a metabolic acidosis exists
   - Is the CO_2 high?
     - If so, a respiratory acidosis exists

b. When the pH is alkalemic (> 7.44), the relevant questions to ask are:
   - Is the bicarbonate high?
     - If so, a metabolic alkalosis exists
   - Is the CO_2 low?
     - If so, a respiratory alkalosis exists

It is a good idea at this point to review the respective causes of the specific primary acid–base disorder diagnosed (**Tables 6.1** through 7)

Table 6.1: Causes of wide anion-gap metabolic acidosis

Lactic acidosis
Type 1 (hypoperfusion) Type 2 (deranged carbohydrate metabolism)
Ketoacidosis
Diabetic ketoacidosis Alcoholic ketoacidosis Starvation ketoacidosis
Renal acidosis
Uremia Acute renal failure
Ingestion of exogenous toxin and drugs
Methanol Ethylene glycol Salicylate

Table 6.2: Causes of normal anion-gap metabolic acidosis

Loss of bases
Loss of bicarbonate-precursors
Recovery phase of diabetic ketoacidosis
Renal lose of bicarbonte
Type 2 RTA-Carbonic inhibitor use
Gastrointestinal loss of bicarbonate
✦ Diarrhea ✦ Loss or drainage of pancreatic secretions ✦ Uretero-sigmoidostomy ✦ Small bowel fistula
Retention of acids
Decreased renal excretion of fixed acids
✦ Type 1 RTA ✦ Type 4 RTA ✦ Chronic renal failure

Depending upon whether the disturbance has turned out to be metabolic or respiratory, one of the two tracks should be selected:

(I) THE METABOLIC TRACK ("ALPHA TRACK")[1]

Remember "(A)-(B)-(C)-(D)-(E)"

(A) 'A' Stands for Anion-Gap (Ag) Analysis

The characterisation of the AG helps to narrow down the differential diagnosis of metabolic acidosis.[2]

The anion gap is based on the Law of Electroneutrality (the sum of all anions is equal the sum of all cations). The AG represents the difference between the sum of the major measured anions (sodium and potassium), and the measured cations (bicarbonate and chloride).

It follows that,

$Na^+ + K^+$ + unmeasured cations = $Cl^- + HCO^-$ + unmeasured anions

Or,

$Na^+ + K^+ - Cl - HCO^-$ = Unmeasured anions – Unmeasured cations+

Or,

Anion gap = unmeasured anions – unmeasured cations.

A widened AG means that unmeasured anions have increased or unmeasured cations have decreased.

One of two formulas are commonly used for the calculation of the Anion Gap

a. $AG = [Na^+] + [K^+] - [Cl^-] - [HCO_3^-]$

   Normal range: 16 ± mEq/L

   This formula is commonly used in renal units, where the value of K^+ is known to fluctuate within a wide range.

b. Alternatively, a simpler formula may be used: $[Na^+] - [Cl^-] - [HCO_3^-]$

Normal range: 12 ± 4 mEq/L

This formula understandably has greater application outside of renal units, which is to say, it is the most used formula for the calculation of the AG.

The next question has to do with the 'width' of the AG. Metabolic acidosis can exist both with a wide or narrow AG, and classification into one or the other not only provides insight into the underlying cause but also impacts upon the treatment.

Is the AG wide?

This happens when the sum of measured cations ($[Na^+] + [K^+]$) exceeds the sum of the measured anions ($[HCO_3^- + [Cl^-]$) due to an increase of unmeasured anions in the blood. If so, a WAGMA is present.[2]

(*See* causes of WAGMA—**Table 6.1**).

Is the AG narrow?

Frequently, the anion gap may remain within normal limits ("narrow" AG) in the presence of a metabolic acidosis. This happens when the bicarbonate is replaced by chloride. Because of the increase in the chloride normal anion-gap metabolic acidosis (NAGMA) is also known as hyperchloremic acidosis.

(*See* causes of NAGMA—**Table 6.2**).

(B) 'B' Stands for Bicarbonate Gap (BG; Syn: Delta gap, Delta-Delta gap, Deviation from the 1:1 correlation)[3]

In WAGMAs it is mainly a decrease in bicarbonate that accounts for the widening of the AG. Depending upon the magnitude of this decease, an additional acid–base disorder (a NAGMA or a metabolic alkalosis) may be surmised to exist. The bicarbonate gap is the difference between the increase in the anion gap (ΔAG) and the decrease in the bicarbonate (ΔHCO_3^-):

$$BG = \Delta AG - \Delta HCO_3^-$$

The next question has to do with the 'range' of the BG.

i. Is the BG > + 6 mEq/L? (If so, an associated metabolic alkalosis is present)
ii. Is the BG < + 6 mEq/L? (If so, an associated narrow-anion gap metabolic acidosis is present)

(C) 'C' stands for Colloid gap (CG; or, the Osmolar gap)

Essentially, the CG is the measured osmolality minus calculated osmolarlity[4]

Osmolarlity can be calculated as: $(2 \times Na) + glucose/18 + BUN/2.8$

The utility of the CG is to make a presumptive diagnosis of toxin ingestion.[5] Thus, the CG is considered when when the anion gap is high and the common causes of a wide AG (DKA, lactic acidosis, uremia and salicylate poisoning) have been ruled out. Other less common conditions that may widen the CG are administration of mannitol, IV immune globulin in maltose (especially against the background of renal failure), and severe hyperlipidemia.

(D) 'D' Stands for Disorders that may be Associated with the Metabolic Acidosis (such as respiratory acidosis or respiratory alkalosis).

This assessment relies on formulas that predict the level of $PaCO_2$ for the measured bicarbonate.

A. When the primary condition is Metabolic Acidosis, the formula used is:

Predicted $PaCO_2 = (1.5 \times HCO^-) + 8 \pm 2$

(this is also referred to as Winter's formula or Winter's equation)

The questions that arise then are:

i. **Is the measured $PaCO_2$ higher than the predicted $PaCO_2$ by >2 mmHg?** If so, an associated primary respiratory acidosis is present.

ii. **Is the measured $PaCO_2$ lower than the predicted $PaCO_2$ by >2 mmHg?** If so, an associated primary respiratory alkalosis is present.

B. When the primary condition is Metabolic Alkalosis[6], the formula used is:

Predicted $PaCO_2 = (0.7 \times HCO^-) + 21 \pm 2$

The questions that arise then are:

i. **Is the measured $PaCO_2$ higher than the predicted $PaCO_2$ by >2 mmHg?** (If so, an associated primary respiratory acidosis is present).

ii. **Is the measured $PaCO_2$ lower than the predicted $PaCO_2$ by >2 mmHg?** (If so, an associated primary respiratory alkalosis is present).

(E) 'E' stands for Electrolytes in the urine, in other words, the Urinary Anion-Gap (UAG)

The urinary anion gap (UAG) is useful when a hyperchloremic metabolic acidosis exists[7], and helps to clarify the causative mechanisms.[7] The UAG is calculated as follows:

$$UAG = [Na^+] + [K^+] - [Cl^-]$$

The questions that then arise then are:

i. Is the UAG negative? (If so, this implies loss of bicarbonate from the bowel).

ii. Is the UAG positive? (If so, this implies loss of bicarbonate from the kidney).

(*See* causes of NAGMA associated with a negative and positive urine anion gap—**Table 6.3**).

Table 6.3: Causes of narrow-anion gap metabolic acidosis (nagma) by urinary anion gap
The differential diagnosis of Narrow-Anion Gap Metabolic Acidosis may be further narrowed down by assessing the urinary anion gap (*see* text):
Increased urine anion gap (Suggestive of low urinary ammonium) Predominantly renal cause (e.g, renal tubular acidosis)
Decreased urine anion gap (Suggestive of high urinary ammonium) Predominantly gastrointestinal cause (e.g, diarrhoea)

In metabolic alkalosis as well, urinary electrolytes are useful in elucidating the underlying cause and predicting response to therapy.

i. Is the urinary chloride low, that is to say, <20 mEq/L?
If so, metabolic alkalosis associated with chloride depletion, either through the gut, kidney or in sweat, and may be expected to improve with saline administration (saline contains chloride). Hypokalemia and/or hypochloremia is often a pointer to this condition.

ii. Is the urinary chloride high, that is to say, >20 mEq/L?
If so, this may reflect significant depletion of total body K^+ stores or urinary K^+ wasting). The matter can be resolved by measuring the urinary potassium levels:
  a. Is the urine K^+ <30 mEq/L? (If so, this reflects depletion of total body K^+ stores due to gastrointestinal loss, e.g, laxative abuse).
  b. Is the urine K^+ >30 mEq/L? (If so, this reflects urinary K^+ wasting due to recent diuretic use, hyperaldosteronism (primary and secondary), Bartter and Gitelman syndromes and other hypokalemic hypertensive syndromes.

Table 6.4: Common causes of mixed disorders

High anion-gap metabolic acidosis (WAGMA) with respiratory acidosis
In a patient with chronic renal failure—is there LRTI or pneumonia*
In a patient with diabetic ketoacidosis—is there LRTI or pneumonia*
In a patient with diabetic ketoacidosis and Kussmaul's breathing—is there espiratory muscle fatigue?
Normal anion-gap metabolic acidosis (NAGMA) with Respiratory Acidosis
In a patient with renal tubular acidosis (RTA)—is there respiratory muscle weakness?
In a patient with diarrhea—is there dyselectrolytemia?
Metabolic acidosis with respiratory alkalosis
In a patient with diabetic ketoacidosis—is there sepsis (e.g, pneumonia)?*
In a patient with chronic renal failure—is there LRTI or pneumonia*
Is there salicylate toxicity
Septic shock
Hepatorenal syndrome
Metabolic alkalosis with respiratory acidosis
In cor pulmonale—check for diuretic use and dyselectrolytemia
Vomiting against the background of chronic respiratory failure of any cause
Metabolic alkalosis with respiratory alkalosis
Severe vomiting in pregnancy
Vomiting against the background of hepatic cirrhosis
Diuretic use in hepatic cirrhosis
Ryle's tube drainage and sepsis

(II) THE RESPIRATORY TRACK ("ALPHA TRACK")[1]

Remember "(O)—(.1)–(.2)–(.3)–(.4)–(.5)"

(O) 'O' here Stands not for Zero, but for the Alphabet O (as in 'O'xygen)

The assessment of oxygenation can be done by the following means:

i. PaO_2: PaO_2 stands for the partial pressure of blood in the systemic arteries. It is used as surrogate measurement for oxygenation of the blood in the peripheral circulation. The PaO_2 directly appears on the ABG printout and requires no calculation. In an individual with healthy lungs, the approximate predicted the PaO_2 is arrived at multiplying the fractions of oxygen (FiO_2) the patient is breathing into 5. It bears emphasis that this value is at best an approximation.

ii. PaO_2/FiO_2 ratio (P/F ratio)

The PaO_2/FiO_2 ratio makes a meaningful assessment of PaO_2 in relevance to the different FiO_2 being inhaled by the patient.

With normal lungs assuming a normal PaO_2 of ~100 mmHg (for ease of calculation) an individual breathing room air (FiO_2 0.21), would have a PaO_2/FiO_2 ratio of (100/0.21) ≈500. A PaO_2/FiO_2 ratio (with a CPAP or PEEP value of at least 5 cmH_2O)[9] of less than 250 implies a major compromise in gas exchange (In ARDS, values of <100, 100–200 and 200–300 represent severe, moderate and mild ARDS respectively.[9]

This formula, despite the conscious incorporation of FiO_2 into it, must still be regarded as an approximation; it is particularly unreliable when the FiO_2 is either very low or very high.[10]

iii. The alveolo-arterial diffusion of oxygen A-DO_2

The capital 'A' represents the partial pressure of O_2 in the alveolar air, and the 'a' in small case represents the partial pressure of O_2 in the arterial blood. The A–aDO_2 is the difference between the alveolar O_2 tension (PAO_2) and the arterial oxygen tension (PaO_2) and thus a measure of the capacity of the lungs to oxygenate blood.

The normal A–a DO_2 is not constant at all values of FiO_2. Normal values range from 7 to 14 mmHg on room air to (less than) 70 mmHg on a FiO_2 of 1.0. Since the normal A–a DO_2 gradient in relation to the FiO_2 describes a bell-shaped curve assessments between the extremes of FiO_2 (0.21 and 1.0) are difficult and unpredictable. Thus, for convenience, the A–aDO_2 is conventionally assessed at either room air or on an FO_2 of 1.0.[10]

The A–aDO_2 helps elucidate mechanism of hypoxemia (it is widened when a V/Q mismatch, right to left shunt or diffusion defect exists; importantly it is normal when hypoventilation is the cause for the hypoxemia (*see* causes of respiratory acidosis, **Tables 6.5 and 6.7**).

Unfortunately, calculation of the A–a DO_2 requires knowledge of the value of PAO_2, which is not directly measurable. PAO_2 itself can however be calculated from from the simplified form of the alveolar gas equation ($PAO_2 = FiO_2 (P_b–P_w)–PaCO_2/R$)*.

Abbreviations: PAO_2 = alveolar oxygen tension; PaO_2 = ; FiO_2 = fraction of inspired oxygen; P_b = atmospheric pressure in mmHg; P_w = partial pressure of water (47 mmHg at body temperature); $PaCO_2$ = arterial CO_2 tension; R = respiratory quotient.

The values of A–aDO_2, he rises physiologically with age, and can be predicted from the following equation:

$$A–aDO_2 = 2.5 + (0.25 \times \text{Age in years}).$$

Nevertheless, like the other 'formulae' listed here, the A–aDO_2 is not foul proof. For one thing, the respiratory quotient is often assumed to be 0.8; in a critically ill individual this is not always the case. For another, estimates of FiO_2 are seldom precise, especially so if the pattern of breathing is irregular. Thus, between the two extremes of inhaled

FiO_2 (0.21 and 1.0), the expected A–aDO_2 level even in the normal subject is difficult to predict. There exists no reliable reference value for the A–aDO_2 when a patient is on intermediate levels of FiO_2.

(.1) '.1' Represents the correction factor applied in acute respiratory acidosis[11]

The question, 'What is the expected compensation for the rise in CO_2 in acute respiratory acidosis?' is answered by the formula:

$$\Delta HCO^- = \Delta CO_2 \times 0.1,$$

since HCO_3^- increases by 0.1 mEq/L for every 1 mmHg rise in CO_2.
Delta (Δ) of course stands for 'change in'

Is the HCO_3^- level greater than expected by the formula? If so, a primary metabolic alkalosis is associated.

Is the HCO_3^- level lower than expected by the formula? If so, a primary metabolic acidosis is associated.

Table 6.5: Causes of acute respiratory acidosis
Central depression of respiratory drive *Drugs* (sedatives, opiates, anaesthetic agents) *CNS lesions* (cerebrovascular events, CNS trauma, encephalitis)
Neuromuscular High spinal cord lesions or trauma (at or above level of C4) High central neural blockade Infection (tetanus, poliomyelitis, botulism) Dyselectreolytemias Amyotrophic lateral sclerosis Myasthenia gravis Organophosphate poisoning Muscular relaxants
Airways Proximal airway obstruction (aspiration, foreign body, tumors) Asthma or COPD
Chest wall Flail chest Diaphragmatic dysfunction (diaphragmatic paralysis, muscle splinting due to pain, rupture)
Pleura Pneumothorax (large primary, or even a relatively small secondary pneumothorax) Pleural effusion (especially when large/rapidly accumulating)
Lung parenchyma Pulmonary edema (cardiogenic) ARDS Pneumonia

Box 6.1: Respiratory acidosis to metabolic alkalosis: Post-hypercapnic status

A patient with chronic respiratory acidosis compensates for the acidosis by retaining bicarbonate over time. A high bicarbonate with a near-normal pH is thus a sign of renal compensation. If such a patient is commenced on artificial respiratory support (invasive or noninvasive mechanical ventilation) with inappropriately high minute ventilation, the washout of CO_2 drops the $PaCO_2$ acutely and thereby raises the pH. The bicarbonate initially remains elevated since the kidney is relatively slow to act. The combination of a high pH and a high bicarbonate thus presents a picture of metabolic alkalosis, whereas in reality it is a respiratory acidosis that has been too-rapidly corrected. Post-hypercapnic metabolic alkalosis is also a low urinary chloride state, owing to acute hypocapnia-related chloride shifts.[12]

(.2) '.2' Represents the correction factor applied in acute respiratory alkalosis[10]

The question, 'What is the expected compensation for the rise in CO_2 in acute respiratory alkalosis?' is answered by the formula:

$$\Delta HCO_3^- = \Delta CO_2 \times 0.2,$$

since HCO_3^- decreases by 0.2 mEq/L for every 1 mmHg fall in CO_2.

Is the HCO_3^- level greater than expected by the formula? If so, a primary metabolic alkalosis is associated.

Is the HCO_3^- level lower than expected by the formula? If so, a primary metabolic acidosis is associated.

(.3) To us, the .3 in the approach presents something of a difficulty.

The modified Henderson-Hasselbalch equation states that,

$$H^+ = 24\ (PaCO\ /HCO_3^-)$$

Using the ratio $\Delta H^+/\Delta CO_2$, acute, acute-on-chronic and chronic respiratory acidosis can be differentiated from each other.[13]

When the value of $\Delta H^+/\Delta CO_2$ falls above **0.3** (but is less than 0.7), an acute-on-chronic respiratory acidosis may be presumed to exist. Unfortunately this formula requires the application of H+ concentration, which is somewhat labour-intensive. Therefore, the '**.3**' in this approach may be considered optional.

(.4) '.4' represents the correction factor applied in chronic respiratory acidosis.[11]

The question, 'What is the expected compensation for the rise in CO_2 in chronic respiratory acidosis?' is answered by the formula:

$$\Delta HCO_3^- = \Delta CO_2 \times 0.4,$$

(since HCO_3^- increases by 0.4 mEq/L for every 1 mmHg rise in CO_2).

Is the HCO_3^- level greater than expected by the formula? If so, a primary metabolic alkalosis is associated.

Is the HCO_3^- level lower than expected by the formula? If so, a primary metabolic acidosis is associated.

(.5) '.5' represents the correction factor applied in chronic respiratory alkalosis.[11]

The question, 'What is the expected compensation for the rise in CO_2 in chronic respiratory alkalosis?' is answered by the formula:

$$\Delta HCO_3^- = \Delta CO_2 \times 0.5,$$

(since HCO_3^- falls by 0.5 mEq/L for every 1 mmHg fall in CO_2).

Is the HCO_3^- level greater than expected by the formula? If so, a primary metabolic alkalosis is associated.

Is the HCO_3^- level lower than expected by the formula? If so, a primary metabolic acidosis is associated.

Table 6.7: Chronic respiratory acidosis
✦ Depression of central respiratory drive ✦ Primary alveolar hypoventilation
Lung parenchyma Longstanding and severe ILD
Airways ✦ Persistent asthma ✦ Severe ✦ COPD ✦ Bronchiectasis
Pleura Chronic large effusions
Chest wall ✦ Kyphoscoliosis ✦ Obesity
Neuromuscular ✦ Dyselectrolytemias ✦ Malnutrition ✦ Chronic neuro-myopathies ✦ Poliomyelitis

Table 6.8: Differentiating the various causes of hypoxemia from each other

	V/Q mismatch	Shunt	Diffusion defect	Hypoventilation
PaO_2	Low	Low	Low	Low
Response to administration of 100% O_2 (FiO_2 1.0)	Responsive	Unresponsive	Responsive	Responsive
$A\text{–}aDO_2$	Wide	Wide	Wide	Normal
$PaCO_2$	Normal*	Normal*	Normal*	Raised

* Unless another mechanism of hypoxemia is present as well **(see Box 6.2)**

Box 6.2: Other points to keep in mind while interpreting blood gases

- **Has the syringe been iced immediately after drawing the sample?**
  A 15 min period is allowable[14] but failure to ice the ABG syringe for a longer time than this can result in falsely low PaO_2 readings due to consumption of the PaO_2 by the blood cells in the sample.
- **Has the ABG sample been drawn after an adequate time has elapsed after making a change in the FiO_2?**
  After any change in FiO_2, a minimum of 5–7 min is considered acceptable in patients with normal lungs[15] and a minimum of 20–25 min in a patient with significant lung disease.
- **Is there a need to factor in a high leucocyte count into the interpretation of the ABG sample?**
  Very high numbers of white cell (as in leukaemia) or platelet counts (as in thrombocytosis) can consume O_2 in spite of icing the sample and result in falser low PaO_2s ("pseudohypoxemia"). As well, cells may physically coat the surface of the O_2 electrode preventing proper measurement.[16]
  Immediate centrifugation of the blood and analysis of the supernatant plasma may circumvent this problem.[17]
- **Has the syringe been properly heparinized (and not over-heparinised)?**
  Physical dilution by the excess fluid represented by the heparin can result in lowering of the PaO_2 and $PaCO_2$ giving spuriously low readings. Heparin is acidic, and if the pH of the blood is initially alkaline or normal, it will be spuriously lowered. On the other hand if the initial pH of the blood is highly acidic, the mildly acidic heparin will cause it to rise.
- **Has care been taken to eliminate air bubbles from the syringe?**
  The partial pressure of O_2 in the ambient air at sea level (and therefore in an air bubble drawn at sea level) is ~160 mmHg. If the PaO_2 of the blood is lower than 160 mmHg, it will rise; if lower, it will fall.[18] An air bubble, containing virtually no CO_2, will reduce the $PaCO_2$ of the blood, and by doing so, raise pH.
- **Is there a difference in the readings depending upon whether a glass or a plastic syringe is used?**
  Plastic syringes are relatively porous. When the PaO_2 of blood is very high (e.g. >220 mmHg), O_2 may diffuse out, thereby spuriuosly lowering the measured PaO_2.[19] As well, the greater suction used in drawing out the piston of a plastic syringe can potentially draw gas 'out of solution.' A spurious fall in PaO_2 by as much as 12 mmHg[20] might then result.

At the beginning of the ABG analysis, the clinical history and manifestations should be kept in mind to give the analysis context; at the end, of the analysis, the conclusions drawn from the blood-gas analysis should be once again correlated with the clinical condition.

References

1. Hasan A. The Analysis of Blood Gases. In: Handbook of Blood Gas and Acid–Base Interpretation, Second Edition (2013) Springer-Verlag London. P 253–66.
2. Hasan A. Metabolic Acidosis. In: Handbook of Blood Gas and Acid–Base Interpretation, Second Edition (2013) Springer-Verlag London. P 189–236.
3. Wren K. The delta gap: an approach to mixed acid–base disorders. Ann Emerg Med. 1990;19:1310.
4. Gennari FJ. Serum osmolality. Uses and limitations. N Engl J Med. 1984;301:102.
5. Glasser L, Sternglanz PD, Combie J, Robinson A. Serum osmolality and its applicability to drug overdose. Am J Clin Pathol. 1973;60:695.

6. Hasan A. Metabolic Alkalosis. In: Handbook of Blood Gas and Acid–Base Interpretation, Second Edition (2013) Springer-Verlag London. P 237–52.
7. Battle DC, Hizon M, Cohen E, Gutterman C, Gupta R. The use of the urinary anion gap in the diagnosis of hyperchloremic metabolic acidosis. New Eng J Med. 1988;318:594–9.
8. Oh MS. Carroll HJ. "Value and Determinants of Urine Anion Gap." Nephron 90 (2002): 252 –55.
9. Fanelli V, Vlachou A, Ghannadian S, Simonetti U, *et al.* Acute respiratory distress syndrome: new definition, current and future therapeutic options. J Thorac Dis. 2013 Jun; 5(3): 326–34.
10. Hasan A. Gas Exchange. In: Handbook of Blood Gas and Acid–Base Interpretation, Second Edition (2013) Springer-Verlag London. P 1–50.
11. Hasan A. Respiratory Acidosis. In: Handbook of Blood Gas and Acid–Base Interpretation, Second Edition (2013) Springer-Verlag London. P 171–180.
12. Schwartz WB, Hays RM, Polak A, Haynie G. Effects of chronic hypercapnia on electrolyte and acid–base equilibrium. II. Recovery with special reference to the influence of chloride intake. J Clin Invest. 1961;40:1238.
13. Demers RR, Irwin RS. Management of hypercapnic respiratory failure: a systematic approach. Rev Resp Care. 1979;24:328
14. Hansen JE. Arterial blood gases. In: Mahler DA, editor. Pulmonary function testing. Clin Chest Med. 1989;5:227–37
15. Cugell DW. How long should you wait? [editorial] Chest. 1975;67:253.
16. Hess CE, Nichols AS, Hunt WB, *et al.* Pseudohypoxemia secondary to leukemia and thrombocy- tosis. N Engl J Med. 1979;301:361–3.
17. Charan NB, Marks M, Carvalho P. Use of plasma for arterial blood gas analysis in leukemia. Chest. 1994;105:954–5.
18. Mueller RG, Lang GE, Beam JM. Bubbles in samples for blood gas determinations: a potential source of error. Am J Clin Pathol. 1976;65:242.
19. Winkler JB, Huntington CG, Wells DE, Befeler B. Influence of syringe material on arterial blood gas determinations. Chest. 1974;66:518.
20. Ansel GM, Douce FH. Effect of needle syringe material and needle size on the minimum plunger- displacement pressure of arterial blood gas syringes. Respir Care. 1982;27:127.

CHAPTER 7

Hypoxemic Respiratory Failure (Prevention and Management)

Srinivas Samavedam

Hypoxia is a state in which oxygen is not available in adequate amounts at the tissue or cellular level. Hypoxemia is low oxygen content in the blood which can be either due to reduced oxygen in inspired air or reduced blood supply, i.e. decreased perfusion or due to defect in diffusion along the alveolar-capillary membrane

Acute respiratory failure is an emergency condition and prompt address of all of the underlying etiology and early initiation of treatment can save the patient

Before understanding the etiology and management we need to understand the basic physiology of oxygen transport.

OXYGEN TRANSPORT

Oxygen is vital for life-sustaining aerobic respiration in humans

Oxygen acts as a terminal electron transport chain in the mitochondrial inner membrane in the electron transport chain (ETC) which helps in ATP formation, which supplies energy to all active metabolic processes.

Types of oxygen transport:

1. **Convective:** It is defined as the building movement of oxygen within the circulation using energy this is an active process.
2. **Diffusive:** It is defined as the oxygen transport by gradient dependent on the partial pressure of oxygen, e.g. diffusion from alveoli to pulmonary capillaries, diffusion from systemic capillaries to cells

   It can be described by Ficks law

Oxygen Cascade

It is defined as the physiological steps for bringing atmospheric oxygen into the body where it is delivered to metabolically active tissue, where it is utilised for energy production.

First step: An initial step of the O_2 cascade is to transport O_2 from the atmosphere to the alveoli

Factors affecting are:

Altitude - partial pressure of O_2

Pulmonary blood flow

Alveolar ventilation

Second step: Transfer of oxygen from alveoli to blood

Factors affecting are:

Alveolar-capillary memberane

Haemoglobin concentration

The partial pressure of O_2 in alveolus —> $PaO_2 = 100$ mmHg

The partial pressure of O_2 in mixed venous blood (SvO_2) = 40 mmHg

Factors helping diffusion of O_2

A large PO_2 gradient

The larger surface area of gas exchange within the diffusion barrier

A favourable diffusion coefficient of O_2

Rapid binding of O_2 to haemoglobin, which helps in near complete equilibration of PO_2 during rapid transit time (0.7 sec) of blood through pulmonary capillaries

Equilibration of PCO_2 is even more rapid than O_2, despite of small pressure gradient (46–40 mmHg), because of the high diffusion coefficient.

Content of oxygen in arterial blood:

CaO_2—the amount of O_2 in each 100 ml of blood

$$CaO_2 = O_2 \text{ bound to haemoglobin} + O_2 \text{ dissolved in plasma}$$
$$= (1.34 \times hb \times SaO_2 \times 0.01) + (0.03 \times PaO_2)$$

1.34 is Hefner's constant (each gram of Hb binds to 1.34 ml of O_2)

Hb-haemoglobin concentration

SaO_2-saturation of HB

0.3-solubility coefficient of O_2 in water

Third step:

DO_2-amount of O_2 delivered to tissues in each minute

$$DO_2 = \text{cardiac output (c.o)} \times CaO_2 \text{ (arterial } O_2 \text{ content)}$$
$$\text{c.o} = \text{heart rate} \times \text{stroke volume}$$

Factors Affecting O_2 Delivery

- Stagnant anoxia = Decreased cardiac output
- Anoxic anoxia = Arterial hypoxemia
- Anaemic anoxia = Reduced HB
- Cytotoxic anoxia = Seconfary to sepsis/inflammation
- Histotoxic anoxia = Cyanide poisoning
- Peripheral causes—Microcircualtion failure
- The reduced affinity of the Hb molecule (**Fig. 7.1**)

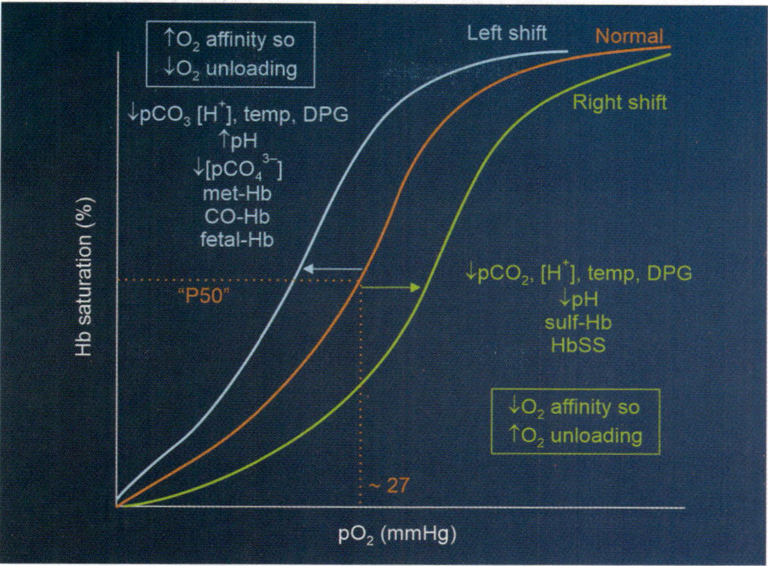

Fig. 7.1: Oxygen dissociation curve

7.1 Oxygen Dissociation Curve

An ODC curve plots the proportion of haemoglobin in its saturated form on the vertical axis, against the prevailing O_2 tension on the X-axis.

It is related to the percentage of the O_2 carrying capacity of HB and partial pressure of O_2

Plateau portion – at pulmonary capillaries

Steep portion – at systemic capillaries

At pressures above 60 mmHg, the curve is relatively flat, the O_2 content of blood does not change significantly even with the larger increase in the O_2 partial pressure

The p50—the partial pressure of O_2 at which 50% of Hb is saturated, typically about 26.6 mmHg for a healthy person

A right shift of the curve implies p50 is increased, larger partial pressure of O_2 is required to maintain 50% O_2 saturation decreased the affinity of O_2 to HB

A right shift of the curve is caused by:

- Increased PCO_2
- Increased H^+ (acidosis)
- Increased diphosphoglycerate
- Increased temperature
- Self-Hb
- Hb-ss

The leftward shift of the curve

Implies lower p50, higher affinity to O_2 to HB

Caused by: Decreased temperature, hydrogen ions (alkalosis), DPG, phosphate

Met-HB
Co-HB
Fetal-HB

Bohr effect: Decrease in oxygen affinity of a respiratory pigment such as haemoglobin in response to decreased Ph, resulting from increased CO_2 concentration in blood

Haldane Effect

Decrease in carbon dioxide affinity of haemoglobin due to increased blood pH resulting from increased oxygen concentration in blood.

Fourth Step

VO_2-oxygen consumed by the tissue per minute

$$VO_2 = c.o \times (CaO_2 - CVO_2)$$

At tissue level $VO_2 = q \times \{(O_{2\,in}) - (O_{2\,out})\}$

$$q = \text{blood flow}$$

$$O_{2\,in} = \text{afferent blood } O_2 \text{ content} = CaO_2$$

$$O_{2\,out} = \text{efferent blood } O_2 \text{ content} = CVO_2$$

Increase VO_2
✦ Exercise
✦ Trauma (surgery, burns)
✦ Shivering
✦ Pain
✦ Agitation
✦ Feeding regimes containing excessive glucose

Decrease VO_2
✦ Sedation/analgesia
✦ Neuromuscular blocking
✦ Hypovolemia/shock
✦ Hypothermia

Oxygen extraction ratio: Oxygen extraction ratio is a ratio of the body's oxygen consumption to the systemic O_2 delivery

$$O_{2\,er} = VO_2/DO_2$$

$$VO_2 = c.o \times (CaO_2 - CvO_2)$$

$$DO_2 = c.o \times CaO_2$$

$$O_{2\,er} = CaO_2 - CvO_2/CaO_2$$

At tissue level $= O_{2\,in} - O_{2\,out}/O_{2\,in}$

In healthy individuals, only 20–30% of the O_2 delivered to the tissue is utilized

In adult $O_{2\,er}$ at rest = 0.26

O_2 consumption is supply independent, and VO_2 is maintained even in the face of decreased DO_2

At criticial DO_2 (approx 4 ml/kg/min) in humans $O_{2\,er}$ is maximum (0.6–0.8), VO_2 is dependent

If DO_2 continue to decrease below the critical value results in tissue hypoxia. Anaerobic respiration (because of an imbalance of ATP supply and demand) sets in and results in lactic acid production.

Hypoxia

It is defined as the reducction of oxygen supply to tissue
It is not directly measured

Hypoxemia

It is defined as decreased arterial oxygen tension/partial pressure of oxygen in the blood
Normal: 80 – 100 mmHg
Mild: 60 – 80 mmHg
Moderate: 40 – 60 mmHg
Severe: <40 mmHg

APPROACH TO HYPOXEMIA

Different types of hypoxia are as follows **(Table 7.1)**:

Table 7.1: Different types of hypoxia

Type	Definition
Hypoxemic hypoxia	Low oxygen tension in the blood
Circulatory hypoxia	Unable to deliver oxygen properly due to pump failure
Anaemic hypoxia	Reduced oxygen-carrying capacity due to low haemoglobin in the blood
Histotoxic hypoxia	Decreased oxygen uptake at a cellular level

Approach to Hypoxemia

Hypoxemia occurs mainly due to 5 causes.

1. Hypoventilation
2. Ventilation-perfusion mismatch
3. Decreased diffusion capacity
4. Reduced inspired oxygen content
5. Shunt

These causes are categorized based on the value of the alveolar-arterial oxygen gradient. Alveolar-arterial oxygen gradient is the difference between partial pressure of oxygen in alveoli and partial pressure of oxygen in arteries.

$$\text{Alveolar-arterial oxygen gradient} = P_AO_2 - P_aO_2$$

The normal alveolar-arterial oxygen gradient is less than 15 mmHg. Alveolar oxygen tension is obtained by the alveolar gas equation. Arterial oxygen tension is obtained by arterial blood gas analysis of the patient (**Fig. 7.2**).

Alveolar gas equation:

$$P_AO_2 = (PB - P_{H_2O})\ FiO_2 - (P_ACO_2/R)$$

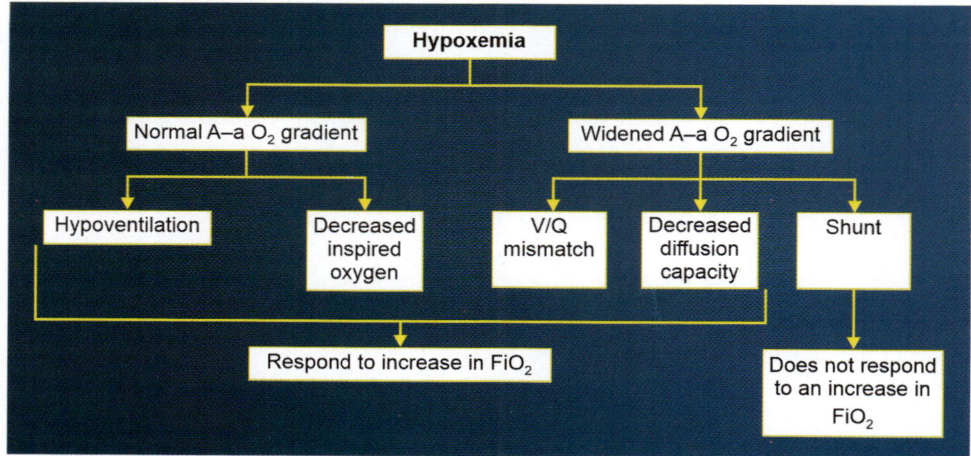

Fig. 7.2: Algorithm to analyze hypoxemia

i. **Decreased inspired oxygen:** It occurs at high altitudes where the alveolar oxygen tension decreases. It can be corrected by an increase in FiO_2.
ii. **Hypoventilation:** It can be caused due to central hypoventilation, neuromuscular disorders, drugs, encephalitis, and obesity. This can be corrected by increased oxygen concentration.
iii. **V/Q mismatch:** It can occur due to a discrepancy between ventilation of the lung and blood flow in the same region. Low V/Q ratio Chronic obstructive pulmonary disease, obstructive airway disease, pulmonary oedema. High V/Q ratio → Emphysematous lung, pulmonary embolism
iv. **Decreased diffusion capacity:** Occurs due to a defect in the alveolar-capillary membrane. Examples include interstitial oedema, interstitial lung disease or pulmonary fibrosis
v. **Shunt:** Anatomic shunt → In case of congenital heart diseases like ASD, VSD, pulmonary arteriovenous malformations. Shunting also occurs when there is blood flow in the region of the non-ventilated alveolar as in the case of atelectasis, ARDS.

Evaluation of Hypoxia

It can be evaluated based on the clinical history of fever, cough, and shortness of breath. Severe hypoxia can cause neurological manifestations like headache, restlessness and confusion.

Physical examination shows tachycardia, tachypnea, dyspnea, and orthopnea. Lung auscultation may reveal wheezing in the case of COPD or crepitations in the case of pulmonary oedema. There may be raised JVP or pedal oedema in case of right ventricular failure.

Hypoxia can be evaluated at the bedside by respiratory rate and pulse oximeter monitoring. Bedside ABG analysis will also help in evaluating the severity of hypoxia and calculating the PaO_2/FiO_2 ratio to grade ARDS. Alveolar and arterial oxygen gradients can also be obtained to differentiate various causes of hypoxemia. Imaging modalities include chest X-ray, lung ultrasound and high-resolution CT. Bedside lung ultrasonography helps in identifying various lung pathologies as per blue protocol.

USG BASED APPROACH

BLUE protocol gives a step-wise approach to identifying the pathology in the lung.

- It emphasises three BLUE profiles
- A profile—A-lines with lung sliding with A lines (A lines are repetitive horizontal artefacts p of pleural line)
- B profile—lung rockets with lung sliding (rockets or B lines are well defined, hyperechoic lines from pleural lines erasing the A lines)
- C profile—represents lung consolidation
- To approach these profiles, we have to keep the linear transducer over the specified points on the anterior chest wall called the BLUE points (**Fig. 7.3**).
- Two hands are placed side by side with thumbs excluded on one side of the anterior chest wall such that the upper hand is touching the clavicle.
- The upper BLUE point is the point corresponding to the middle of the upper hand.
- The lower BLUE point is the point corresponding to the middle of the lower hand.
- PLAPS point is the point corresponding to the intersection of the horizontal line drawn at the level of the lower BLUE point with the vertical line at the posterior axillary line.

The various signs associated are as described

1. **Normal lung:** The pleural line indicates the parietal pleura on B mode and shows a bat sign with the underlying lung showing A-lines.

   On M-mode, it shows a **seashore sign**, therefore, indicating that the pleural line also is the visceral pleura. Above the pleural line, the motionless chest wall displays a stratified pattern. Below the pleural line, the dynamics of lung sliding show this sandy pattern

2. **Pleural effusion:** Below the pleural line, a line parallel to will be seen indicating the visceral pleura (lung line). These two parallel horizontal lines along with ribs are called the quad sign (**Fig. 7.4**)

   M mode shows a movement of the lung line toward the pleural line) on inspiration called the sinusoid sign

3. **Consolidation:** A consolidation which does not invade the whole lobe generates a shredded or broken boundary between the consolidation and the underlying aerated lung. This is called the shred or fractal sign. Such an anterior consolidation generates the C-profile in the BLUE protocol.

   When the consolidation involves the entire lung, no aerated zone is soon and it looks like the liver. This is called a tissue like sign

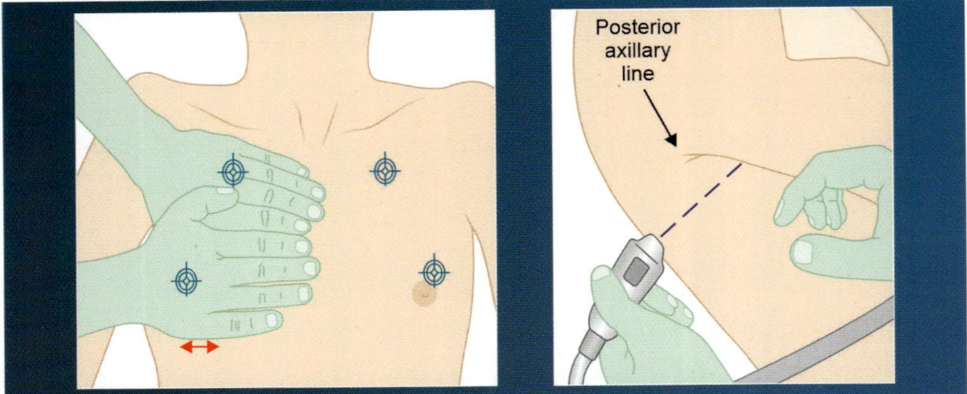

Fig. 7.3A and B: The bedside lung ultrasound in emergency (BLUE)-points. This figure shows the standardized points used in the BLUE-protocol. Two hands (from roughly the patient's size) are applied as follows: upper little finger just below clavicle, fingertips at middle line, and lower hand just below upper hand (thumbs excluded). The point coined "upper BLUE-point" is at the middle of the upper hand the "lower BLUE-point is at the middle of the lower palm. These four points roughly follow the anatomy of the lungs, and avoid the hear as much as possible. The posterolateral alveoar and/ or pleural syndrome (PLAPS)-point is built from the horizontal line continuing the lowe BLUE-point and the vertical line continuing the lower BLUE-point and the vertical line continuing the posterior axillary line. The intersection, rigorously, is the PLAPS-point, but the user can mover the probe in two directions: (1) As posteriorly as possible in order to get more the probe scans the abdomen. Like the six spots of ECG, the six BLUE-points help in reproducible analysis. They were sufficient for providing the 90.5% accuracy of the BLUE-protocol. (Adapted with permission from Lichtenstein)

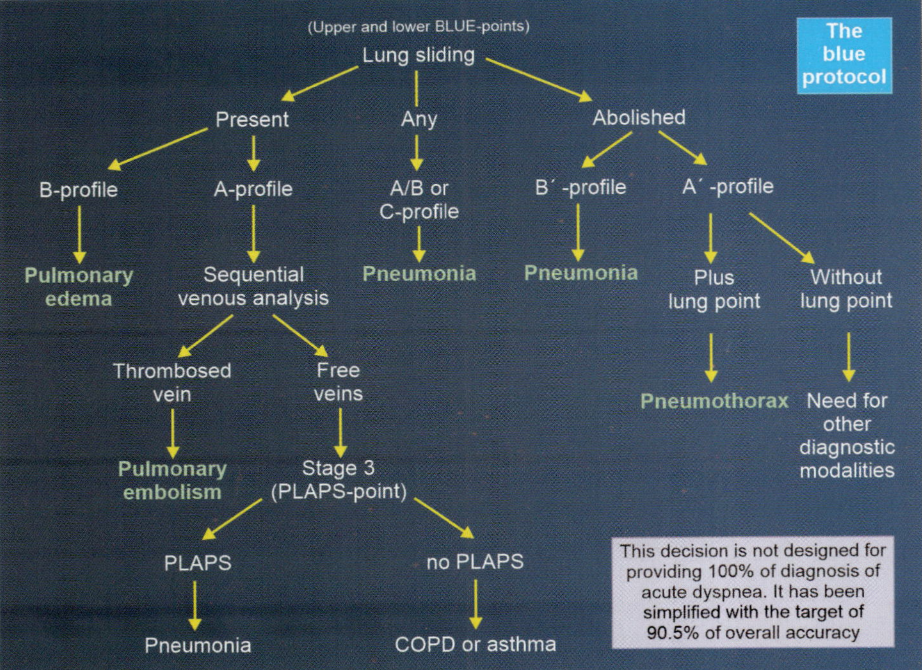

Fig. 7.4: The blue protocol (ultrasound) to evaluate lung pathology

4. **Pneumothorax:** Even with A-lines when sliding are absent, on M mode the normal seashore sign is abolished and it shows a stratosphere sign.
   Sometimes 'A'-lines are seen and at one point shift to the B profile. On M mode, it shows a sudden transition to the stratosphere sign from the seashore sign. This point is called a lung point sign and is more specific for pneumothorax.

OXYGEN DELIVERY DEVICES

Supplemental oxygen is delivered through various devices based on the severity of hypoxia and clinical status. They are classified based on oxygen flow per minute into a low flow and high flow devices. Also classified based on the performance of the device whether they provide a variable or constant FiO_2 into variable or fixed performance devices **(Table 7.2)**.

Table 7.2

Low flow devices	High flow devices
These devices provide oxygen at flow rates less than the patient's ventilatory demands. They provide variable FiO_2 due to the entrainment of room air based on the inspiratory flows.	These devices provide oxygen at higher flow rates ensuring adequate ventilation.
Example: Nasal cannula Simple face mask Partial rebreather facemask Non-rebreather facemask	**Example:** Venturi mask High flow nasal cannula Non-invasive ventilation Invasive mechanical ventilation

Nasal Cannula

A most common device used for oxygen delivery. It can be used to deliver oxygen up to flow rates of 6 liters/min. Inspired oxygen concentration can vary between 24 and 40% based on the flow rate. Beyond the flow rate of 6 liters/min, they can cause drying of the nasal mucosa and nasal bleeding **(Fig. 7.5)**.

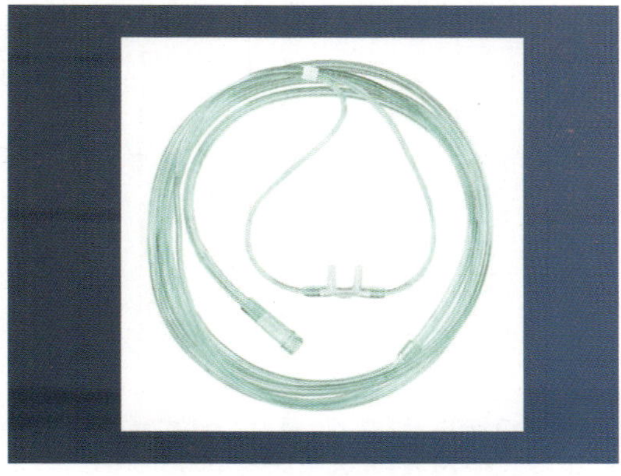

Fig. 7.5: Nasal cannula

Simple Face Mask

Flow rates used through a simple face mask are 6–8 litres/minute. FiO_2 delivered can vary from 40–60% based on flow rate. They also cause dryness of mucosa (**Fig. 7.6**).

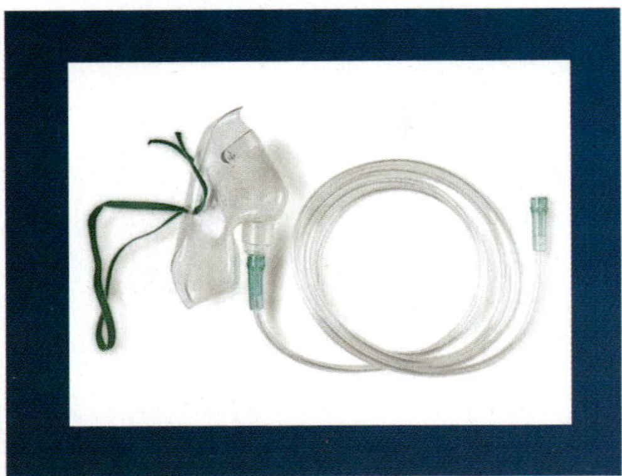

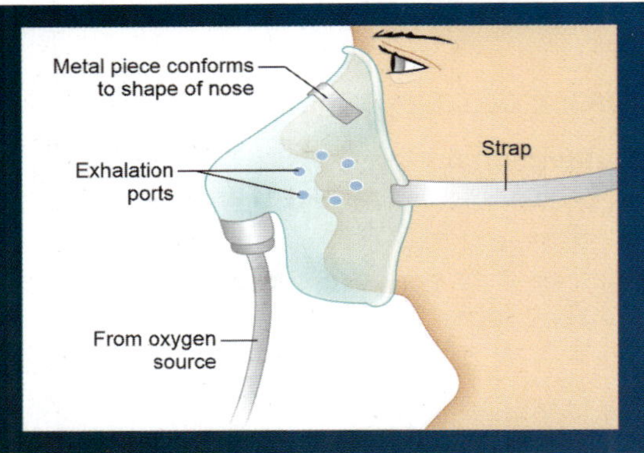

Fig. 7.6: Simple face mask

Partial Rebreather Mask

It has a reservoir bag of 300–500 ml capacity. There is no one-way valve between the mask and reservoir bag allowing the mixture of inspired and expired gas. Flow rates are to be maintained between 6 and 10 liters/minute. FiO_2 delivered varies between 50 and 70%. Flow rates less than the prescribed lead to the collapse of the reservoir.

Non-Rebreather Mask

It has a reservoir bag of 300–500 ml capacity with 2 one-way valves to prevent exhaled air to enter into reservoir bag. Flow rates are to be maintained between 10 and 15 liters/ minutes. FiO_2 delivered varies between 85 and 90%. Flow rates less than the prescribed lead to a collapse of a reservoir (**Fig. 7.7**).

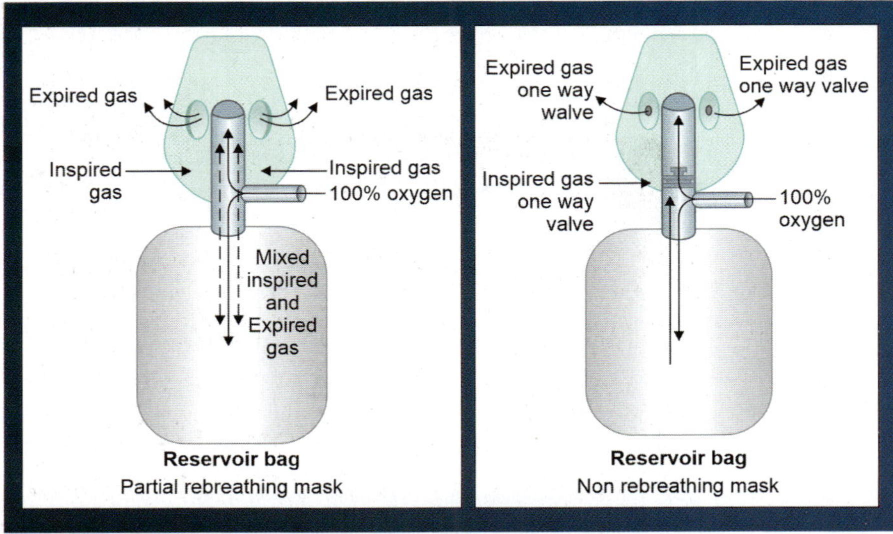

Fig. 7.7: Mask with reservoir bag (two types)

Venturi Mask

It is a facemask with a valve for air entrainment. It works on the Bernoulli principle **(Table 7.3)**.

Table 7.3: Venturi valve

Color	FiO_2	O_2 Flow
Blue	24%	2L/min
White	28%	4 L/min
Orange	31%	6 L/min
Yellow	35%	8 L/min
Red	40%	10 L/min
Green	60%	15 L/min

It is a fixed-performance device. It can also be used during weaning on T-piece.

High Flow Nasal Cannula

It consists of a flow generator, air-oxygen blender, humidifier and a nasal cannula. Flows can be generated up to 60 litres/minute. FiO_2 can be titrated up to 100%. Advantages of HFNC include providing humidified oxygen at high flows to improve FRC by providing a PEEP of 6–8 cm H_2O and reducing the work of breathing **(Fig. 7.8)**.

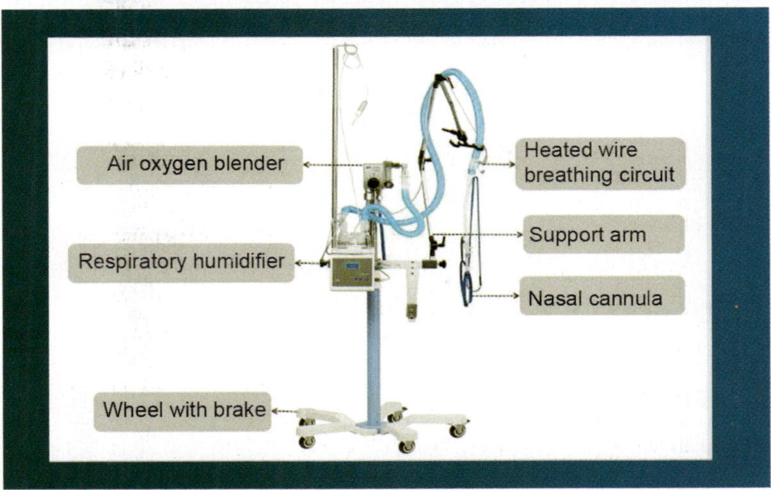

Fig. 7.8

Non-invasive and Invasive Positive Pressure Ventilation

CPAP/BiPAP is used to provide positive pressure ventilation at fixed FiO_2. Used in patients with COPD, ARDS and OSA. Patients who are not maintained with NIV are provided invasive positive pressure ventilation through an endotracheal tube.

CHAPTER 8

Essentials of Ventilator Waveforms

Scan QR code to access additional material on waveform

❐ Vijay Deshpande ❐ Ruben Restrepo

INTRODUCTION

The purpose of this chapter is to provide clinicians with the specific knowledge and interpretive skills necessary to recognize various aspects of patient and ventilator interaction, in both text and graphical formats.

DESCRIPTION

This chapter identifies typical tracings and analysis of commonly encountered waveforms during mechanical ventilation. The following waveforms are described in this module:

Scalars
1. Flow vs Time
2. Pressure vs Time
3. Volume vs Time

Loops
1. Pressure – Volume Loop
2. Flow – Volume Loop

OBJECTIVES

A. General Objectives

1. Identify the variables that make up the scalars and loops.
2. Differentiate between loops and scalars.
3. Recognize the most common modes of ventilation on scalar graphics.

B. Identify on a Flow–Time Curve:

1. Inadequate flow
2. Different Flow Patterns
3. Airway Obstruction vs. Active Exhalation
4. Air trapping

C. Identify on a Volume–Time Curve:

1. Air leak.
2. Active exhalation.

D. Identify on a Pressure–Time Curve:

1. Mechanical vs spontaneous breath.
2. Patient cycled or assisted breath.
3. Components of the pressure curve.
4. PIP, P_{plat} and correlation with airway resistance (R_{aw})

E. Identify on a Pressure–Volume Loop:

1. Controlled, assisted, and spontaneous breath.
2. Opening pressure.
3. Hysteresis.
4. Increased airway resistance.
5. Decreased and increased lung compliance.
6. Components of mechanical WOB.
7. Overdistension.
8. Inspiratory and expiratory inflection points.
9. Air leak.

F. Identify on a Flow–Volume Loop:

1. PIFR/PEFR.
2. Air leak.
3. Air trapping.
4. Airway resistance.
5. β_2 response.
6. Inadequate flow.

Abbreviations and Definitions

Throughout this chapter the following words and abbreviations are used:

PIFR	-	Peak Inspiratory Flow Rate
PEFR	-	Peak Expiratory Flow Rate
PIP	-	Peak Inspiratory Pressure
PEEP	-	Positive End Expiratory Pressure
Pplat	-	Plateau Pressure
Raw	-	Airway Resistance
Paw	-	Airway Pressure
VT	-	Tidal Volume
TI	-	Inspiratory Time, in seconds
TE	-	Expiratory Time, in seconds
TCT	-	Total Cycle Time, in seconds
I–E ratio	-	Inspiratory to Expiratory time ratio
Scalar graphic	-	A single variable plotted against time
Loop	-	Two variables plotted simultaneously

Hysteresis	-	Widening of a pressure–volume loop inflection
Point	-	The point of change in the slope of a line
Tracing	-	Used interchangeably with loop or curve
Opening Pressure	-	The point where pressure delivered begins to induce a corresponding volume change
WOB	-	Work of Breathing
CL	-	Lung Compliance
FRC	-	Functional Residual Capacity

Ventilator Graphics: General Concepts

Ventilator graphics have become an essential tool in managing patients on mechanical ventilators. All newer mechanical ventilators are equipped with a graphic package that displays selected ventilator waveforms facilitating assessment of the patient's condition.

Guidelines for proper interpretation and application of the most common ventilator graphics are described below:

The following waveforms will be described in this module:

Scalars	Loop
1. Flow vs Time	1. Pressure – Volume Loop
2. Pressure vs Time	2. Flow – Volume Loop
3. Volume vs Time	

Any single variable displayed against time is known as a **Scalar** graphic. The three parameters that make up the ventilator graphics, Flow, Volume and Pressure are plotted against Time.

These three scalars are generally referred to as:

Flow Curve | Volume Curve | Pressure Curve

When viewing scalar graphics, time is conventionally shown on the horizontal (x) axis, whereas, flow, volume, and pressure are plotted on the vertical (y) axis.

The tracings indicate typical Flow vs. Time, Pressure vs. Time and Volume vs. Time scalars during mechanical volume cycled ventilation with a constant (preset) flow. The next few frames discuss scalars and their clinical significance (**Figs 8.1 to 8.2**).

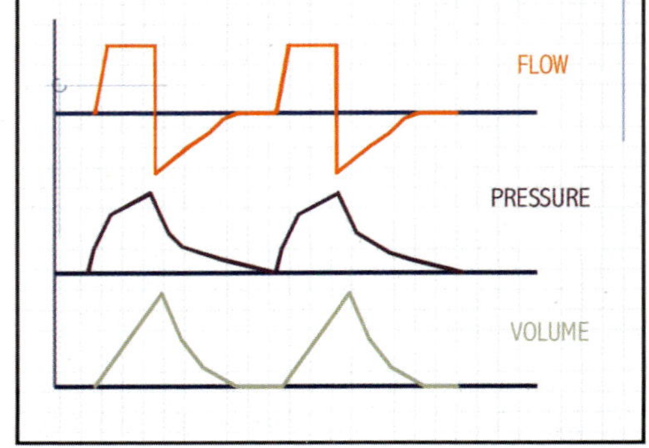

Fig. 8.1

Loops are the two-dimensional graphic displays of two scalar values. There are two loops available for interpretation. They are:

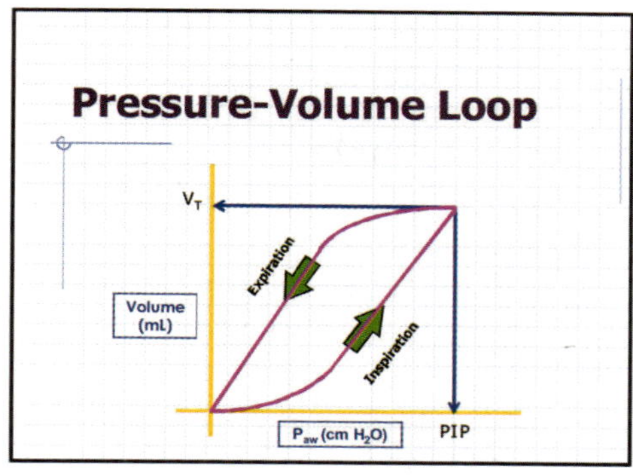

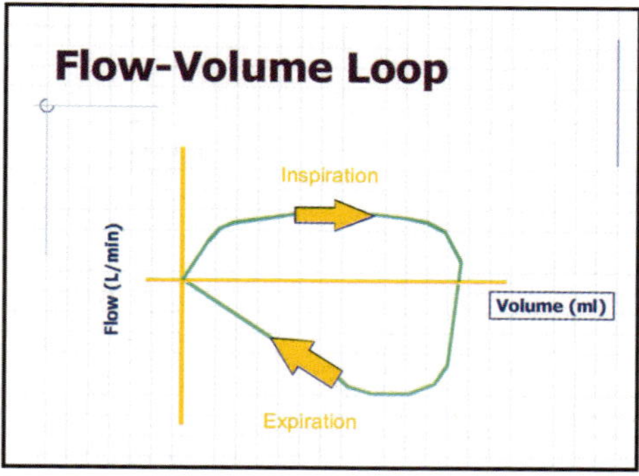

Fig. 8.2

When viewing the Pressure-Volume Loop, pressure is usually displayed on the horizontal (x) axis while volume is displayed on the vertical (y) axis.

When viewing the Flow-Volume Loop, the horizontal (x) axis is used to indicate volume whereas flow is displayed on the vertical (y) axis. As indicated in the flow-volume loop below, the inspiratory curve is plotted above the baseline and expiratory curve is traced below the baseline. However, it is not unusual to see a completely reverse pattern where the inspiratory component is presented below the baseline.

ANALYSIS OF SCALAR GRAPHICS

Each scalar will be discussed individually identifying components of the tracing and commonly observed normal and abnormal patterns.

Flow vs. Time Curve	
Basics of Flow vs. Time Curve	**Recognition of Common Abnormalities**
Spontaneous breath	Obstruction vs. active expiration
Mechanical breath	Response to bronchodilators
Typical flow patterns	Air trapping/auto-PEEP
Inspiratory flow	
Expiratory flow	

Spontaneous Breath

Observe that the inspiratory flow is traced above the baseline whereas expiratory flow is indicated below the baseline. The flow/time curve for a spontaneous breath resembles a SINEWAVE flow pattern (Fig. 8.3).

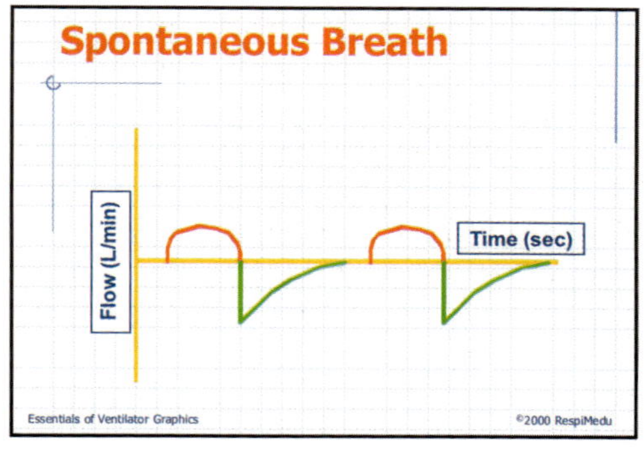

Fig. 8.3

Mechanical Breath

This tracing shows components of a flow vs. time curve for a mechanical volume-targeted breath (Fig. 8.4). Observe the following:

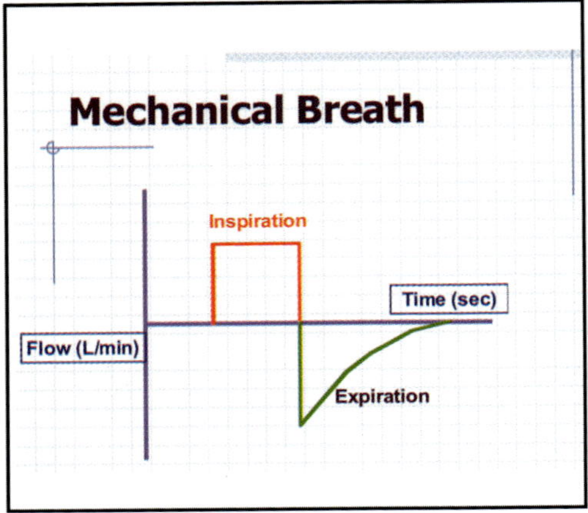

Fig. 8.4

- The inspiratory flow pattern is square, indicating a constant flow delivery. This pattern is selected by the operator on the ventilator
- There is a significant tracing below the baseline representing expiratory flow, which is dependent on the patient's lung characteristics and effort
- Only the Flow vs. Time curve demonstrates a significant tracing below the baseline. The other scalars stay above the baseline except on a Pressure vs. Time curve where a very small deflection occurs below the baseline when the patient initiates inspiration.

Typical Flow Patterns

Most ventilators allow a clinician to select a flow pattern that is most suitable to the patient. Typically a Square Flow, Descending Ramp or Decelerating Flow, Ascending or Accelerating Flow and A Sine Wave (**Fig. 8.5**).

Flow patterns are available. Observe that in each flow pattern illustrated on this frame the maximum flow rate is the same and T_I varies. However, if using a time-cycled ventilator (e.g. Servo 300) the T_I remains constant and flow varies to deliver the preset V_T.

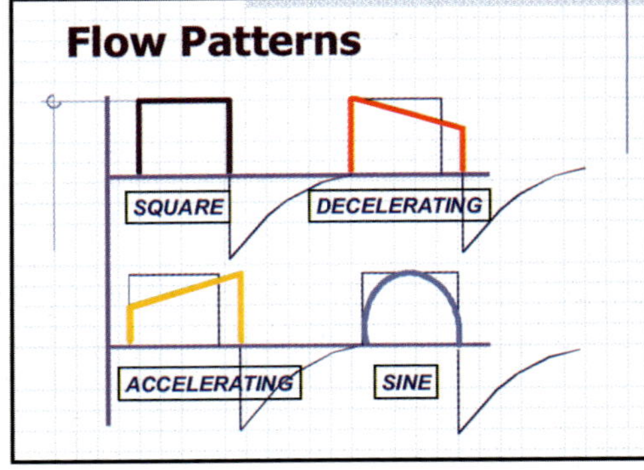

Fig. 8.5

Components of Inspiratory Flow

A Square Flow Pattern is used throughout this part to identify each component during the inspiratory phase of a mechanical volume-targeted breath. Observe each phase of the development of the inspiratory flow. Notice the following points and events on the flow vs. time scalar (**Fig. 8.6**):

- Initiation of flow at the beginning of inspiration: At this time the exhalation valve closes to permit a mechanical breath to deliver volume to the patient's lungs.

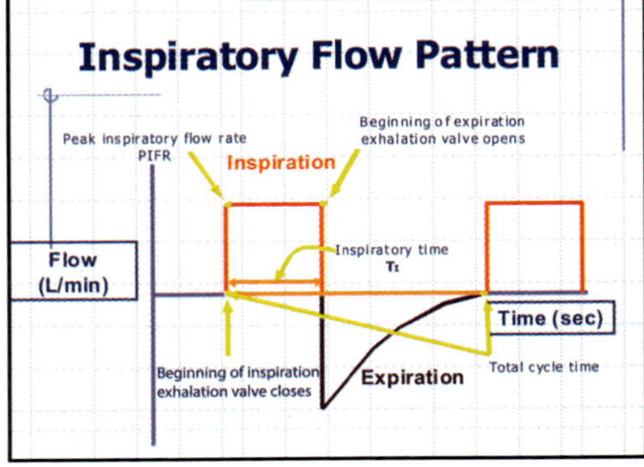

Fig. 8.6

- The peak inspiratory flow (PIFR) level is reached instantaneously during a constant flow pattern. The flow remains at this level until the inspiration is terminated.
- End of inspiratory flow delivery and beginning of expiration: This event occurs when the preset tidal volume is delivered. At this time the exhalation valve opens to allow for passive exhalation.
- Notice Inspiratory Time (T_I), Expiratory Time (T_E) and the Total Cycle Time (TCT) for one mechanical breath.

Components of Expiratory Flow

Expiration, whether from a mechanical breath or a spontaneous breath, is generally a passive maneuver. Both the inspiratory and the expiratory flows reach their peak value instantaneously and both return to the baseline (**Fig. 8.7**).

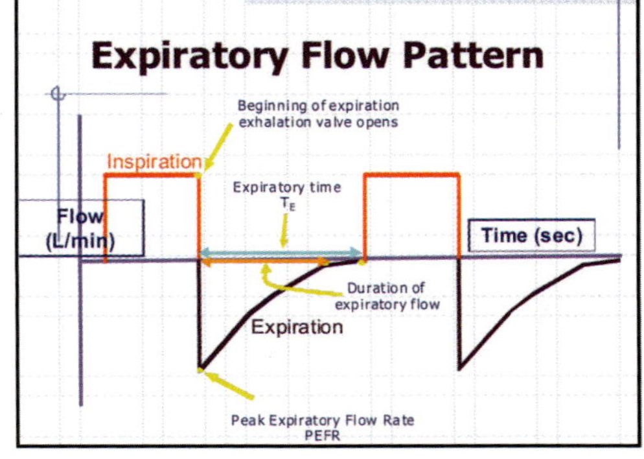

Fig. 8.7

Observe the following points on the expiratory section of the flow/time tracing:

1. Initiation of expiration
2. Peak Expiratory Flow Rate (PEFR)
3. Duration of expiratory flow
4. Expiratory time (T_E)

Notice that the expiratory flow decays to zero before the next mechanical breath is initiated. Thus, the duration of expiratory flow may be shorter than the allocated expiratory time (TCT–T_I).

Recognition of Common Abnormalities

Flow vs. Time scalars help in recognizing certain disorders. Different lung disorders show different flow patterns. These abnormal flow patterns, their causes, and appropriate actions are discussed below:

Airway Obstruction vs. Active Exhalation

Exhalation is normally passive. The expiratory flow pattern and PEFR depend upon the changes in the patient's lung compliance and airway resistance, as well as patient's active efforts to exhale (**Fig. 8.8**).

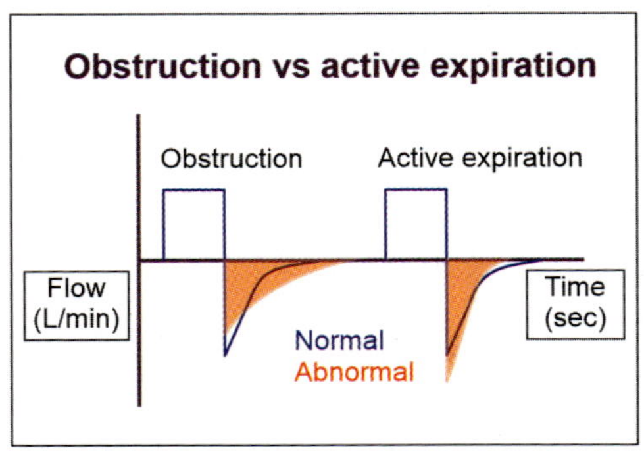

Fig. 8.8

For example, increased airway resistance due to bronchospasm or accumulation of secretions in the airway may result in decreased PEFR and a prolonged expiratory flow. If the patient begins to actively exhale using expiratory muscles, this may result in an increase in PEFR and a shorter duration of expiratory flow.

Response to Bronchodilator

Flow vs. Time tracing can verify clinically suspected bronchoconstriction. In these cases, the PEFR is reduced and expiratory flow returns to the baseline very slowly. Administration of a bronchodilator improves PEFR and allows for an expiratory flow to return to baseline within a normaltime (**Fig. 8.9**).

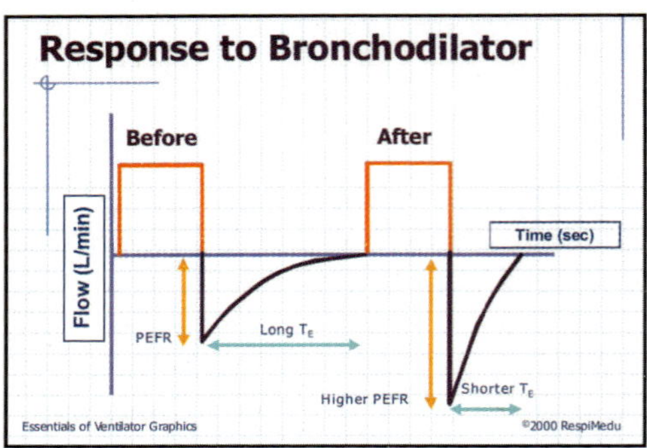

Fig. 8.9

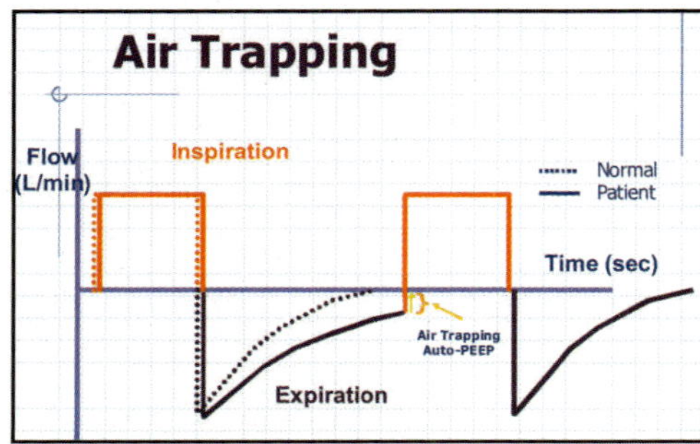

Fig. 8.10

Air-trapping or Auto-PEEP

Normally, expiratory flow returns to the baseline prior to the next breath. In the event that the expiratory flow does not return to the zero line and the subsequent inspiration begins below the baseline, auto-PEEP or air trapping is present (**Fig. 8.10**).

The presence of auto-PEEP or air trapping may result from:

a. Inadequate expiratory time
b. Too high respiratory rate
c. Long inspiratory time
d. Prolonged exhalation due to bronchoconstriction or loss of recoiling force as observed in advanced emphysema patients.

Even though auto-PEEP is best detected from the flow-time waveform, its magnitude is not directly measured from the flow-time scalar. A higher inspiratory flow rate (in volume-cycled ventilators) or short TI (in time-cycled ventilators) allows for a longer TE and may eliminate auto-PEEP.

Volume vs. Time Curve	
Basics of Volume vs. Time Curve: Components of the Volume vs Time	**Recognition of Common Abnormalities:** Air Leak Active Exhalation

Basics of Volume vs. Time Curve

Information obtained from a Volume vs Time scalar graph includes a visual representation of:

- Inspiratory tidal volume (**Fig. 8.11**)
- Inspiratory phase

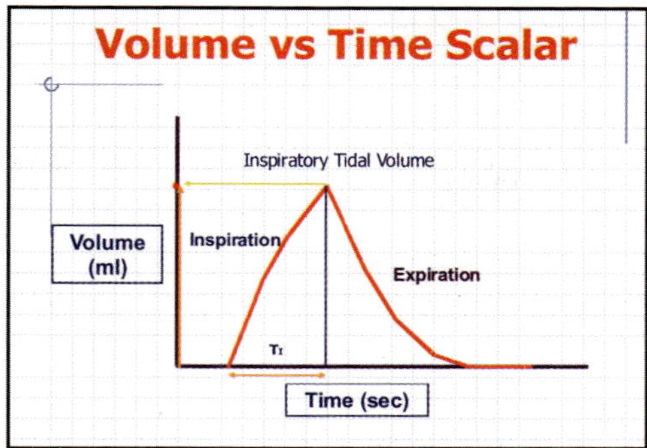

Fig. 8.11

- Expiratory phase
- Inspiratory time

Recognition of Common Abnormalities

The Volume vs. Time scalar can be used to identify the following common abnormalities:

Presence of Air Leak

A leak in the circuit or around the tracheal tube can be detected from the volume/ time curve. If the expiratory tracing smoothly descends, and then plateaus, and abruptly drops to the baseline followed by the next tracing, it indicates the presence of a leak in the system. This pattern mandates that the leak should be located and fixed. The volume of the leak can be easily estimated by measuring the distance from the plateau to the end of the expiratory tracing (**Fig. 8.12**).

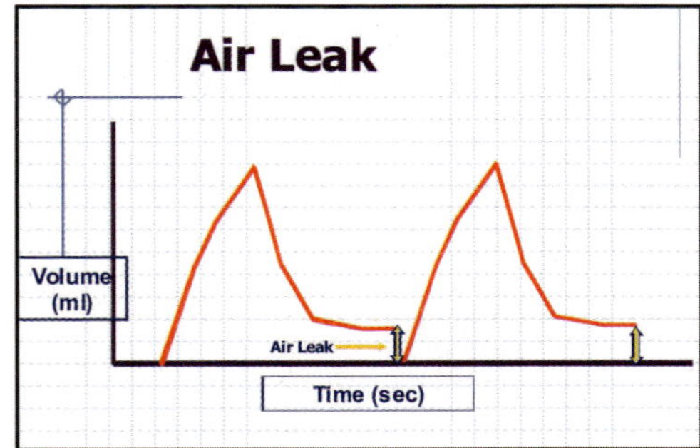

Fig. 8.12

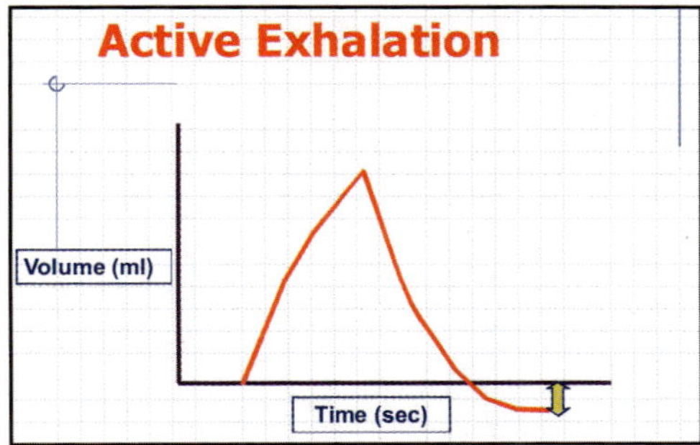

Fig. 8.13

Active Exhalation

Forced exhalation is seen on the volume/ time tracing as a tracing that extends below the zero line. It can also occur if the flow transducer is out of calibration.

Pressure vs. Time Curve	
Basics of Pressure vs. Time Curve	**Recognition of Common Abnormalities**
Spontaneous Breath	Increased Airway Resistance Effect of High Inspiratory Flow
Mechanical Breath	Decreased Lung Compliance Inadequate Inspiratory Flow
Controlled vs Assisted Breath	
Components of Inflation Pressure	

Basics of Pressure vs. Time Curve

Spontaneous Breath

Observe that unlike the Flow vs. Time curve, the Pressure vs. Time scalar indicates inspiration below the baseline and expiration is traced above the baseline which is consistent with the normal spontaneous respiratory pattern. Observe that during the inspiratory phase the pressure curve shows a negative deflection and during exhalation goes above the baseline. Compare this with the adjacent mechanical breath demonstrating inspiration above the baseline and no tracing below the baseline since during exhalation the pressure returns to zero (**Fig. 8.14**).

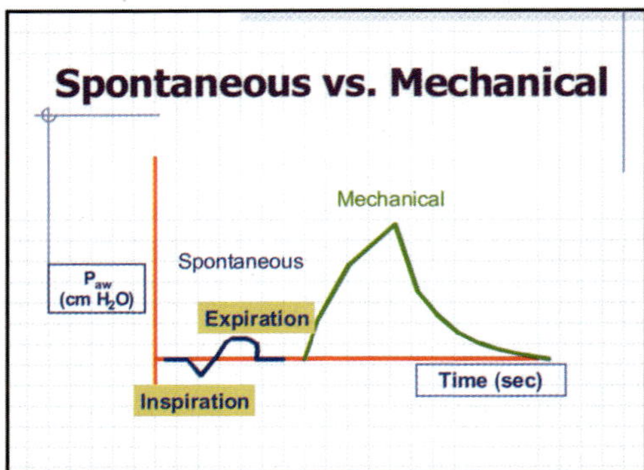

Fig. 8.14

Mechanical Breath

The Pressure vs Time scalar is one of the most useful waveforms in clinical setting. It provides visual representations of the following:

Peak Inspiratory Pressure (PIP) is the maximum pressure achieved during a breath. PIP indicates the pressure required to deliver a set tidal volume during volume ventilation. Increased Airway Resistance (R_{aw}) and/or decreased lung compliance result in an increased PIP (**Fig. 8.15**).

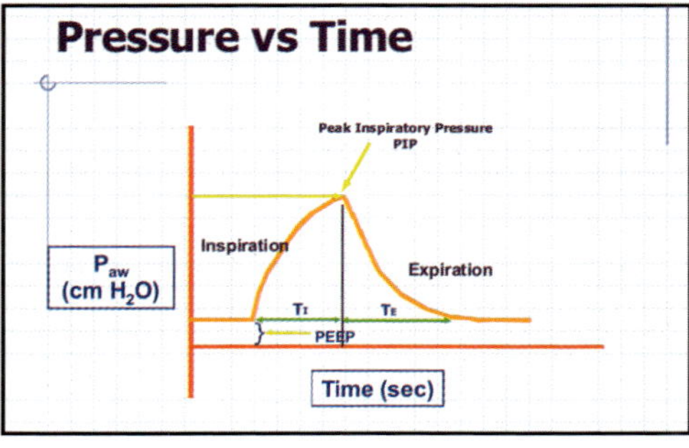

Fig. 8.15

Positive End Expiratory Pressure (PEEP), Since PEEP is a pressure parameter it can be seen only on a Pressure vs Time scalar and a pressure-volume loop. PEEP is present when the baseline pressure is above zero. The tracing also shows the ***Inspiratory time and Expiratory time***.

A Pressure vs. Time scalar verifies the triggering mechanism of the mechanical breath. If the breaths are initiated at the baseline at fixed intervals the mode is time triggered or a control mode. In an assist mode the patient initiates the breath by generating a

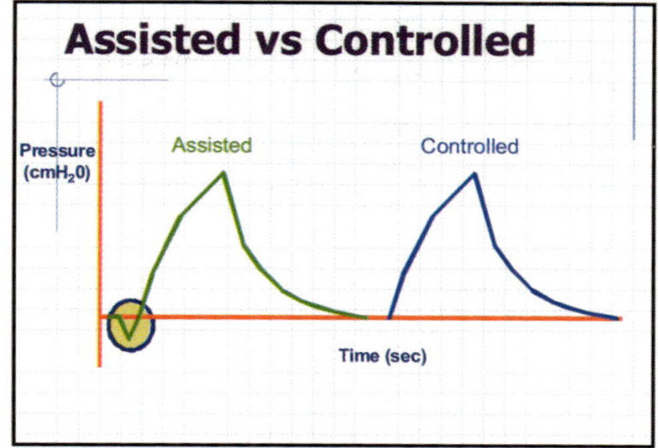

Fig. 8.16

negative pressure. The ventilator sensor recognizes the patient's effort and delivers a mechanical breath. This event can be observed on the Pressure vs. Time scalar where a small negative deflection below the baseline precedes a mechanical breath (**Fig. 8.17**).

Components of Inflation Pressure

Although dynamic lung mechanics can be observed from a Pressure vs. Time curve, the addition of an inspiratory pause or inflation hold provides information to calculate static mechanics (**Fig. 8.17**).

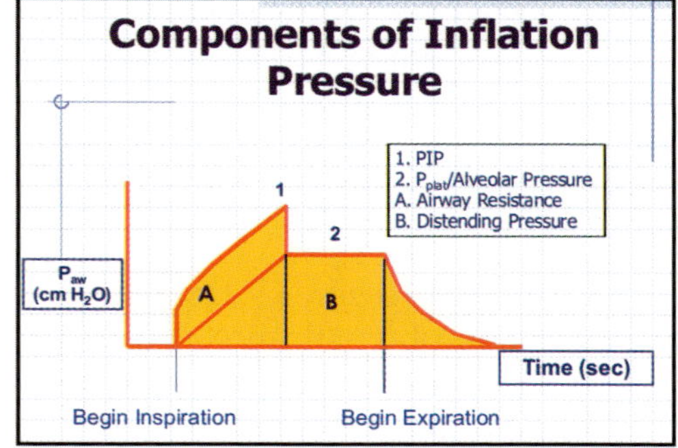

Fig. 8.17

Plateau Pressure (P_{plat}) or Alveolar Pressure is obtained upon activation of an Inflation Hold or Inspiratory Pause control. The exhalation valve is kept in a closed position after the tidal volume is delivered and the volume is held in the lungs.

For clinical purposes, the plateau pressure is the same as the alveolar pressure. This measurement provides a means of measuring static lung compliance.

Transairway Pressure (P_{TA} = PIP – P_{plat}) reflects the pressure required to overcome airway resistance. Bronchospasm, airway secretions, and other types of airway obstructions are verified from an increase in the transairway pressure (PIP-P_{plat}).

With inflation hold, the pressure required to overcome the recoiling force (lung compliance) can be determined. The static lung compliance can be obtained by dividing the tidal volume in the lungs by the plateau pressure minus PEEP, if present.

$$C_{static} = \frac{V_T}{PIP - P_{plat}}$$

Observe the sequence of tracing pressure vs. time curve when the inflation hold (inspiratory pause) is activated. At the beginning, the exhalation valve closes and the ventilator delivers volume to the patient's lungs. During this volume delivery the flow of gas molecules experience frictional resistance. The pressure time curve indicates this pressure generated by flow resistance as initial rise in the pressure. As the gas reaches beyond terminal bronchioles elastic characteristics of the lung oppose the incoming gas. Delivered tidal volume generates pressure required to overcome elastic recoil of the lung. The total pressure is represented by Peak Inspiratory Pressure (PIP). At the end of volume delivery, inspiratory flow stops. Technically, the exhalation valve is supposed to open. However, inspiratory hold activation maintains the exhalation valve in closed position. Thus, the volume in the lungs is balanced by the elastic recoil and the resultant pressure represents Plateau Pressure (P_{plat}) **(Fig. 8.18)**. Clinically this is the alveolar pressure. As shown, PIP is higher than P_{plat}, since P_{plat} represents only the pressure required to oppose elastic recoil to deliver volume to the lungs. Flow resistance is absent since the gas flow is stopped. This pressure is known as Transairway Pressure (P_{TA}). As the time set for inspiratory hold elapses, exhalation valve opens and the pressure returns to the baseline. This graph has significant clinical significance as seen in the next two waveforms.

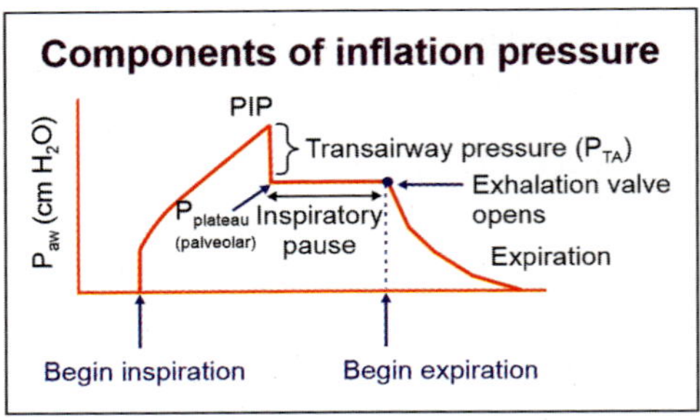

Fig. 8.18

Recognition of Common Abnormalities

PIP vs. P_{plat}

Changes in the pressure vs. time curve have profound clinical significance. Four common clinical situations are demonstrated in the following tracings **(Fig. 8.19)**:

Normalcurve: Indicates PIP, P_{plat}, P_{TA}, and T_I.

High Raw: A significant increase in the P_{TA} is associated with increased airway resistance.

High Flow: Notice that the inspiratory time is shorter than normal, indicating a higher inspiratory gas flow rate.

Decreased Lung Compliance: An increase in the plateau pressure and a corresponding increase in the PIP is consistent with decreased lung compliance.

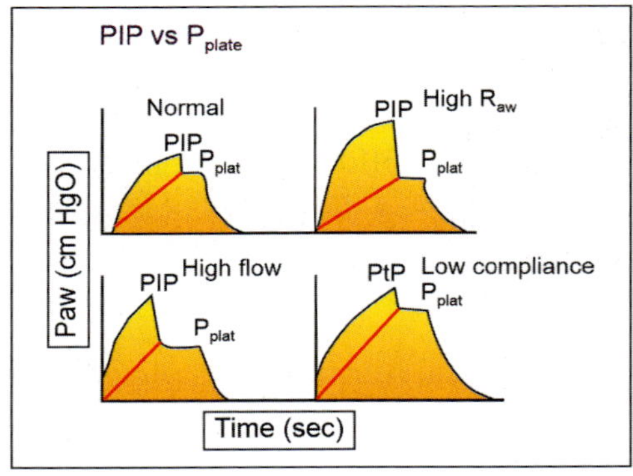

Fig. 8.19

Increased Airway Resistance

As the airway resistance increases due to bronchospasm, secretions or any obstruction, the transairway pressure (PTA) increases as shown by the rise in PIP without any increase in P_{plat}. The gradient PIP–P_{plat} represents PTA **(Fig. 8.20)**.

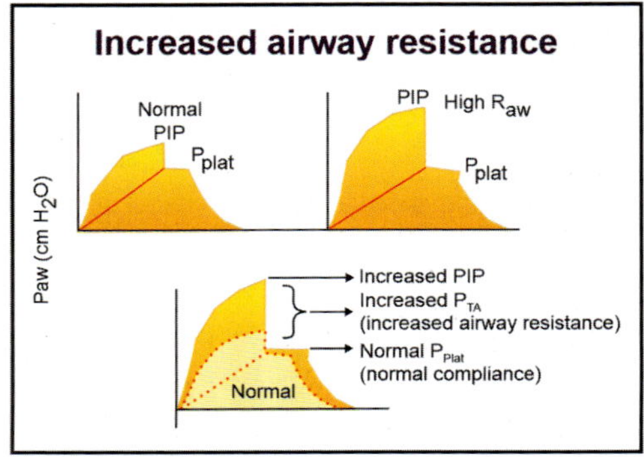

Fig. 8.20

Clinically, this situation requires airway suctioning, administration of bronchodilators or removal of obstruction such as kink in the inspiratory line of the circuit.

Decreased Lung Compliance

PIP can also increase when the lung compliance decreases. In conditions such as small pneumothoraces or blocked chest tube drainage system, lung compliance decreases. Consequently, P_{plat} or Alveolar Pressure increases causing equivalent increase in PIP. Recognize that the difference between PIP and P_{plat} or P_{TA} is unchanged from the original condition. Suctioning the airways serves no purpose since the airways resistance is normal. Identification of the underlying cause and eliminating it is essential in this situation (**Fig. 8.21**).

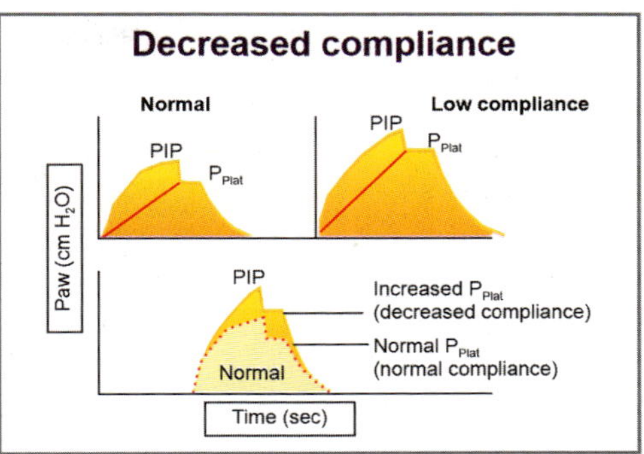

Fig. 8.21

Inadequate Inspiratory Flow

A Pressure vs. Time curve can also detect inadequate flow that is indicated when the Inadequate Inspiratory Flow pressure rises very slowly or sometimes is indicated when there is a depression in the inspiratory limb of the pressure contour (**Fig. 8.22**).

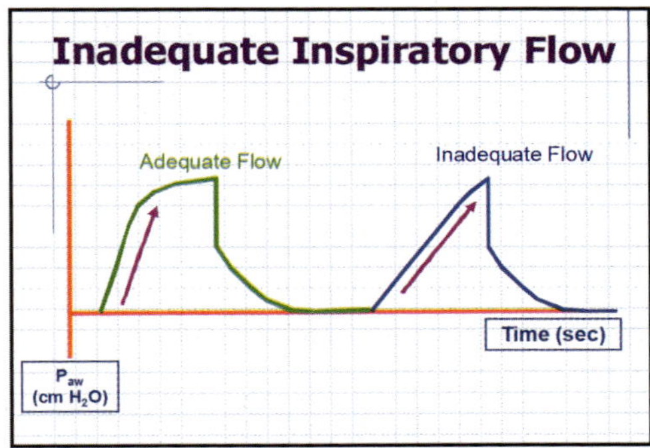

Fig. 8.22

LOOPS

Loops are the two-dimensional graphic displays of two scalar parameters.

Pressure-Volume Loop	
Basics of a Pressure-Volume Loop	**Recognition of Common Abnormalities**
Type of Breath	Decreased Lung Compliance
Spontaneous-Assisted-Controlled	Increased Airway Resistance
FRC andPressure-Volume Loop	Alveolar Overdistension
Components of a Pressure-Volume Loop	Increased Work of Breathing
PEEP and the P-V Loop	Inappropriate Sensitivity
Inflection Points (Upper and Lower)	Inadequate Inspiratory Flow
Type of Breath	Air Leak
Work of Breathing	

Observe the direction of the tracing of the loop. When the tracing is counterclockwise, the breath delivered is a mechanical breath. On the other hand, a clockwise tracing indicates a spontaneous breath. The angle, shape and size of the loop impart pertinent information to the clinician. In an assisted mechanical breath the tracing begins clockwise indicating patient's spontaneous effort and resumes in counterclockwise fashion for the mechanical delivery (**Fig. 8.23**).

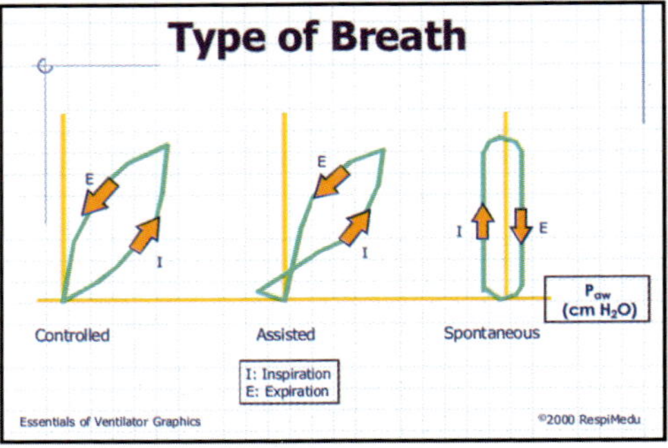

Fig. 8.23

FRC and P-V Loop

It is important to recognize that the beginning point on a Pressure-Volume loop is the FRC level since, the breath is delivered at end-expiratory level (FRC). When PEEP is added, the FRC level increases or moves up the compliance curve (**Fig. 8.24**).

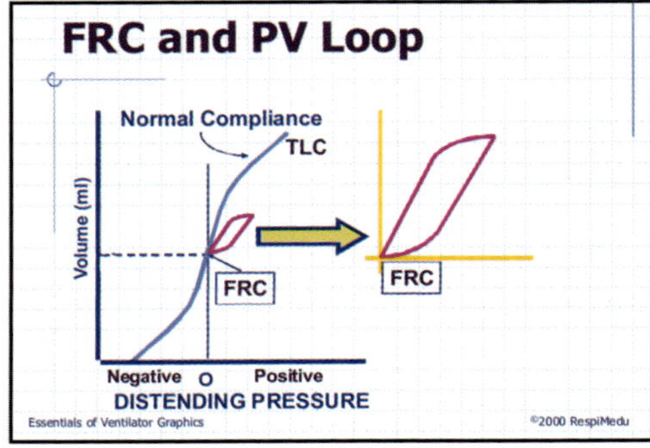

Fig. 8.24

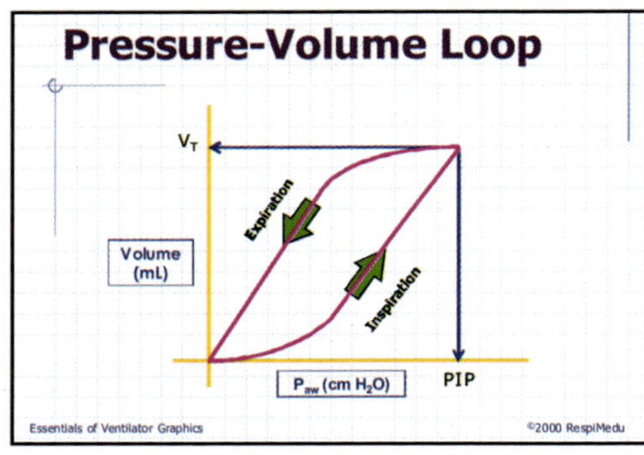

Fig. 8.25

Component of a P-V Loop

A Pressure-Volume loop traces changes in pressures and corresponding changes in volume. Inspiration begins from the FRC level and terminates when the preset parameter (volume or pressure) is achieved. The tracing continues during expiration and returns to FRC at end of exhalation. PIP and delivered tidal volume can readily be obtained from the Pressure-Volume loop (**Fig. 8.25**).

PEEP

When PEEP is applied, the Pressure-Volume curve shifts to the PEEP level on the horizontal scale (Pressure scale) (**Fig. 8.26**).

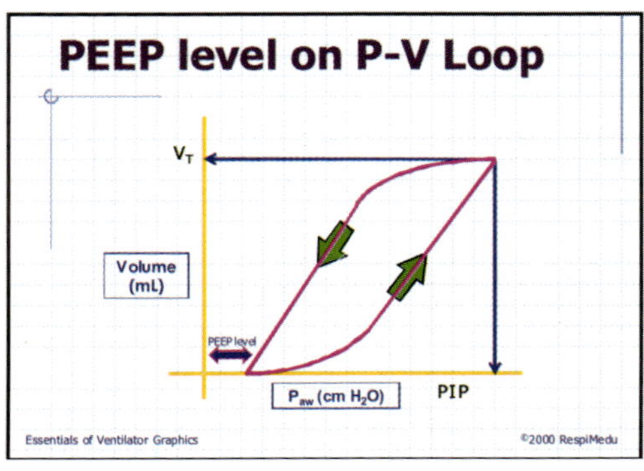

Fig. 8.26

Inflection Point

Inflection point, in geometry, represents sudden change of direction in a graphical tracing **(Fig. 8.27)**.

Physiologically, the inflection points on P-V loop are associated with sudden changes in alveolar opening and closing. The lower inflection point represents the opening pressure, whereas the upper inflection point, in this graph, represents recoiling characteristics.

The higher the opening pressure, the stiffer the lung, as indicated by the curve moving laterally to the right along the pressure axis. Setting PEEP levels at the level of the lower inflection point is recommended to optimize alveolar recruitment and prevent repeated opening and closing of alveoli.

Fig. 8.27

Work of Breathing

The major advantage of a Pressure-Volume loop is that it provides a quick assessment of the elastic as well as resistive work of breathing.

Since, work of breathing is calculated from the product of pressure and volume (WOB = Pressure × Volume). The shaded area represents elastic work of breathing **(Fig. 8.28)**.

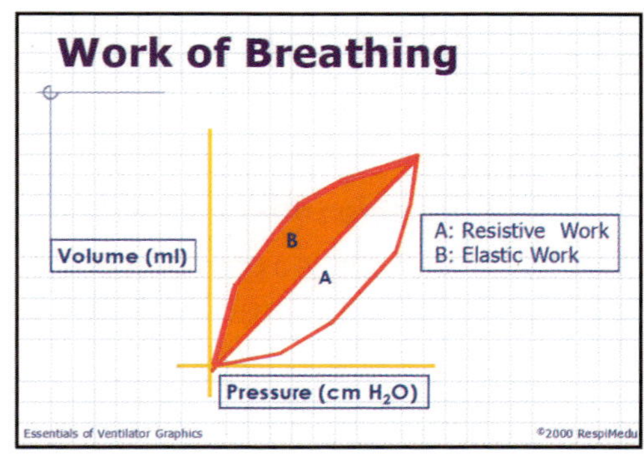

Fig. 8.28

Decreased Lung Compliance

A shift of the curve to the right of a Pressure-Volume loop indicates decreased lung compliance and a shift to the left is associated with an increased compliance. Observe the pressure required to deliver the same tidal volume in the three graphs.

Notice that in Volume-Targeted Ventilation the PIP is the changing variable **(Fig. 8.29)**.

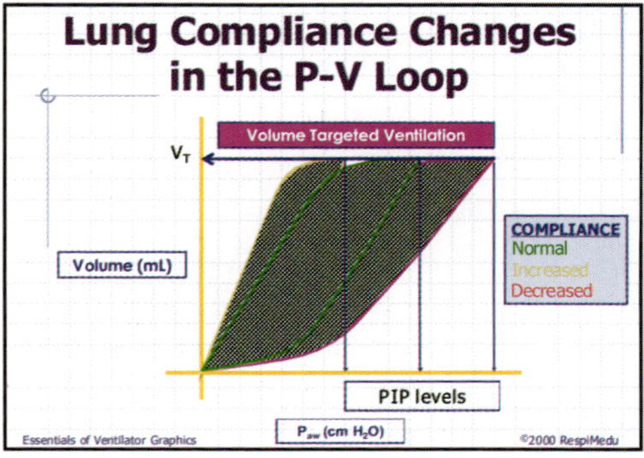

Fig. 8.29: Volume targeted ventilation

Pressure-Targeted Ventilation

In Pressure-Targeted Ventilation where the PIP is kept constant and V_T is the changing variable (**Fig. 8.30**).

Observe as dynamic compliance varies, so does the delivered volume. Essentially, as lung becomes stiffer, the delivered volume decreases for the given present pressure.

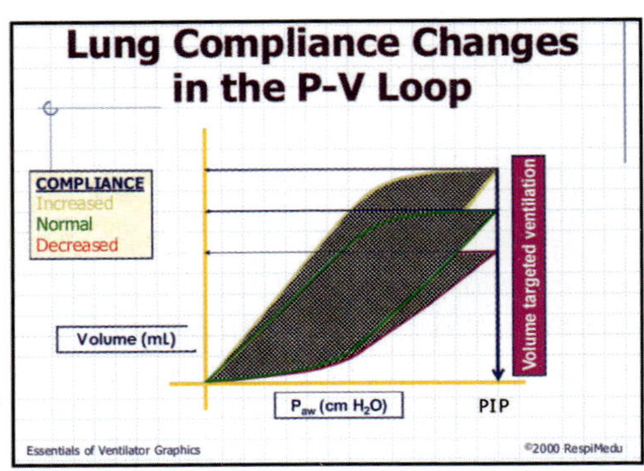

Fig. 8.30

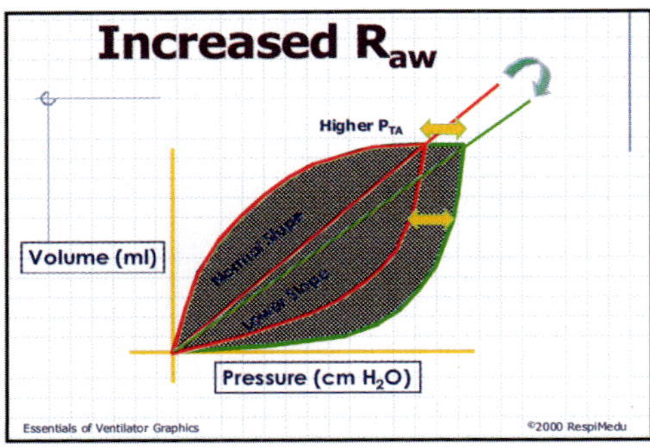

Fig. 8.31

Increased Airways Resistance

An increased airway resistance is associated with the abnormal widening of the inspiratory tracing. Patients with obstructive disorders exhibit a wide Pressure-Volume loop. This abnormal widening of the shape of the P-V loop is referred to as an increased "Hysteresis" (**Fig. 8.31**).

Alveolar Overdistension

Alveolar distension is a common observation made during ventilation of patients with ARDS on a volume-targeted mode. Alveolar overdistension is detrimental to patients. The classic sign, known as "Beak Effect" or "Duckbill" shows an increase in airway pressure without any appreciable increase in volume. A switch to pressure targeted ventilation, at appropriate safe pressure level, or a reduction in VT are indicated (**Fig. 8.32**).

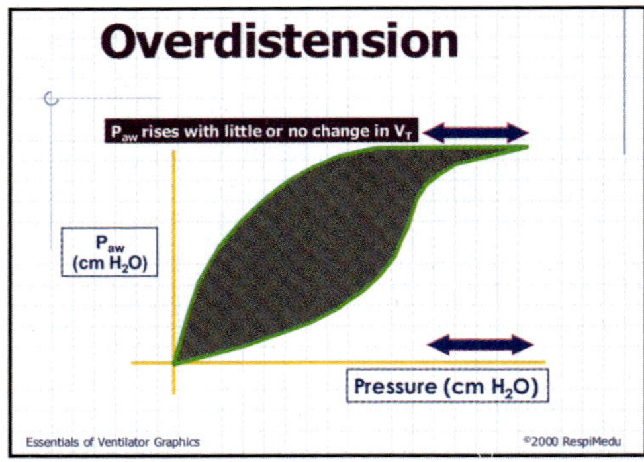

Fig. 8.32

Increased WOB

Inadequate Sensitivity

Normally the Pressure-Volume loop traces in a counterclockwise direction. A clockwise tracing prior to the initiation of a mechanical breath indicates patient's effort (**Fig. 8.33**). Adjusting the sensitivity can minimize this effort. Inadequate sensitivity setting promotes increased triggering WOB. On the P-V loop it exhibits a significant clockwise

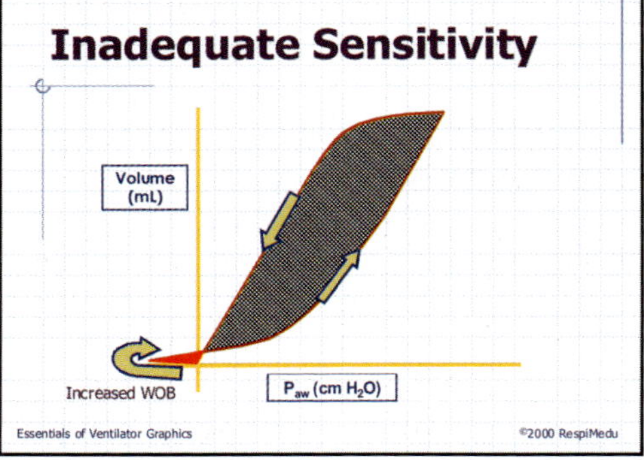

Fig. 8.33

deflection of the tracing with the pressure decreasing significantly (>5 cm H_2O) below the baseline pressure.

Inadequate Inspiratory Flow Rate

Inappropriate inspiratory flow rates are recognized from a scooped out pattern. In some situations, the patient makes inspiratory effort in the middle of the mechanical breath exhibiting a "notch" on the inspiratory curve **(Fig. 8.34)**.

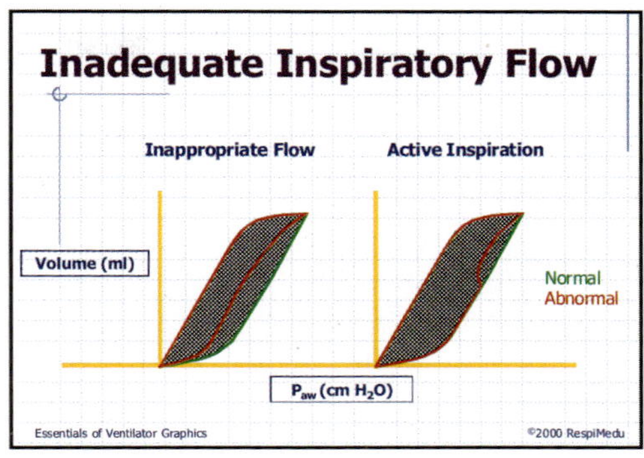

Fig. 8.34

Air Leak

On Volume/Time scalar when the expiratory curve does not return to the baseline, a leak in the system is present **(Fig. 8.35)**.

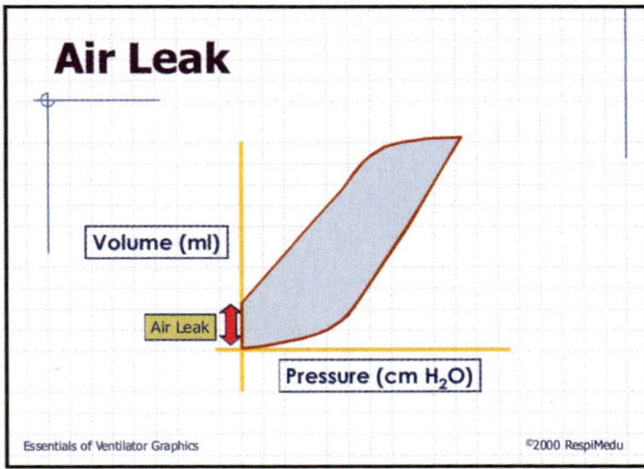

Fig. 8.35

Flow-Volume Loop	
Basics of Pressure-Volume Loop	**Recognition of common Abnormalities**
Components of a Flow-Volume Loop	Air Leak Auto-PEEP/Air Trapping Increased Airway Resistance Airway Secretions/Accumulation of Condensate

Basics of Flow-Volume Loop

Components of a Flow-Volume Loop

There is no set convention in assigning the inspiratory and expiratory quadrants on a Flow-Volume loop. Some ventilators produce flow-volume loop with inspiration on the upper half and expiration on the lower half. Other ventilators plot inspiration on the lower side of the volume axis and expiration on the upper side. A flow-volume loop provides the following information **(Fig. 8.36)**.

1. PIFR
2. PEFR
3. Tidal Volume
4. End Expiration and Beginning of Inspiration

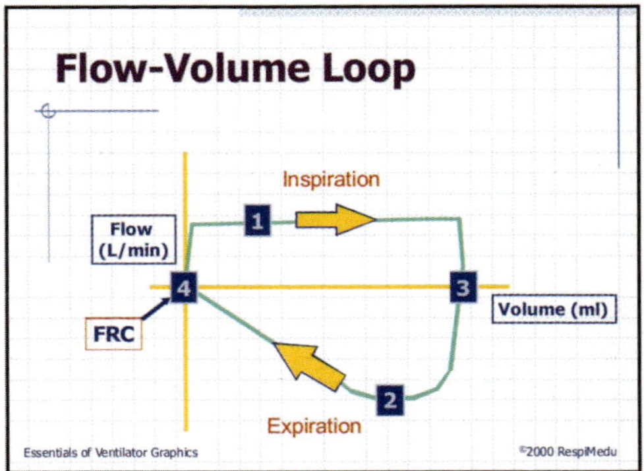

Fig. 8.36

Recognition of Common Abnormalities

Air Leak

Ideally, expired volume should be equal to the inspired volume. With an air leak, however, expired volume is less than inspired volume. This is commonly observed in situations such as leak around the endotracheal tube, and in the ventilator circuit. A leak can be identified from a flow-volume loop when the volume does not return to the FRC (zero volume level). The deficit of volume indicates the magnitude of air leak (Fig. 8.37).

Auto-PEEP

In an air trapping or auto-PEEP situation the flow does not return to the zero level. Since the next inspiration must begin from the zero flow level, the tracing jumps abruptly, from the trapped level to the zero level and proceeds with next breath.

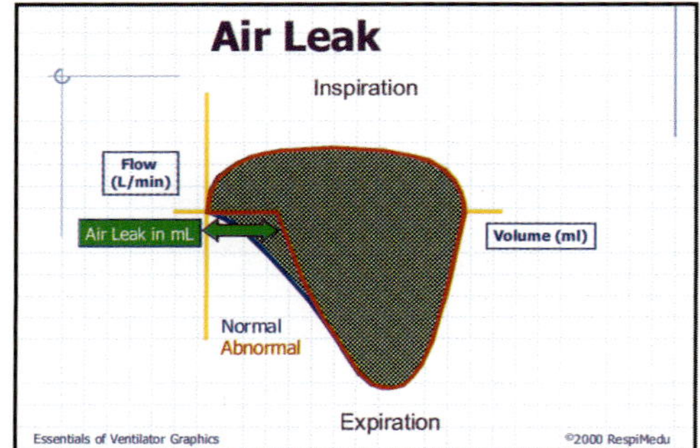

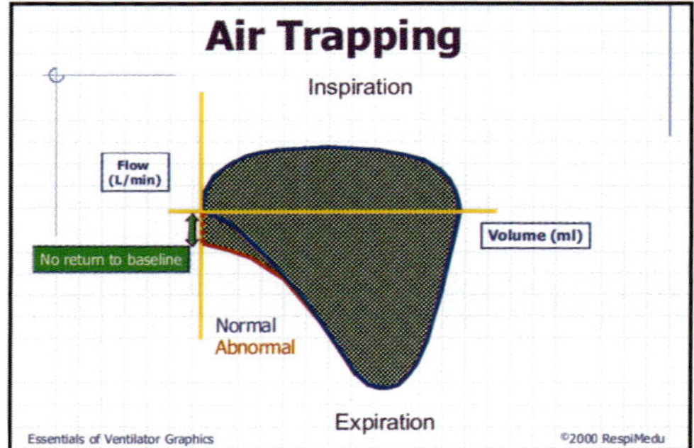

Fig. 8.37

Increased Airway Resistance

An increased airway resistance due to broncho-spasm, such as in asthma, is shown on a flow-volume loop as a scooped out pattern on the expiratory tracing and a decreased PEFR. Effective administration of bronchodilator will show an improvement on both the configuration of the expiratory tracing and the PEFR. A continued scooped out appearance and a low PEFR indicates ineffectiveness of the broncho-dilator therapy.

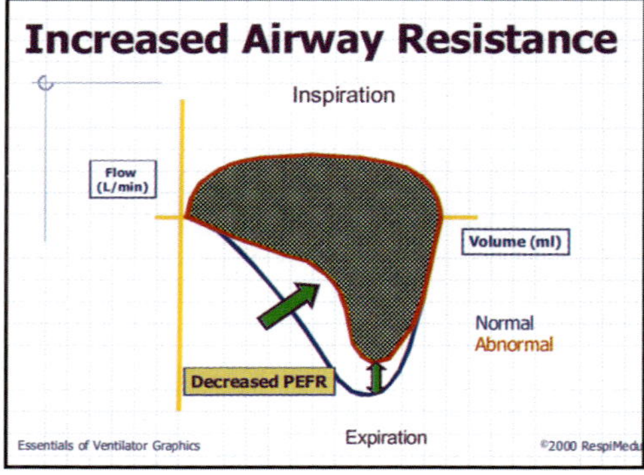

Fig. 8.38

Airway Secretions and Accumulation of Condensate in the Tubing

The presence of secretions in the large airways, as well as excessive fluid condensation in the ventilator circuit, appear as a distinctive pattern in the flow-volume loop known as a "saw-tooth" pattern, which occurs mostly on the expiratory component of the curve. However, if the situation is not corrected this pattern will also appear on the inspiratory curve.

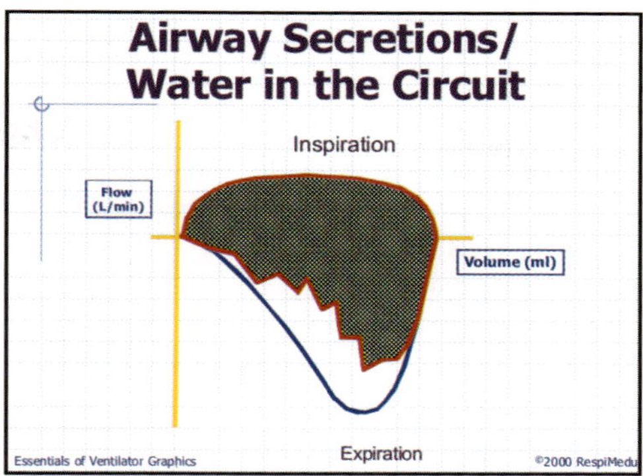

Fig. 8.39

Recognition of Different Modes of Ventilation		
Spontaneous Modes	**Modes of Mechanical Ventilation**	
Spontaneous Breath CPAP PSV CPAP + PS	Volume-Targeted Controlled Assisted SIMV SIMV + PS SIMV + PS + CPAP	Pressure-Targeted Controlled Assisted SIMV SIMV + PS SIMV + PS + CPAP

Spontaneous Modes

Spontaneous Breath

Observe the difference between the Flow vs. Time, the Pressure vs. Time and the Volume vs. Time scalars. Only the pressure curve shows a negative or below baseline tracing during inspiration; however, flow and volume are positive during inspiration **(Fig. 8.40)**.

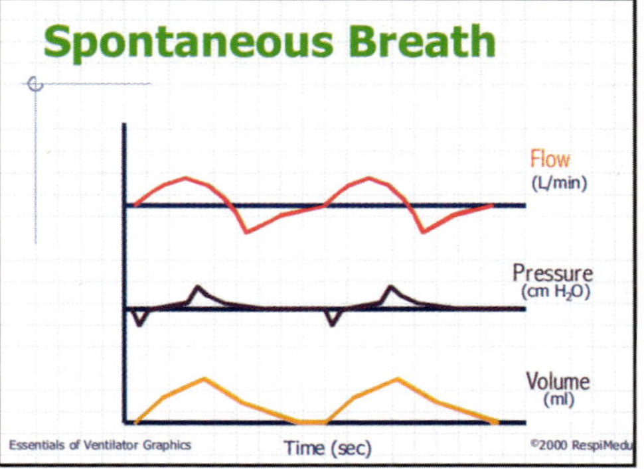

Fig. 8.40

CPAP

A CPAP mode is identical to a spontaneous breath except that the baseline in the Pressure vs. Time curve is at a higher level. CPAP can be verified fromthe P vs. T curveand P-V loop only **(Fig. 8.41)**.

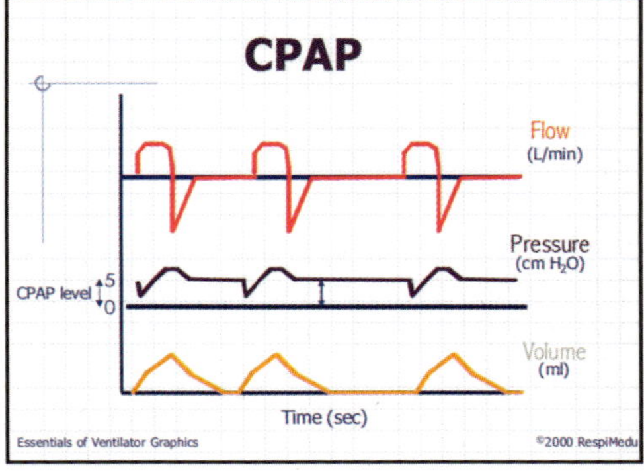

Fig. 8.41

Pressure Support Ventilation

Pressure Support Ventilation is designed to augment spontaneous breath. It provides a higher volume with a lower inspiratory effort. Patients with neuromuscular disorders, COPD, and postoperative patients benefit from PSV. It is also used during weaning from mechanical ventilation (**Fig. 8.42**).

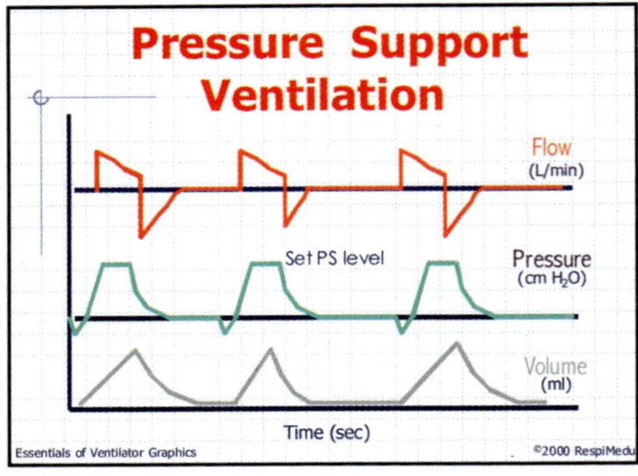

Fig. 8.42

Observe the scalars: The key waveform for recognition of PSV is the Flow *vs*. Time curve. PSV terminates inspiration when the flow reaches a predetermined value (generally 25% of the peak flow). It is a flow-cycled mode. The Pressure vs. Time curve indicates a constant pressure tracing at the set pressure support level. Also notice the negative deflection on the Pressure vs. Time curve indicating that PSV is strictly an assist mode of ventilation. The delivered volume is dependent on the patient's lung compliance, airway resistance, patient's inspiratory effort and the pressure support level.

CPAP + PS

This mode is used to facilitate weaning from mechanical ventilation.

Observe the flow/time and pressure/time scalars confirm pressure support (PSV) mode. Also, the pressure/time scalar indicates that the baseline is at a higher level consistent with CPAP (**Fig. 8.43**).

Fig. 8.43

Modes of Mechanical Ventilation

Volume Targeted Ventilation

NOTE: A square flow pattern will be used to identify the inspiratory phase of the mechanical breaths in the Flow vs. Time curve.

Controlled Mode

In a controlled mode the ventilator provides the entire breathing. The ventilator exclusively performs the work of breathing. The ventilator initiates inspiration when a preset time elapses (Time-triggered) (**Fig. 8.44**).

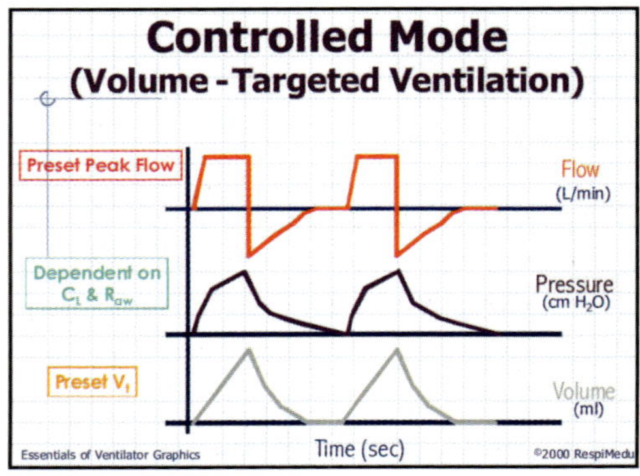

Fig. 8.44

It terminates inspiration when the preset tidal volume is delivered (volume cycled). Flow level is set by the clinician and remains constant throughout the inspiratory phase. Even in the event that the lung characteristics (resistance and compliance) change the flow rate remains constant. The flow parameter is termed as "limiting" parameter. Thus, volume controlled breath is classified as "Time triggered, flow limited, volume cycled".

Assisted Mode

An assisted mode is identical to a controlled mode except that the Pressure *vs*. Time curve shows a negative deflection just prior to the mechanical breath. This negative deflection indicates patient triggering. An Assisted mode is termed as "Patient triggered, flow limited, volume cycled" **(Fig. 8.45)**.

SIMV

This is the one of the common modes used in the clinical settings. It is primarily used to provide partial mechanical support. The patient's spontaneous breathing is supported with periodic assisted mechanical breaths. Observe small volume spontaneous breaths interposed between mechanical breaths **(Fig. 8.46)**.

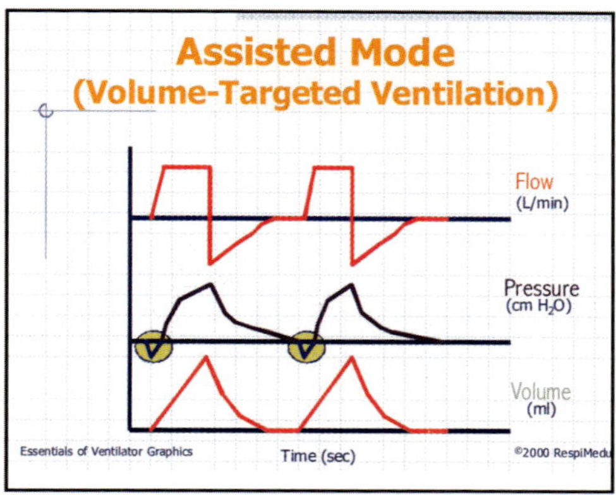

Fig. 8.45

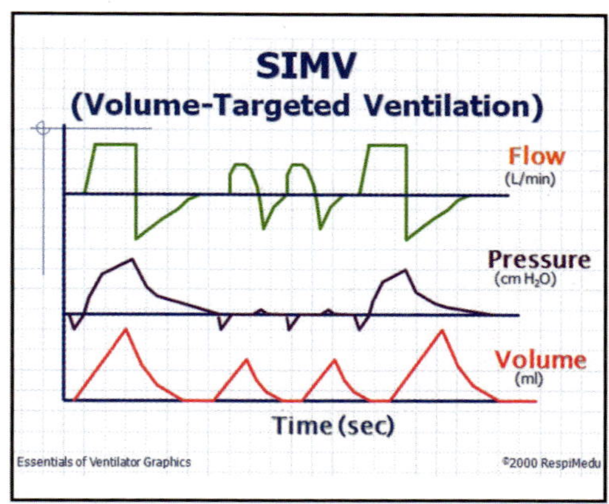

Fig. 8.46

SIMV + PS

It is recommended that PS be added to SIMV to provide augmentation of unsupported spontaneous breath through the endotracheal tube. Each breath is a patient triggered breath. Volume delivered during mechanical breaths is preset. However, the volume delivered by the pressure supported breath is dependent on the level of pressure support, patient's lung compliance, airway resistance, and patient's inspiratory effort **(Fig. 8.47)**.

SIMV + PS + CPAP

The only difference in this waveform from the previous (SIMV + PSV) is that CPAP is added to the circuit as indicated on the Pressure/Time scalar.

Remember, the Pressure vs. Time curve and Pressure-Volume loop can be used to verify the use of CPAP. No other waveforms show CPAP **(Fig. 8.48)**.

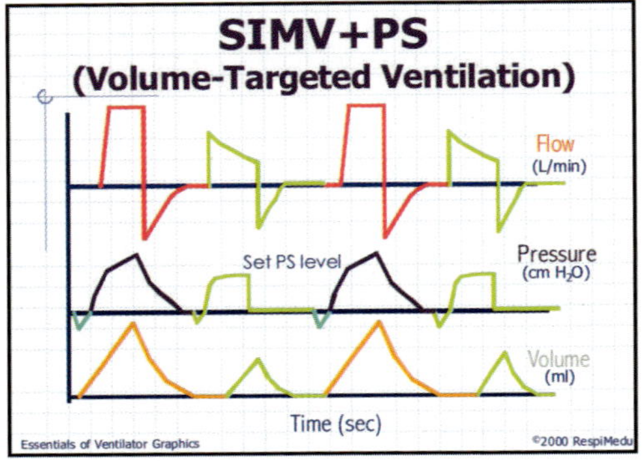

Fig. 8.47

Fig. 8.48

Pressure-Targeted Ventilation

Controlled Mode

A pressure targeted control breath is a pressure-limited (Preset pressure control level), time-cycled breath. The peak flow is a result of the set pressure level, the patient's lung characteristics and patient's inspiratory effort. Observe that the flow curve is decelerating and the flow decreases to zero at the end of preset inspiratory time (**Fig. 8.49**).

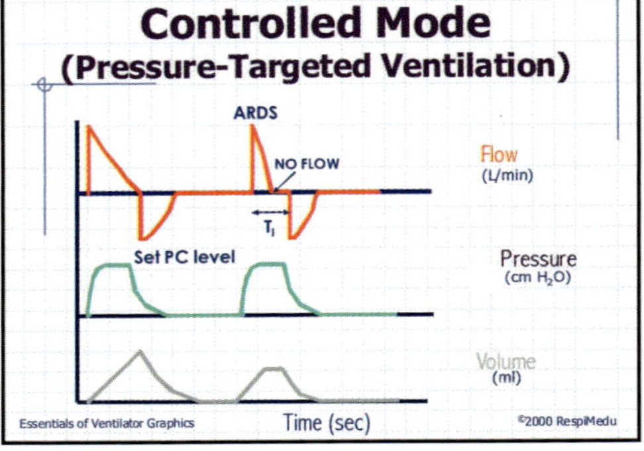

Fig. 8.49

In specific situations, such as decreased compliance (ARDS) the flow may return to baseline prior to termination of inspiratory time and a state of zero flow exists until the inspiratory time elapses. The Pressure vs. Time curve exhibits a square pattern indicating that the pressure remains at the preset level throughout the inspiratory phase. The Volume vs. Time curve shows an initial sharp rise due to higher flow. However, the slope then tapers, indicating lesser amount of volume delivered as the lungs fill.

Assisted Mode

An assisted mode is identical to a controlled mode except that the Pressure vs. Time curve shows a negative deflection just prior to the mechanical breath. This negative deflection indicates patient triggering (**Fig. 8.50**).

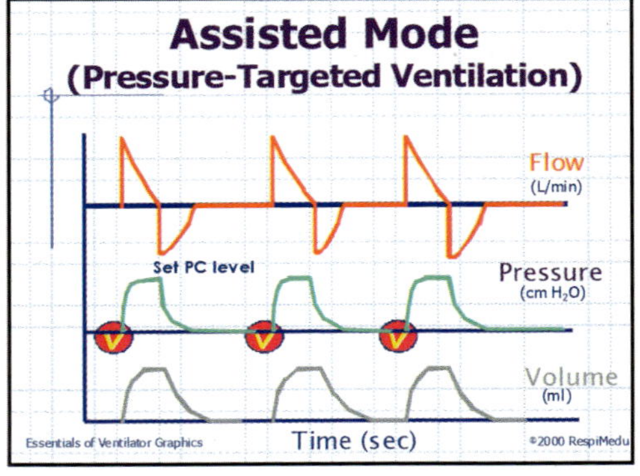

Fig. 8.50

SIMV

The patient's spontaneous breathing is supported with periodic assisted, pressure-targeted mechanical breaths (Fig. 8.51).

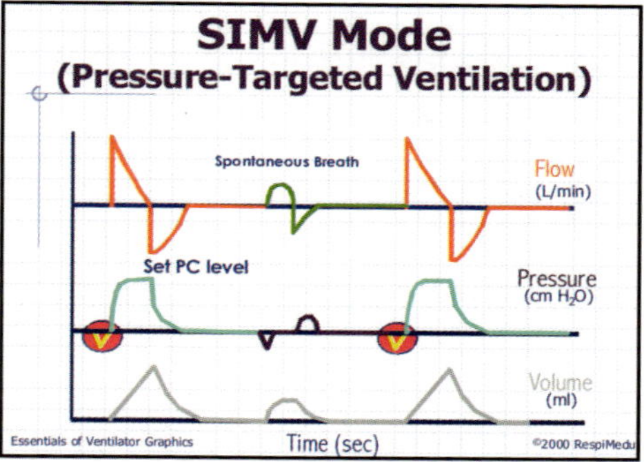

Fig. 8.51

SIMV + PS

Exactly the same SIMV + PS mode as in volume-targeted ventilation, except the mechanical breaths are pressure-controlled breaths and PS augments the spontaneous breaths. The Pressure vs. Time curve is constant pressure curve since both the PCV and PS breaths are pressure limited and exhibit a square wave pressure pattern at their respective set levels. The Flow vs. Time curve shows the flow rate decaying to zero level for PC breaths; whereas PS breaths are flow cycled (Fig. 8.52).

SIMV + PS + CPAP

Similar patterns as SIMV + PS with an addition of CPAP as shown on the Pressure vs. Time curve (Fig. 8.53).

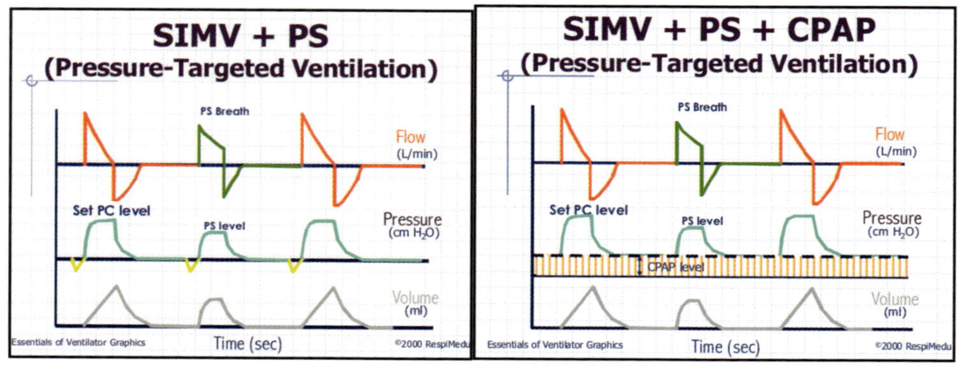

Fig. 8.52

Fig. 8.53

The figures in this chapter may look different since they are reproduced directly from the QR Codes which is provided in the back cover pocket.

"Essentials of Ventilator Graphics" developed by Vijay Deshpande, MS, RRT, FAARC and Ruben Restrepo, MD, RRT, FAARC and FCCP for Respimedu, Inc. in 2000.

CHAPTER 9

Positive End Expiratory Pressure (PEEP)

❐ Anitha Shenoy ❐ Shwethapriya R

INTRODUCTION

From the time of inception of PEEP in the treatment of acute respiratory failure till the 1980's, PEEP was mainly used to improve oxygenation of the patient. In 1980's, with the introduction of the concept of atelectrauma as the leading cause of ventilator-induced lung injury, the main role of PEEP changed from improving oxygenation to protecting the lung from ventilator-induced lung injury. The exact mechanism of lung protection is not known but it is presumed that PEEP acts by recruiting the alveoli thereby preventing the cyclical collapse and opening of alveoli and also by protecting the lung surfactant.

DEFINITION

Positive end expiratory pressure is the pressure above atmospheric pressure in the alveoli at the end of expiration in mechanically ventilated patients. It is often used interchangeably with the pressure during expiration (EPAP) in a patient who is on bilevel positive airway pressure (BiPAP) and continuous positive airway pressure (CPAP) in a patient who is breathing spontaneously.

PEEP is of two types: Extrinsic and Intrinsic. When PEEP is set externally through the ventilator during mechanical ventilation as a therapeutic parameter, it is called **extrinsic** PEEP. When airway pressure becomes positive in the airways during expiration because of incomplete exhalation, it is called intrinsic PEEP (also called auto-PEEP). Total PEEP refers to the sum of extrinsic and intrinsic PEEP in a given patient.

PEEP set during mechanical ventilation can be represented on a pressure-time scalar as shown in **Fig. 9.1**.

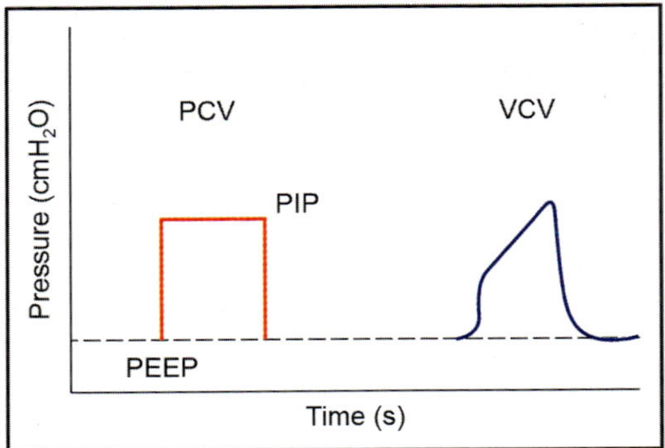

Fig. 9.1: Pressure time scalar showing PEEP during pressure controlled ventilation (PCV) and volume controlled ventilation (VCV)

BENEFITS OF THE USE OF EXTRINSIC PEEP

Application of PEEP opens up the closed alveoli and results in better distribution of the tidal volume to larger areas of the lung resulting in better oxygenation, overall reduced peak airway pressure, improved compliance.

During inspiration, the alveoli expand and during exhalation, they contract but do not collapse completely due to the presence of surfactant which reduces the surface tension in the alveoli. Initiation of mechanical ventilation can cause inactivation of the surfactant leading to collapse of the alveoli. Injury to the lung can also result in activation of neutrophils and other inflammatory cells, and release of cytokines. This increases alveolocapillary permeability and flooding of the alveoli with edema fluid causing alveolar collapse. Ventilation of such a 'wet' lung causes repeated cyclical opening and closing of the alveoli. In the areas of the lung with collapsed and consolidated alveoli, significant pressure is required to open these alveoli. This results in shear force on the thin wall of the adjacent normal alveoli and disruption of its epithelial lining. This causes further lung injury. By opening up the alveoli and preventing their collapse, PEEP reduces ventilator-induced lung injury.

Furthermore, PEEP drives out the edema fluid from the alveoli into the interstitium which is then absorbed by the lymphatics. In the presence of alveolar edema, PEEP may prevent airway flooding by working as a deterrent to entry of fluid into the alveoli. This helps in better diffusion of oxygen across the alveolocapillary membrane. Thus, PEEP reduces oxygen requirements and risk of oxygen toxicity.

PEEP is useful even in patients undergoing short-term mechanical ventilation as during administration of general anesthesia. Airways start closing during expiration as a result of increasing pleural pressure. The volume that is above residual volume at which airway closure starts is called the closing volume (CV). Residual volume and closing volume together constitute the closing capacity. Usually this is lesser than the functional residual capacity (FRC). In supine position, especially after induction of general anesthesia, the FRC decreases but the closing capacity does not change. If the FRC drops below the closing capacity, the airways may remain closed continuously. Application of PEEP results in increase in FRC and this increase in FRC above closing capacity keeps the airways open **(Fig. 9.2)**. In any condition that increases the CC, higher PEEP has to be provided to prevent collapse of the airways. Increased FRC increases the surface area for gas exchange by opening collapsed alveoli leading to improved oxygenation.

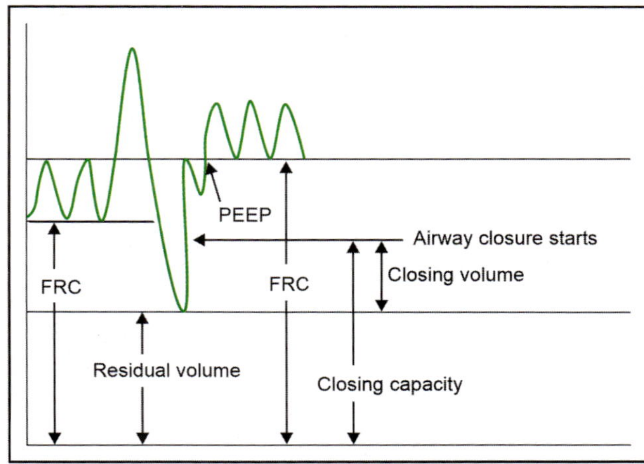

Fig. 9.2: Relationship of closing capacity, functional residual capacity at baseline and after application of PEEP

ADVERSE EFFECTS OF PEEP

- Since PEEP increases intrathoracic pressure, it impairs venous return and can reduce cardiac output, especially in hypovolaemic patients. This can impair blood supply to various organs, especially the abdominal viscera.
- Excessive PEEP can cause overdistention of alveoli and cause volutrauma and barotrauma (**Fig. 9.3**).

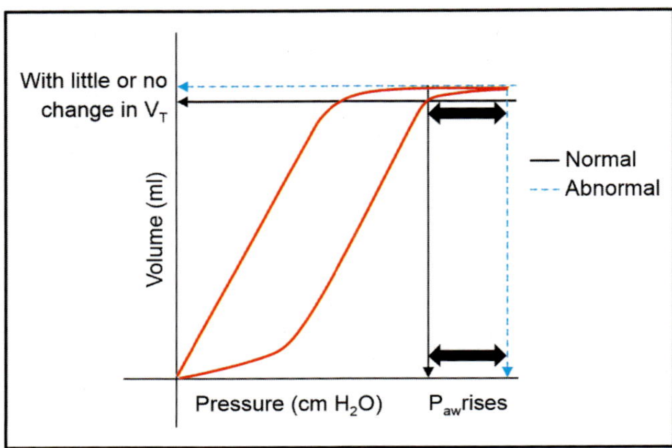

Fig. 9.3: Overdistension of alveoli showing beaking effect on the pressure volume curve

INDICATIONS FOR THE USE OF PEEP

The use of PEEP is universal. About 3–5 cm H_2O PEEP is believed to be exerted by vocal cords during spontaneous ventilation through the natural airway, primarily to reduce basal airway collapse (a physiological mechanism). This is also called physiological PEEP. When this mechanism is bypassed by endotracheal intubation, airways are exposed to atmospheric pressure at ZEEP and the alveoli can collapse, especially in patients with factors that can produce alveolar collapse. Hence, unless contraindicated, a minimum of 5 cmH_2O is applied during mechanical ventilation even in healthy lungs.

In diseased lungs, use of PEEP is indicated in all conditions that result in hypoxia consequent to intrapulmonary shunt or alveolar atelectasis. The amount of PEEP needed will depend on the disease condition as well as whether the patient is a responder or a nonresponder (*vide infra*).

CONTRAINDICATIONS FOR THE USE OF PEEP

- PEEP is contraindicated in a patient with pneumothorax as it can enlarge producing a worsening or even tension pneumothorax. PEEP should also be used carefully in patients with hyperinflated lungs such as emphysema or bronchial asthma as it can cause barotrauma.
- PEEP increases the intrathoracic pressure which reduces the venous return to the heart. This results in decreased cardiac output which will be more profound in patients with hypovolemic or cardiogenic shock. PEEP can be introduced after correction of hypovolemia in patients with hypovolemic shock if hypoxia is present.

- PEEP reduces venous return from the head and neck. This can increase intracranial pressure and hence, is contraindicated in patients with raised intracranial pressure (ICP). If these patients are hypoxic, PEEP can be used but ICP has to be monitored carefully.

EFFECT OF PEEP ON VARIOUS ORGAN SYSTEMS

Effect on Cardiovascular System

PEEP increases the intrathoracic pressure and reduces venous return. Right ventricular (RV) filling is reduced. Pressure in the pulmonary vasculature increases as a result of hypoxia (hypoxic pulmonary vasoconstriction) as well as collapse of the pulmonary capillaries due to high airway pressure. The right ventricular pressure increases as pulmonary arterial pressure increases. This causes bulging of the interventricular septum to the left side decreasing LV filling. The combined effect of decreased venous return and increased RV pressure decreases LV output (**Fig. 9.4**). This response is exaggerated in patients with hypovolemia or cardiac failure. To counter the effects of PEEP on cardiovascular system, ensure euvolaemia and add vasopressors as necessary, if the use of PEEP is essential to improve oxygenation in that patient.

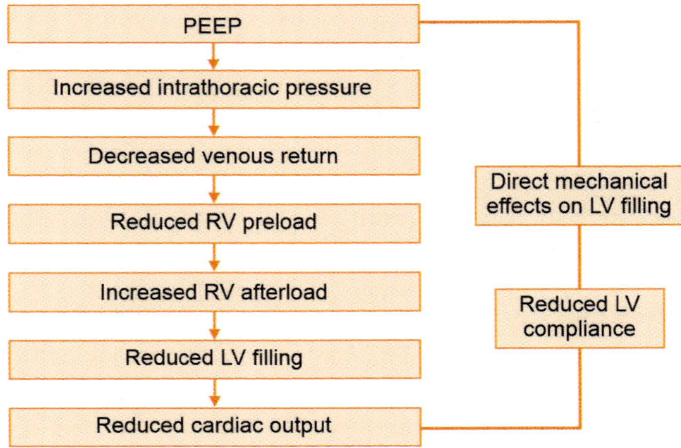

Fig. 9.4: Hemodynamic effects of PEEP

Effect on Cerebral Perfusion

The increased intrathoracic pressure decreases venous return from the head and neck area. This causes elevation of the intracranial pressure. High levels of PEEP have to be avoided in patients with elevated intracranial pressure and increments or decrements of PEEP have to be done gradually and carefully.

Effects on Hepatobiliary System

PEEP causes decrease in hepatic perfusion by reducing the cardiac output. Liver has dual blood flow from hepatic artery and portal vein. Mechanical ventilation decreases both hepatic arterial and portal blood flow. Higher PEEP also causes congestion of the liver by reducing venous return which acts by increasing pressure in the inferior vena cava (IVC) which in turn increases pressure in the hepatic vein. This congestion can cause elevation of aminotransferases in patients who are critically ill. Increased PEEP levels also increase the resistance to bile flow through the bile duct.

Effects on Renal System

Renal and pulmonary systems are largely interconnected. Decreased cardiac output caused by increased PEEP can reduce the blood flow in renal arteries reducing renal perfusion. Increased intrathoracic pressure increases the back pressure on IVC which in turn results in congestion of the renal veins. It reduces urine output by decreasing glomerular filtration rate (GFR), increasing antidiuretic hormone level and decreasing the level of atrial natriuretic peptide.

Effects on Gastrointestinal (GI) System

Requirement of PEEP for >48 hours has been shown to be an independent risk factor for GI bleeding in critically ill patients. PEEP produces splanchnic hypoperfusion due to decrease in mean arterial pressure (MAP) and increase in resistance in GI vascular bed. Activation of the renin angiotensin system and circulating catecholamines (both exogenous and endogenous) further worsens the vasoconstriction and redistributes blood away from the splanchnic vascular bed.

Gut is more prone to ischemic injury because it has no autoregulation. Vascular architecture of gut mucosa is similar to renal medulla. Hypoxia is common at the tips of villi even during normal conditions because O_2 diffuses out of arterioles directly into adjacent venules without ever being carried in the blood to tips of the villi (counter current blood flow). Furthermore, oxygen content in gut mucosal vessels is low because of dilution by absorbed fluids and nutrients. All these lead to relative O_2 deficit resulting in GI complications such as mucosal damage and altered GI motility. In addition to this, there is reperfusion injury and the cytokines involved may affect many organs.

Humoral Responses to PEEP

The main neurohormonal mechanisms thought to cause increased systemic and renal sympathetic nervous system activity are increased activity of renin-angiotensin-aldosterone system, increased secretion of vasopressin, and decreased release of atrial natriuretic peptide (ANP). The net effect of salt and water retention is intravascular volume expansion which can alleviate the negative hemodynamic and neurohormonal consequences of PEEP on renal function. However, it may be detrimental in many patients especially those with poor underlying cardiac function or ARDS.

HOW MUCH PEEP SHOULD WE USE?

PEEP requirements vary between patients and one value of PEEP will not fit all. PEEP settings have to be individualized as requirements may differ between patients as a result of variable chest wall compliance, abdominal content, lung weight, etc. Many clinicians find it difficult to distinguish overdistention from underinflation while trying to determine an optimal value of PEEP.

Optimal PEEP

Optimal PEEP is the level of PEEP at which end-inspiratory overdistention as well as end-expiratory atelectasis are minimal. It is the PEEP level at which maximal beneficial effect is observed, i.e. improvement in oxygenation, increase in FRC, reduction in shunt and improvement in compliance. At optimum PEEP, the adverse effects of PEEP are minimal.

Tissue oxygen delivery is a cardiorespiratory function. The improved oxygenation effect of PEEP can be offset by reduced oxygen delivery. Oxygen delivery declines, if the drop in cardiac output caused by PEEP outweighs the rise in arterial oxygen content. Whenever augmentation of PEEP is done, it is mandatory to follow the adequacy of tissue oxygen delivery by monitoring cardiac output (or its surrogates) as well as SaO_2. Whenever feasible, the determinants of tissue O_2 sufficiency such as central venous oxygen saturation ($ScVO_2$) and serum lactate levels, should be tracked.

There are numerous ways to measure optimal PEEP. The best method of determination of optimal PEEP is still elusive and controversial. Which method to follow is up to the discretion of the clinician. The following methods have been used commonly:

PEEP by best Oxygenation

Set PEEP at 25 cm H_2O with fixed driving pressure ensuring delivery of tidal volume of 6 ml/kg of ideal body weight at a FiO_2 of 60%. Decrease PEEP in decrements of 4 cm H_2O every 10 minutes until a PEEP of 5 cm H_2O is reached. In each step, monitor static lung compliance, total lung compliance, arterial blood gas, cardiac output and mixed venous oxygen saturation. Optimal PEEP is defined as the PEEP below which PaO_2/FiO_2 ratio drops by at least 20%. If PaO_2/FiO_2 ratio does not drop by 20% or more, then the PEEP at which best PaO_2/FiO_2 ratio is obtained is considered as the optimal PEEP.

PEEP by Best Compliance

In this method, a recruitment manoeuvre is done and PEEP is set either at 10 or 20 cm of H_2O. In incremental PEEP method, PEEP is set at 10 cmH_2O. PEEP is then increased in steps of 1 or 2 cm of H_2O. Breath-by-breath compliance is estimated. It may first increase to a maximum and then decrease again. The PEEP at which compliance starts to decrease is the overdistending pressure. At this juncture, a new recruitment maneuver is performed and PEEP is set about 1 cmH_2O below this value.

In decremental PEEP method, PEEP can be set at 20 cmH_2O. PEEP is then decreased in steps of 1 or 2 cm of H_2O. Breath-by-breath compliance is estimated. It may first increase to a maximum and then decrease again. The PEEP at which compliance starts to decrease is similar to the collapse pressure. At this juncture, a new recruitment maneuver is performed and PEEP is set about 1 cm H_2O above this value. Decremental PEEP trial is the method more commonly used in ARDS patients **(Table 9.1)**.

Parameters such as position, tidal volume, pressure control (with P_{plat} <30 cm H_2O), appropriate sedation levels to tolerate high PEEP and/or hypercarbia and FiO_2 (<60%) should be constant when PEEP trial is being carried out to assess PEEP induced recruitment.

Table 9.1: An example of decremental PEEP trial using oxygenation and compliance as indicators

PEEP (cmH_2O)	PaO_2/SpO_2	Compliance (cmH_2O)
18	43/70%	26
16	67/92%	33
14	77/96%	37
12	83/98%	43
10	70/92%	38

PEEP by Esophageal Pressure

Here, an esophageal balloon is inserted to measure esophageal pressure which is a reflection of pleural pressure. Transpulmonary pressure is the difference between airway pressure and the pleural pressure. The end-inspiratory and end-expiratory transpulmonary pressures are measured. PEEP is titrated to target end-expiratory transpulmonary pressure between 0–10 cm H_2O to prevent cyclical alveolar collapse. Tidal volume will be titrated to maintain end-inspiratory transpulmonary pressure <25 cm H_2O to prevent cyclical alveolar overdistention.

Use of ARDS Net PEEP/FiO_2 Table

PEEP can also be set according to ARDSNet PEEP/FiO_2 table, where the PEEP is changed along with FiO_2 as per the oxygen requirement of the patient **(Table 9.2)**.

Table 9.2: ARDSNet PEEP/FiO_2 table

High PEEP/Low FiO_2														
FiO_2	0.3	0.3	0.3	0.3	0.3	0.4	0.4	0.5	0.5	0.5 – 0.8	0.8	0.9	1.0	1.0
PEEP	5	8	10	12	14	14	16	16	18	20	22	22	22	24

Limitations of PEEP/FiO_2 table: The PEEP/FiO_2 table is easy to use but has limitations. It has fixed pairings of PEEP and FiO_2. Patients can be either PEEP responders and PEEP nonresponders. PEEP nonresponders recruit little (and arterial PaO_2 improves little) in response to higher levels of PEEP. In these patients, an FiO_2 rise which is optimal will result in higher PEEP and risk of overdistension. Whereas, in PEEP responders who recruit well in response to higher levels of PEEP, the PEEP rise which is required, comes along with higher FiO_2 and risk of oxygen toxicity.

Use of Pressure–Volume Loop Analysis

A pressure-volume curve of the lung can be constructed using slow inflation method. If the lower and higher inflection points are clear, PEEP can be set slightly above the lower inflection point on the inspiratory limb **(Fig. 9.5)**.

Setting PEEP using Stress Index Method

Stress index is a method adopted in new generation ventilators (Maquet Servo-I) which helps in monitoring PEEP induced recruitment and avoids over distension. Stress index is measured on a passive patient on volume controlled ventilation with constant flow and

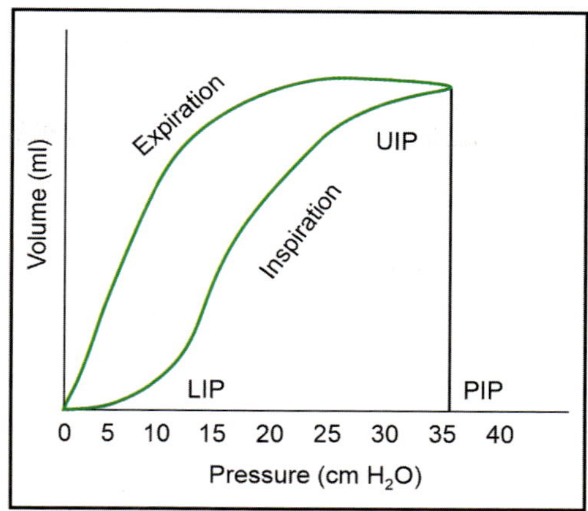

Fig. 9.5: Setting PEEP using pressure-volume curve. LIP: Lower inflection point; UIP: Upper inflection point; PIP: Peak inspiratory pressure

observing pressure over time graph. This method is based on the observation that during constant-flow insufflation, the rate of change of pressure at the airway corresponds to the rate of change in respiratory-system compliance. Accordingly, if the graph is linear, it is considered as normal and stress index is equal to one. If the graph shows upward concavity it indicates decreased compliance due to lung over distension and stress index is more than one. If the graph shows downward concavity, it indicates increased compliance and potential for alveolar recruitment and the stress index is less than one (**Fig. 9.6**).

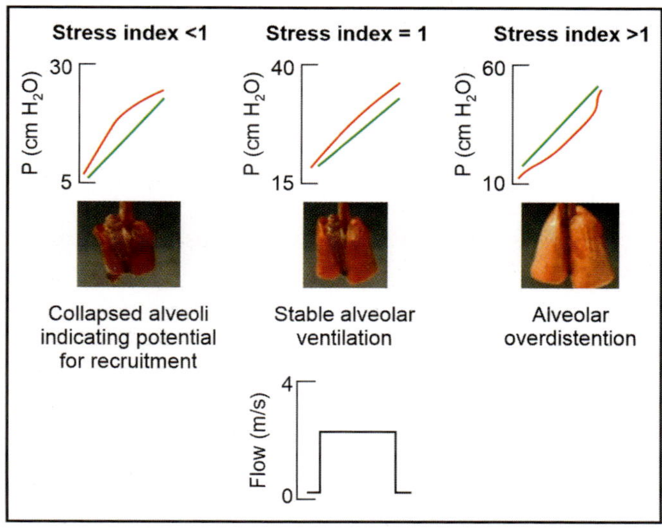

Fig. 9.6: Stress index and setting PEEP

Limitations: Stress index merely considers the inspiratory part of the breath. There may also be some doubts as to whether airway resistance is constant during inspiration.

The other Methods used to set PEEP are:

- Adjusting PEEP to optimize driving pressure
- PEEP at which $PaCO_2$ to $ETCO_2$ gradient is minimal (minimal dead space)
- Optimal PEEP can also be determined by electrical impedance tomography and sequential CT imaging.

MEASUREMENT OF PEEP-INDUCED ALVEOLAR RECRUITMENT

The goal of PEEP therapy is to ensure that PEEP recruits "recruitable" alveoli but not over distend alveoli that are already open. This depends on the recruitability potential of the diseased alveoli. The question is, can it be measured at the bedside? Research is on and experts have proposed the following methods for doing this:

1. CT scan
2. P-V curve
3. Volumetric capnography
4. Dynamic estimation of FRC
5. Electrical impedance tomography
6. Positron emission tomography (PET) scan

'Gold standard' measurement of recruitment is end-expiratory CT scan, which is done by obtaining end-expiratory spiral CT scan of whole lung at ZEEP and set PEEP. Then the respective volumes are compared. This method is cumbersome and carries a high risk of hypoxemia when PEEP is reduced to zero. There is additional risk involved in transporting the patient to radiology unit.

Electrical impedance tomography, volumetric capnography, dynamic FRC estimation and positron emission tomography scan are being popularised for clinical practice. Performing these measurements at bedside is difficult.

LOW PEEP VS HIGH PEEP

Most clinicians use PEEP levels of 5–12 cm H_2O for ventilating patients with acute respiratory distress syndrome to balance between the beneficial effects of PEEP and adverse effects. In patients with ARDS, few studies had shown that higher than traditional PEEP levels may be advantageous in terms of reducing mortality and lower levels of inflammatory mediators. However, these studies had also used low tidal volumes and low airway pressures making it difficult to predict whether the benefits are attributable to PEEP alone. Recent literature has shown with low to moderate level evidence that outcomes are similar between patients who receive lower or higher PEEP levels with the use of low tidal volumes and low inspiratory plateau pressures. In patients without ARDS, studies have shown that low PEEP strategy is non-inferior to high PEEP strategy.

PEEP AND RECRUITMENT MANEUVER

Recruitment is application of a high level of sustained airway pressure to open up collapsed alveoli and then application of appropriate PEEP to prevent the collapse of those recruited alveoli. Experimental studies have shown that recruitment results in temporary improvement in oxygenation but mortality benefit is not observed. It has to be used with caution in selected patients.

Various methods are used for recruitment. Following methods are commonly used.

Method 1

Keep the patient in CPAP mode and hold at 40 cm H_2O pressure for up to 30 sec at FiO_2 of 1.

Method 2

- Using PCV, adjust FiO_2 to target SaO_2 90–92%.
- Set inspiratory pressure (Pi) to 15 cm H_2O above the PEEP and maintain this difference.
- Increase PEEP in a stepwise manner to 20, 30 and then 40 cm H_2O with adjustments made every two minutes (i.e. Pi will reach 55 cmH_2O).
- Reduce PEEP progressively to 25 cmH_2O, 22.5, 20, 17.5 and then to minimum of 15 cm H_2O every three minutes until a decrease in SaO_2 ≥1% from maximum SaO_2 is observed (the derecruitment point).
- Increase PEEP to 40 cm H_2O for one minute then return to a PEEP level 2.5 cm H_2O above the derecruitment point (the optimal PEEP).
- Then adjust to tidal volume ≤6 ml/kg ideal body weight and a plateau pressure 30 cm H_2O, tolerate permissive hypercapnia if pH >7.15.

The patient is considered a responder, if a recruitment test proves that PEEP manipulation leads toaddition of new alveoli and not overdistention of normal alveoli. Recruitment results in decreased plateau pressure and PCO_2. These patients are suitable for decremental PEEP trial. In non-responders, PEEP manipulation leads to over-distension of normal alveoli causing increased plateau pressure and PCO_2. These patients are candidates for incremental PEEP trial.

Additional selection criteria for incremental and decremental PEEP trials

Decremental PEEP trial: Decremental PEEP trials should be used in patients with lower inflection point (LIP) on PV curve, ground glass appearance on image studies (interstitial edema) and recruitment test producing decreased plateau pressure/PCO_2.

Incremental PEEP trial: Incremental PEEP trial should be used if the patient has no LIP on PV curve and has consolidation radiologically (alveolar edema) and if recruitment test produces increase in plateau pressure and PCO_2.

PEEP is manipulated in small installments whilst monitoring oxygenation and/or lung compliance.

WEANING PEEP

Weaning from PEEP should be considered only when there is partial or complete reversibility of the disease process. Weaning from PEEP should not be attempted unless the patient is on a FiO_2 of <0.5. PEEP should be gradually reduced by 2 cm H_2O at a time with monitoring of saturation and arterial blood gases at each step. Abrupt withdrawal of PEEP can result in worsening of oxygenation, lung oedema and overloading of the cardiovascular system. Spontaneous breathing trials can be tried once the PEEP level is below 10 cm H_2O.

AUTOPEEP

Intrinsic PEEP or AutoPEEP is generated when exhalation is incomplete. Air gets trapped in the alveoli and with continued respirations, the pressure builds up. This happens due to shift of the equal pressure point from the better-supported proximal airways to the distal airways with no cartilaginous support. In these patients, the pleural pressure exceeds the pressure inside the airways leading to collapse of those airways trapping the residual gas inside the alveoli (air-trapping) **(Fig. 9.7)**.

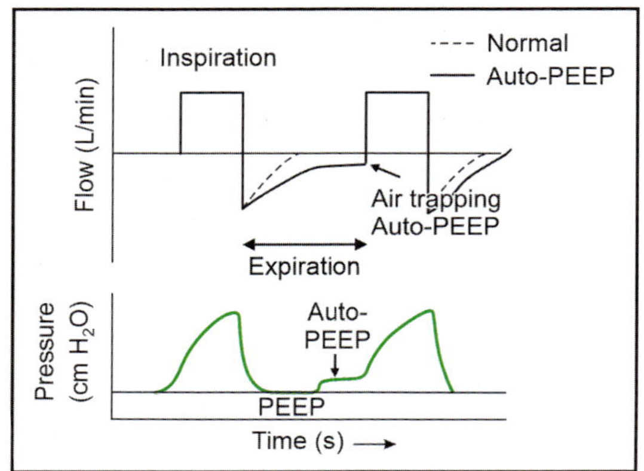

Fig. 9.7: Flow time scalar showing failure of the expiratory flow curve to reach baseline indicating air-trapping. Pressure time scalar shows the development of AutoPEEP over and above the set PEEP due to air-trapping

This can be prevented by ensuring complete exhalation. This can be done by:

1. Increasing expiratory time
2. Increasing inspiratory flow to ensure adequate tidal volume delivery in the reduced inspiratory time
3. Reduce respiratory rate and tidal volume
4. Ensure bronchodilatation
5. Ensure effective removal of secretions
6. Use larger endotracheal tubes
7. Use of extrinsic PEEP to reduce intrinsic PEEP

CONCLUSION

Even though, PEEP is one of the most important parameters to be set on the ventilator for patients requiring mechanical ventilation, there is considerable controversy regarding the best way to choose the optimum PEEP for the patient. PEEP has been shown to improve oxygenation and also reduce ventilator induced lung injury. An optimum PEEP level that improves oxygenation with minimum cardiovascular function impairment has to be carefully chosen for the patient. Clinicians must watch carefully for the development of complications in a patient who requires high level of PEEP.

TAKE-HOME POINTS

- Positive end expiratory pressure is the pressure above atmospheric pressure in the alveoli at the end of expiration in mechanically ventilated patients. It can be extrinsic or intrinsic.
- Extrinsic PEEP is PEEP set by the clinician during mechanical ventilation. PEEP improves oxygenation and reduces lung compliance by recruiting collapsed alveoli.
- PEEP protects the lung from ventilator-induced lung injury by protecting the surfactant, reducing inflammation and preventing alveolar edema.
- PEEP increases intrathoracic pressure, reduces venous return, increases right ventricular afterload and reduces cardiac output. Splanchnic hypoperfusion affects hepatic and renal circulation. Impaired venous return can raise intracranial pressure.
- Optimum PEEP is the PEEP level at which the beneficial effects are maximum and the adverse effects are minimal. Optimum PEEP can be set by various methods: Best oxygenation, best compliance, incremental PEEP or decremental PEEP, using pressure volume curve, PEEP/FiO_2 table, stress index, etc.
- It is important to recognise that not all patients respond to PEEP. They may be responders or nonresponders and PEEP has to be set appropriately. A carefully applied recruitment maneuver may help distinguish between the two.
- Whether to use high PEEP or low PEEP has been a matter of study. Recent literature has shown with low to moderate level evidence that outcomes are similar between patients who receive lower or higher PEEP levels with the use of low tidal volumes and low inspiratory plateau pressures.
- Intrinsic PEEP or AutoPEEP is seen when exhalation is incomplete in patients with air-trapping (e.g. emphysema). This may add onto extrinsic PEEP and can be monitored using flow time scalar.
- Weaning PEEP is done slowly, in small decrements, and only after oxygenation is adequate and the FiO_2 requirement is <60% unless a complication such as pneumothorax or hemodynamic instability warrants its immediate reduction.
- PEEP is an important parameter to be set during mechanical ventilation and must be used judiciously for the best benefit to the patient.

Recommended Reading

1. Brower RG, Lanken PN, MacIntyre N, Matthay MA, Morris A, Ancukiewicz M, Schoenfeld D, Thompson BT; National Heart, Lung, and Blood Institute ARDS Clinical Trials Network. Higher versus lower positive end-expiratory pressures in patients with the acute respiratory distress syndrome. N Engl J Med. 2004;351(4):327–36. doi: 10.1056/NEJMoa032193. PMID: 15269312.
2. David J Dries, John J Marini. Finding Best PEEP: A Little at a Time. Respiratory Care May 2020; 65 (5):722–4; DOI: 10.4187/respcare.07799.
3. Gattinoni L, Collino F, Maiolo G, Rapetti F, Romitti F, Tonetti T, Vasques F, Quintel M. Positive end-expiratory pressure: how to set it at the individual level. Ann Transl Med. 2017;5(14):288. doi: 10.21037/atm.2017.06.64. PMID: 28828363; PMCID: PMC5537121.

4. Mercat A, Richard JM, Vielle B, et al. Positive End-Expiratory Pressure Setting in Adults With Acute Lung Injury and Acute Respiratory Distress Syndrome: A Randomized Controlled *Trial*. JAMA. 2008;299(6):646–55. doi:10.1001/jama.299.6.646
5. Writing Committee and Steering Committee for the RELAx Collaborative Group, Algera AG, Pisani L, Serpa Neto A, den Boer SS, Bosch FFH, Bruin K, Klooster PM, Van der Meer NJM, Nowitzky RO, Purmer IM, Slabbekoorn M, Spronk PE, van Vliet J, Weenink JJ, Gama de Abreu M, Pelosi P, Schultz MJ, Paulus F. Effect of a Lower vs Higher Positive End-Expiratory Pressure Strategy on Ventilator-Free Days in ICU Patients Without ARDS: A Randomized Clinical Trial. JAMA. 2020;324(24):2509–20. doi: 10.1001/jama.2020.23517. PMID: 33295981; PMCID: PMC7726701.

CHAPTER 10

Volume versus Pressure Ventilation

❐ Manimala S Rao ❐ Vijay Deshpande

Defining these two important aspects of mechanical ventilation is not an easy task. However to simplify, the volume control favours to control ventilation, where as the pressure control is to improve oxygenation.

If we can keep this simple rule in mind one can easily categorize them and use them where and when necessary. They have distinct advantages and disadvantages which are mainly related to flow and pressure patterns of gas delivery.[1] When one understands the advantages and disadvantages of these two modes of ventilation, the differences and uses can be sorted out correctly to the needs of a patient.

Volume Control

The most important advantage is that a guaranteed tidal volume produces a more stable minute volume. This remains stable even with some changes in pulmonary characteristics. The initial flow rate is lower therefore a high resistance is not encountered. The mean airway pressure is lower with volume control so that it may not be able to recruit the alveoli well when the compliance is low. In the presence of a leak the Mean Alveolar Pressure (MAP) can become unstable. Insufficient flow can give rise to patient ventilatory dissynchrony.

Pressure Control

This mode increases the Mean Alveolar Pressure (MAP). Therefore it increases the duration for alveolar recruitment, thereby protecting against the barotrauma. The work of breathing and patient comfort on the ventilator is improved. The disadvantages are the Tidal Volume (TV) may be variable. Increase in volume may result in volutrauma. High inspiratory flow in the very beginning may breach the pressure limit if airway resistance is high.

In this mode the pattern is like a square. Therefore the mean pressure is high for a set period of time, there by it is useful to recruit non-compliant alveoli. This in turn improves the oxygenation. This is an ideal mode to start in moderate to severe ARDS patients.

The Volume Control Ventilation (VCV) and Pressure controlled Ventilation (PCV) are not really different modes but are different control variables within a mode. As the debate continues as which is the best mode so does for the Control Variables. In VCV we have a set TV and MV but requires a set inspiratory flow, inspiratory flow wave form and inspiratory time. During this ventilatory method the airway pressure increases in response to decrease in the compliance or increase in the airway resistance. For example, in a patient with low compliance as in ARDS, the airway Pressure increases and this could lead to barotrauma or VALI. (ventilator associated lung injury).

The PCV by design limits the maximum or the peak pressure to develop in the airways. However, it may result in variable tidal volume. The inspiratory flow and wave form are determined by the ventilator as it maintains a square wave inspiratory pressure profile (**Figs 10.1 and 10.2**).

However the PCV may not offer any advantages over VCV in patients who do not have any spontaneous respiration except when the oxygenation is very poor and have

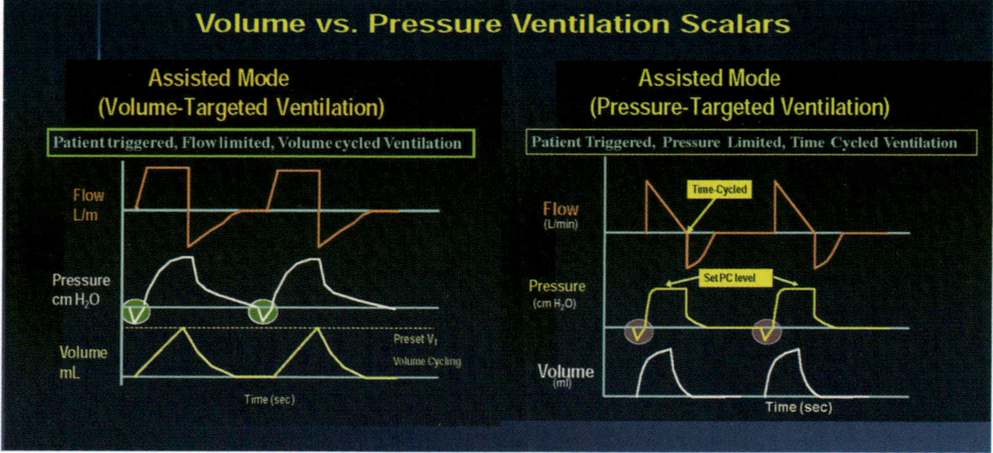

Fig. 10.1: The scalars represent the volume and pressure graphics which have their own features in flow volume pressure and time

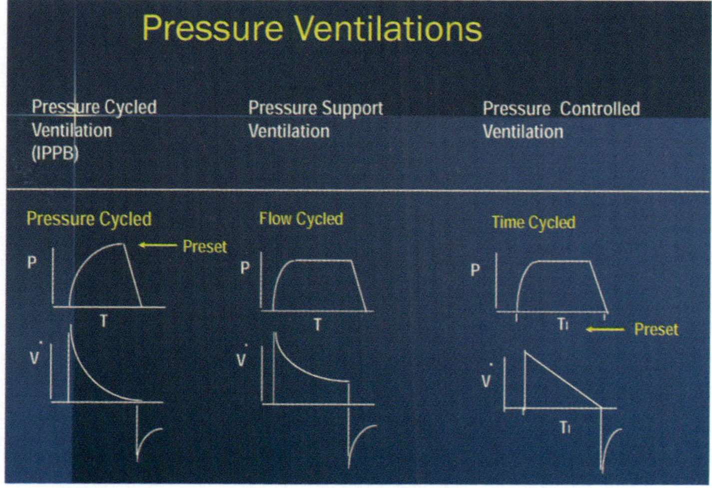

Fig. 10.2: The lower graph represents the different types of pressure variables used in day to day management of patients on pressure modes

low compliance like in ARDS. PCV could be the mode in this particular settings as it offers lower work of breathing and improves patient comfort and oxygenation.

With advent of dual modes, which can deliver lower tidal volumes and limit the pressure have become the order of the day to tide over the disadvantages of both VCV and PCV to an extent unless, of course if it is used for recruitment and oxygenation.

Most of the studies comparing VCV and PCV were really not very well controlled or designed and offer little to our understanding as to when and how to use each of them.[2]

Work of Breathing (WOB)

The patients work of breathing (WOB) in assisted ventilation is reduced when the inspiratory flow from the ventilator exceeds patients flow demand. Patients with ARDS often have unstable breathing patterns and their requirement of inspiratory flow may change from breath to breath. In the volume control the flow is preset in contrast to pressure control ventilation. This comprises a variable decelerated wave form with a high inspiratory flow is available as the controlled breath starts.

In a prospective randomized cross over study R.H. Callet et al measured work of breathing with BICORE CP-100 monitor and found that WOB was much less in PCV compared to VCV.[3]

Table 10.1

VCV Ventilation	PCV Oxygenation
Flow is decreased as pressure increases	Work of breathing is reduced
Adequate MV to drive out CO_2	Flow is better as there is a square wave pattern
Pressure increases as the compliance decreases or resistance ++ Barotrauma	Ventilation is variable as volume is not controlled Minute ventilation has to be maintained by increasing respiratory rate Volutrauma
Adequate ventilation CO_2 is driven out the possibility of Barotrauma	Adequate flow Adequate Mean alveolar pressure Better oxygenation CO_2 retention Increase in RR to reduce CO_2 Better oxygenation

The most common primary initial mode is VCV. One has to also answer some questions like why would we like to ventilate every breath with same volume? Does it happen in our normal spontaneous breaths? Can we inflate with set pressure PCV?

Now how would we inflate the lung with pressure or volume is an important question. It may not be the correct choice to every situation. The car tires are inflated with pressure than volume not to cause over inflation with volume. But the tire is made of rubber and the lung is made of elastic fibers. So there are some patients who will benefit with Pressure Ventilation where you can avoid volutrauma, particularly when the lung volume is small.

The main reason one prefers volume ventilation over pressure is to have adequate minute ventilation to drive out the CO_2 which is the main metabolic activity of the lung. This requires adequate minute ventilation. If one does not do it properly more complications will follow.

In the VCV mode, the bugbear was the rise in peak and plateau pressures which can cause barotrauma. The newer dual modes have solved this problem to a great extent by limiting the pressure. The minute ventilation is calculated by tidal volume and the respiratory rate which are set on the ventilator according to the patients gender, height and weight.

The Pressure Control mode will limit the pressure and prevent volutrauma, as well as barotrauma but may not give the correct minute ventilation to drive out the CO_2. Therefore, for all practical purposes one can set up VCV as a common mode but in circumstances where oxygenation is the primary end point, one can directly start the PCV to achieve the results and allow some permissive hypercapnia as is done in patients with ARDS. The volume and MV must be constantly checked and should not allow to go down or up. Continuous checking these two parameters will avoid the hypercapnia. At this juncture continuous monitoring of end tidal CO_2 will be an ideal back up.

In conclusion one has to wonder to understand how to use either pressure or volume ventilation in mechanically ventilated patient. There are four main types of lung conditions which one encounters when we ventilate patients.

Normal Lungs

The first one is a normal lung. It has no pathology. Our endeavour is to see that we do not cause any type of damage either by Volume or Pressure, or ventilator associated events.

Therefore one can use 7 ml/kg. TV and limit the plateau pressures to less than 30 cm H_2O. To achieve this we can safely use volume controlled pressure limited mode, which gives both ventilation and oxygenation to the normal lung and prevents any ventilator associated injury.

Fibrosed Lungs

The second variety is consolidated and fibrotic lung with low compliance and has difficulty to oxygenate. This lung when it has moderate or severe disease like in ARDS, one can safely use pressure controlled ventilation which limits the pressure and allows the Mean Pressure is for a longer time period and, therefor, results in better oxygenation. As the pressure is regulated one has to watch the volume and flow constantly so that better oxygenation is achieved along with institution of positive and expiatory pressures. Keeping in mind not to allow the tidal volume to go up more than 6 ml/kg. In this way even an increase in the inspiratory time will give longer Mean Pressure, thereby improving oxygenation. Some permissive hypercapnia is allowed. The ventilation can improved by increasing the respiratory rate.

Lungs in Emphysema

The third type of lung is non-elastic as we see in the emphysematous patient. In this particular disease one cannot drive out the CO_2 Leading to respiratory acidosis and surviving on hypoxic drive. The lung volume is tremendously increased leading to pneumothorax due to rupture of either bullae or septa. The tidal volume may be kept below 7–8 ml/kg with a respiratory rate towards normal range (14/min). The CO_2 levels to be kept slightly above normal ranges and the bicarb levels should be to an extent compensated. Volume ventilation with pressure limit is fairly suited for these patients.

Lungs in Asthma

10% of patients admitted with asthma go to intensive care and 2% of them get intubated and mechanically ventilated. The most difficult problem is to deal with gas trapping which leads to dynamic hyperinflation leading to intrinsic positive end expiatory pressure or PEEPi or Auto-PEEP. The air trapping occurs due to bronchoconstriction, airway edema and mucus plugging. Work of breathing increases due to high airway resistance. The normal process of passive expiration, becomes an active process. If the volume at the end of expiration is more than 20 ml/kg predicts the complication of barotrauma and hyper inflation. For these patients the ventilation mode should be pressure controlled with a setting pressure which will achieve a tidal volume of 6–8 ml/kg and a PH of 7.2 one has to deligently watch for the volume of dynamic hyperinflation.[4]

Finally one has to choose the ventilatory mode which is best suited to the acuteness of the disease,with least percentage of complications and should be very patient centric and should be watched on a regular basis for any problems that will be encountered and change the variables if and when necessary. The modes and variables are the tools available on ventilator and they should be set and carefully monitored to get the best outcomes.

References

1. https//deranged physiology.com
2. Robert.S. Canbel, et al. Resp Care 2002 April. Pressure control *vs* Volume control. Ventilator does it mater.
3. RLH. Callet, *et al.* Respiratory care 2000 Sep. The effect of PCV vs VCV on patient work of breathing in acute lung injury and ARDS .
4. David R Stather, *et al.* Critical Care 2005 9(6) 581–87. Regn. No. PMID 16356242.

CHAPTER 11

Dual Controlled Modes of Ventilation

❒ Manjush Karthika ❒ Sanjay Sasikumar

ABSTRACT

The conventional modes of ventilation are reported to have many limitations. Although they are routinely used and the mechanism is well-understood, they often fail to match the patient specific requirements. Over the period, many modifications are incorporated in various modes of ventilators to improve the patient outcome. The new generation ventilators available are equipped with feedback system to respond to the patient's demands. In this chapter, we will discuss the popular dual modes of ventilation that have been accepted into the clinical practice.

INTRODUCTION

The process of ventilator to initiate, maintain, and terminate an artificial breath is derived from the concept, "Equation of motion" (**Fig. 11.1**).[1, 2] The equation of motion states that to deliver a breath, there are two components of pressure; the pressure needed to overcome elastic recoil of the chest wall and the lungs; and the pressure required for flow through the airways.

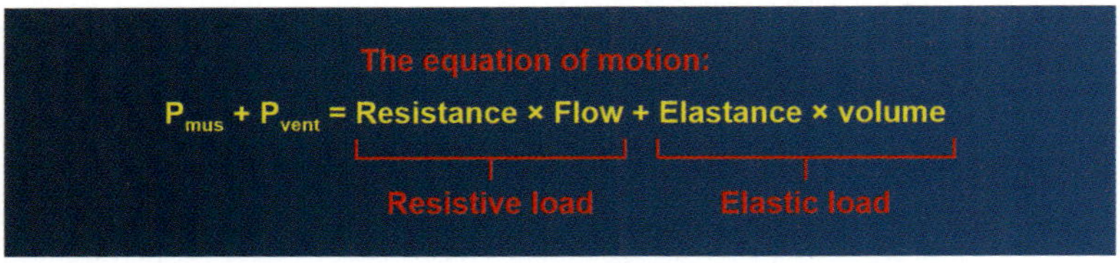

The equation of motion:

$P_{mus} + P_{vent}$ = Resistance × Flow + Elastance × volume

Resistive load (Resistance × Flow); Elastic load (Elastance × volume)

Fig. 11.1: Application of equation of motion in respiratory system

The above equation is expanded as:

$$P_{mus} + P_{vent} = P$$

$$P_{mus} + P_{vent} = (R \times \dot{V}) + (E \times V)$$

Where P = The total pressure required

P_{mus} = Pressure generated by the inspiratory muscles

P_{vent} = Paw (airway pressure) = Pao (pressure at the airway opening)

R = Resistance of the respiratory system

E = Elastance of the respiratory system

V = Change in volume from baseline (e.g. tidal volume)

$\dot{V}$ = Flow rate

The left side of the equation describes the total pressure required to generate a certain level of ventilation. This is the sum of the total pressure delivered by the ventilator (P_{vent}) and the pressure generated by the patient's respiratory muscles (P_{mus}). Important to note that, the relative contribution of P_{vent} and P_{mus} varies based on the clinical scenarios, e.g. in a paralyzed patient, P_{mus} is zero. If the ventilator is disconnected, P_{vent} becomes zero and the required pressure must be generated by the patient's respiratory muscles. In a day-to-day practice, we observe the combined effect of P_{mus} and P_{vent}.

The right side of the equation describes how the pressures mentioned on the left side is utilized. As can be seen from the equation, this is also a sum of two components of pressure.

a. Resistive (dynamic) load, which mathematically is the product of resistance and flow. Before the inspired air reaches the alveoli, it passes through several levels of airways. Resistive pressure is the pressure generated due to the friction caused by any source of resistance from the airway opening to the alveoli. Resistive pressure increases with an increase in resistance (e.g. asthma) and/or flow (e.g. high flow set on the ventilator).
b. Elastic (static) load is mathematically expressed as the product of elastance of respiratory system and tidal volume. Elastic load increases with increased lung and/or chest wall elastance.

In the acute care settings, all the parameters of equation of motion changes, as respiratory mechanics is always dynamic. The ventilator parameters set at one point of time may not be the ideal when the patient deteriorates or improves.[3]

The conventional old-generation ventilators are categorized under open-loop system, considering their limitation of continuously delivering the set parameters without sensing any feedback from patient variables or respiratory mechanics. Some of the newer modes aim to make changes in the set parameters with the dynamic respiratory pattern, with the feedback from patient parameters, thus completing the feedback loop and are known as "Closed loop" modes.[4,5]

In the new modes, the control variables and phase variables such as cycle and limit variables undergo self-adjustment with the feedback from the patient. Some ventilators offer special modes that control both the control variables. However, there is only one single variable (pressure or volume/flow) that is controlled at a given part of inspiration. These variables are not limited to a single set parameter but if the threshold of one component is reached, they shift to the other alternate set parameter. This has led to the name "Dual control" modes of ventilation. Dual control modes operate "within a breath" or on a "breath to breath" basis. Dual control within a breath refers to a technique in which the ventilator switches from pressure to volume control in the middle of a breath. On the other side, during the dual control breath to breath, all the breaths are pressure control breaths, but the level of pressure varies from breath to breath to maintain a constant tidal volume.

Dual Control: Within the Breath

In 'dual-control within the breath' modes of ventilation, the ventilator can automatically switch between pressure and volume control during a single breath. However, the ventilator can only control either pressure or volume at any given time, but not at the same time. The proposed advantage of this mode is to reduce work-of-breathing while maintaining a minimum minute volume and tidal volume. Such modes are operational during mandatory breaths or pressure-supported breaths to combine the high initial flow of a pressure-controlled breath with the constant volume delivery of a volume-controlled breath. The examples of such 'dual-control within a breath' modes are volume-assured pressure support and pressure augmentation. These modes are not commonly available in the newest generation of ICU ventilators.

Pressure Augmentation/Volume Assured Pressure Support

Pressure augmentation mode (Paug) provides pressure-limited ventilation with targeted tidal volume delivery in every breath. The functional concept of this mode is like that of volume-assured pressure support (VAPS) mode, which is available on the Bird 8400ST ventilator. This is a modified pressure control mode of ventilation, where the ventilator to switches from pressure control to volume control mode if a minimum set tidal volume is not achieved (**Fig. 11.2**).[6] With this mode, the ventilation initiates with a patient triggered- pressure set breath, as in case of a pressure support breath, but it delivers the volume as set by the clinician.[6]

The patients are expected to trigger inspiratory efforts, as this mode will not work in patients whose respiratory centers are compromised due to sedation or due to any neurological impairments. The clinician-set parameters are as in conventional pressure control mode, such as pressure limit, peak flow rate, minimum respiratory rate, and positive end-expiratory pressure alongside a desired tidal volume, an inspiratory gas flow, and sensitivity setting. When the patient triggers a breath, the ventilator delivers the set pressure level and monitors the flow and volume. If the tidal volume is attained before the drop in inspiratory flow to the pre-set value, the breath cycles into expiration. Cycling occurs when the measured flow drops to 25 to 30% of the patient's peak

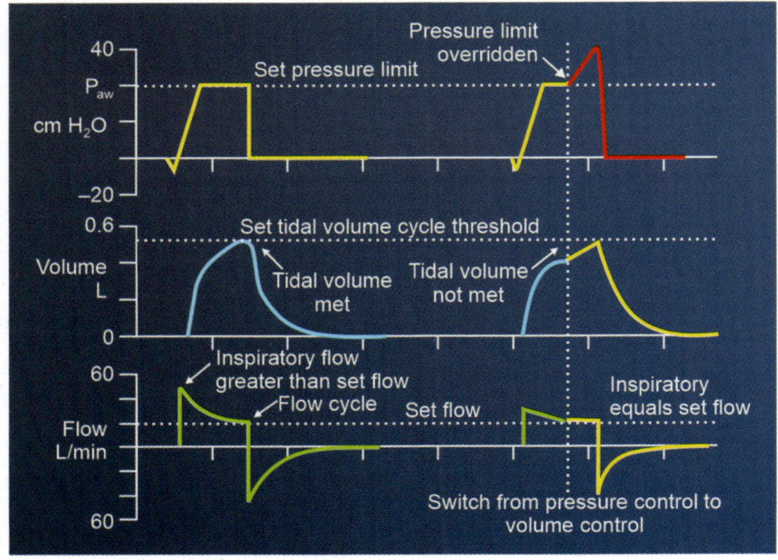

Fig. 11.2: Graphical representation of VAPS

inspiratory flow. If tidal volume is not achieved before the flow drops to the set value, the ventilator maintains a constant flow at the set value until the volume is delivered (volume cycled). In case if the patient's inspiratory flow requirement is high and the pressure starts to drop below the pre-set pressure level, the machine provides additional flow to the patient. Here, the Paug mode targets a minimum volume, but the breath is not limited to that volume, and the patients receive more than the set tidal volume if demands a high inspiratory flow.

In patients with low lung compliance this mode is found to be useful against increasing blood CO_2 levels by maintaining minimal minute ventilation. The operator must understand that, if the set pressure limit is too high it will not only result in barotrauma but also will result in higher tidal volume than set tidal volume, thereby negating the effect of volume guarantee. If the set flow rates are very low, and the minimal tidal volume is not delivered, it may cause a delay in switching from pressure control to volume control and resulting in prolongation of inspiratory time. However, this mode is proven to decrease the work of breathing and lowers the intrinsic PEEP. [7,8]

Dual Control: Breath-to-Breath

Breath-to-breath dual control modes takes feedback from the output parameters of initial breaths and automatic adjustments will be made to set the targets in the subsequent breaths.

Pressure-Regulated Volume Control

Pressure-regulated volume control (PRVC) is a dual mode of ventilation earlier in 1990 on Siemens 300A Servo Ventilator, and subsequently with its successor brands such as Servo-i and Servo-s by Maquet, Inc, Wayne, N.J. The working principle of PRVC mode is similar to that of other manufacturer modes such as AutoFlow on the Dräger ventilators, VC+ on the Covidien PB 840, and Adaptive Pressure Ventilation on the Hamilton ventilators.

PRVC delivers pressure control breaths that are patient- or time-triggered, volume-targeted, and time cycled. Here the clinician determines the inspiratory time and volume. Ventilation begins with volume-controlled breaths of set volume to identify the plateau pressure as the starting value for the inspiratory pressure of the following pressure control ventilation. Then during the pressure control mode, the ventilator measures the tidal volume achieved and compares it to the targeted tidal volume set. If the volume delivered is less than the set tidal volume, the ventilator increases the pressure over many breaths until the set and the targeted tidal volumes becomes equal (**Fig. 11.3**).

If the measured volume is too high, the pressure is decreased to reach the targeted tidal volume. However, the ventilator does not allow the pressure to rise more than 5 cm H_2O below the upper pressure limit setting, i.e. if the upper pressure limit is 35 cm H_2O and the ventilator requires more than 30 cm H_2O to deliver a tidal volume of 500 mL, it alarms, and the pressure delivery is limited to 30 cm H_2O. Various causes of high-pressure alarms such as secretions in the airway, bronchospasms, or changes in lung compliance needs to be addressed by the clinician. As the patient's lung mechanics improves, less pressure is required to achieve the set tidal volume, and the ventilator gradually lowers the pressure to balance the set volume.[9–11]

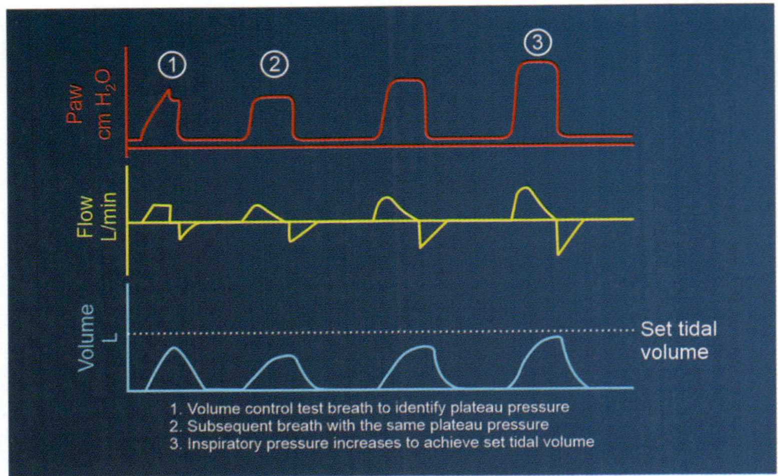

Fig. 11.3: Incremental pressure control in PRVC to meet set tidal volume

Volume Support

Volume support mode is functionally alike PRVC. It is a modification of pressure support mode where the pressure support is automatically titrated by the ventilator to achieve the minimal set tidal volume **(Fig. 11.4)**.[12] The clinician needs to be aware that the patient must have spontaneous breathing activity to activate this mode, and the ventilator will automatically shift to backup mode if the patient turns apnoeic.

The clinician sets the respiratory rate, minimal tidal volume, and PEEP. During this mode of ventilation, the machine measures the delivered tidal volume in the initial breaths and if the minimal volume set is higher than this, it automatically increases the pressure support in the next breaths to achieve the set volume.[13]

This mode offers the benefits of pressure support mode ensuring the adequate tidal volume despite of the changes in lung compliance. Volume support is a useful in weaning, as once the patient starts to achieve a desired tidal volume it automatically

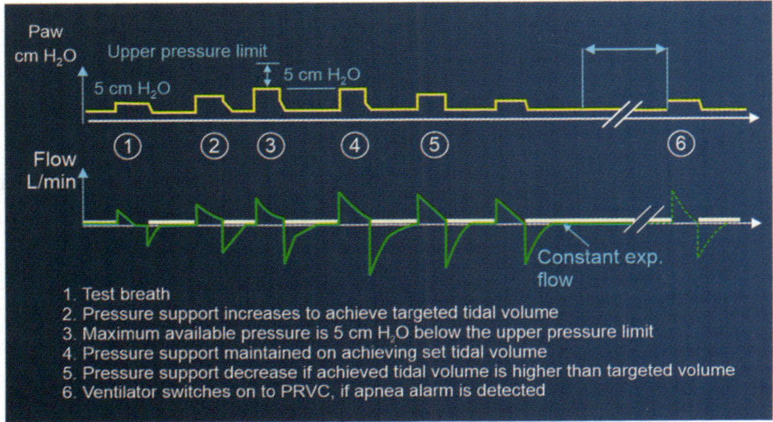

Fig. 11.4: Incremental pressure support in VS to meet set tidal volume

decreases the pressure support, thereby gradually allowing the respiratory muscles to facilitate the work of breathing. Unlike PRVC, volume support mode is flow cycled, when the flow drops to a set percentage of peak flow. In some scenarios, it will be time cycled, if the inspiratory time is extended for any reason or pressure cycled, if the pressure rises too high. Like the pressure support mode patient controls the I:E (Inspiratory time: Expiratory time) and the total inspiratory time, which improves the ventilator-patient synchrony. If the set tidal volume is too high, the ventilator will raise the pressure support level to achieve the volume and may result in barotraumas and hemodynamic compromise. Contrary, lower set tidal volume may result in inadequate pressure support thereby increased respiratory rate resulting in increased work of breathing.[14] If apnea alarm is detected, the ventilator switches on to PRVC mode.

Adaptive Support Ventilation

Adaptive Support Ventilation (ASV) mode is a closed loop pressure targeted mode that selects and continuously adapts the respiratory rate, tidal volume, and inspiratory time depending on the patient's lung mechanics and effort, as per the Otis equation.[15] ASV incorporates various ventilatory modes in its working principle, i.e. pressure support mode, pressure controlled mode, and synchronized intermittent mandatory ventilation mode, when patient's RR is lower than target. Depending on the patient's spontaneous respiratory rate; ASV can work as pressure control ventilation if there is no spontaneous breathing; it acts as pressure control SIMV (PC-SIMV), if the spontaneous respiratory rate is lower than target; and it acts as pressure support ventilation, if the patient's respiratory rate is higher. Hence it is also known as "integrated mode" or "three in one mode".[16] Pressure level is then adapted to attain the set tidal volume within limits imposed by pressure alarms. Cycling is flow based in the case of assisted ventilation and time-based cycling for mandatory breaths.

ASV automatically determines the tidal volume and respiratory rate that best maintains the peak pressure below the target level. The clinician set parameters include patient's ideal body weight, high pressure limit, PEEP, FiO_2, inspiratory rise time, flow cycle percentage, and % of predicted minute volume desired. The % of minute volume varies from 25–350%, i.e. normal 100%, asthma 90%, acute respiratory distress syndrome (ARDS) 120%, others 110%; Add 20% if body temperature is >38.5°C (101.3°F), as a corrective factor. Once ventilation starts, ASV provides a series of test breaths in which it measures the expiratory time constant (compliance × resistance) for the respiratory system and uses this along with the estimated dead space and normal minute ventilation to calculate an optimal respiratory rate in terms of mechanical work. During this test breaths, the ventilator measures compliance, expiratory time constant, tidal volume and respiratory rate based on selected inspiratory time, mandatory respiratory rate, and inspiratory pressure, according to the height (adult or pediatric age range) that the clinician sets. Hence, the pressure limit is automatically adjusted to achieve an average delivered VT equal to the targeted tidal volume. The mode adjusts the I:E ratio and inspiratory time of the mandatory breaths by calculation of the expiratory time constant to maintain sufficient expiratory time The ventilator periodically monitors the dynamic compliance and expiratory time constant to adjust the settings accordingly.[17,18]

Conclusion

The dual modes integrating closed loop technology are shown to improve patient ventilator synchrony and facilitate optimal weaning. Some of these modes are found to be tailored for patient specific requirements and demands. Conventional modes are routinely in use in intensive care settings globally; however, proper understanding of the working principles of dual modes may enhance case-based care and most importantly improved patient outcomes.

References

1. Lucangelo U, Bernabè F, Blanch L. Lung mechanics at the bedside: Make it simple. Curr Opin Crit Care. 2007; 13:64–72.
2. Lucangelo U, Bernabé F, Blanch L. Respiratory mechanics derived from signals in the ventilator circuit. Respir Care. 2005; 50:55–65.
3. Mireles-Cabodevila E, Hatipoglu U, Chatburn RL. A rational framework for selecting modes of ventilation. Respir Care. 2013; 58:348–66.
4. Chatburn RL, Mireles-Cabodevila E. Closed-loop control of mechanical ventilation: Description and classification of targeting schemes. Respir Care. 2011; 56:85–102.
5. Branson RD, Johannigman JA, Campbell RS, Davis K., Jr Closed-loop mechanical ventilation. Respir Care. 2002; 47:427–451.
6. Amato MB, Barbas CS, Bonassa J, Saldiva PH, Zin WA, De Carvalho CR. Volume-assured pressure support ventilation (VAPSV). A new approach for reducing muscle workload during acute respiratory failure. CHEST. 1992; 102:1225–34.
7. Oscroft NS, Smith IE. A bench test to confirm the core features of volume-assured non-invasive ventilation. Respirology. 2010; 15:361–4.
8. Okuda M, Kashio M, Tanaka N, Fujii T, Okuda Y. Positive outcome of average volume-assured pressure support mode of a Respironics V60 Ventilator in acute exacerbation of chronic obstructive pulmonary disease: A case report. J Med Case Rep. 2012; 6:284.
9. B.D. Singer, T.C. Corbridge, Pressure modes of invasive mechanical ventilation, South. Med. J. 2011; 104 (10): 701–709.
10. RD Branson, RL Chatburn. Should adaptive pressure control modes be utilized for virtually all patients receiving mechanical ventilation? Respir Care 2002; 52 (4): 478–488.
11. DJ Pierson Invasive mechanical ventilation, in: R.K. Albert, S.G. Spiro, J.R. Jett (Eds.), Clinical Respiratory Medicine, second ed., Philadelphia Saunders, London, 2004; 189–209.
12. Sottiaux TM. Patient-ventilator interactions during volume-support ventilation: Asynchrony and tidal volume instability - a report of three cases. Respir Care. 2001; 46:255–262
13. McGough EK, Banner MJ, Boysen PG. Pressure support and flow-cycled, assisted mechanical ventilation in acute lung injury. Chest. 1990; 98:458–62
14. Donn SM, Sinha SK. Newer modes of mechanical ventilation for the neonate. Curr Opin Pediatr. 2001; 13:99–103.
15. Tehrani FT. The origin of adaptive support ventilation. Int J Artif Organs. 2005; 28:1051–1052
16. Wysocki M, Brunner JX. Closed-loop ventilation: An emerging standard of care? Crit Care Clin. 2007; 23:223–40.
17. Thompson BT, Hayden D, Matthay MA, et al: Clinicians' approaches to mechanical ventilation in acute lung injury and ARDS. Chest 120:1622–27, 2001.
18. Hamilton Medical: Adaptive support ventilation. www.hamilton-medical.com, accessed November 2022.

CHAPTER 12

Patient Monitoring and Abnormal Waveforms

❒ Vijay Deshpande

Once the patient is connected to mechanical ventilator the clinician records initial ventilator parameters. The first assessment of the patient after connecting to the mechanical ventilator is very thorough and crucial. It gives a baseline record to compare with similar assessments later during ICU stay.

INITIAL ASSESSMENTS FOR THE "VENTILATOR RECORDS DOCUMENT"

Figure 12.1 identifies the three major areas of parameter monitoring, typically done on all mechanically ventilated patients. The parameters, Mode of Ventilation, Tidal Volume, Respiratory frequency, Minute Volume, PIP, P_{plate}, FiO_2, PEEP/CPAP and alarm settings, must be recorded on a "Ventilator Record Sheet" designed by the ICU clinicians. While recording the ventilator parameters, the clinicians should also record the basic patient evaluation findings such as vital signs, initial chest physical examination including inspection of chest wall expansion, absence of uneven expansion, auscultation, SpO and ABG and if needed a chest radiogram. It is imperative that the clinician 2 inspects the ET tube position and stability **(Fig. 12.2)**.

Since Volume Ventilation is used most often, especially in short term mechanical support as well as in other situations except ALI/ARDS, it is vital that the clinicians understand all aspects of associated pressures and significance of changes in these

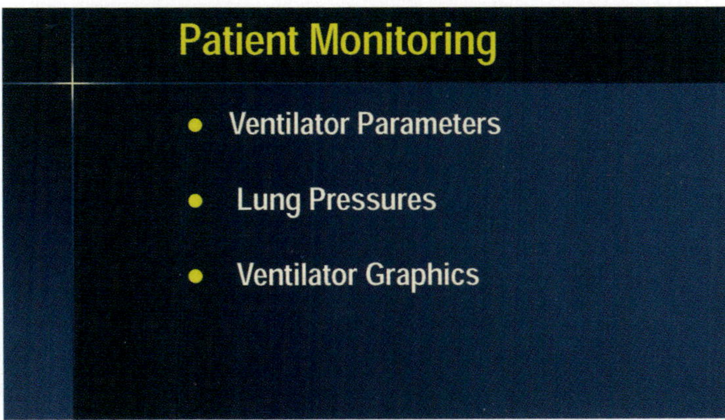

Fig. 12.1

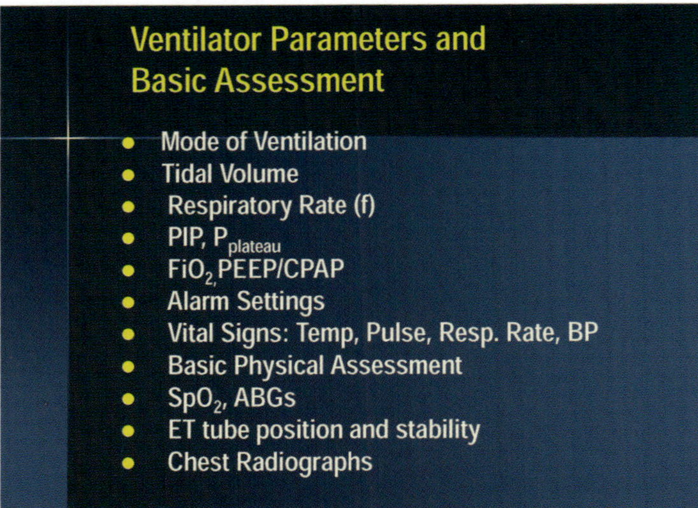

Fig. 12.2

pressures. **Figure 12.3** identifies these pressures. The waveform of inflation pressure (**Fig. 12.4**) traced when inspiratory pause control is activated, identifying PIP, P_{plat} and transairway pressure (P_{TA}), was discussed in this chapter.

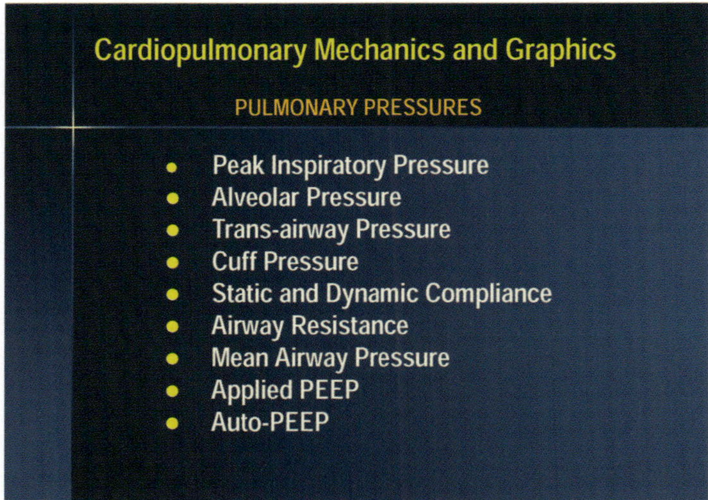

Fig. 12.3

Peak Inspiratory Pressure and Alarms

PIP is the total pressure measured by the ventilator and incorporates resistive and elastic pressures (**Fig. 12.5**). PIP is always recorded as a yardstick to compare later during management of the ventilated patient. It gives a quick view of dynamic compliance. It should be noted that PIP includes PTA and Palv. The High Pressure Alarm is set at a 5–10 cm H_2O above the PIP level. During mechanical ventilation when the high pressure

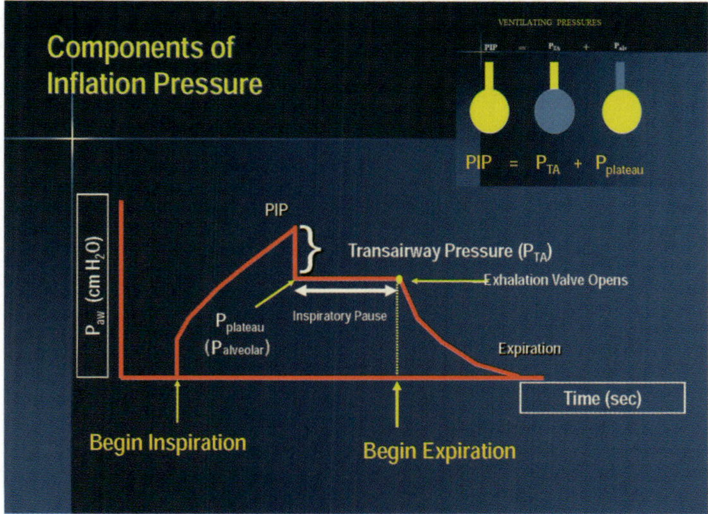

Fig. 12.4

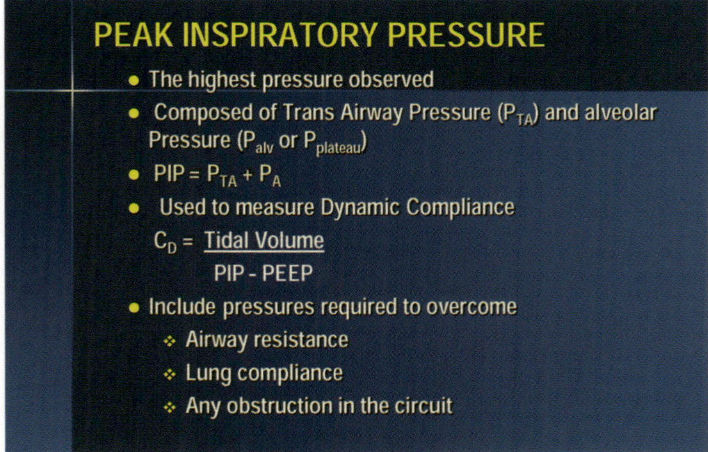

Fig. 12.5

alarm is activated, an audio sound and a visual display on the ventilator screen, the clinician should quickly identify the cause of the increased PIP.

Generally, increased airway secretions, bronchospasm, kinking of the ET tube or any obstruction in the inspiratory limb results in high pressure and alarm sounds **(Fig. 12.6)**. It is important to address the situation immediately to prevent barotrauma. In case the clinician cannot identify the underlying cause, the patient should be disconnected and hand ventilated with a resuscitation bag until the reason for high pressure is ascertained. Setting the Low Pressure Alarm is equally important to detect disconnection, leaks in the system or occasionally, leak around the ET tube cuff **(Fig. 12.7)**.

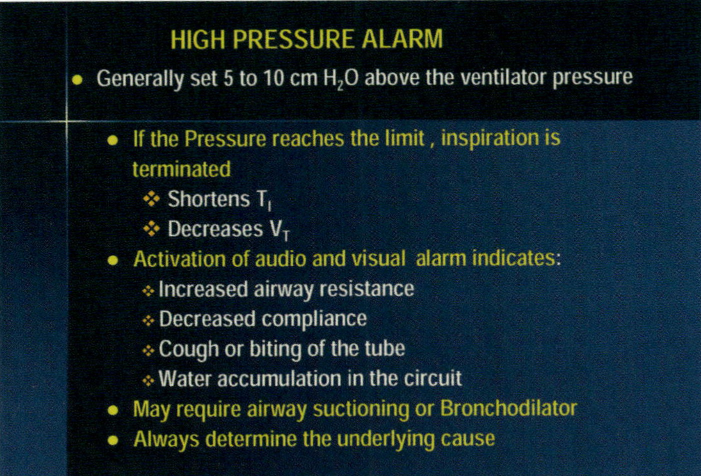

Fig. 12.6

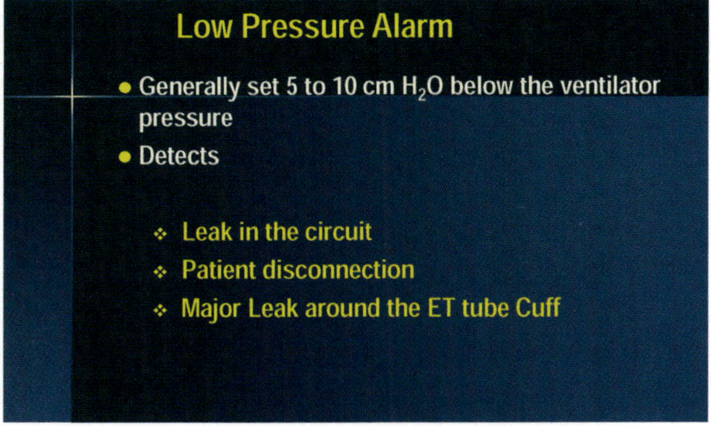

Fig. 12.7

Plateau Pressure (P_{plat})

During volume breath when the Inflation Hold or Inspiratory Pause is activated, at the end of inspiration, inspiratory flow stops and the ventilator keeps the exhalation valve closed for the duration of the pause time set by the clinician. Plateau pressure should be measured during each ventilator check. It is the pressure generated by the recoil of the lung in the closed system.

Plateau Pressure is generally considered as equivalent to Alveolar Pressure (PAlv). It gives the direct measure of Static Lung Compliance. Increase in Plateau pressure is indicative of decreased lung compliance (**Fig. 12.8**).

Transairway Pressure (P_{TA})

Frictional resistance to gas flow during its transit through the airways results in transairway pressure. This pressure exists only in the airways during gas flow. In absence of gas flow there is no PTA.

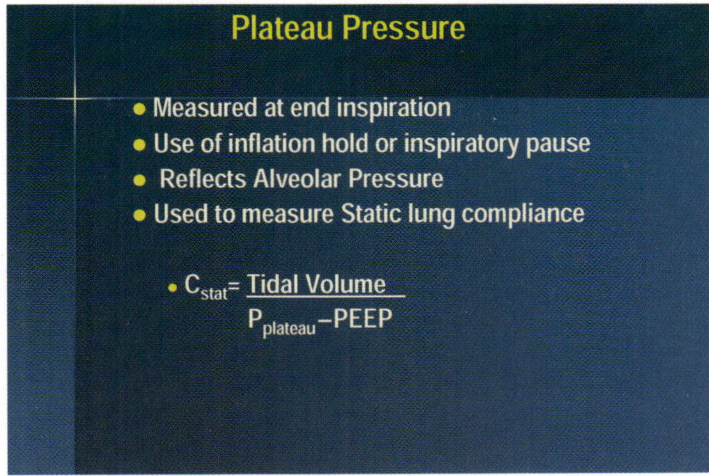

Fig. 12.8

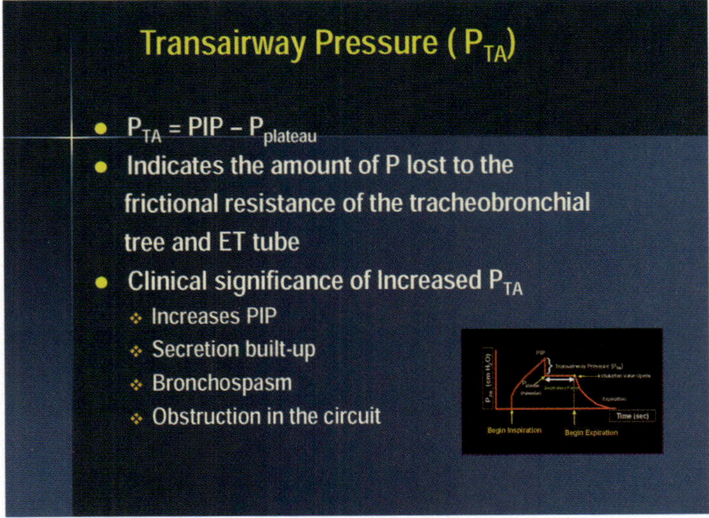

Fig. 12.9

When gas flows from the mouth to alveoli, the pressure at the mouth cascades down the airways influenced by airway caliber and gasflow.

At the terminal bronchioles the remaining pressure is delivered to the alveoli (to deliver tidal volume). Changes in airway caliber secondary to increased secretions, bronchospasm and any obstruction in the circuit increases PTA and thus PIP. It is vital that the patient should be protected from high airway pressures by setting the high pressure alarm (**Fig. 12.9**).

Dynamic and Static Lung Compliance

Compliance is defined as ease of distensibility and in pulmonary medicine it is simply measured as volume delivered per unit pressure or $\Delta V/\Delta P$. In Mechanical ventilation

∇V is the tidal volume and ∇P is either PIP or P_{plat}. Dynamic compliance, as the term reflects, includes pressure generated by gasflow.

It also includes pressure resulting from volume delivery against recoiling force of the alveoli. Dynamic compliance is calculated as:

$$C_D = \frac{\text{Exhaled Tidal Volume}}{\text{PIP} - \text{PEEP}}$$

Clinically dynamic compliance reflects Static Compliance provided RAW is constant (**Fig. 12.10**). Static Compliance is the amount of volume delivered to alveoli per unit of alveolar pressure.

$$C_S = \frac{\text{Exhaled Tidal Volume}}{P_{plat} - \text{PEEP}}$$

Dynamic Lung Compliance

- $C_{dynamic} = \frac{\text{Exhaled Tidal Volume}}{P_{plat} - \text{PEEP}}$
- Influenced by R_{aw}
- A serial Measurements (trend) than spot checking is Clinically useful
- Factors that decrease Dynamic lung compliance:
  - All causes of increased R_{aw}
  - All causes of decreased C_S
  - During unchanging, airway resistance decreased C_D is associated with decreased C_S

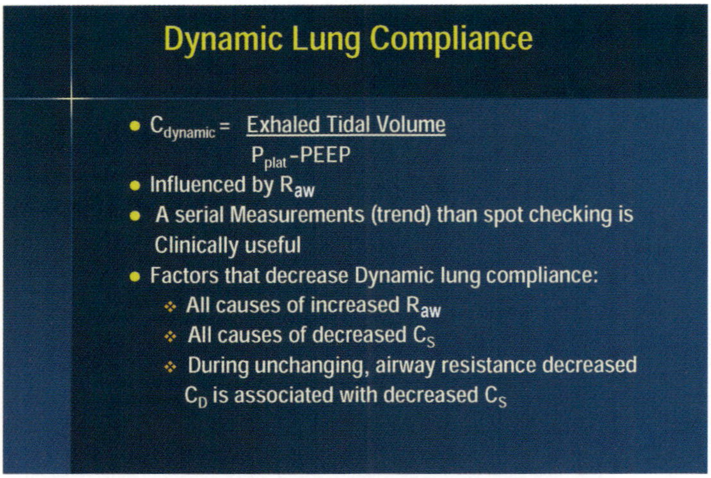

Fig. 12.10

PEEP being a constant pressure applied during inspiration and expiration is subtracted from PIP and Plateau pressures. A spontaneously breathing individual has a Static Complianceof ~ 100 ml/cm H_2O. Compliance value of 50–60 ml/cm H_2O is considered as normal for intubated patients. Thus, when a patient on mechanical ventilation with severe decrease in compliance (20–25 ml/cm H_2O) improves to a compliance of 50 ml/cm H_2O, weaning should be strongly considered. All restrictive disorders have low lung compliance. Incidentally, Emphysema is the only disease where Static Lung Compliance is increased due to loss of recoiling force (**Fig. 12.11**).

Interrelationship between PIP, P_{TA}, P_{plat} and Lung Compliances

The total ventilating pressure during a mechanical breath depends on transairway pressure and alveolar pressure. P_{TA} results from airway resistance and the gas flow, whereas, Alveolar pressure is dependent on tidal volume and lung compliance (**Fig. 12.12**). Increased R_{aw} and gas flow result in increased P_{TA} (**Fig. 12.13**).

Static Lung Compliance

- $C_{dynamic} = V_T / P_{plat}$-PEEP
- Normal ~ 100 mL/cmH_2O
- In intubated patients C_S = 50-70 mL/cmH_2O
- Factors that decrease static lung compliance:
  - Atelectasis
  - Pneumonia
  - Restrictive disorders- ARDS,
  - Pleural Disorders – Pneumothorax, Pleural Effusion

Fig. 12.11

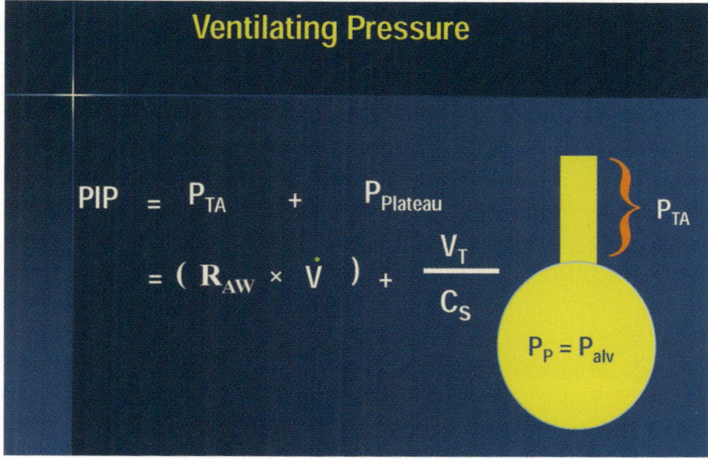

Fig. 12.12

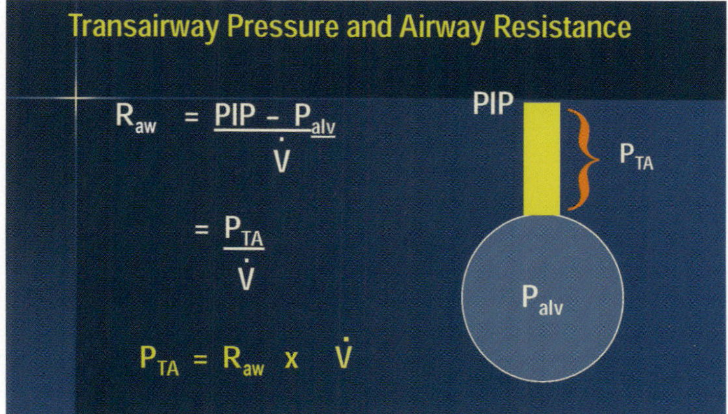

Fig. 12.13

The relationship between Tidal Volume, Static Complianceand Plateau Pressure (Alveolar Pressure) is demonstrated in **Fig. 12.14**. During mechanical ventilation situations occur where the R_{aw} increases suddenly as a consequence of Mucus Plug in large bronchi or severe asthmatic episode.

The PIP increases **(Fig. 12.15)**. Notice that there is no change in plateau pressure indicating that the lung compliance is not affected, only the airways are experiencing partial occlusion (increased P_{TA} and PIP).

The PIP can also increase when the lung compliance decreases. **Figure 12.16** demon-strates the effect of decreased lung compliance (increased P_{plat} and PIP). PTA is unchanged indicating that the problem originated in the lungs and did not affect airways.

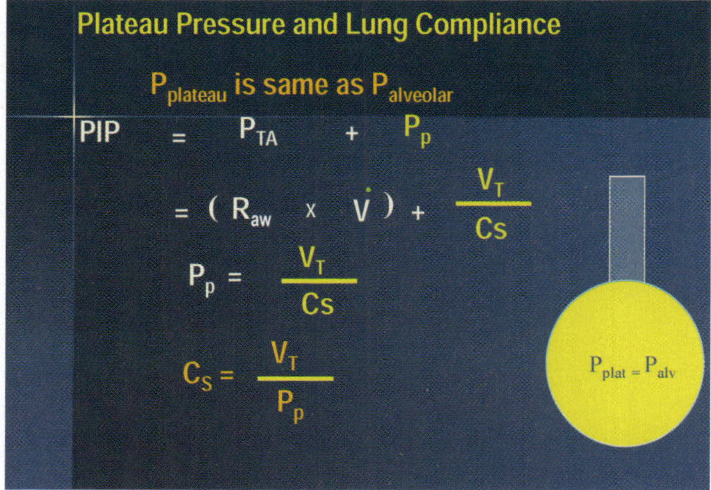

Fig. 12.14

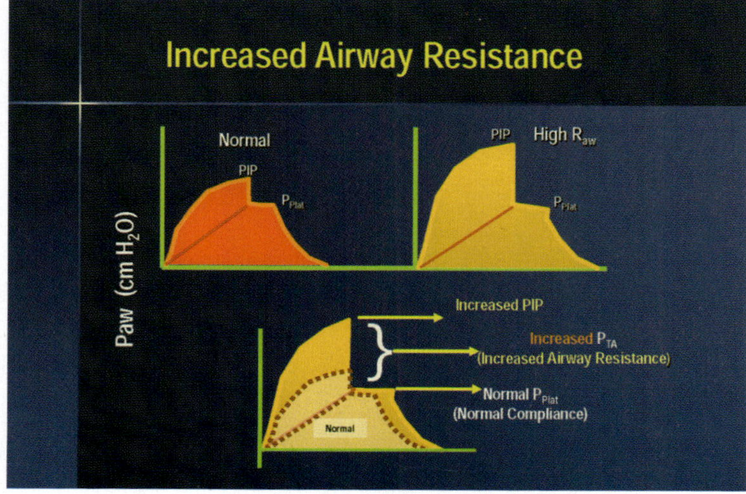

Fig. 12.15

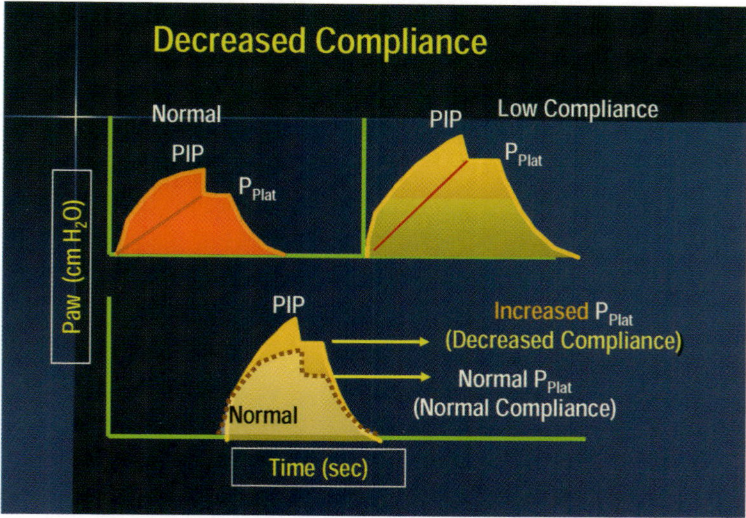

Fig. 12.16

Cuff Pressure

During initial evaluation the clinician is expected to check the position and security of the ET tube as well as the cuff pressure. It is argued by some clinicians that high cuff pressures result in damage to tracheal wall due to tracheal necrosis, mucosal edema and ischemia.

The cuff pressure is recommended not to exceed 25 mm Hg. **Figure 12.17** shows the effect of increased cuff pressures on the blood flow and lymphatic flow to tracheal mucosa. Cuff pressure-measuring devices, cuffalators, also allow the clinician to add or remove air from the cuff. To protect the airways from high cuff pressures, the minimal leak techniques is recommended.

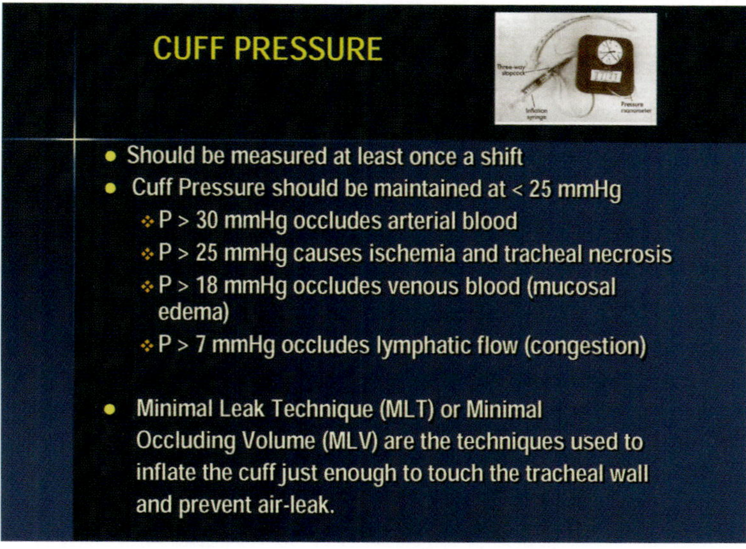

Fig. 12.17

Mean Airway Pressure

Finally, it is desirable to monitor Mean Airway Pressure which the clinicians manipulates to open recruitable lung in ALI and ARDS. **Figure 12.18** shows the basic formula for estimating Mean Airway Pressure. Since the pressure is applied only during inspiratory phase the first equation indicates Mean airway pressure = ½ PIP × T_I / TCT, where, T_I is the inspiratory time and TCT is the total cycle time. If PEEP is added, then the equation incorporates PEEP recognizing that it is applied throughout the respiratory cycle, PEEP is subtracted from PIP and added at the end of the equation. Getting a little more academic the equation expands to the final version where values for PTA and PAlv, the two components of PIP, are substituted. This equation provides all the factors that can be manipulated by the clinician to increase or decrease Mean Airway Pressure. **Figure 12.19** identifies parameters, V_T, T_I, TCT and PEEP that are readily available for changing mean airway pressure whereas R_{aw} and C are lung characteristics and cannot be manipulated.

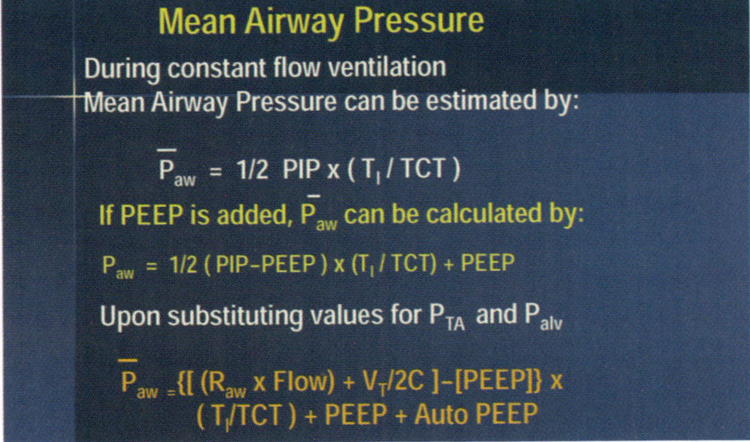

Fig. 12.18

Practical Methods to Increase $\bar{P}_{AW}$ in ARDS patients

$\bar{P}_{aw}$ = {[(R_{aw} x Flow) + V_T/2C]-[PEEP]} x (T_I/TCT) + PEEP

- Increasing T_I
- Increasing V_T
- Increasing PEEP
- Increasing f (decreases TCT)

Fig. 12.19

In ALI/ARDS patients increasing Mean Airway Pressure by increasing tidal volume may be detrimental for the patient as it can promote overdistension and volutrauma **(Fig. 12.20)**. However, in clinical practice, mean airway pressure is increased by manipulating T_I (inverse ratio ventilation-IRV) and by decreasing total cycle time (TCT) via increased frequency. Application of PEEP has been a cornerstone in managing ALI/ARDS patients. PEEP, not only increases Mean Airway Pressure but it also prevents decruitment. Increased Mean Airway pressure increases alveolar ventilation by opening recruitable alveoli and improves gas exchange **(Fig.12.21)**. It must be recognized that in lungs that are not stiff, increased Mean Airway Pressure may decrease cardiac output and can also promote barotrauma.

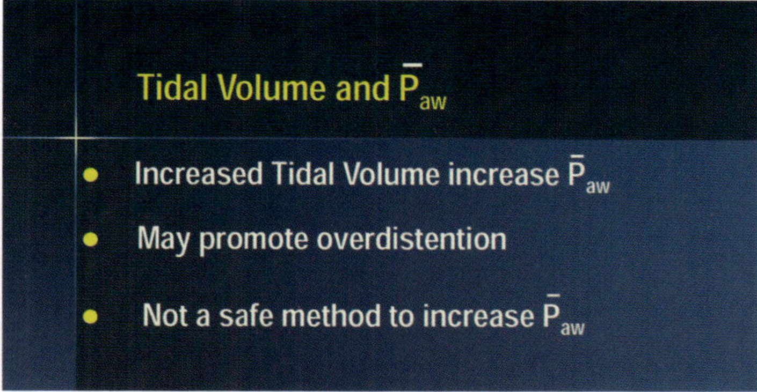

Fig. 12.20

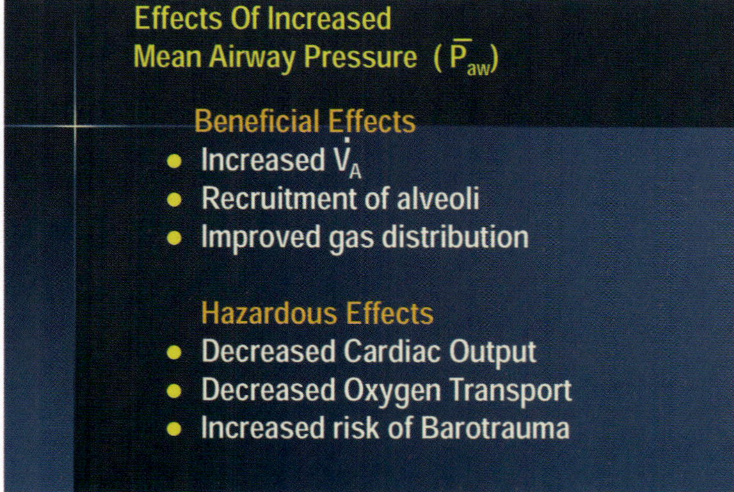

Fig. 12.21

Commonly Encountered Abnormal Ventilator Waveforms

Ventilator waveforms have opened the door for evaluating clinical situations by observing changes in ventilator graphics. Nuances in abnormal waveforms are published in literatures identifying waveforms indicating different types of dissynchrony. This section will identify only three commonly observed abnormal waveforms—Auto-PEEP, Air Leak and Inadequate Inspiratory Flow (**Fig. 12.22**). These abnormalities are very common in most ICUs and can be fixed easily. Identification of Auto-PEEP, small leak and especially inadequate inspiratory flow is missed in most cases. Ventilator waveforms are the best tool to verify these correctable situations.

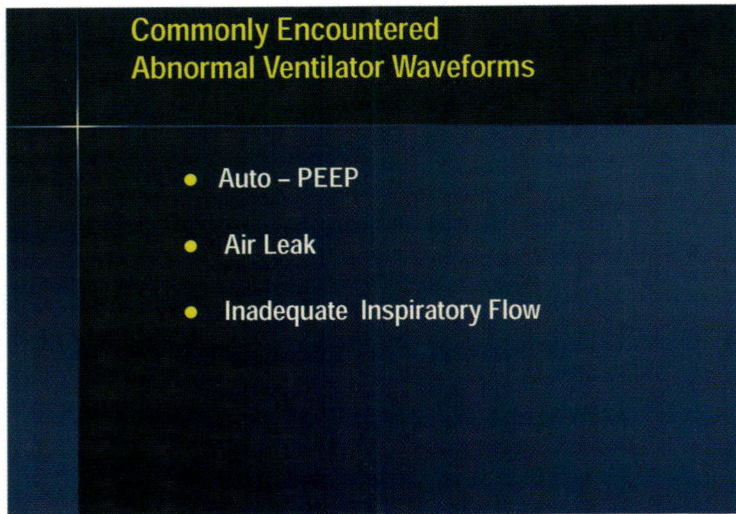

Fig. 12.22

Auto-PEEP or Air Trapping

PEEP set on the ventilator by the clinician is termed as Extrinsic PEEP. Auto-PEEP is referred to as Intrinsic PEEP, since it occurs from altered intrinsic function of the lung leading to inadequate expiratory time. Technically, at end exhalation the pressure in the lungs should be at atmospheric. In situations such as premature bronchiolar collapse (COPD), high minute ventilation and expiratory flow limitation due to increased airway resistance (Asthma) or decreased recoiling force (Emphysema), the lung pressure does not return to the baseline (atmospheric). The pressure remaining in the lung is called Auto-PEEP. Unfortunately, in normal circumstances, Auto-PEEP is not indicated on ventilator pressure manometer (**Fig. 12.23**). Current ventilators are able to close inspiratory and expiratory ports and not only identify presence of auto-PEEP but also quantify the magnitude of Auto-PEEP.

Ventilator graphics provide an avenue to detect Auto-PEEP. **Figure 12.24** shows that the expiratory flow for the ventilator cycle does not have adequate time to complete exhalation and the next breath is delivered before the expiratory flow returns to the baseline. The dotted line on expiratory limb represents normal expiratory time returning to the baseline. Auto-PEEP can also be detected on a Flow-Volume loop (*see* Chapter 8). Another way to detect Auto-PEEP is to add extrinsic PEEP on the ventilator until the PIP begins to increase. The PIP does not increase until the applied PEEP has exceeded auto-PEEP level.

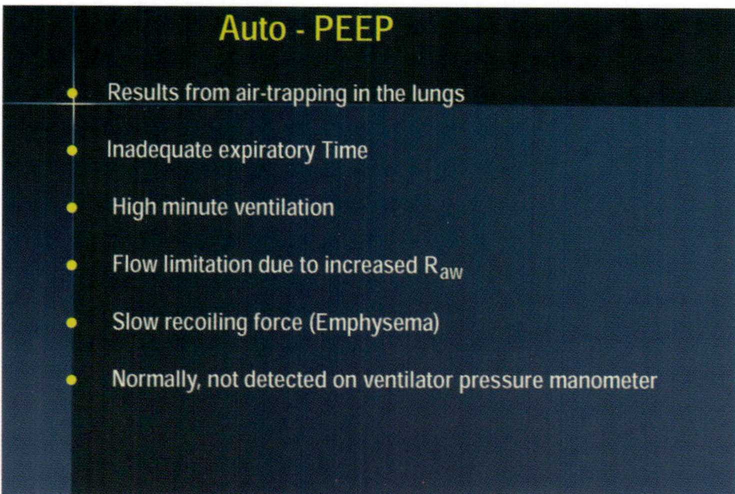

Fig. 12.23

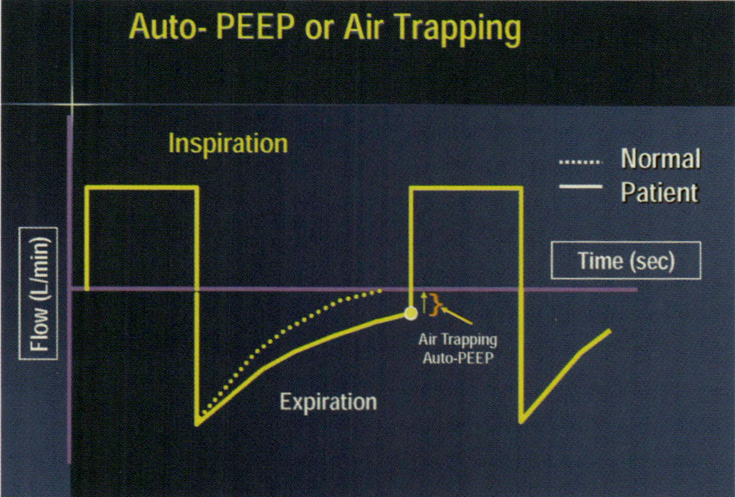

Fig. 12.24

Auto-PEEP is undesirable in ventilated patients, since it can increase work of breathing, hyperinflate the lung and most importantly, auto-PEEP can interfere with triggering the ventilator breath (**Fig. 12.25**). Missed breaths in assisted ventilation are commonly seen in patients with auto-PEEP. In presence of Auto-PEEP, the patient on A/C mode has to make an inspiratory effort greater than the auto-PEEP level, to trigger the ventilator and in many cases the patient is incapable of creating negative pressure of that magnitude, missing the breath (**Fig. 12.25**).

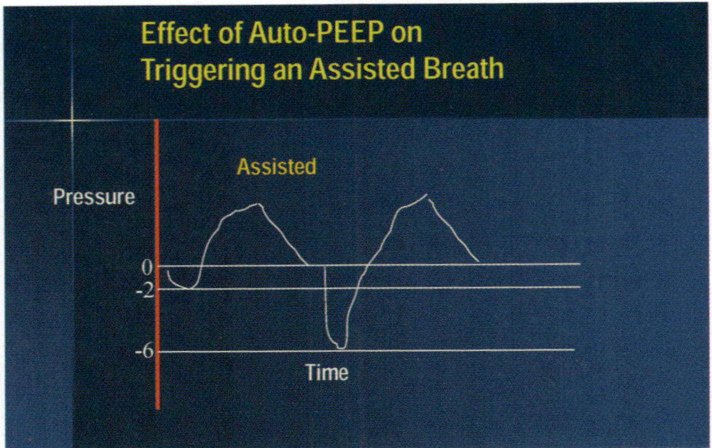

Fig. 12.25

Elimination of auto-PEEP is essential in managing ventilated patients. This can be accomplished by suctioning the airways, increasing expiratory time by decreasing inspiratory time or add extrinsic PEEP (**Fig. 12.26**). In spontaneously breathing patients such as COPD and those unable to trigger the ventilator, auto-PEEP can be reduced by applying extrinsic PEEP. Up to 80% of auto-PEEP can be nullified by extrinsic PEEP decreasing effort needed to trigger ventilator breath (**Fig. 12.27**).

Elimination of Auto-PEEP

- Suction the ET tube
- Increase inspiratory flow rate to decrease inspiratory time and allow for longer expiratory time
- Add PEEP to off-set auto-PEEP

Fig. 12.26

Air Leak

Volume vs. Time Scalar detects leaks in the ventilator circuit. Normally, the volume tracing descends to the baseline at end exhalation. In presence of air leak the tracing does not return to the baseline. It stagnates at the level of leaked volume and for the next breath abruptly drops to the baseline and proceeds with the next inspiratory tracing (**Fig. 12.28**). Occasionally the patient makes an extra expiratory effort and the exhaled volume tracing goes below the baseline (**Fig. 12.29**).

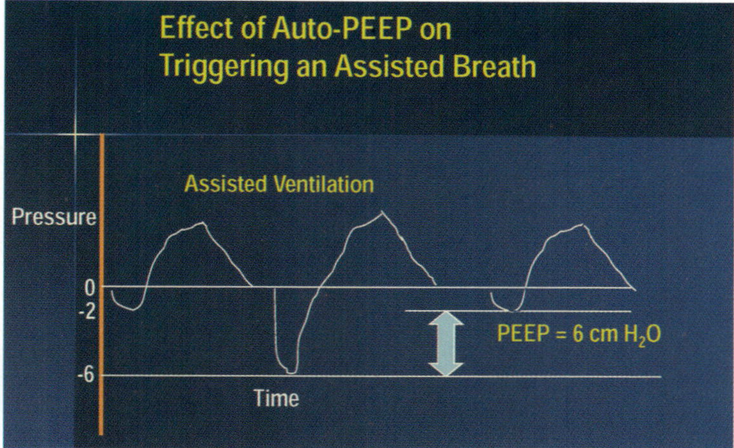

Fig. 12.27

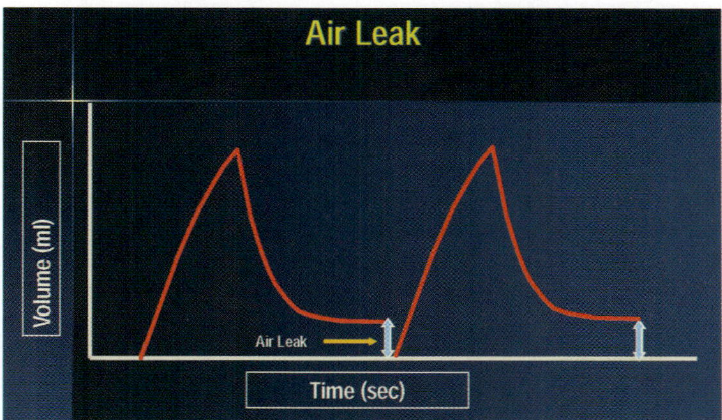

Fig. 12.28

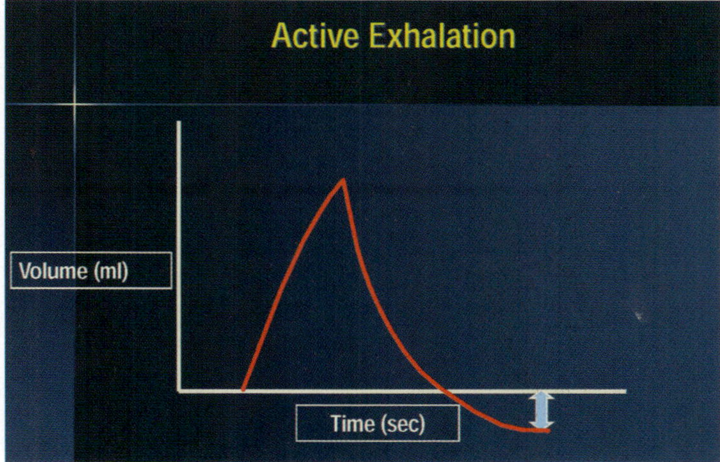

Fig. 12.29

Inadequate Inspiratory Flow

It is claimed that inadequate inspiratory time is most commonly observed in ICUs. Clinicians are reluctant to give high flows to patients. A most standard setting is 30 L/min flow for all patients. This can promote flow dissynchrony demonstrated on Flow/Time, Pressure/Time, and most profoundly on Pressure/Volume loop. On Flow/Time scalar an uneven pattern is observed in place of square flow (Volume Ventilation) indicating patient's effort to add more flow **(Fig. 12.30)**. On pressure/Time scalar the smooth contour of the pressure waveform shows concavity **(Fig. 12.31)** caused by patient's inspiratory effort.

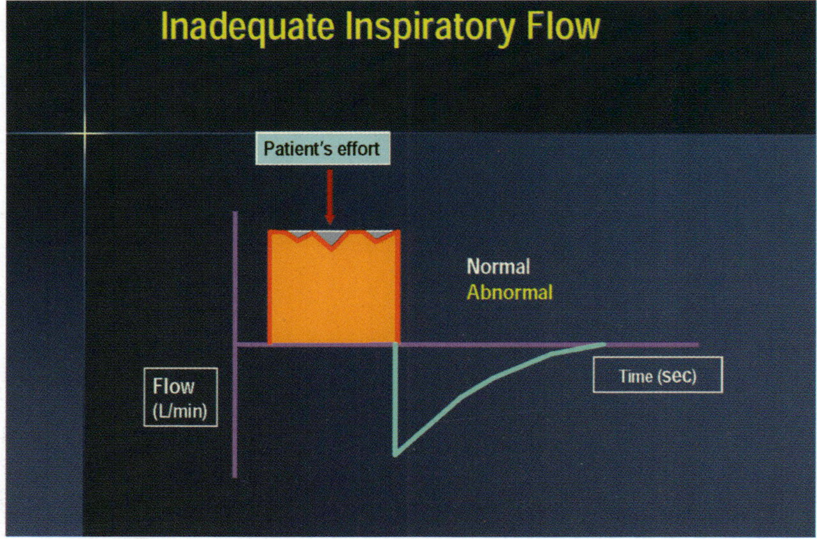

Fig. 12.30

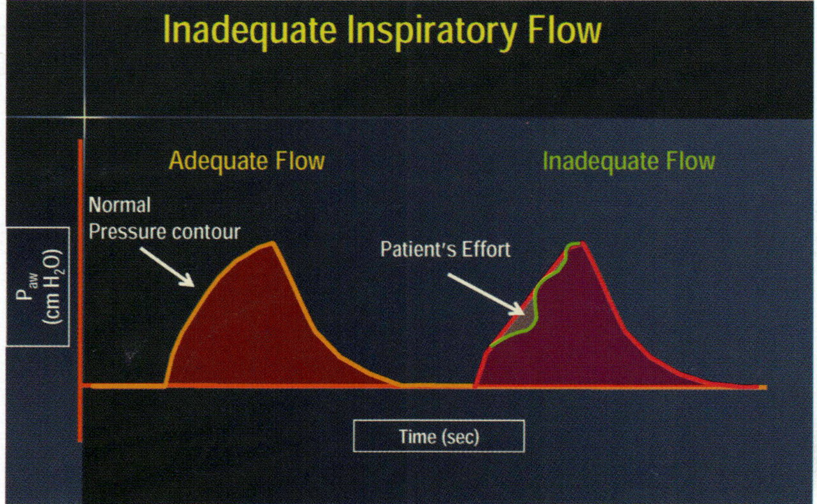

Fig. 12.31

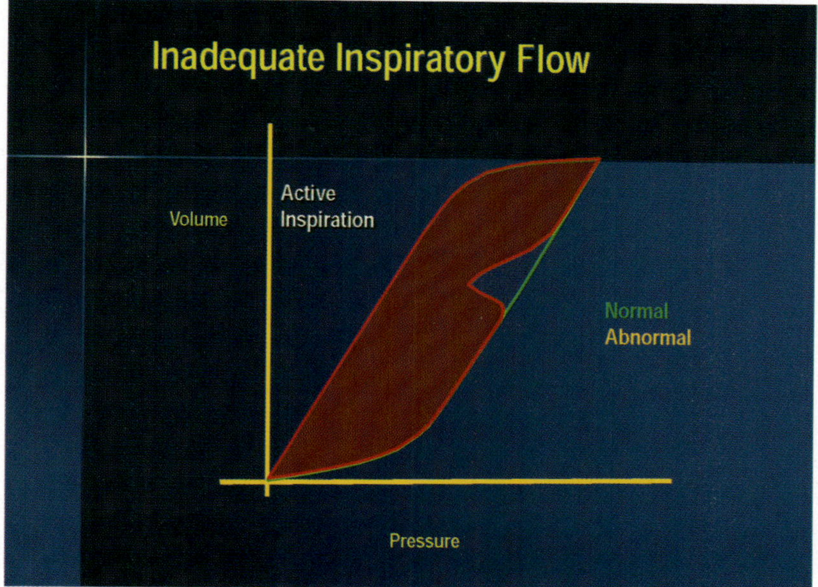

Fig. 12.32

Pressure-Volume loop shows a sudden depression in the inspiratory tracing signifying patient's inspiratory activity while the ventilator breath is in progress (Fig. 12.32). Upon encountering these waveforms the clinician, simply increases inspiratory flow (decreased T_I, or T_I % or manipulating I–E ratio).

In later chapters more complex ventilator graphics are discussed.

CHAPTER 13

Aerosol Therapy and Humidification

Saumy Johnson

Keywords: Nebulization, Humidifiers, Particle Deposition, Inhalation Devices, Therapeutic Aerosols, Humidity Control, Aerosolized Medications

INTRODUCTION

The foremost goal of aerosol therapy is maintaining a high concentration of drug in the lung. Aerosolized drug has been used for the treatment of respiratory disorders .This also aids in delivery of aerosol therapy to systemic diseases which are not completely a respiratory cause. There are many aspects that makes inhalational route a preferred one such as the huge surface area, thin alveolocapillary membrane, epithelium which are well vascularized, presence of a diminished low pass metabolism combined with the functions of the enzyme produces increased bioavailability. Other factors in favor of aerosol therapy are that it gives the chance of attaining high concentrations of the local drug at the treatment site for the respiratory diseases, fast onset of action and less side effects, all these together increased the interest of aerosolized drug therapy in the Intensive care Unit.

Side effects are that the efficacy depends on the optimal delivery of the technique and there can be a decision-making problem for the non-respiratory care professionals in selecting the correct inhalation device and right technique of administration.

THE AEROSOL SYSTEM

An aerosol is defined as the suspension of liquid or solid in gaseous medium. Aerosol droplet size is most commonly characterized by the mass median aerodynamic diameter (MMAD). MMAD is that diameter around which the mass of particles is equally distributed. The drug deposition in the lower respiratory tract of mechanically ventilated patients is more efficient with devices generating aerosols with a MMAD of 1–3 µ. Optimal technique of administration, lead to deposition of the drug in the lower respiratory tract of ventilated patients. Pressurized metered dose inhalers (pMDIs) with spacer result in deposition of around 10 to 11% of nominal dose and 6 to 10% of nominal dose for nebulizer. Efficiency of drug deposition in the lower respiratory tract of ventilated patients is lower with nebulizers than with pMDIs. This is offset by the higher drug dose used by the nebulizers.

The aerosol system typically has the drug, the aerosol device, the target site and the respiratory system of the individual receiving the medication. In a ventilated patient, ventilator would be an added factor. Essential factors of the aerosols are:

- Drug deposition
- Absorption
- Metabolism
- Elimination

There are some fundamental differences in aerosol delivery in spontaneously breathing and mechanically ventilated patients which are mentioned in **Table 13.1**. These differences can have impact on amount of drug deposited at the target site of action. Most of the discussion in this chapter will be about aerosol therapy in mechanically ventilated patients.

Table 13.1: Aerosol delivery in spontaneously breathing versus mechanically ventilated patients

	Spontaneously breathing patient	Mechanically ventilated patient
Position of the patient	Sitting or standing	Supine or semi-recumbent
Aerosol device	PMDI/PMDI and spacer/ nebulizer/dry powder inhaler	PMDI and spacer/nebulizer
Mode of delivery	By mouthpiece or facemask	Connected to endotracheal tube or inspiratory limb of ventilator circuit
Humidity	Ambient humidity	Humidified (approximately 96% to 97% relative humidity)
Temperature	Room or ambient	Warmed to approximately 35°C
Inspiratory airflow	Sinusoidal	Constant or ramp flow
Breath configuration	Patient controlled	Ventilator controlled (in assisted mode it is influenced by patient)
Aerosol administration	Administered by patient	Administered by staff or respiratory therapist
Airway	Oral or nasal cavity and upper airway	Endotracheal or tracheostomy tube

Types of aerosol delivery devices

There are three classes of aerosol delivery devices nebulizers:

- Jet nebulizers [also known as small volume (SVN) or pneumatic nebulizers]
- Ultrasonic nebulizers
- Vibrating mesh nebulizers
- Metered dose inhalers
- Dry powder inhalers

Metered dose inhalers (MDIs), nebulizers, and dry powder inhalers (DPIs) are the aerosol-generating devices of choice in ambulatory patients. In mechanically ventilated patients pressurized MDIs and nebulizers are preferred for inhalation therapy. Vibrating mesh nebulizer (expensive and requires disassembly and thorough cleaning) and dry powder inhalers (not very suitable for mechanically ventilated patients) are not commonly used. Therefore, it will not be discussed in detail.

Nebulizers

SVN uses the Bernoulli principle to produce an aerosol. It produces a broad range of particle size, from 0.5 to 15 µm MMAD. Usually, more than 50% of the drug volume is not released from the nebulizer and is trapped on the baffles and internal walls at the completion of nebulization. This quantity of residual drug is referred to as dead volume. Jet nebulizers are placed in the inspiratory limb of the ventilator circuit during mechanical ventilation and may be run continuously by pressurized gas from outside source or intermittently by using a separate line to provide driving pressure and gas flow from the ventilator. The nebulizer generates aerosol only during the inspiratory phase during intermittent operation, and the ventilator compensates for the flow to the nebulizer to maintain a constant tidal volume. It is important to know whether the ventilator takes into account the extra volume of gas used to drive the nebulizer otherwise it can result in lung injury due to excess tidal volume and pressure.

Intermittent operation is more efficient for aerosol delivery than continuous aerosol generation because drug is deposited only in the lower respiratory tract only during inspiration. Some ventilators provide driving pressure which is lower compared to the external source (compressed air or oxygen sources) which could change aerosol characteristics and affect the efficiency of the nebulizer.

SVN-position in the Ventilator Circuit

The SVN position in the ventilator circuit significantly influences the efficiency of aerosol delivery. It is found to be least effective when it is placed proximal to the patient, between the ventilator circuit and the endotracheal tube.

Aerosol delivery is most effective: When placed closer to the endotracheal tube in the inspiratory limb

The advantages and disadvantages of SVN are summarized in **Table 13.2**.

Table 13.2: SVN

Advantages	Disadvantages
✦ Patient co-ordination not required	✦ Not very portable
✦ Effective with tidal breathing	✦ Pressurized gas source is required
✦ Modification of drug dose and high doses is possible	✦ Prolonged treatment time
✦ No risk of chlorofluorocarbons	✦ Regular cleaning is required
✦ Supplemental oxygen can also be given simultaneously	✦ Risk of contamination
✦ Combination therapies can be delivered if compatible	✦ Non-availability of all medications in solution form
✦ No rise in temperature during operation and hence meditation is not altered	✦ Suspensions are not aerosolized well
	✦ Preparation of device required
	✦ Variation in the perfomance

Ultrasonic nebulizer: Uses a piezoelectric crystal to convert electrical energy to high-frequency sound waves. These sound waves cause disruption of the solution surface resulting in aerosol formation. The aerosol particle size and drug output are influenced by the frequency and amplitude of vibration of the piezoelectric crystal, respectively.

Ultrasonic Nebulizers (USN)-Position in the Ventilator Circuit

When the USN is placed in the inspiratory limb of the ventilator circuit, close to the patient wye, it delivers significantly more medication to the airway than SVN and it is less efficient when placed closer to the ventilator.

The advantages and disadvantages of USN are summarized in **Table 13.3**:

Table 13.3: Advantages and disadvantages of USN

Ultrasonic Nebulizers	
Advantages	**Disadvantages**
✦ Patient co-ordination not required	✦ Expensive
✦ Modification of drug dose and high doses is possible	✦ Requires electrical power source(wall outlet or batteries)
✦ No risk of chlorofluorocarbons	✦ Risk of contamination
✦ Small dead volume	✦ Non-availability of all medications in solution form
✦ Silent operation	✦ Preparation of device required
✦ Earlier models were bulky, newer designs are small and portable	✦ Suspensions are not nebulized well
✦ Less time require because of quicker delivery than jet nebulizer	✦ Because of increase in solution temperature by 10° to 15°C there is denaturation and degradation of the drug
✦ Drug loss is not there during exhalation (breath actuated devices)	

Metered Dose Inhalers (MDI)

Pressured MDIs contain the drug in the form of micronized crystals, suspended with a surfactant in a mixture of two or three chlorofluorocarbon (CFC) propellants. Preservatives and antioxidants are added to improve the shelf-life of the inhaler. Aerosol suspension is released from the tip of the canister at a very high velocity (around 60 mph) when MDI is actuated.

The aerosol may exceed 30–40 µm MMAD initially, but as the particles slow down and the propellants evaporate, size of the aerosol particles decrease to around 2–5 µm. Previously, most pMDIs used chlorofluorocarbon (CFC) propellants. Due to environmental concerns CFC (causes damage to ozone layer) are being phased out and being replaced by hydrofluoroalkane (HFA) propellants.

MDI-position in the Ventilator Circuit

Immediately after MDI actuation the MMAD of aerosol is large but decrease rapidly as the propellant evaporates. The larger particles which are traveling at high speed are lost by impaction when MDI is directly connected to the endotracheal tube.

On the contrary, if MDI is actuated into a spacer device placed at a distance from endotracheal tube the particle size decreases as a result of propellant evaporation which in turn increases the delivery of aerosol into the patient 's lungs. Therefore, it is advisable to actuate MDI into a spacer device with a chamber placed at a distance (around 15 cm) from the endotracheal tube for optimum aerosol delivery in mechanically ventilated patients.

The advantages and disadvantages of MDI are summarized in **Table 13.4**.

Table 13.4: MDI

Advantages	Disadvantages
✦ Compact/Portable ✦ Short treatment time ✦ Drug preparation is not required ✦ No risk of contamination ✦ Dose-dose reproducibility high	✦ Needs to be co-ordinated with inspiration during actuation ✦ Device has to be actuated ✦ Upper limit to unit dose content ✦ Difficult to determine remaining doses ✦ Abuse potential ✦ All medications are not available in MDI form ✦ CFC propellants used in many MDIs is a environmental hazard

Spacer or Adapter Devices

Many commercially available adapters or actuators **(Fig. 13.1)** are used to connect the pMDI canister to the ventilator circuit. The efficiency of drug delivery is greatly affected by the type of adapter used. Many varieties of adapters are available for clinical use like elbow adapters, inline devices that may be unidirectional or bidirectional, and chamber or reservoir (collapsible and non collapsible) adapters. A chamber spacer with a pMDI in a ventilator circuit results in better aerosol drug delivery, compared with either an elbow adapter or a unidirectional inline spacer.

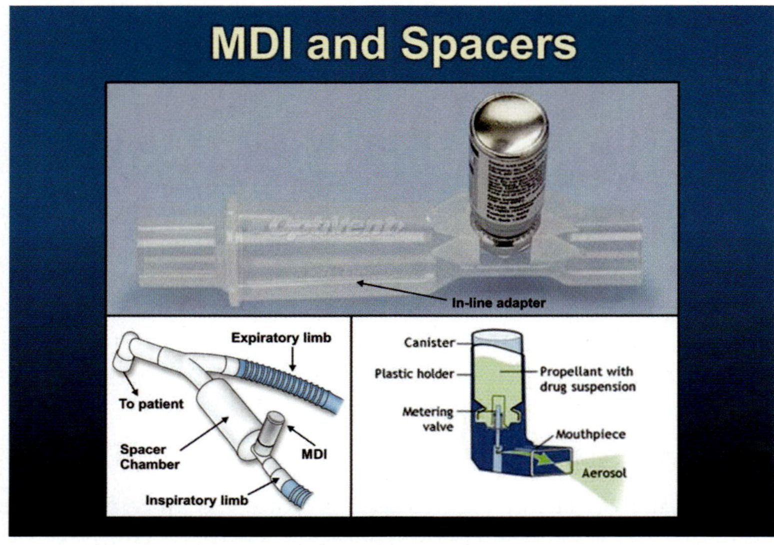

Fig. 13.1

Factors Effecting Aerosol Therapy during Mechanical Ventilation (Table 13.5) Aerosol Particle Size

The deposition of aerosol particles is determined by three mechanisms:

1. Inertial impaction
2. Sedimentation
3. Diffusion-having little therapeutic effect

The ventilator circuit and endotracheal tube in mechanically ventilated patients, act as baffles that trap particles with larger diameter en route to the bronchi. The MMAD of aerosols produced by different brands of nebulizer vary widely. Nebulizers producing <2 μm aerosols are more likely to result in greater deposition in the lower respiratory tract of ventilated patients. When MDI is actuated into a spacer at the beginning of inspiration, a sizeable proportion of aerosol emerging from the distal end of the endotracheal tube was in the respirable range, with a MMAD of 1–2 μm. Hence, deposition in the lower respiratory tract of mechanically ventilated patients is more likely with devices that generate aerosols with a MMAD of 1–3 μm.

Table 13.5: Possible factors influencing aerosol deposition and efficacy in the ventilated patient

Ventilator-related factors ✦ Spontaneous breathing pattern ✦ Mechanism of airway obstruction ✦ Severity of airway obstruction ✦ Presence of dynamic hyperinflation ✦ Patient-ventilator synchrony ✦ Presence of secretions ✦ Airway edema	**Aerosol device-related factors** **MDI** ✦ Timing of actuation ✦ Type of spacer or adapter ✦ Type of MDI **Nebulizer** ✦ Size of particle generated by brand of nebulizer ✦ Degree of variability within brand of nebulizer ✦ Gas flow rate for driving nebulizer ✦ Volume of fill
Ventilator-related factors ✦ Model of ventilator ✦ Gas flow rate and driving pressure of ventilator nebulizer system ✦ Continuous versus intermittent delivery by ventilator **Ventilator settings** ✦ Respiratory rate ✦ Tidal volume ✦ Mode of ventilation ✦ Duty cycle ✦ Use of inspiratory pause ✦ Inspiratory flow rate ✦ Inspiratory flow waveform	**Circuit-related factors** ✦ Amount of drug administered ✦ Location of aerosol device in circuit ✦ Diameter of endotracheal tube ✦ Presence of humidification device

Heating and Humidification

Due to increased particle loss in the ventilator circuit, humidification of inspired gas decreases aerosol deposition with MDIs and nebulizers by approximately 40%. When MDI (four puffs at 20–30 second intervals) is used to deliver aerosol therapy, the absence of humidification during that brief period does not cause much problem. Some nebulizers take a very long time sometimes up to 30–40 minutes to deliver the medication and inhalation of dry air for such long time causes damage to the airway. Therefore, it is not advisable to switch off the humidifier for aerosol therapy. Also disconnection of the ventilator circuit interferes with the ventilation sometimes resulting in de-recruitment, fatal hypoxemia (ARDS) and accidental disconnection later.

If HME is being used it should be removed before administering aerosol therapy because drug gets trapped in HMEs. If a patient requires multiple or continuous aerosol therapy (status asthmaticus or severe COPD), it is better to use MDI with spacer or nebulizer with heated humidifier in a ventilator circuit.

Density of the Inhaled Gas

Because of the turbulence in the airway during high inspiratory flows, the impaction of aerosol particles is increased. This loss of aerosol particles due to impaction can be reduced by preserving the laminar flow by decreasing the density of inspired gas (i.e. helium–oxygen). Therefore, breathing helium–oxygen may improve aerosol deposition.

Studies in ambulatory patients with airway obstruction have revealed higher lower respiratory tract aerosol delivery when breathing helium–oxygen compared with air. Helium–oxygen mixtures improved aerosol deposition during *in vitro* studies from a MDI during continuous mandatory ventilation (CMV) of a simulated adult patient.

On the contrary, helium–oxygen with pneumatic nebulizer produces less respirable mass of drug per liter of operating flow compared to when air or oxygen is used necessitating increased flow rate to produce similar nebulizer output.

Endotracheal Tube Size

Endotracheal tube reduces aerosol delivery in mechanically ventilated patients due to aerosol impaction and is inversely related to the airway diameter. However, no difference in drug deposition has been shown between endotracheal tubes with 9.0–7.0 mm internal diameter (ID). As airway ID gets smaller (6.0–3.0 mm ID) aerosol delivery to the lower respiratory tract is reduced. With an adult-sized endotracheal tube, ≥7.0 mm, the loss of aerosol during mechanical ventilation appears to be more in the ventilator circuit, between the aerosol generator and the artificial airway, than in the endotracheal tube itself.

Ventilator Mode and Settings

The characteristics of the breath used to deliver aerosol therapy in mechanically ventilated patients, is influenced by mode, tidal volume, inspiratory flow rate and respiratory rate. Actuation of an MDI into a spacer needs to be synchronized with the precise onset of inspiration for optimal aerosol delivery.

The tidal volume of the ventilator-delivered breath must be more than the volume of the ventilator tubing and endotracheal tube for better efficiency of aerosol delivery to patient's lungs. Tidal volumes of 500 ml or more in adults are associated with satisfactory aerosol delivery. But, at the same time one should keep in mind that higher airway pressures associated with higher tidal volume can worsen lung injury. Aerosol delivery is better with lower inspiratory flows and higher inspiratory time (higher duty cycle).

Aerosol delivery is affected by flow patterns, with decelerating flow pattern delivering around 20% more drug to the lower respiratory tract than square wave patterns. The significance of inspiratory hold on aerosol deposition has not been determined.

Aerosol delivery from nebulizers has been shown to decrease by as much as 80% by continuous flow through the ventilator circuit, whereas reductions in delivery from MDIs were not statistically significant.

The technique for using nebulisers and MDIs in ventilated patients has been summarized in **Boxes 13.1 and 13.2**.

Box 13.1: Technique for using nebulizers in mechanically ventilated patients

1. Place drug solution in nebulizer to optimal fill volume (2–6 ml)
2. Place nebulizer in inspiratory line at least 30 cm from the patient wye
3. Ensure airflow of 6–8 L/min through the nebulizer
4. Ensure adequate tidal volume (500 mL in adults). Attempt to use duty cycle >0.3, if required.
5. Adjust minute volume to compensate for additional airflow through the nebulizer, if required.
6. Turn off flow-by or continuous flow mode on ventilator
7. Observe nebulizer for adequate aerosol generation throughout use
8. Disconnect nebulizer when all medications are nebulized or when no more aerosol is being produced
9. Reconnect ventilator circuit and return to original ventilator setting

Box 13.2: Technique for using MDIs in mechanically ventilated patients

1. Ensure VT >500 mL (in adults) during assisted ventilation.
2. Aim for an inspiratory time (excluding the inspiratory pause) >0.3 of total breath duration
3. Ensure that the ventilator breath is synchronized with the patient's inspiration
4. Shake the MDI vigorously
5. Place canister in actuator of a cylindrical spacer situated in inspiratory limb of ventilator circuit
6. Actuate MDI to synchronize with precise onset of inspiration by the ventilator
7. Allow a breath hold at end-inspiration for 3–5 seconds
8. Allow passive exhalation
9. Repeat actuations after 20–30 seconds until total dose is delivered

Care of Spacers and Nebulizers

Contamination of nebulizers placed in-line in the ventilator circuit can result in microorganisms being delivered as microaerosols directly to the lower respiratory tract. Therefore, the Centers for Disease Control and Prevention recommended that nebulizers should be sterile at the start of aerosol therapy and should be detached from the ventilator circuit after each use and either replaced or disassembled, cleaned with sterile water, rinsed, and air dried. Also, it is preferable to use single-dose ampoules of drug compared to multidose vials, which can become contaminated easily. Condensate collects inside chamber spacer when it is left in the ventilator circuit between aerosol therapy which can be reduced by using collapsible chamber actuators and the heated wire type of circuits. Even though, no data suggest that contamination in the spacer results in pathogens being delivered by aerosol to the patient, care must be taken to prevent the condensate in the spacer from being drained down into the patient's respiratory tract when the spacer is manipulated during use.

Assessing Bronchodilator Response

β2-agonists are effective in improving respiratory mechanics in mechanically ventilated patients. Following changes in peak airway pressures, transairway pressure ($P_{ta} = P_{peak} - P_{plat}$) and auto-PEEP are useful in assessing the efficacy of bronchodilator therapy. Improvement in clinical signs and symptoms like reduced wheezing, decreased sensation of dyspnea and work of breathing, improvement in hemodynamics and patient-ventilator synchrony are also important. Bronchodilator therapy could assist weaning in patients with limited cardiopulmonary reserve.

Aerosol Delivery during Noninvasive Positive Pressure Ventilation (NPPV)

NPPV is being more and more preferred for treatment of patients with acute and chronic respiratory failure. NPPV is often used as a first line mode of ventilatory support in as much as 50% of patients with hypercapnic respiratory failure. If NPPV is successful then it will avert the need for endotracheal intubation and all its associated complications and improve mortality. Inhaled bronchodilators are often being used in patients with acute or acute-on-chronic hypercapnic respiratory failure who are receiving NPPV.

Although it seems that during NPPV, inhaled drugs (e.g. bronchodilators) could be efficiently delivered via either nebulizer or MDI spacer, there is a lacunae in medical knowledge about the ventilator features best suited for this application. Some studies have shown optimum drug delivery is achieved if nebulizer position is between the leak port and patient connection, administering high inspiratory pressure, low expiratory pressure, and a breath rate of 20/min.

Devices used for aerosol therapy during NPPV (Fig. 13.2).

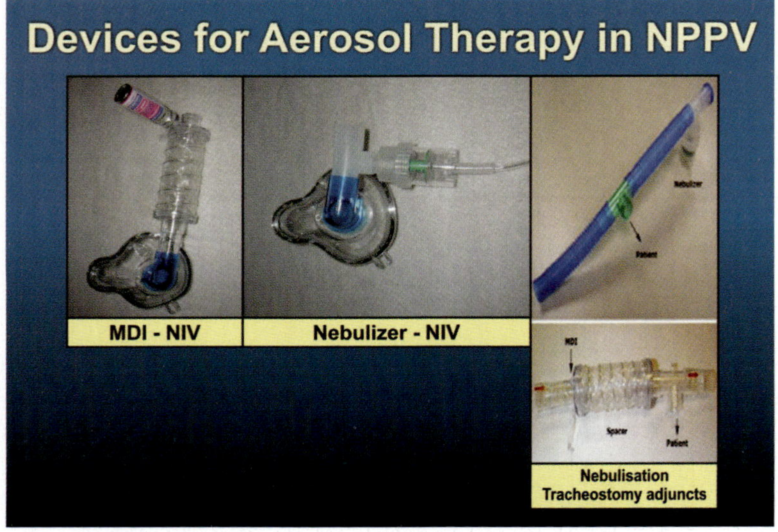

Fig. 13.2

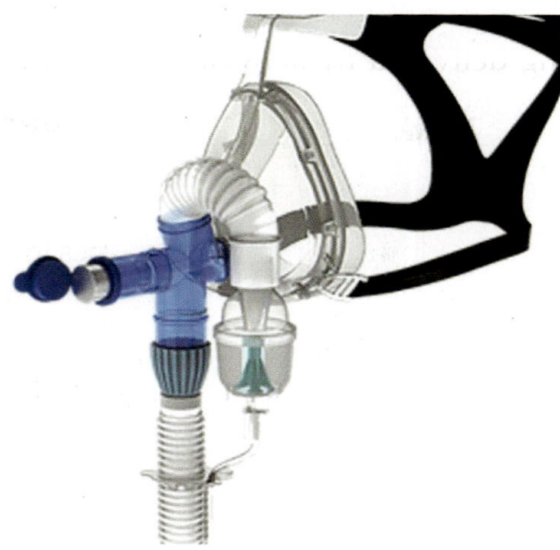

Fig. 13.3: Easy 2 neb mask is NIV full face mask with universal nebulization port (*Courtesy:* Pneumocare Health Pvt. Ltd.)

Aerosolized Drugs

Bronchodilators

Aerosolized bronchodilators are one of the most frequently used drugs in ventilator-supported patients with asthma or chronic obstructive pulmonary disease (COPD). The goals of bronchodilator therapy are to reverse bronchoconstriction, decrease tachypnoea and the work of breathing, or alleviate dyspnea. Both aerosolized β-adrenergic or anticholinergic bronchodilators are used for bronchodilator therapy. But, the combination of β-adrenergic and anticholinergic bronchodilators (ipratropium) is found to be more effective than ipratropium alone in a group of ventilator-supported patients with COPD.

In mechanically ventilated patients, considerable bronchodilator effects occur after administration of 2.5 mg of albuterol (or salbutamol) with a standard nebulizer or four puffs (400 µg) with a pMDI. Usually 2.5 ml of salbutamol respules contain around 2.5 mg of salbutamol which is diluted with another 2.5 ml of sterile water and used in jet nebulizer. 2.0 ml of ipratropium respules contains 500 µg which is diluted with sterile water to a final volume of 4 to 5 ml and used in the jet nebulizer. Each puff from pMDI (salbutamol) delivers 100 µg of salbutamol.

So, around 4 puffs are given at 20 to 30 seconds interval. Each puff from pMDI (ipratropium) delivers 20 µg of ipratropium bromide. So, around 2 puffs are given at 20 to 30 seconds interval. Higher doses result in negligible therapeutic advantage, whereas the potential for side-effects was increased. However, in certain clinical settings, higher doses of bronchodilators may be needed in patients especially with severe airway obstruction or if the technique of administration is not optimal. In stable mechanically ventilated patients with COPD the duration of bronchodilator response appears to be shorter than that in ambulatory patients (2–3 hr versus 4–6 hr, respectively). Hence, patients on ventilator support require scheduled administration of short-acting β-agonist bronchodilator (albuterol) every 3–4 hr.

Inhaled steroids are used in conjugation with bronchodilators to suppress inflammation in COPD and asthma.

Toxicity

Administration of very high doses of β-agonists is associated with an increased risk of arrhythmias, tremors, restlessness and hypokalemia. When pMDIs are used in excessive doses or when pMDI aerosol is delivered directly beyond the endotracheal tube by attaching a catheter to the canister nozzle, propellants in the formulation could cause local ulceration.

Surfactant

In surfactant deficiency (ARDS) disease states, surfactant replacement therapy (SRT) has been evaluated. The viscosity of exogenous surfactants makes them difficult to administer in aerosol form and they tend to foam and form stable bubbles during nebulization. Therefore, surfactant delivery to the lower respiratory tract by nebulisation is inefficient and the bulk of the aerosol is lost in the delivery system and the ventilator circuit. It may deposit and get in the way of the functioning of valves and monitoring devices of the ventilator which can be avoided to some extent by placing filters in the expiratory limb of the circuit to trap any aerosol before it reaches the ventilator. Further developments in the design of exogenous surfactants and better delivery systems and studies supporting surfactant therapy in ARDS patients are desirable for aerosolized surfactant to become an effective treatment for ARDS.

Other Drugs

Aerosolized antibiotics are used for treatment of cystic fibrosis and multi-drug resistant ventilator associated pneumonia. Prostanoids and mucolytics are not commonly used in ICU. The inhalation route of drug delivery is also being evaluated for a variety of anti-inflammatory, immunoregulatory agents, and for gene therapy. Some of these therapies may become available for treatment of patients receiving mechanical ventilation in future.

Choice of Aerosol-Generating Device: MDIs vs. Nebulizers

Studies have established that nebulizers and MDIs are equally effective in the treatment of airway obstruction in ambulatory patients and in mechanically ventilated patients. The use of MDIs for aerosol therapy in mechanically ventilated patients is preferred because of numerous problems associated with the use of nebulizers.

- The rate of aerosol production and particle size of aerosol is highly unpredictable, not only in nebulizers of different brands but also in different batches of the same brand. Also the operational efficiency of a nebulizer varies with the pressure of the driving gas and with different fill volumes. Hence, it is essential to characterize the efficiency of nebulizer in a ventilator circuit before using.
- Risk of contamination with bacteria is also possible with nebulizer use unless the nebulizers and solutions are meticulously cleaned and disinfected.
- Tidal volume and inspiratory flow needs to be monitored and adjusted. The additional gas flow driving the nebulizer can lead to lung injury due to excess tidal volume. Additional flow leads to lack of triggering in assisted mode resulting in hypoventilation.

MDIs are easy to administer, portable, require less personnel time, are free from the risk of bacterial contamination and provide a reliable dose of the drug. Also, ventilator circuit need not be disconnected if a spacer is used minimizing the risk of airway contamination and de-recruitment.

Conclusion

Use of MDIs for bronchodilator therapy instead of nebulizers is an economical and time-saving measure especially when cost of medical treatment is going up. There is inadequate evidence to guide the choice of MDI or nebulizer for NPPV support.

References

1. Brewis BCRA, Geddes DM, Gibson GJ. Respiratory medicine. 2nd ed. London: W.B. Saunders; 1995
2. Skyler JS, Cefalu WT, Kourides IA, Landschulz WH, Balagtas CC, Cheng SL, Gelfand RA. Efficacy of inhaled human insulin in type 1 diabetes mellitus: a randomised proof-of-concept study. Lancet. 2001;357(9253):331–5.
3. Lipworth BJ. Pharmacokinetics of inhaled drugs. Br J Clin Pharmacol. 1996;42(6):697–705.
4. Ari A, Areabi H, Fink JB. Evaluation of aerosol generator devices at 3 locations in humidified and non-humidified circuits during adult mechanical ventilation. Respir Care. 2010;55(7):837–44.
5. Inhalation therapy in invasive and noninvasive mechanical ventilation: Rajiv Dhand. Current Opinion in Critical Care 2007: 13:27–38
6. Aerosol Therapy in Mechanically Ventilated Patients: Recent Advances and New Techniques: James B. Fink, and Rajiv Dhand. Seminars in respiratory and critical care medicine 2000: vol. 21, no. 3
7. Bronchodilator Aerosol Delivery in Mechanical Ventilation: Jantz MA, Collop NA. Intensive Care Med 1999: 14: 166-183
8. Device Selection and Outcomes of Aerosol Therapy: Evidence-Based Guidelines, American College of Chest Physicians/ American College of Asthma, Allergy, and Immunology. Myrna B. Dolovich, Richard C. Ahrens, Dean R. Hess *et al.* Chest 2005; 127:335–371
9. How Best to Deliver Aerosol Medications to Mechanically Ventilated Patients. Rajiv Dhand, VamP. Guntur, Clin Chest Med 2008: 29: 277–296

HUMIDIFICATION

During invasive ventilation, upper airway of the patient is bypassed, so humidification is needed to avoid hypothermia, bronchoconstriction, atelectasis, airway obstruction and destruction of the airway epithelium.

Humidification is an essential part of any successful ventilatory strategy. The importance of this strategy and its impact on control of bronchial secretions, gas exchange, weaning and complications such as ventilator-associated pneumonia (VAP), are under-recognized by clinicians. Understanding pathophysiology and techniques of humidification is important for instituting safe mechanical ventilation.

Water in vapour form (gaseous state) is humidity and process of conditioning inspired air to body temperature and 100% relative humidity is termed as humidification. To understand humidification some basic understanding of physical aspects of humidity and process of humidification and various devices of humidification is essential which will be discussed in this chapter.

Basic Definitions

Humidity is the amount of water vapor present in the air. It can be expressed in several ways:

- **Relative humidity (RH)** is a ratio of the actual water vapor content of air to the amount of water vapor needed to reach saturation at a particular temperature.
- **Absolute humidity (AH)** is the mass of water vapor contained in a given volume of air. It is commonly expressed in milligrams of water per liter of gas.

Alveolar gas has a temperature of 37°C, relative humidity 100% and contains 43.9 mg H_2O/L of water vapor.

Relationship between Gas Temperature, Absolute Humidity and Water Vapor Pressure (Figs 13.4 and 13.5)

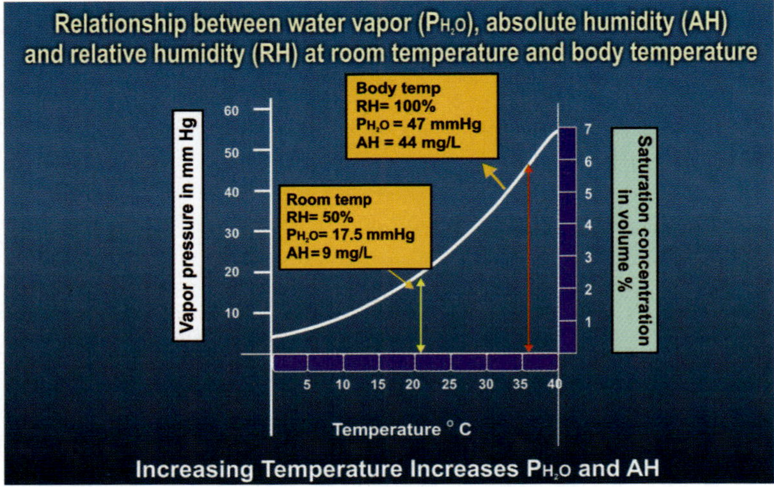

Fig. 13.4

Gas Temperature °C	Absolute humidity mg H_2O/L	Water vapor pressure P_{H_2O}
0	4.85	4.6
5	6.8	6.5
10	9.4	9.2
15	12.8	12.8
20	17.3	17.5
25	23.0	23.7
30	30.4	31.7
32	33.8	35.5
34	37.6	39.8
36	41.7	44.4
37	43.9	46.9
38	46.2	49.5
40	51.1	55.1
42	56.5	61.3
44	62.5	68.1

The relationship of Gas temperature, Absolute Humidity & Water Vapor pressure

Fig. 13.5

Hotter gas can hold more amount of water vapor therefore absolute humidity and water vapor pressure increases. As the inspired air leaves the humidifier and moves towards the patient, it cools.

This results in condensation as the capacity to hold the water vapor decreases with the drop in temperature. This can be reduced by using heated wire circuit. A water trap will be necessary to collect the condensed water.

Physiologic and Thermodynamic Basics

Usually respiration occurs through nose when inspired air is warmed and humidified by evaporation of water from the surface of mucous membranes. Ambient air at a temperature of 37°C has a moisture content of 10 mg/L. Therefore, 34 mg of water has to be added to each liter of inspired air along with warmth to achieve physiologic saturation condition (100% relative humidity at body temperature). Part of this (around 20 to 30%) is recovered during subsequent expiration by condensation. This exchange of warmth and moisture mainly occurs in the nasopharyngeal region.

Therefore, effective moisture loss from nasopharyngeal region is around 17 mg/L and from the lower respiratory tract it is around 7 mg/L leading to a total water loss of around 24 mg/L. Hence, the process of conditioning the inspired gas is an active one (**Figs 13.6 and 13.7**).

Humidity of Medical Gas and Ambient Air

	Medical Gases	Ambient Air	Lungs
Temperature	15 °C	22 °C	37 °C
Relative humidity	2%	35%	100%
Absolute humidity	0.3 mg/L	7 mg/L	44 mg/L

Fig. 13.6

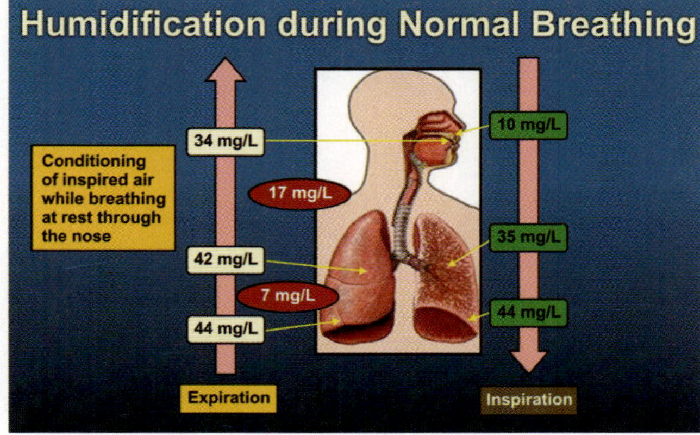

Fig. 13.7

Intubation bypasses the nasopharyngeal region which results in isothermic saturation boundary (point in the respiratory tract at which inspired air attains 100% relative humidity at 37°C and this is normally at or just below the carina) being shifted down towards the lung's periphery. The process of humidification of inspired air is now shifted to lower respiratory tract which is exposed to dry air for long periods. This problem is further worsened by the fact that medical gases are drier when compared to ambient air. Increased water loss from the lower respiratory tract is around 32 g/L (**Fig. 13.8**). This results in impaired function of the mucociliary elevator.

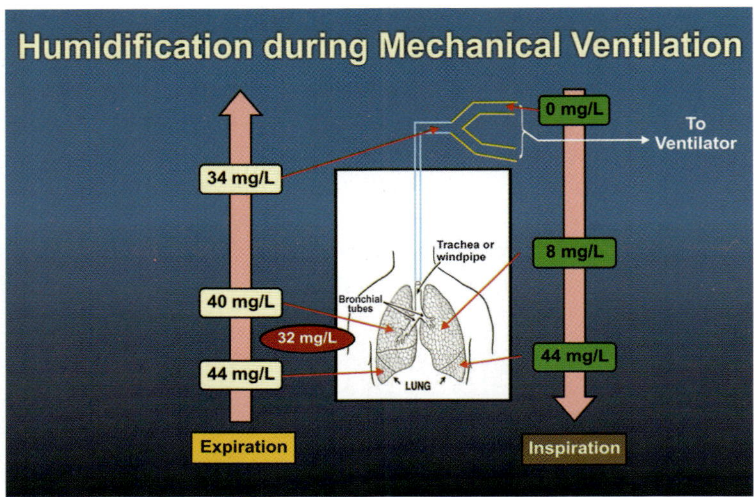

Fig. 13.8

Mucociliary Escalator (Fig. 13.9)

Respiratory mucous consists of a thick superficial (gel) layer and a deep watery (sol) layer. This allows the tips of the cilia to 'grip' mucous and push it cranially on a forward

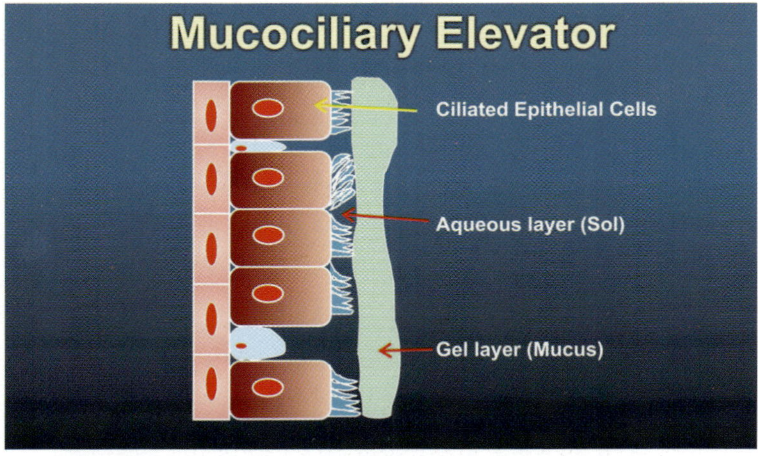

Fig. 13.9

stroke, yet pass back through it on the recovery stroke. This is the basic unit of the mucociliary elevator. Loss of water leads to lowering of the liquid sol layer, which does not allow cilia to function optimally. Therefore, micro-organisms are not cleared which predisposes the patient for respiratory infections. The relationship between the mucociliary transport system's performance and the humidity of the inspired gas has been studied extensively. At any given level of temperature and humidity, mucosal dysfunction is expected to worsen serially through four steps as listed below:

- Thickened mucus (or thinned mucus, in the case of overhydration)
- Slowed mucociliary transport
- Mucociliary stasis
- Cell damage

The rate of worsening through these steps is proportional to the humidity deficit. Humidity-related mucosal dysfunction may be further compromised by the presence of lung disease.

Complications of Mechanical Ventilation with Suboptimal Humidification

Due to dry medical gases and shifting of ISB downward towards the periphery of lungs, mechanical ventilation without appropriate humidification results in various complications as discussed in Fig. 13.10.

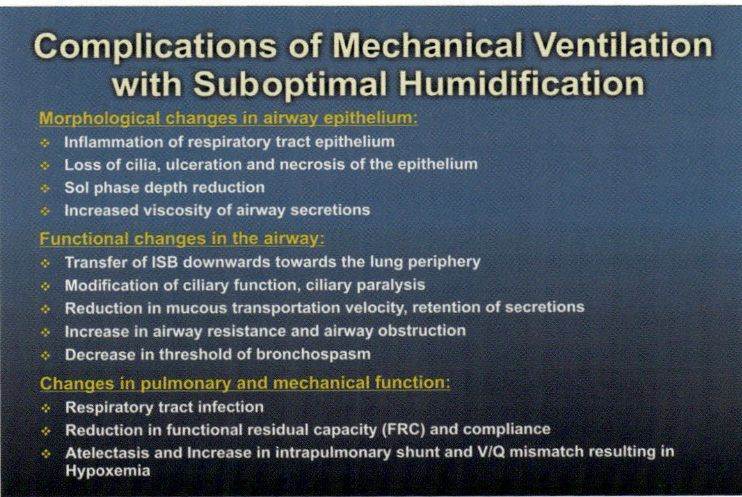

Fig. 13.10

Types of Humidifiers

Humidification of respired gases during mechanical ventilation is a standard of care. The humidification of respiratory gases should be started as early as possible and should not be dispensed with, even during short-term postoperative mechanical ventilation, patient transport or other emergency room situations.

Two systems are commonly used to humidify and warm inspired gases:

1. Heated humidifiers (HHs) also known as active humidifiers and
2. Heat and moisture exchangers (HMEs) also known as passive humidifiers

There is one more type of humidifier which tries to combine the features of both heated humidifiers and HMEs known as active heat moisture exchanger (not commonly used).

Passive Humidifiers/Heat Moisture Exchangers (HMEs)

In passive humidifiers (**Fig. 13.11**), the heat and moisture in expired air is trapped and transferred to inspired air during subsequent respiratory cycle. There is no external source for addition of heat and moisture. These are provided by the patient.

Types of HMEs

1. Condenser humidifier which is unsuitable for mechanical ventilation
2. Hygroscopic condenser humidifier
3. Hydrophobic condenser humidifier
4. Hygroscopic condenser humidifier filters (provide both humidification and filtration)
5. Hydrophobic condenser humidifier filters (provide both humidification and filtration)

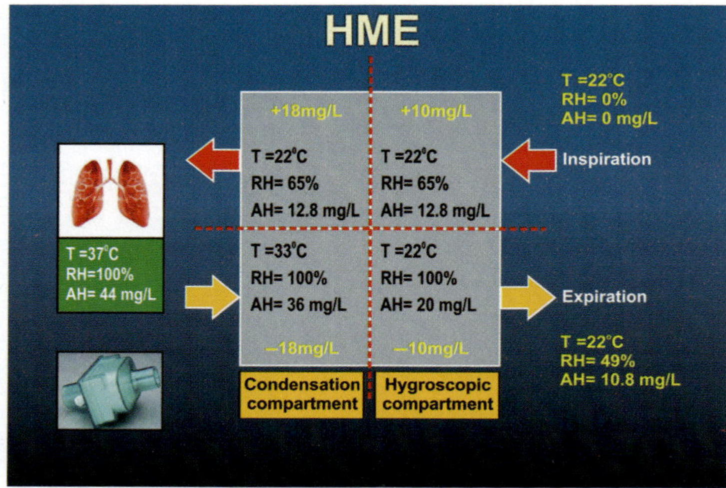

Fig. 13.11

Mechanism

Heat and moisture in the expired air are absorbed by the hygroscopic or hydrophobic material in HME, trapped, stored and transferred to the dry gas during subsequent inspiration. The efficiency of each device varies. HMEs that provide an AH <26 mg/L should not be used. The use of HMEs that deliver an AH of at least 30 mg H_2O/L are recommended, as they are associated with a lower incidence of endotracheal tube (ETT) blockage.

Usage

- It should visible and accessible in order to detect contamination or disconnection
- It should be positioned next to the tracheal tube, mask or supraglottic airway device
- If a nebulizer or metered dose inhaler is used to deliver medication, it should be inserted in between the HME and the patient or preferably the HME should be removed from the circuit during aerosol therapy.

Contraindications

There are no contraindications to providing humidification of inspired gas during mechanical ventilation. But HME is contraindicated under some circumstances.

- In patients with frank bloody or thick, copious secretions as HME can get blocked and the resistance is increased.
- In patients with an expired tidal volume less than 70% of inspired tidal volume (e.g. large bronchopleural fistula, endotracheal tube cuff defect, etc.) as HME uses heat and moisture in expired air to humidify inspired air.
- In ARDS/ALI and obstructive airway disease, because HMEs add additional dead space, resistance and cause increased work of breathing and $PaCO_2$
- In patients with body temperatures <32°C because HMEs use patients own body heat to warm inspired gas
- In patients with high spontaneous minute volumes (>10 l/ min)
- It should be removed from the ventilator circuit during aerosol therapy or should be bypassed **Heated humidifiers (HH)**

In heated humidifiers, heat and moisture is added to inspired gas from an external source by active process.

Types of heated humidifiers

1. Cascade humidifier
2. Bubble through humidifier
3. Surface-contact humidifier
4. Wick humidifier

Mechanism

Heated humidifiers add moisture and heat to the inspired air from temperature-regulated water reservoirs. Based on the mode of temperature control there are two types servo controlled unit and non-servo controlled unit. A servo controlled unit automatically controls power to the heating element in the humidifier in response to the temperature sensed by a probe near the patient connection or the humidifier outlet. A non-servo controlled unit provides power to the heating element according to the setting of a control, irrespective of the delivered temperature (**Fig. 13.12**).

Usage

- It should be placed in the inspiratory limb
- To avoid the risk of water entering into patient's airway it should be at a lower level than the patient
- Periodically the condensate must be drained or a water trap must be inserted in the most dependent part of the tubing to prevent blockage or aspiration. Since condensate is considered as infectious waste, it should not be drained back into humidifier reservoir.
- The heater wire in the ventilator circuit should not be bunched, but strung evenly along the length of the circuit.
- One should not fill the chamber above the maximum level as liquid could enter the ventilator circuit and then the patient's airway, if the chamber is overfilled.

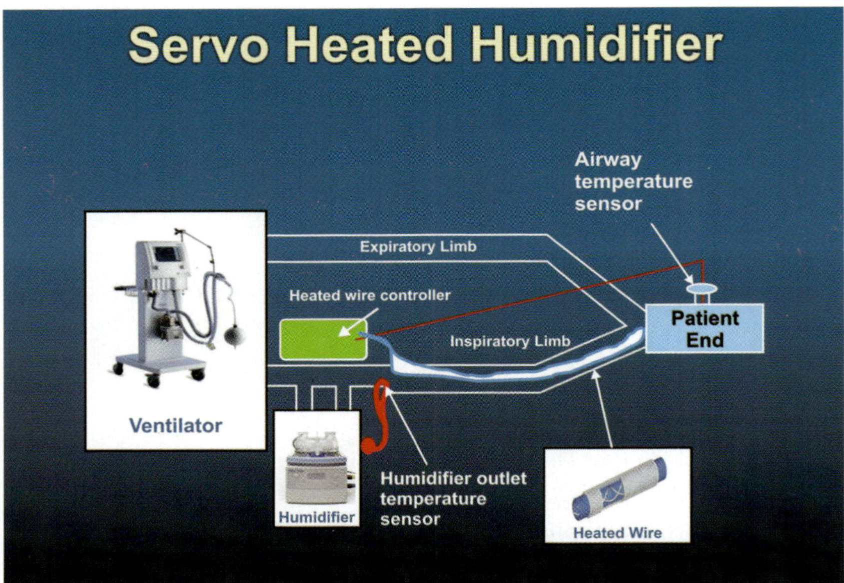

Fig. 13.12

Contraindications

Heated humidifiers have no contraindications and can be used on any patient requiring ventilatory assistance or supplemental oxygen.

Advantages and Disadvantages of Various Humidification Devices (Fig. 13.13)

Advantages and Disadvantages of Humidification devices

	Advantages	Disadvantages
HH with heated wire circuit	• Wide range of temperatures • Universal application • Reliable • Temperature monitoring • Alarms • Elimination of condensate	• Potential for reduced relative humidity and airway obstruction • Cost if used<48 hrs • Lack of portability • Complexity
HME	• Passive operation • Portable • Lightweight • Simple • Low cost	• Net water loss from respiratory tract • Not suitable for all patients • Dead space • Resistance • Potential for occlusion • Must remove to administer aerosol therapy
Active HME	• Universal application • Low water consumption • Elimination of condensate • Temperature monitoring • Alarms • Continued passive operation if water or electricity is lost • Elimination of water traps / heated wires	• Dead space • Weight • Potential for occlusion • Limited temperature range • Heat source near patient • Must remove to administer aerosols

Fig. 13.13

Complications of Humidification Devices

Complications of HME

- Hypothermia
- Hypercapnia due to hypoventilation caused by the increase in dead space
- Low-pressure alarm may become ineffective during disconnection, due to resistance through the HME

Complications of Heated Humidifiers

- Potential for electrical shock
- Hyperthermia
- Risk of burns to the patient and health staff, thermal injury to the airway, and tubing meltdown
- Unintentional tracheal lavage because of overfilling, tilting of the water reservoir or draining of condensate
- The condensation in the circuit may cause patient ventilator dyssynchrony and triggering issues and may affect ventilator performance.
- May cause dehydration of the airway if temperature is set to body temperature, yet the RH is low.
- Risk of over hydration with associated complications like pulmonary edema, hyponatremia, etc.

Complications common to both HME and Heated humidifier

- If AH is <26 mg H_2O/l, it can lead to dehydration and thickening and impaction of mucus secretions
- Insufficient AH can lead to mucus plugging of airways resulting in hypoventilation, gas trapping, increase airway resistance causing increase in work of breathing
- Increased resistance through the humidifier (more in HME) could result in elevated airway pressures and possible disconnection
- When humidifier (more so in heated humidifier) is disconnected from the patient, some ventilators generate a high flow through the ventilator circuit that may aerosolize contaminated condensate, increasing risk of nosocomial infection for both the patient and clinician.
- Compressible volume loss (more in heated humidifier) can lead to inaccurate effective tidal volume and possible hypoventilation (if not calculated)

Mechanical Effects of Heated Humidifier and HME

There are some mechanical effects due to usage of heated humidifier and HME which are summarized in **Fig. 13.14**.

Selecting the type of Humidifier (Fig. 13.15)

As HMEs are less expensive, light weight and portable they are preferred for short-term use (≤96 hr) and also during transport. HH should be used for patients who exhibit contraindications for HME use. There is no major difference in the incidence of ventilator-associated pneumonia in patients humidified with HMEs versus HHs.

Mechanical Effects of HH and HME

	Heated Humidifier	HME
Compressible volume	+++	+
Dead space	0	++
Inspiratory resistance	±	+
Expiratory resistance	0	++
Intrinsic PEEP	0	+
Ventilatory load	0	++

Fig. 13.14

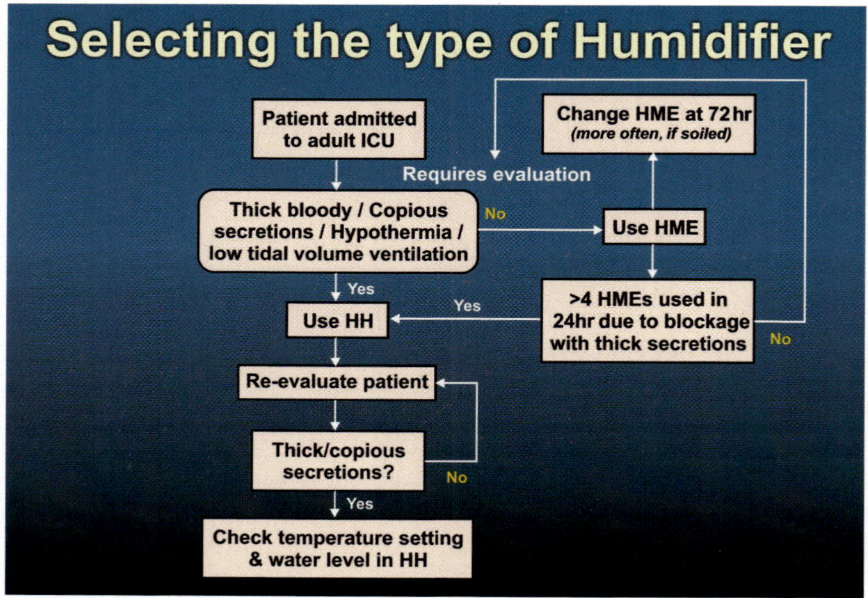

Fig. 13.15

Assessing the Adequacy of Humidification

It is difficult to objectively measure humidification. Therefore, humidification should be assessed clinically and it is understood to be appropriate if the patient exhibits none of the complications of under- or over-humidification listed above. The presence of condensate in the ET connector implies that RH is 100%.

Infection Control

- Heated humidifiers should be thoroughly disinfected. Aseptic technique should be used when filling the water reservoir and only medical grade sterile water should be used.
- The water left over in the water feed reservoir remains sterile and need not be discarded when the ventilator circuit is changed. Nevertheless, the water feed system should be used for single patient only.
- Condensation from the ventilator circuit should be considered infectious waste and disposed of according to hospital policy, using strict universal precautions. Condensate should never be drained back into the humidifier reservoir.
- There is no need to change the circuits on a timely basis. But it should be changed when they are visibly soiled or not functioning properly.
- There is no need to change HME daily for reasons of infection control. They should be changed only when they are visibly soiled, blocked or damaged. HME can be safely used for at least 48 hours, and sometimes for up to 1 week.

Recommendations for Humidification are Summarized in Fig. 13.16

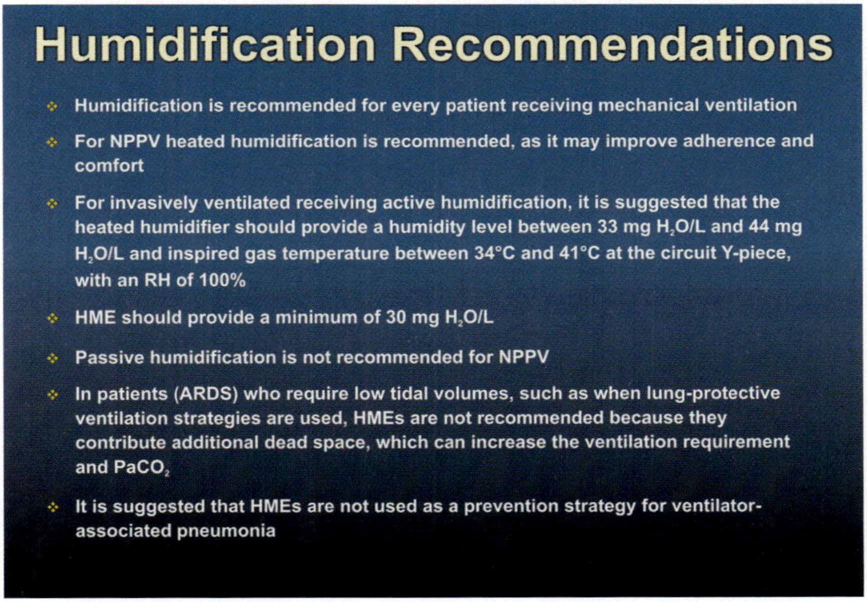

Humidification Recommendations

- Humidification is recommended for every patient receiving mechanical ventilation
- For NPPV heated humidification is recommended, as it may improve adherence and comfort
- For invasively ventilated receiving active humidification, it is suggested that the heated humidifier should provide a humidity level between 33 mg H_2O/L and 44 mg H_2O/L and inspired gas temperature between 34°C and 41°C at the circuit Y-piece, with an RH of 100%
- HME should provide a minimum of 30 mg H_2O/L
- Passive humidification is not recommended for NPPV
- In patients (ARDS) who require low tidal volumes, such as when lung-protective ventilation strategies are used, HMEs are not recommended because they contribute additional dead space, which can increase the ventilation requirement and $PaCO_2$
- It is suggested that HMEs are not used as a prevention strategy for ventilator-associated pneumonia

Fig. 13.16

Humidification for NPPV

From a pathophysiological view point, spontaneously breathing patients without an endotracheal tube or tracheostomy tube do not necessarily require additional strategies for conditioning respiratory gases. In NPPV there are large leaks around the mask and high inspiratory flow (sometimes up to 120 L/min) of dry medical gases.

These overwhelm the mucosal humidification capacity. Added to these, there may be worsening of secretions and fluid depletion. It is, therefore, advisable to use active humidifier as they have a large capacity to produce heated and humidified air.

Well humidified air at a temperature between 25–30°C is one of the factors for success in NPPV therapy. This improves both secretion clearance and the tolerance of the NPPV therapy. Passive humidification is not recommended for NPPV.

Conclusion

All mechanically ventilated patients should receive adequate humidification of inspired gases to avoid the hazards of under- and over-humidification. The selection of type of humidifying device depends on many factors like patient's temperature, quantity and quality of secretions, history of chronic lung disease, duration of ventilatory support, etc.

In patients requiring short term ventilation considering the cost advantage of HME, it can be preferred over heated humidifier provided there are no contraindications. Humidification should not be considered in isolation but as part of total airway management.

It should be associated with careful fluid balance, physiotherapy, bronchial hygiene therapy and appropriate drug therapy.

References

1. Restrepo RD, Walsh BK, American Association for Respiratory Care. Humidification during invasive and noninvasive mechanical ventilation: 2012. Respir Care 2012;57(5):782–88.
2. Devices used to humidify respired gases. Dr. Jorg Rathgeber. Respir Care Clin 2006: 12: 165–82.
3. Humidification during mechanical ventilation: Current Trends and Controversies. Tim Op't Holt
4. Humidification during invasive and noninvasive mechanical ventilation: 2012, Restrepo RD, Walsh BK. Respir Care 2012 May; 57(5):782–8.

CHAPTER 14

Sedation, Analgesics, and Neuromuscular Blockers

❒ Venkat Raman Kola ❒ Ravi Krishna M

ICU is a foreign environment for patients. It is an environment which they have not chosen and they do not have family members around them for comfort. These patients often experience pain and physical discomfort resulting from invasive procedures, surgery, and monitoring devices, as well as more direct stimuli from injury, inflammation, and immobility (**Fig. 14.1**). Performing routine nursing care, such as airway suctioning, physical therapy, dressing changes, and patient mobilization, can also be painful.

PREDISPOSING AND CAUSATIVE FACTORS OF PAIN (Fig. 14.1)

One-third patients in intensive care units (ICUs) worldwide are mechanically ventilated and require sedation and analgesia frequently to enhance comfort.[1] Assessment of the problem, sound knowledge of medications used and an understanding of disease pathology help in preventing the adverse effects of over- or under-sedation (**Fig. 14.2**).

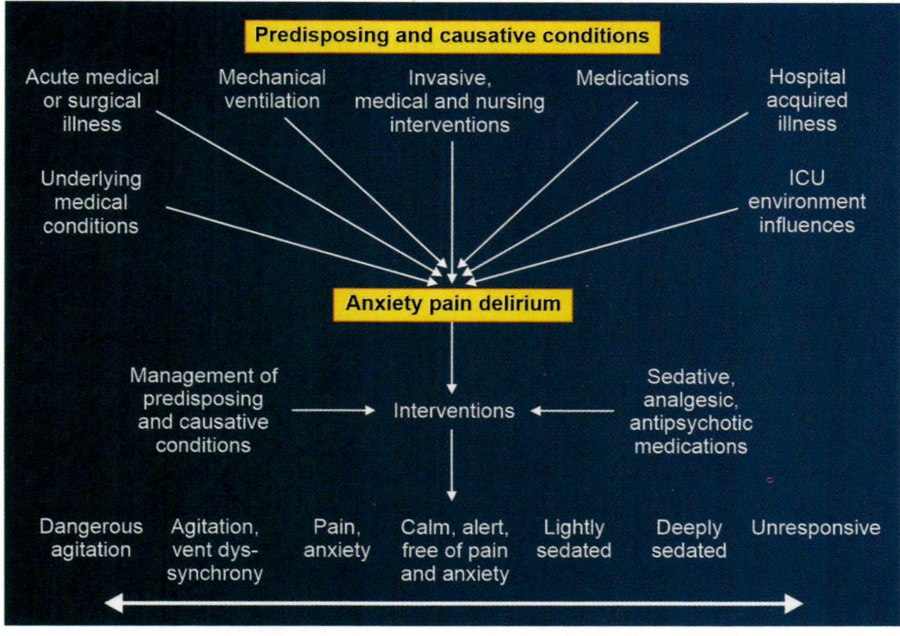

Fig. 14.1: Predisposing and causative factors of pain

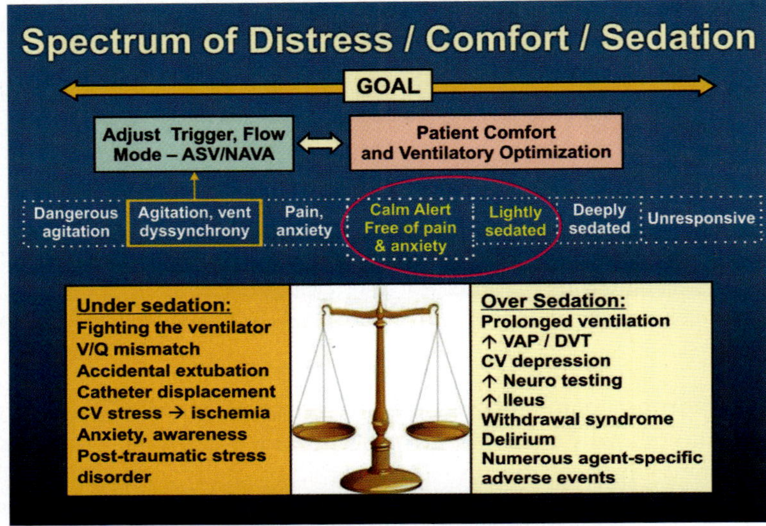

Fig. 14.2: Spectrum of distress/comfort

The term "Sedation" in a mechanically ventilated patient first encompasses the component of adequate pain management. Studies in agitated patients in the ICU have found that after analgesia wasgiven, more than half the patients did not require sedation. Analgesics have to be administered first to agitated patients (analgosedation strategy or AFS (analgesia first).[2] This should be based on patient-centred assessment, enabling patients to be comfortable, calm, cooperative and communicative. 'Optimum sedation' has to be tailored to individual patient's needs.

Sedation and analgesics in mechanically ventilated patients help in:

- Prevention of pain and anxiety
- Amnesia during neuromuscular blockade
  - Reduced response to stimulation resulting in decreased metabolic demand and oxygen consumption
  - Control of delusional agitation and delirium
  - Improving patient-ventilator synchrony
  - Avoid adverse neurocognitive sequelae like depression and post-traumatic stress disorder (PTSD)
  - Avoiding PICS (postintensive care syndrome)

Pain and anxiety lead to stimulation of the autonomic nervous system and the release of humoral factors. This leads to increased heart rate, increased blood pressure and increased myocardial oxygen consumption resulting in myocardial ischemia or infarction. An altered humoral response can lead to hypercoagulability as a result of increased levels of clotting factors, fibrinogen, platelet activity and inhibition of fibrinolysis. Stress hormones produce insulin resistance, increase metabolic rate and cause protein catabolism. Decreased gastric and bowel motility and increased risk of gut bacterial translocation are seen in these patients. Pain and anxiety result in immunosuppression with reduction in number and function of lymphocytes and granulocytes.[3]

Clinical Approach to Sedation and Analgesia use in a Mechanically Ventilated Patient

Approach to these patients involves evaluation of the cause-effect of the problem, quantifying it and formulating a protocol for its management.

All sedation strategies should start with assessing for and ensuring adequate pain control. The 2018 PADIS guidelines recommend adequately treating pain before considering initiation of sedation.[4]

Ideally, pain should be described regarding location, duration, type, exacerbating and relieving factors, and intensity. Pain is sometimes conceptualized by subtypes, including somatic, visceral, and neuropathic because manifestations and management can differ.

Detailed verbal communication by ICU patients is often limited; however, the use of simple tools such as the numerical rating scale or a series of cartoon faces ranging from smiling to crying can facilitate communication by pointing or nodding in the nonverbal but cognitively intact patient.

Other techniques to enhance the use of self-reporting of pain include adding descriptive words to the numerical scale, carefully explaining the tool and correct use with each encounter, providing glasses and hearing aids if necessary, and allowing adequate time for instructions and patient response.

Many ICU patients are cognitively impaired and self-reporting pain intensity is not feasible. Accordingly, clinicians must rely on observed behaviours that correlate with self-reported pain or are associated with noxious stimuli.

Pain observation tools for adults in ICU care include the Critical-Care Pain Observation Tool (CPOT), the Behavioral Pain Scale (BPS), the Nonverbal Pain Scale (NVPS) **(Fig. 14.3)**.

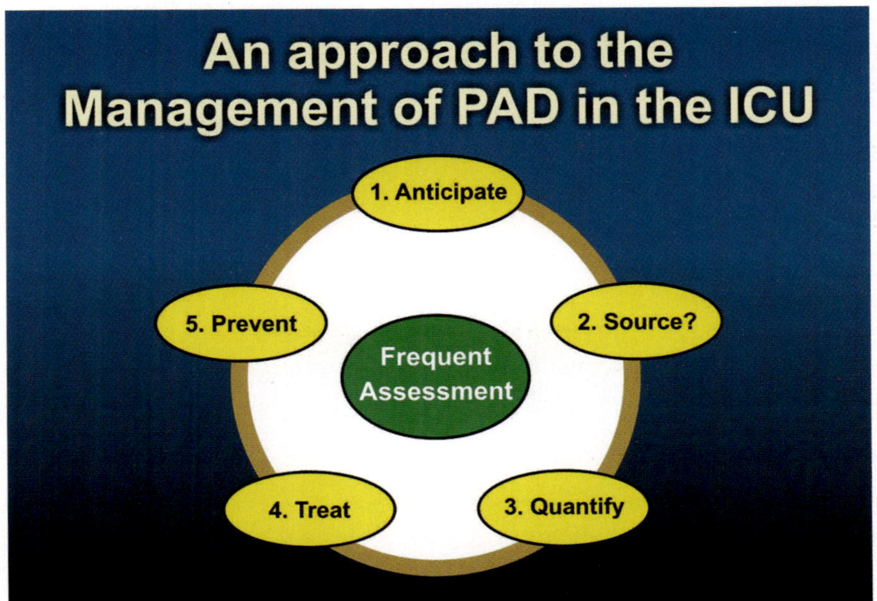

Fig. 14.3: Approach to management of PAD in ICU

Analgesic First Strategy (AFS)

Pain is defined as an unpleasant sensory and emotional experience associated with actual or potential tissue damage, or described in terms of such damage. For a clinician pain should be considered to be "whatever" the experiencing person says it is, existing "whenever" the experiencing person says it does.

Assessment of Pain in a Mechanically Ventilated Patient

No patient should be allowed to 'fight' the ventilator in the ICU. An optimal sedation protocol in mechanically ventilated patients can prevent this. Although modern ventilators that allow synchronized spontaneous breathing have reduced the need for sedation, some sedation is usually needed, particularly following the initiation of assisted ventilation.

Vital signs (increased heart rate, blood pressure and sweating) may be used as a cue to begin further assessment of pain in these patients. However, changes in vital signs are inconsistently associated with pain, with many confounding factors that can mask anticipated changes, such as the administration of β-blockers, as well as lack of specificity with many other causes of tachycardia, hypertension, and tachypnea.[5] Hence guidelines suggest that vital signs alone should not be used for pain assessment in adult ICU patients.

Patients on ventilators can either be communicative or they may be drowsy and unable to communicate pain. Hence assessment in these two categories of patients is different and is discussed below.

Pain Assessment

Communication is the best way of assessing pain in patients who can self-report. A simple question-answer interaction can solve the problem. A writing board can be used for patients who can write. Many patients in ICU are too weak to write.

In such cases an alphabetical chart in the language understood by the patient can be used by nurses to construct what the patient is trying to communicate. New guidelines recommend that pain be routinely monitored in all ICU patients.

Communicative Patients

Numerical Rating Scale (NPS)

The numeric pain scale (NPS) employs a verbal rating of pain on a scale from 0 to 10, with 10 being the worst pain ever experienced. This is broadly used in a variety of clinical settings. Self-reported pain is considered to be the standard and NPS is recommended by PAD guidelines (UNGRADED) (**Fig. 14.4**).[4]

Non-communicative Patients

The behavioural pain scale (BPS) and critical-care pain observation tool (CPOT) are the most valid and reliable behavioural pain scales for monitoring pain in medical, postoperative or trauma cases (except in head injury). These tools are used in patients who are unable to self-report, in whom the motor function is intact and behaviours are observable.

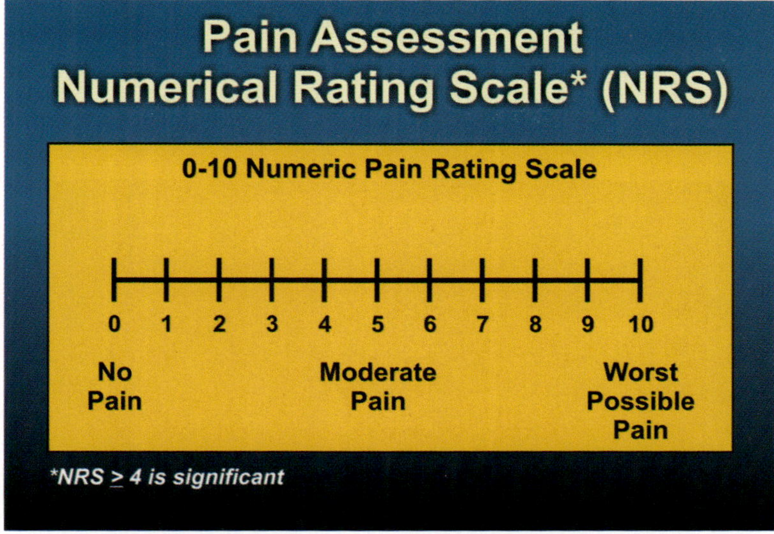

Fig. 14.4: Self reported numerical pain scale

Among critically ill adults unable to self-report pain and in whom behaviours are observable, the Behavioral Pain Scale (BPS) in intubated patients and the Critical-Care Pain Observation Tool (CPOT) demonstrate the greatest validity and reliability for monitoring pain and are recommended by PADIS guidelines (UNGRADED).[4,6]

The behavioural pain scale (BPS) is based on a sum score of three components:

1. Facial expression,
2. Movements of upper limbs, and
3. Compliance with mechanical ventilation.

Based upon the assumption that a relationship exists between the score and pain intensity, each pain indicator is scored from 1 (no response) to 4 (full response), with a maximum score of 12. A BPSscore of more than 6 is considered significant. One limitation of BPS is that responsiveness of the patient decreases substantially with deepening levels of sedation. Compliance with mechanical ventilation may be considered to be a separate parameter from other behaviors. Some intensivists therefore only score facial expression and movements of upper limbs to assess the individual pain state.

Another behavior pain tool, critical-care pain observation tool (CPOT), has four components:

1. Facial expression
2. Body movement
3. Muscle tension and
4. Compliance with the ventilator for intubated patients or vocalization for extubated patients.

Each of these behaviors is assigned a rating of 0 to 2 (CPOT range = 0 to 8, CPOT > 3 is significant).Current practice for adult ICU patients commonly includes a combination of NPS or a similar self-reported pain quantification tool plus an instrument designed to identify pain using behavior and physiologic parameters in the non-communicative patient (e.g. the CPOT).

BEHAVIOURAL PAIN SCALE (BPS)

Sub-scale	Description	Score
Facial expression	Relaxed	1
	Partially tightened	2
	Fully tightened	3
	Grimacing	4
Upper limbs	No movement	1
	Partially bent	2
	Fully bent with finger flexion	3
	Permanently retracted	4
Compliance with ventilation	Tolerating movement	1
	Coughing but tolerating ventilation For most of the time	2
	Fighting ventilator	3
	Unable to control ventilation	4

Fig. 14.5: Behavioural pain scale (BPS)

BPS is illustrated in **Fig. 14.5**.

Tenets to Managing Pain

- Usually, simple non-pharmacological interventions decrease or even alleviate the need for drugs. An empathetic and thorough explanation, perhaps combined with a visit from a family member, may be all that is required.
- Determine the underlying cause(s) and reverse what is treatable/modifiable.
- Perform structured pain assessments with a consistent tool.
- Work with an interdisciplinary team to understand and treat the emotional, psychological, social, and existential/spiritual aspects of pain.
- Start low and go slow with medications in patients with altered absorption, metabolism, and excretion due to serious illness.
- Use the IV route for pain crises, and premedicate before procedures.
- Understand the pharmacokinetics of opioids and how to dose for continuous pain (based on the half-life of the drug) and breakthrough pain (based on time to maximum concentration in the serum).

- Utilize multimodal analgesia, including adjuvants (paracetamol, nefopam, ketamine), interventional modalities and nonpharmacologic approaches.
- Consider strategies to treat multiple symptoms simultaneously to minimize polypharmacy (i.e. corticosteroids for bone pain and nausea, antidepressants for neuropathic pain and mood).
- It is recommended that either enterally administered gabapentin or carbamazepine, in addition to intravenous opioids, should be considered for the treatment of neuropathic pain and patients after cardiovascular surgery.
- Thoracic epidural anaesthesia or analgesia should be considered in patients with rib fractures and for postoperative analgesia in patients with post thoracotomy.
- Monitor closely and adjust medications based on analgesic response and side effects.
- Coordinate a plan of care for pain management with outside providers if a patient will be discharged from the ICU.
- Full bladder, distended bowels and other irritants such as an itch from a plaster cast are all causes of discomfort in critically ill patients. These are best relieved by dealing with the cause rather than treating pharmacologically.
- Music and massage have also been shown to reduce opioid requirements.[7]
- Ice pack therapy and relaxation techniques also help in procedural pain management.[7]

Regional Anesthesia and Analgesia

Although systemic administration of opioids for pain management in the ICU is typically by the IV route, regional approaches can offer advantages in selected cases like traumatic ARDS. These options include continuous epidural analgesia and/or anaesthesia (central neuraxial techniques) and continuous peripheral nerve or plexus block.

Pain management is summarized in **Fig. 14.6**.

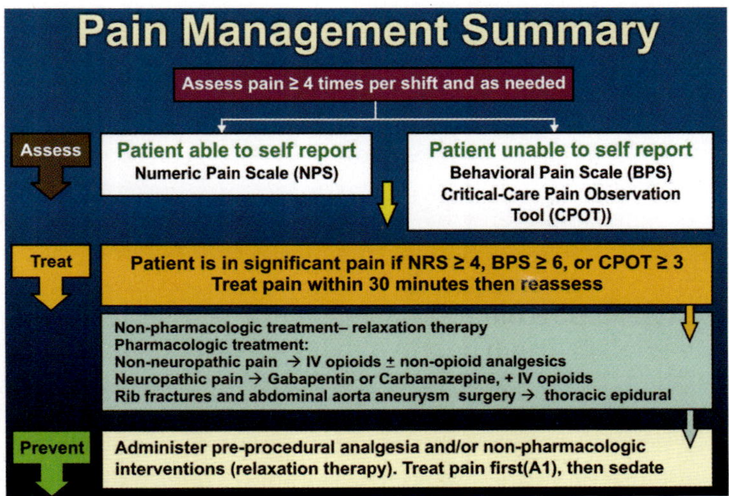

Fig. 14.6: Pain management summary

Commonly used analgesic doses and side effects are given in Fig. 14.7.

Commonly used analgesic doses and side effects

Opioid drug	Approximate Equivalent Single IV Dose	Typical Infusion Rate	Onset to Peak Effect	Duration
Fentanyl	100–200 mcg	50–200 mcg/hr	2–5 min	0.5–2 hours
Morphine	10 mg	2–10 mg/hr	20–30 min	3–4 hours
Hydromorphone	1.5 mg	7–15 mcg/kg/hr	30–60 min	2–3 hours
Remifentanil	Bolus doses are not usually recommended	0.05–0.2 mcg/kg/hr	1–2 min	10–20 min

Fig. 14.7: Commonly used analgesic doses

SEDATION IN MECHANICALLY VENTILATED PATIENTS

Although the importance of non-pharmacologic approaches such as comfortable positioning in bedand verbal reassurance may be adequate at times, anxiety is common in mechanically ventilated patients and sedation to a point of coma may seem like an attractive option for some patients.[8]

Some patients may require no sedation with proper pain control. Although amnesia is important during surgical procedures, its importance in mechanically ventilated patients during critical illness is far less certain. Indeed, complete amnesia for extended periods during mechanical ventilation in the ICU has never been proven to confer a benefit and thereis data to suggest that light sedation will shorten the time to extubation and reduce ICU length of stay.

A scoring scale that assesses the level of sedation should be used in the management of allmechanically ventilated ICU patients.

The Richmond Agitation-Sedation Scale (RASS) and Sedation Agitation Scale are the most extensively evaluated. RASS has been shown to have excellent inter-rater reliability.[9] It is the first scale to be validated to detect changing levels of sedation and correlate it to the level of consciousness and delirium over consecutive days of ICU care (Figs 14.8 and 14.9).

The amount of sedation preferred by patients is likely variable; some patients or families may prefer deeper sedation, but this preference may not be considered appropriate by clinicians given the adverse outcomes associated with deep sedation.

New PADIS guidelines recommend maintaining light levels of sedation in adult ICU patients. It is associated with improved clinical outcomes (e.g. shorter duration of mechanical ventilation and a shorter length of ICU stay).[10] Maintaining light levels of sedation increases the physiologic stress response but is not associated with an increased incidence of myocardial ischemia.

Despite the wide use of various validated sedation scales like RASS and SAS there is still no consensus on the definition of light, moderate and deep sedation. Further studies on the concept of wakefulness and light sedation are required.

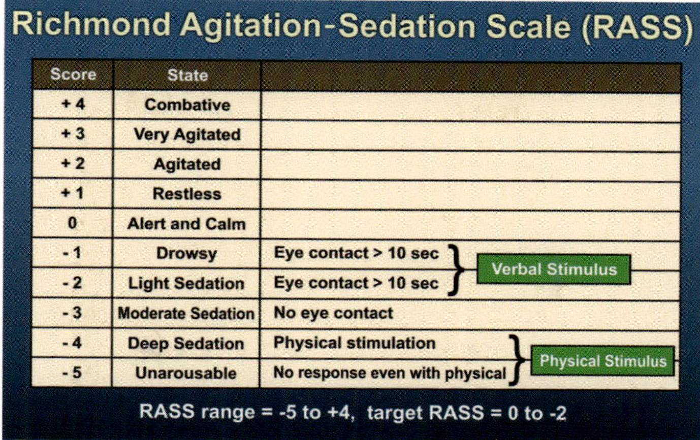

Richmond Agitation-Sedation Scale (RASS)

Score	State		
+ 4	Combative		
+ 3	Very Agitated		
+ 2	Agitated		
+ 1	Restless		
0	Alert and Calm		
- 1	Drowsy	Eye contact > 10 sec	Verbal Stimulus
- 2	Light Sedation	Eye contact > 10 sec	
- 3	Moderate Sedation	No eye contact	
- 4	Deep Sedation	Physical stimulation	Physical Stimulus
- 5	Unarousable	No response even with physical	

RASS range = -5 to +4, target RASS = 0 to -2

Fig. 14.8: Richmond agitation-sedation scale

Sedation-Agitation Scale (SAS)

Score	State	Behaviors
7	Very Agitated	Pulling at ET tube, climbing over bedrail, striking at staff, thrashing side-to-side
6	Very Agitated	Does not calm despite frequent verbal reminding, requires physical restraints
5	Agitated	Anxious or mildly agitated, attempting to sit up, calms down to verbal instructions
4	Calm and Co-operative	Calm, awakens easily, follows commands
3	Sedated	Difficult to arouse, awakens to verbal stimuli or gentle shaking but drifts off
2	Very Sedated	Arouses to physical stimuli but does not communicate or follow commands
1	Unarousable	Minimal or no response to noxious stimuli, does not communicate or follow commands

SAS range = 1 to 7, target SAS = 3 to 4

Fig. 14.9: Sedation agitation scale

Daily Sedative Interruption/Nurse-Protocolized Sedation

A DSI (daily sedation interruption) or an SAT (spontaneous awakening trial) is defined as a period, each day, during which a patient's sedative medication is discontinued and patients can wake up and achieve arousal and/or alertness, defined by objective actions such as opening eyes in response to a voice, following simple commands, and/or having a Sedation-Agitation Scale (SAS) score of 4–7 or a RASS score of –1 to +1. Nurse-Protocolized Sedation is defined as an established sedation protocol implemented by nurses at the bedside to determine sedative choices and to titrate these medications to achieve prescription-targeted sedation scores.

Respiratory Drive and Sedation

A given respiratory drive might result in very different efforts depending on the respiratory muscle strength or the diaphragmatic conformation. For example, some patients with emphysema and flattening of the diaphragm have respiratory drives out of proportion to their ability to generate inspiratory pressure. Conversely, some conditions are associated with respiratory drives higher than their metabolic demand would require. In situations such as delirium and altered pulmonary mechanoreceptors, excessive ventilatory efforts can lead to hyperventilation and, possibly, patient self-inflicted lung (P-SILI) or respiratory muscle injury.[11]

Propofol and benzodiazepines both cause respiratory depression, principally by reducing the amplitude of respiratory effort.[12]

Cardiovascular Effects of Sedation

Sedatives have important cardiovascular effects. An understanding of the physiologic effects of each agent is important, to tailor the sedation strategy.

Commonly used Sedatives and their Cardiovascular Effects (Fig. 14.10)

Sedation and Neurological Effects

The association between the depth of sedation and psychological stress in these patients remains unclear. Subjective sedation scoring systems are better than objective measures such as auditoryevoked potentials (AEP), bispectral index (BIS), narcotrend index (NI), patient state index (PSI), state entropy (SE), etc. in monitoring depth of sedation in non-comatose, non-paralyzed critically ill adult patients. The use of electroencephalogram derived parameters (e.g. BIS), is not recommended in routine in the ICU setting, either in paralysed and non-paralysed patients, because of the high proportion of false positive and false negative measurements of sedation.[13]

The objective measures of brain function may be used as an adjuvant to subjective sedation assessment in patients receiving neuromuscular blocking agents as subjective sedation assessments may be unobtainable.[14]

To enhance the electrophysiological measurement of the stress response, related to pain or other stressful factors (e.g. anxiety, fear), new devices have been developed recently. All these devices are based on the measurement of surrogate markers of the adrenergic response: an increase of the pupillary diameter (measured by videopupillometry),[15] a decrease of physiological Heart Rate Variability (HRV) related to a decrease of parasympathetic tone (meaning an increase of sympathetic tone), or other parameters.

Sedation strategies using non-benzodiazepine sedatives (either propofol or dexmedetomidine) arepreferred over sedation with benzodiazepines (either midazolam or lorazepam) to improve clinicaloutcomes. In general, the choice of sedative agent used in ICU patients should be driven by:

1. Indications for sedation
2. Goals of sedation
3. Effect and side effects of the drug
4. Cost of medication

Drug class	Mechanism of action	Blood pressure	Heart rate	Respiratory rate	Tidal volume	Comments
Propofol	GABA receptor agonist	↓	↓/↔	↓	↓	Hypotensive effects may be exacerbated in those with cardiac dysfunction. Avoid use in cardiogenic shock
Opioids	μ receptor agonist	↓	↓	↓	↓	Often used in combination with other agents, potentiating their haemodynamic effects
Benzodiazepines	GABA receptor agonist	Mild ↓	↔	↓/↔/↑	↓	Not recommended by current guidelines for continuous infusion due to risk of delirium. Respiratory effects are dose dependent, with higher doses increasing risk of respiratory depression.
Ketamine	NMDA receptor anatgonist	↓/↔/↑	↓/↔	↔	↔	Haemodynamic effects depend on overall volume status, sympathetic tone
Dexmedetomidine - bolus	α_2 receptor agonist	↑	↓	↔	↔	Initial bolus can cause hypertension due to stimulation of peripheral vasoconstrictor receptors,
Dexmedetomidine - no bolus	α_2 receptor agonist	↓	↓	↔	↔	A third of patients still experience significant bradycardia without a bolus
Etomidate	GABA receptor agonist	↔/↓	↔	↔	↔	Used for induction of anaesthesia, risk of adrenal insufficiency and resultant hypotension
Volatiles	GABA receptor agonist, AMPA and NMDA receptor antagonist	↓	↑	↓/↑	↓	Decrease in tidal volume may be compensated for by an increase in respiratory rate.

Physiological effects of sedation

GABA = gamma-aminobutyric acid, NMDA = N-methyl-D-aspartate, AMPA = α-amino-3-hydroxy-5-methyl-4-isoxazolepropionic acid

Fig. 14.10: Commonly used sedatives and their cardiovascular effects

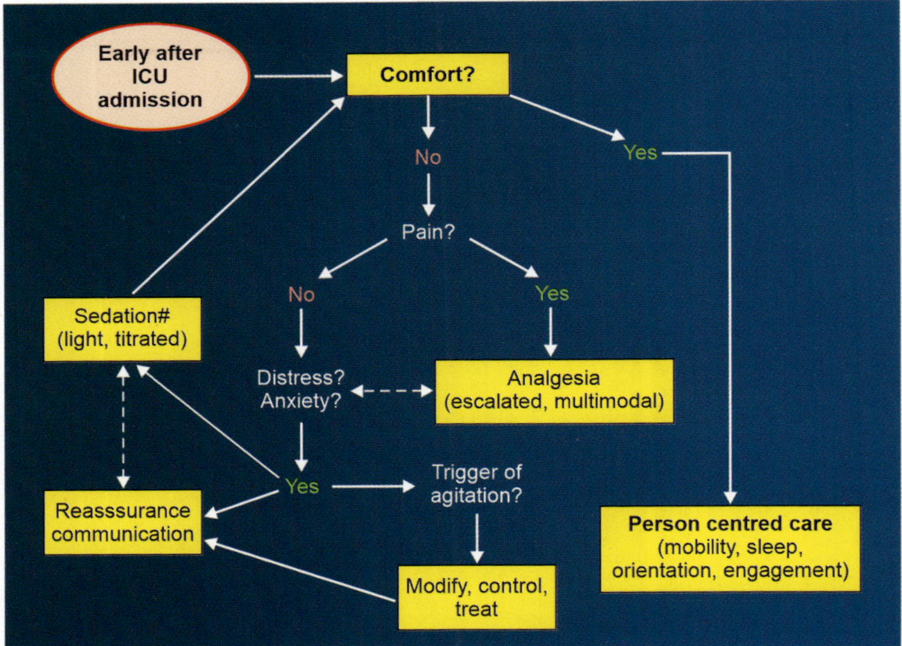

Fig. 14.11: eCASH concept

eCASH Concept (Fig. 14.11)

eCASH aims to establish optimal patient comfort with minimal sedation as the default presumption for intensive care unit (ICU) patients in the absence of recognised medical requirements for deeper sedation.

Sedation is secondary to pain relief and where possible should be based on agents that can be titrated to a prespecified target level that is subject to regular review and adjustment; routine use of benzodiazepines should be minimised. From the outset, the objective of sedation strategy is to eliminate the use of sedatives at the earliest medically justifiable opportunity.

Sedation Management Summary (Fig. 14.12)

Dexmedetomidine offers a cost advantage over midazolam infusions, especially in healthcare institutions that are efficient in transferring patients out of the ICU.

Dexmedetomidine and ketamine are attractive agents for use in mechanically ventilated patients. Unlike other agents, they provide sedation, anxiolysis (ketamine may cause rebound agitation), and analgesia with more limited occurrences of respiratory depression.

Despite some apparent advantages in using either propofol or dexmedetomidine over benzodiazepines for ICU sedation, benzodiazepines remain the most commonly prescribed sedatives in mechanically ventilated patients.

It is advised to have institution-specific sedation and weaning algorithms to achieve a shorter duration of mechanical ventilation and/or shorter ICU length of stay. Other benefits include more 'on-target' sedation, less pain, reduced direct costs, less patient-ventilator asynchrony and decreased incidence of ventilator-associated pneumonia.

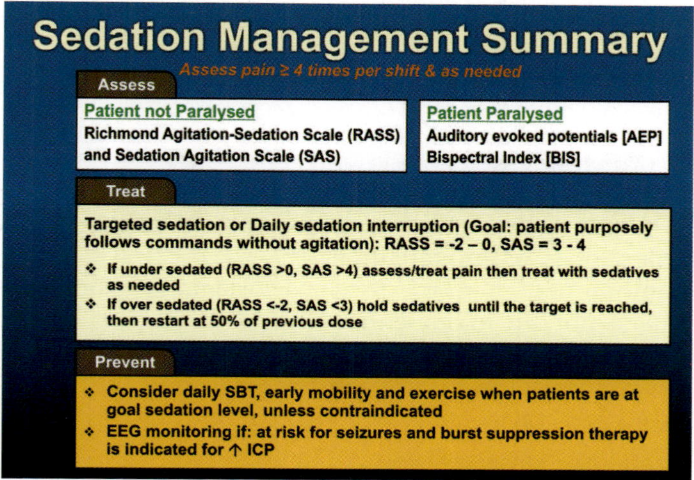

Fig. 14.12: Sedation management summary

Commonly used sedatives and their doses are given in Fig. 14.13D.

A patient's need for sedation will vary from time to time. Factors responsible for this change are:

a. Variation in severity of illness
b. Need for surgical interventions
c. Changes in the mode of ventilatory support
d. Tolerance to drugs
e. Changes in renal and liver function resulting in altered drug elimination and volume of distribution
f. Toxicity of the sedative agent or its solvent
g. Need for patient transfer (e.g. MRI scan)

Commonly used Sedatives and their doses

Drug	Typical IV Bolus Dose	Typical Infusion Rate	Onset to Peak	Duration
Propofol	0.03–0.15 mg/kg (max 20 mg)	5-80 mcg/kg/min	1–2 min	< 20 min
Midazolam	1–6 mg	1–10 mg/hr	5–10 min	1.5–2 hours
Lorazepam	1–3 mg	1–5 mg/hr	15–20 min	2–4 hours
Dexmedetomidine	Not recommended	0.2–1.5 mcg/kg/hr	30 min	2–4 hours

Fig. 14.13: Commonly used sedatives and their doses

Delirium in a Mechanically Ventilated Patient

Delirium is defined as a change in cognition or the development of a perceptual disturbance that is not accounted for by pre-existing established or evolving dementia.

Delirium incidence, once reported in 60–80% of mechanically ventilated patients, is down by about 25% in many ICUs worldwide.[16]

Diagnostic Criteria for Delirium

- Alteration of consciousness and attention
- Change in cognition (e.g. memory deficit, disorientation, language or perceptual disturbance) that is not due to dementia
- Development over a short period of time and fluctuates
- Not explained by other neurocognitive disorders
- Disturbance is a direct consequence of a medical condition or its treatment.

Sub-Syndromal Delirium

It refers to acute cognitive changes that are compatible with delirium but do not fulfill all delirium criteria

Causes of Delirium (Fig. 14.14)

We can also attempt to categorise the delirium spectrum into subphenotypes, using psychomotor subtypes (known as hypoactive, hyperactive, and mixed).[17]

Another subtype seen in mechanically ventilated patients is a rapidly reversible sedation-related delirium, defined as delirium while receiving sedation that resolved within two hours after stopping sedation during a spontaneous awakening trial.

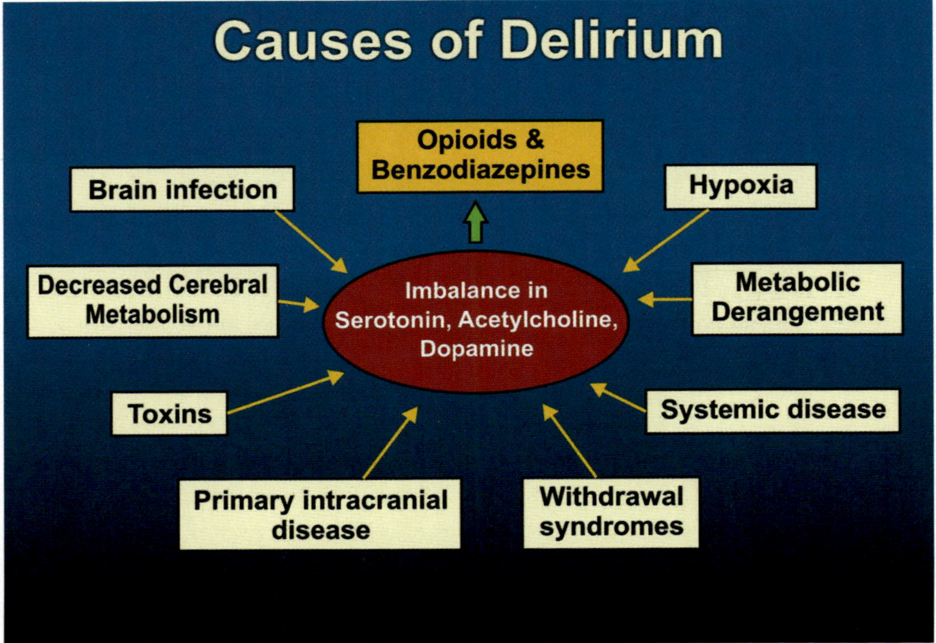

Fig. 14.14: Causes of delirium

The majority of patients suffering from delirium present with the hypoactive subtype. Withdrawn and psychometrically retarded, the patient with hypoactive delirium is frequently thought by caretakers and family to be depressed.

Although these patients cause little disruption to the ICU environment and provoke less acute distress in their caregivers, they are no less subject to the adverse outcomes of altered sensorium. Although the immediate threat to safety may be less apparent in these cases, hypoactive delirium can rapidly and unpredictably evolve into acute agitation as a result of unchecked, upsetting delusions.

Diagnosis

The confusion assessment method for the ICU (CAM-ICU) and the intensive care delirium screening checklist (ICDSC) are the most valid and reliable delirium monitoring tools in adult ICU patients (**Fig. 14.15**).

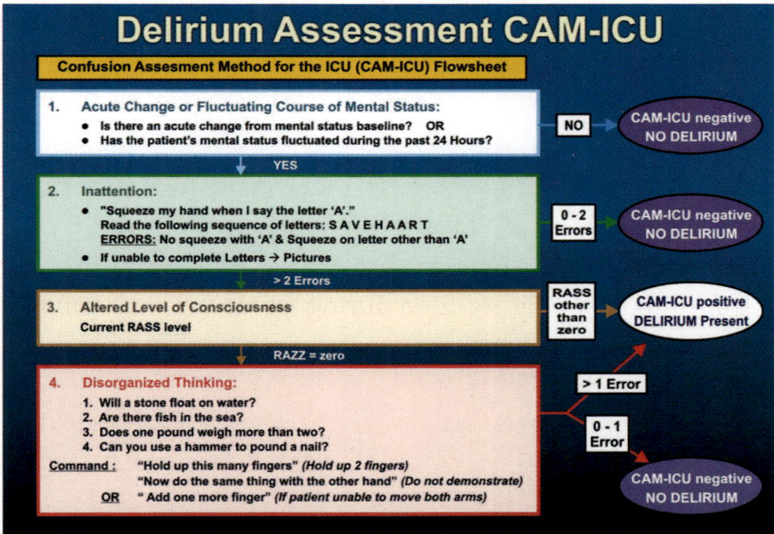

Fig. 14.15: CAM-ICU score

Several other scales have been developed and validated to diagnose delirium in ICU patients (Delirium Detection Score [DDS], Cognitive Test for Delirium [CTD]), Abbreviated Cognitive Test for Delirium.

In recent years, several models have been developed to predict the risk of ICU delirium based on known risk factors for this condition. PRE-DERILIC, E-PRE-DERILIC models have demonstrated moderate predictive ability.[18]

Delirium development is associated with multiple complications (especially in the hypoactive motoric subtype): increased mortality, longer duration of mechanical ventilation, higher reintubation rate, increased hospital stay, higher early instrumental activities of daily living dependence scores, and worse long-term cognition.

Delirium patients show an increased risk of developing post-ICU syndrome, already known to affect patients' perceived quality of life profoundly.

Non-pharmacologic Interventions in Delirium Management

Pain, if any, should be monitored and managed using an objective scale. The patient should be orientated to the date, place and reason for hospitalization.

Whiteboards should be updated with caregiver names. Clocks and calendars should be provided in the room. Current events should be discussed with the patients. The need for hearing aids and/or eyeglasses should be ascertained. Good quality sleep should be assured. Patient-ventilator synchrony should be maintained. Promote comfort and relaxation (e.g. back care, oral care, washing face/hands and daytime bath, massage).

ABCDEF bundle for Management of Delirium (Fig. 14.16)

Recently, an expert panel proposed to update the bundle by adding an "R" for respiratory drive control. The objectives are:

1. Reducing sedatives (especially benzodiazepines and opioids)
2. Preferring more participative ventilation modes, and
3. Optimising management of patient's associated factors of high respiratory demand (metabolic acidosis, fever, pain, anxiety, dyspnoea). Optimisation of ventilator settings should be a priority.

There is conflicting data surrounding the relationship between the use of opioids and the development of delirium in patients. Benzodiazepines may be a risk factor in the development of delirium in patients. There is insufficient data to determine the relationship between the use of propofol and the development of delirium.

Symptoms Pain, agitation, delirium guidelines	Monitoring tools	Care ABCDEF boundle	Done
Pain	Critical care pain observation tool (CPOT) NRS numeric rating scale BPS behavioral pain scale	A: Assess, prevent and manage pain	☐
		B: Both sportaneous awakening trials (SAT) and spontaneous breathing trials (SBT)	☐
Agitation	Richmond agitation-Sedation scale (RASS) Sedation-agitation scale (SAS)	C: Choice of analgesia and sedation	☐
		D: Delirium: Assess, prevent and manage	☐
Delirium	Confusion assessment Method for the intensive Care unit (CAM-ICU) Intensive care delirium Screening checklist (ICDSC)	E: Early mobility and exercise	☐
		F: Family engagement and empowerment	☐

Fig. 14.16: ABCDEF bundle for management of delirium

Dexmedetomidine may be associated with a lower prevalence of delirium compared to benzodiazepines in mechanically ventilated patients.[19] Guidelines recommend that early mobilization of adult ICU patients should be performed whenever feasible to reduce the incidence and duration of delirium.

Guidelines also recommend against the usage of antipsychotics for treating subsyndromal delirium.[4]

Although guidelines do not recommend either haloperidol or atypical antipsychotics, many centres in the world use haloperidol with starting dose of 2–10 mg (5 mg over 5–10 minutes) in treating delirium. This is repeated every 20 minutes till the end point is achieved.

Guidelines also recommend administering dexmedetomidine for delirium in mechanically ventilated adults where agitation is precluding weaning/extubation. Sleep should be promoted by optimizing the patient's environment, using strategies to control light and noise, clustering patient care activities and decreasing stimuli (disturbances) at night.

Guidelines also suggest using a multicomponent, nonpharmacologic intervention that is focused on (but not limited to) reducing modifiable risk factors for delirium, improving cognition, and optimizing sleep, mobility, hearing, and vision in critically ill adults.

Guidelines provide no recommendation for the use of a combined non- pharmacological and pharmacological delirium prevention protocol in adult ICU patients, as this has not been shown to reduce the incidence of delirium.

Summary of Delirium Management (Fig. 14.17)

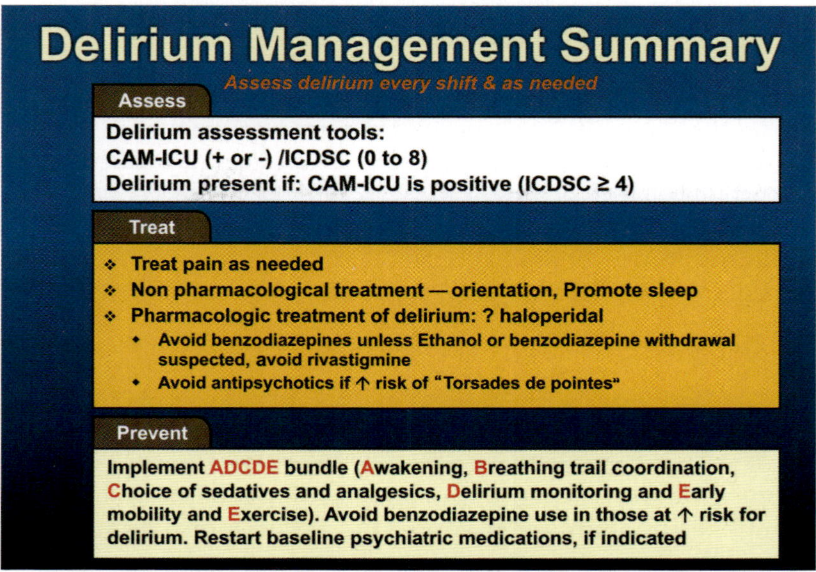

Fig. 14.17: Summary of delirium management

Conclusion

Routinely and separately assess pain, sedation, agitation and delirium using validated tools. Avoid deep sedation. Let patients be interactive. Integrate PAD management with SBT, early mobility and environmental sleep management. Implement the PAD care bundle using an interdisciplinary, team-based approach.

Finally, the overall management of delirium in critically ill patients should not lag. We should try to seek new tools in the new and promising technologies.

Neuromuscular Blockers in Mechanically Ventilated Patients

A better understanding of hazards associated with the use of neuromuscular blockers (NMB) has led to a substantial decline in the use of these drugs in patients on ventilator support. An occasional scenario still demands the use of NMB. Hence, a sound knowledge of these drugs is essential. It should be emphasized that all other modalities to improve the clinical situation must be tried before using

NMBs as a last resort. In the rare patient where NMBs are used, patients should be adequately sedated before initiation of neuromuscular blockade.

Indications for the use of NMBs Include

1. Tracheal intubation
2. Ventilatory modes that are difficult for the patient to tolerate (such as high PEEP, prolonged I:E ratio)
3. Extreme hypoxia/hypercarbia
4. To treat muscle spasms as a last resort when all other means have failed
5. To decrease oxygen consumption
6. Raised intracranial pressure
7. Ventilator/patient dyssynchrony, where appropriate sedation and analgesia have failed
8. To facilitate short procedures

Sometimes boluses of NMBs before and during transportation might increase safety. The use of neuromuscular blockers in mechanically ventilated patients is sometimes inevitable as there is an increased respiratory drive secondary to low tidal volume ventilation and resulting permissible hypoxia and hypercapnia. Studies have shown mortality benefits when NMBs are used in the early management of moderate to severe ARDS.

NMB Drugs

NMBs are structurally related to acetylcholine (ACh) and act by interfering with the binding of ACh to the motor endplate. They are divided into depolarizing (succinylcholine used only for securing the airway) or non-depolarizing (pancuronium, cisatracurium, pipecuronium, rocuronium, and vecuronium) agents based on their mechanism of action. Succinylcholine is the only available depolarizing neuromuscular blocker. It is characterized by rapid onset of effect and ultra-short duration of action because of its rapid hydrolysis by butyrylcholinesterase.

Non-depolarizing neuromuscular blockers available can be classified according to chemical class (steroidal, benzylisoquinolinium, or other compounds) or according to onset or duration of action (long, intermediate, and short-acting drugs) for equipotent doses. The ideal NMB agents for use in intensive care produce an early, titratable paralysis and have a moderately rapid offset of action (less than 15 minutes) to allow for repeated neurologic assessment. No adverse hemodynamic or other adverse physiologic effects should exist. Elimination should be independent of hepatic or renal function. Metabolites produced should be inactive. There should be no propensity to accumulate. It should be stable over 24 hours to allow for continuous infusion. The cost should be modest.

Doses of commonly used NMB (Fig. 14.18)

Doses of commonly used NMB

Drug	Intubating Dose (mg/kg)	Time to Maximum Block (min)	Clinical Duration (min)	Maintenance dose
Succinylcholine	1	1–2		
Rocuronium	0.6	1.7	25–30 min	0.2–0.5 mg/kg/ hour
Vecuronium	0.1	2.4	25–40 min	0.05–0.1 mg/kg/ hour
Pancuronium	0.1	2.4	40–60 min	0.03–0.1 mg/kg/ hour
Atracurium	0.5	3.2	20–40 min	0.3–1.0 mg/kg/ hour
Cisatracurium	0.2	7.7	25–35 min	0.03–0.2 mg/kg/ hour
Mivacurium	0.15	3.3	10–20 min	9–10 μg/kg/min

Fig. 14.18: Doses of commonly used neuromuscular blockers

Suxamethonium produces a large increase in plasma potassium levels that could produce cardiac arrest and hence should be used with caution in certain situations. Suxamethonium is contraindicated in patients with renal failure, neuromuscular disease, and paraplegia and those with muscular atrophy due to long-term ICU or hospital stays. Suxamethonium-induced fasciculations may lead to increased intracranial pressure and should therefore be avoided in patients with pre-existing raised ICP.

Rarely, suxamethonium may cause malignant hyperthermia. In all such circumstances, the use of a rapid onset non-depolarising agent such as rocuronium is preferred. The usual dose of suxamethonium is 1–2 mg/kg.

The majority of patients in an ICU who are prescribed an NMB agent can be managed effectively with pancuronium. For patients for whom vagolysis is contraindicated (e.g. those with cardiovascular disease), NMB agents other than pancuronium may be used. Because of their unique metabolism (Hofmann elimination), cisatracurium or atracurium is recommended for patients with significant hepatic/renal disease.

For patients on corticosteroids, every effort should be made to discontinue NMBs as soon as possible.

Drugs which may potentiate/antagonize the action of non-depolarizing NMB are listed below (Fig. 14.19):

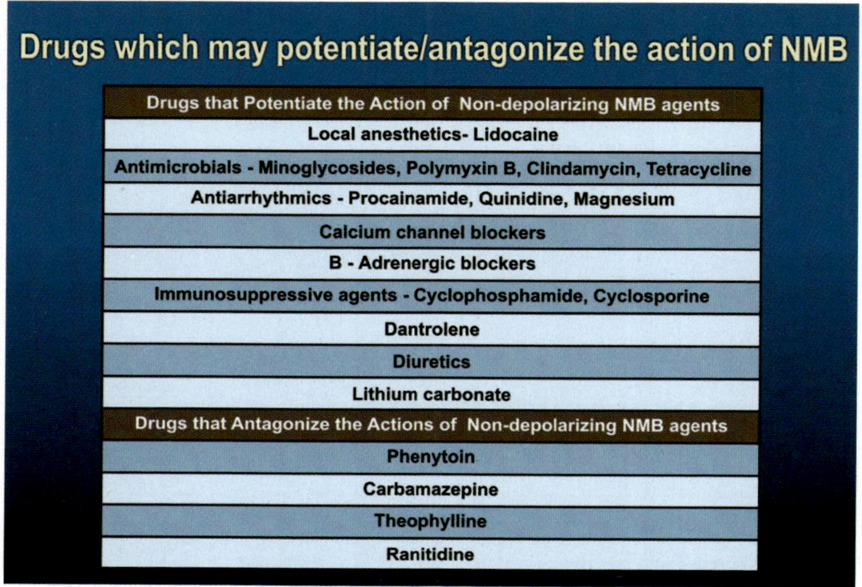

Drugs which may potentiate/antagonize the action of NMB

Drugs that Potentiate the Action of Non-depolarizing NMB agents
Local anesthetics- Lidocaine
Antimicrobials - Minoglycosides, Polymyxin B, Clindamycin, Tetracycline
Antiarrhythmics - Procainamide, Quinidine, Magnesium
Calcium channel blockers
B - Adrenergic blockers
Immunosuppressive agents - Cyclophosphamide, Cyclosporine
Dantrolene
Diuretics
Lithium carbonate
Drugs that Antagonize the Actions of Non-depolarizing NMB agents
Phenytoin
Carbamazepine
Theophylline
Ranitidine

Fig. 14.19: Drug interactions with neuromuscular blockers

Monitoring of Neuromuscular Blockade

Current guidelines recommend the routine monitoring of the depth of neuromuscular blockade in critically ill patients.

Careful clinical monitoring of the patient for signs consistent with inadequate sedation or analgesia—such as tachycardia, hypertension, salivation, and lacrimation—while receiving NMBAs is important.

The modality of choice to monitor the depth of nondepolarizing neuromuscular blockade at present is train-of-four (TOF) monitoring. A value <0.7 is considered adequate paralysis.

In a recent study that compared three strategies for using NMB (a fixed dose of cisatracurium; titration based solely on TOF and a ventilator synchrony protocol), it was shown that a protocol using ventilator synchrony for cisatracurium titration required significantly less drug compared to TOF-based titration and a fixed dosing regimen

Adverse Effects of using Neuromuscular Blockers

There will be life-threatening hypoxia in the event of accidental tracheal airway extubation. Neuromuscular blockers contribute to ICU-acquired weakness in some patients. Steroid-based neuromuscular blocking agents (pancuronium and vecuronium especially) are most commonly implicated. Protective reflexes are reduced resulting in an increased risk of micro-aspirations and the development of ventilator-associated pneumonia (VAP).

Measures to prevent corneal abrasion like artificial tears should be instilled every two to four hours and eyelids should be taped shut. Neuromuscular blockers exacerbate complications related to immobility. There is probably an increased risk of deep vein thrombosis (DVT), muscle wasting and peripheral nerve injury.

All paralyzed patients require the following precautions to prevent complications. Ensure adequate sedation and analgesia before paralyzing the patient. Back up ventilation rate and settings have to be properly set. Supervise patients closely, as interruption of the ventilator circuit can be fatal.

Patients require frequent posture changes and specialized mattresses to prevent skin breakdown and decubitus ulcers. Prophylactic deep venous thrombosis therapy with either low-dose subcutaneous heparin or mechanical compression devices is mandatory. The head end of the bed should be elevated to 450 to reduce the risk of aspiration, particularly during enteral feeding. Pupillary reflexes should be closely monitored to assess neurologic status (unreliable if pancuronium is used as it has antimuscarinic effects).

The majority of patients hospitalized in an ICU will undergo postsynaptic upregulation of nAChRs due to immobility, upper and/or lower motor neuron lesions, and/or pharmacologic denervation (such as NMBAs and aminoglycoside antibiotics). This will lead to increased sensitivity to depolarizing NMBAs and decreased sensitivity to nondepolarizing NMBAs. Furthermore, these changes in receptor distribution and physiology put the patient at a heightened risk of succinylcholine-induced hyperkalemia.

Intensive Care Unit-acquired Weakness

Intensive care unit-acquired weakness (ICUAW) is a term used to describe all weaknesses developed in critically ill patients after the onset of illness and in the absence of any identifiable causes. ICUAW is further classified into three entities: critical illness polyneuropathy (CIP), critical illness myopathy (CIM), and critical illness neuromyopathy.[20]

Nondepolarizing muscle relaxants of both classes, aminosteroids and benzylisoquinoliniums, have been associated with the development of these neuromuscular disorders.

Atrophy and weakness are observed primarily in muscles of the trunk and extremities, and functional denervation of muscle with NMBAs in conjunction with corticosteroid therapy seems to heighten the risk of myopathy.

Conclusion

NMB use in mechanically ventilated patients has substantially declined over a time. Except for intubation and initial 48 hours of Severe ARDS ventilation, NMB is usually avoided.[21] Clinicians should be aware of adverse effects, associated with their use. Institution-based protocols for sedation, NMB use and weaning should be in place to minimize the use of NMB.

TAKE HOME POINTS (Fig. 14.20)

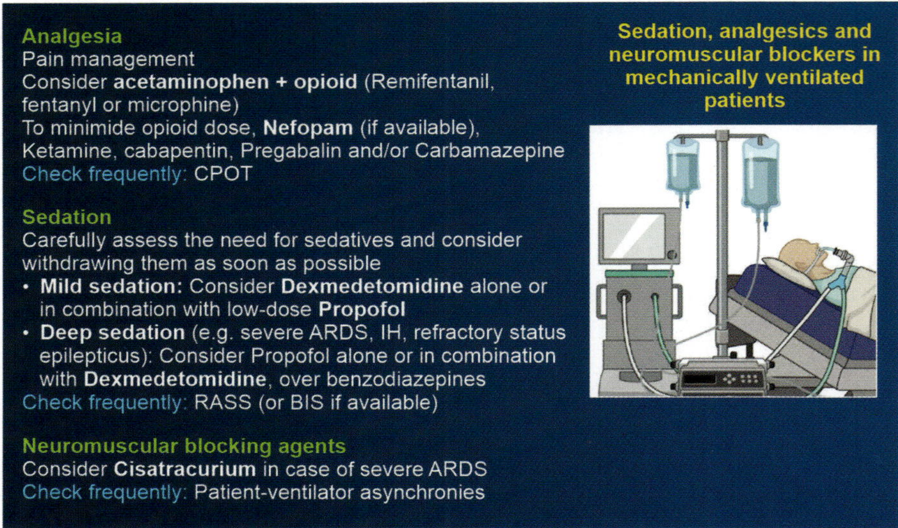

Fig. 14.20: Take home points

References

1. Brush DR, Kress JP. Sedation and Analgesia for the Mechanically Ventilated Patient. Clin Chest Med. 2009 Mar 1;30(1):131–41.
2. Devabhakthuni S, Armahizer MJ, Dasta JF, Kane-Gill SL. Analgosedation: a paradigm shift in intensive care unit sedation practice. Ann Pharmacother. 2012 Apr;46(4):530–40.
3. Dhabhar FS, Malarkey WB, Neri E, McEwen BS. Stress-induced Redistribution of Immune Cells-from Barracks to Boulevards to Battlefields: A Tale of Three Hormones-curt Richter Award Winner. Psychoneuroendocrinology. 2012 Sep;37(9):1345.
4. Devlin JW, Skrobik Y, Gélinas C, Needham DM, Slooter AJC, Pandharipande PP, *et al.* Executive Summary: Clinical Practice Guidelines for the Prevention and Management of Pain, Agitation/Sedation, Delirium, Immobility, and Sleep Disruption in Adult Patients in the ICU. Crit Care Med. 2018 Sep 1;46(9):1532–48.
5. Use of Sedatives, Analgesics, and Neuromuscular Blockers | Clinical Gate [Internet].
6. Severgnini P, Pelosi P, Contino E, Serafinelli E, Novario R, Chiaranda M. Accuracy of Critical Care Pain Observation Tool and Behavioral Pain Scale to assess pain in critically ill conscious and unconscious patients: Prospective, observational study. J Intensive Care. 2016 Nov 7;4(1):1–8.
7. Tick H, Nielsen A, Pelletier KR, Bonakdar R, Simmons S, Glick R, *et al.* Evidence-Based Nonpharmacologic Strategies for Comprehensive Pain Care: The Consortium Pain Task Force White Paper. EXPLORE. 2018 May 1;14(3):177–211.
8. Olsen HT, Nedergaard HK, Strøm T, Oxlund J, Wian K-A, Ytrebø LM, *et al.* Nonsedation or Light Sedation in Critically Ill, Mechanically Ventilated Patients. New England Journal of Medicine. 2020 Mar 19;382(12):1103–11.
9. Sessler CN, Gosnell MS, Grap MJ, Brophy GM, O'Neal P v., Keane KA, *et al.* The Richmond Agitation–Sedation Scale. https://doi.org/101164/rccm2107138. 2012 Dec 20;166(10):1338–44.

10. Girard TD, Kress JP, Fuchs BD, Thomason JW, Schweickert WD, Pun BT, *et al.* Efficacy and safety of a paired sedation and ventilator weaning protocol for mechanically ventilated patients in intensive care (Awakening and Breathing Controlled trial): a randomised controlled trial. The Lancet. 2008 Jan 12;371(9607):126–34.
11. Jonkman AH, de Vries HJ, Heunks LMA. Physiology of the Respiratory Drive in ICU Patients: Implications for Diagnosis and Treatment. Crit Care. 2020 Mar 24;24(1):104–104.
12. Vaschetto R, Cammarota G, Colombo D, Longhini F, Grossi F, Giovanniello A, *et al.* Effects of propofol on patient-ventilator synchrony and interaction during pressure support ventilation and neurally adjusted ventilatory assist. Crit Care Med. 2014;42(1):74–82.
13. Chanques G, Constantin JM, Devlin JW, Ely EW, Fraser GL, Gélinas C, *et al.* Analgesia and sedation in patients with ARDS. Intensive Care Med. 2020 Dec 1;46(12):2342–56.
14. Gélinas C, Joffe AM, Szumita PM, Payen JF, Bérubé M, Shahiri ST, *et al.* A Psychometric Analysis Update of Behavioral Pain Assessment Tools for Noncommunicative, Critically Ill Adults. AACN Adv Crit Care. 2019;30(4):365–87.
15. Vinclair M, Schilte C, Roudaud F, Lavolaine J, Francony G, Bouzat P, *et al.* Using Pupillary Pain Index to Assess Nociception in Sedated Critically Ill Patients. Anesth Analg. 2019 Dec 1;129(6):1540–6.
16. Pandharipande P, Cotton BA, Shintani A, Thompson J, Pun BT, Morris JA, *et al.* PREVALENCE AND RISK FACTORS FOR DEVELOPMENT OF DELIRIUM IN SURGICAL AND TRAUMA ICU PATIENTS. J Trauma. 2008 Jul;65(1):34.
17. Bowman EML, Cunningham EL, Page VJ, McAuley DF. Phenotypes and subphenotypes of delirium: a review of current categorisations and suggestions for progression. Crit Care. 2021 Dec 1;25(1).
18. Linkaité G, Riauka M, Bunevičiūté I, Vosylius S. Evaluation of PRE-DELIRIC (PREdiction of DELIRium in ICu patients) delirium prediction model for the patients in the intensive care unit. Acta Med Litu. 2018 May 14;25(1):14.
19. Flükiger J, Hollinger A, Speich B, Meier V, Tontsch J, Zehnder T, *et al.* Dexmedetomidine in prevention and treatment of postoperative and intensive care unit delirium: a systematic review and meta-analysis. Ann Intensive Care. 2018 Dec 1;8(1):1–15.
20. Jolley SE, Bunnell AE, Hough CL. ICU-Acquired Weakness. Chest. 2016 Nov 1;150(5):1129.
21. Early Neuromuscular Blockade in the Acute Respiratory Distress Syndrome. New England Journal of Medicine. 2019 May 23;380(21):1997–2008.

CHAPTER 15

Suctioning

❐ Anitha Patil GK ❐ Narasimha Murthy T

Removing of secretions from the airway by mechanical aspiration is known as **suctioning.**

Airway Obstruction can be Caused by Retained Secrections

It can cause hypoxemia, hypercapina, atelectasis and infection. Suctioning is performed when the patient is unable to effectively move secretions from the respiratory track. Other reason for suctioning is to maintain the patency of artificial airways such as endotreacheal tube or tracheostomy tube. ***Suctioning is the application of negative pressure to the airways through a suction catheter.*** Suctioning can be done either orally with rigid yankauer/suction catheter for upper airways or through aritifical airway for lower airways (**Fig. 15.1**).

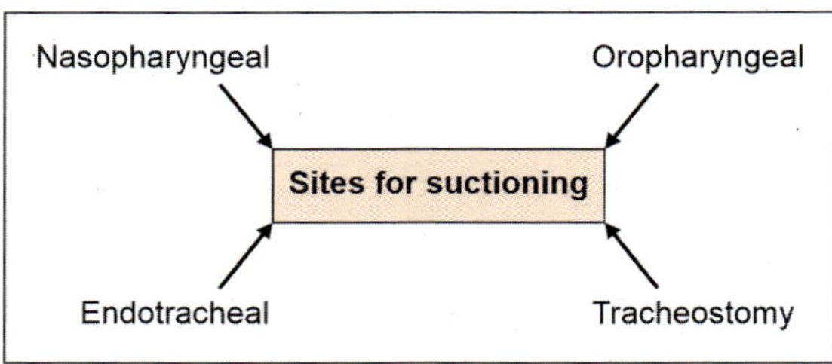

Fig. 15.1: Sites for suctioning

Endotracheal Suctioning (ETS)

ETS is one of the most common bronchial hygiene therapy done in patients with mechanical ventilation to prevent airway obstuction. ***It should be done on need basis not as routine procedure and it should be done cautiously.***

There are 2 types of ETS: **Open and Closed suction**. In open suctioning technique requires disconnecting the patient from the ventilator whereas in closed suction patient remains connected to the ventilator and sterile in-line catheter is used which allows passage of a suction catheter through the artifical airway (**Fig. 15.2**).

There are 2 types of suctioning based on how far the catheter depth should be during the procedure: **Deep and Shallow. Deep suctioning** is insertion of the catheter until resistance is felt followed by withdrawal of the catheter by 1 cm before application of

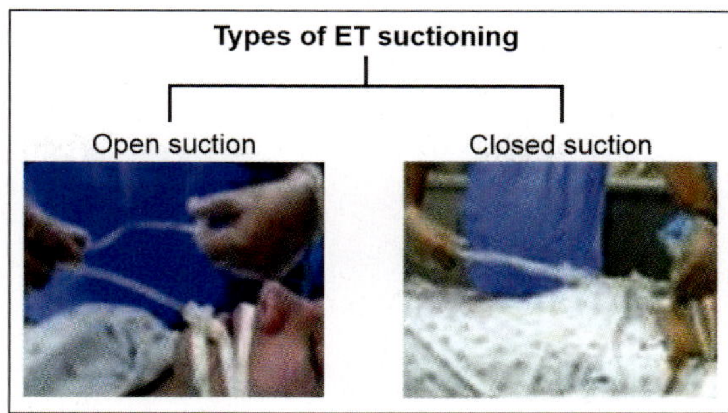

Fig. 15.2: Types of ET suctioning

negative pressure. **Shallow suctioning** is insertion of a catheter to a predetermined depth usually the length of the artifical airway.

Indication

1. Patient's inability to generate effective cough
2. Coarse breath sounds during auscultation
3. Visible secrections in the ET tube
4. Sawtooth pattern on flow-volume loop on ventilator monitor
5. Increased peak pressure on volume control ventilation and decrease tidal voulme on pressure control ventilation
6. Falling saturation (hypoxia)
7. Need to obtain a tracheal aspirate for microbiological examination

Complications

1. Cardiac arrhythmias
2. **Pulmonary atelectasis:** Intrapulmonary pressure becomes negative due to suction, which in turn cause removal of gases from the lung
3. Hypoxemia
4. Vagal stimulation
5. Hypertension, hypotension
6. Bronchospasm
7. Infection
8. Increase intracranial pressure
9. **Mucosal trauma:** Occurs if the suctioning is done more vigorously. Trauma results in small hemorrhagic areas seen in aspiration as blood steaks.

Contraindications

There is no absolute contraindication for ETS. Patient with increased ICP and with severe hypertrnsion should be avioded.

Suction Catheter

A suction catheter is a long flexible tube made up of polyvinylchloride material, which makes it easier to inspect the secretions for quantity, color and thickness. The distal end of the catheter is open with one lateral eye. When distal end is blocked with thick secrections then through lateral eye secrections will come out. It is recommended to choose smaller size suction catheter for suctioning. Diameter of the suction catheter should be approximately half of the diameter of the ETT which allows gases to flow around the catheter during suctioning (**Figs 15.3 and 15.4**).

To calculate the French (Fr) suction catheter size is:

Fr = (ETT size in mm – 2) × 2

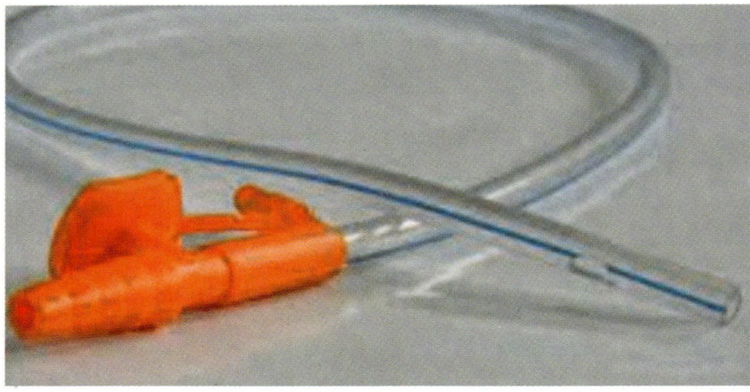

Fig. 15.3: Suction catheter

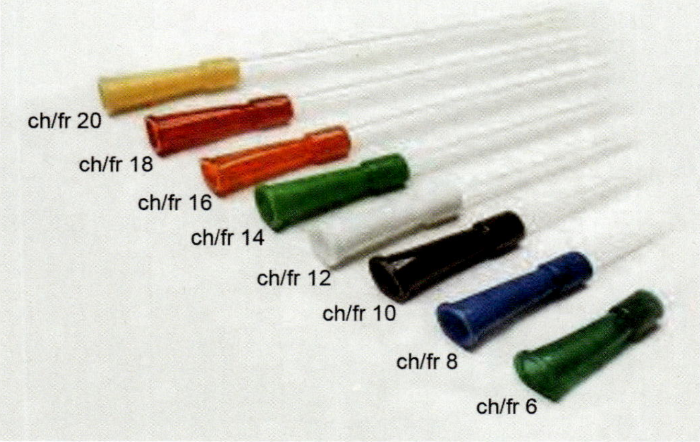

Fig. 15.4: Different colours and sizes of suction catheter

Closed Suctioning

Facilitates continous mechanical ventilation and oxygenation during the suctioning event. It may prevent lung derecruitment assosicated with the use of open suction system. Closed suctioning should be considered in patients requiring high FiO_2 and PEEP. Daily changing the in-line catheter will not decrease the risk of VAP. The closed suction catheter is protected inside the sterile sleeve (**Fig. 15.5**).

Suctioning the patients airway should be based on a **clinical assessment, not on routine basis**. Hyperinflation and hyperoxygenation via the respirator could minimise suctioning induced hypoxemia and result in less hemodynamic alteration.

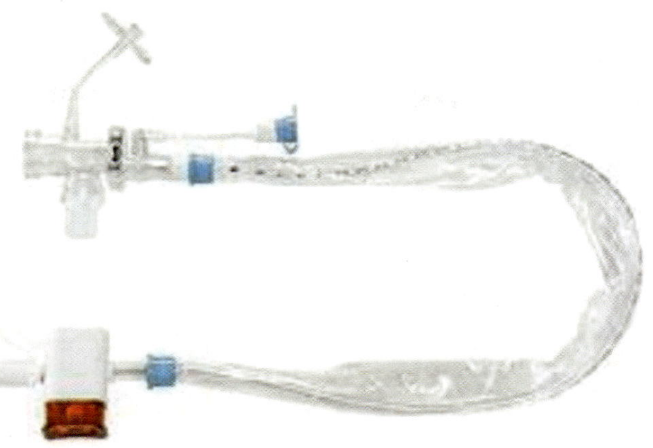

Fig. 15.5: Closed suction catheter

Equipment Required for Suctioning

1. Vacuum source
2. Calibrated, adjustable regulator
3. Collection bottle and connecting tubing
4. Gloves: Sterile (open suction)
   Clean (closed suction)
5. Goggles, mask
6. Sterile suction catheter
7. Sterile saline
8. Manual resuscitation bag for ventilation
9. Continuous monitoring equipment for pulse oximetry and heart rate

Recommended Negative Pressure for Suctioning

1. Adult: 100 to 120 mmHg
2. Children: 80 to 100 mmHg
3. Infants: 60 to 80 mmHg

Technique

1. Assemble all the neccessary equipment and check their functioning before starting the procedure.
2. Wash hands before and after the procedure.
3. Eye protection to the person who is doing the procedure should be done with the help of goggles .
4. Preoxygenate the patient with 100% oxygen for at least 3 minutes before and after suctioning.
5. No suction while inserting the catheter into the ETT. Insert gently. Apply suction while withdrawing the catheter using a rotating motion
6. Duration of each suction event should be approx. 10–15 secs

7. 20–30 seconds interval should be given in between the 2 insertions
8. Rinse the catheter with sterile saline after ETT suctioning and use the same catheter for oral suctioning and finally dispose off both catheter and gloves
9. Use of normal saline while suctioning is not recommended due to increase in nosocomial pneumonia by displacing bacteria from the walls of the airways .
10. If secrections are tenacious instill acetylcysteine which is more effective than normal sailne

References

1. American Association for Respiratory Care (AARC). Clinical Practice Guidelines. Endotracheal suctioning of mechanically ventilated patients with artificial airways 2010. Respir Care. 2010 Jun;55(6):758–64. [PubMed]
2. Pritchard M, Flenady V, Woodgate P. Preoxygenation for tracheal suctioning in intubated, ventilated newborn infants. Cochrane Database Syst Rev. 2001;(3):CD000427. [PMC free article] [PubMed]
3. Wilińska M, Zielińska M, Szreter T, Lesiuk W, Wilkowski J, Ziółkowski J, Swietliński J. [Endotracheal suctioning in neonates and children]. Med Wieku Rozwoj. 2008 Oct-Dec;12(4 Pt 1):878-84. [PubMed]
4. Stoller JK, Orens DK, Fatica C, Elliott M, Kester L, Woods J, Hoffman-Hogg L, Karafa MT, Arroliga AC. Weekly versus daily changes of in-line suction catheters: impact on rates of ventilator-associated pneumonia and associated costs. Respir Care. 2003 May;48(5):494–9. [PubMed]
5. Pedersen CM, Rosendahl-Nielsen M, Hjermind J, Egerod I. Endotracheal suctioning of the adult intubated patient–what is the evidence? Intensive Crit Care Nurs. 2009 Feb;25(1):21–30. [PubMed]
6. Boo NY, Suhaida AR, Rohana J. Frequent nasopharyngeal suctioning as a risk factor associated with neonatal coagulase-negative staphylococcal colonisation and sepsis. Singapore Med J. 2015 Mar;56(3):164–8. [PMC free article] [PubMed]
7. Muthu V, Sehgal IS, Prasad KT, Agarwal R. Iatrogenic pneumothorax following vigorous suctioning of mucus plug during flexible bronchoscopy. BMJ Case Rep. 2019 Oct 05;12(10) [PMC free article] [PubMed].
8. Singh NC, Kissoon N, Frewen T, Tiffin N. Physiological responses to endotracheal and oral suctioning in paediatric patients: the influence of endotracheal tube sizes and suction pressures. Clin Intensive Care. 1991;2(6):345–50. [PubMed]
9. Stille CJ, Honigfeld L, Heitlinger LA, Kuo DZ, Werner EJ. The Pediatric Primary Care-Specialist Interface: A Call For Action. J Pediatr. 2017 Aug;187:303–08. [PubMed]
10. Oberwaldner B, Eber E. Tracheostomy care in the home. Paediatr Respir Rev. 2006 Sep;7(3):185–90. [PubMed]

CHAPTER 16

Strategies and Protocols to Prevent and Manage Hospital Acquired Infections in Patients on Mechanical Ventilator

❒ Monalisa Sahu ❒ Sudipta Mukherjee

INTRODUCTION

Mechanical ventilator is an advance respiratory support in intensive care. It has been used for acute or impending cardiorespiratory failure or to protect unsecured airway in an unconscious patient. During its inception at the time of polio pandemic, it had started its journey as negative pressure ventilation when the whole body was inside an iron chamber.[1] Nowadays, we have shifted fully to positive pressure ventilation when a cuffed endotracheal tube (ETT) is inserted inside the trachea and connected with ventilator. With the cuff of ETT inflated via a pilot balloon, the internal circuit of the ventilator, external circuit, endotracheal tube and patient's airway and lung will become a closed system, making positive pressure ventilation feasible. But at the same time, we are bypassing our upper airway protective mechanisms by putting the ETT in the lower airway. So, once a pathogenic bacteria get access to the lower airway around the endotracheal tube, it can get colonized there and depending on local immunity, can cause infection–tracheobronchitis or pneumonia. Besides, as the patient is critically ill and mostly restricted to the bed to begin with; usually central vascular access for medications, nasogastric tube for enteral feeding and urinary catheter are present. All these invasive or semi-invasive catheters and lines make the patient more vulnerable to infection. Strict infection control protocols are recommended to minimize the risk of ventilation and hospital acquired (hospital associated infection or HAI will be a more appropriate term) infections in every critical care unit. All these infection rates are important quality indications for any hospital.

Airway Defense Mechanisms

Human beings have different protective mechanism in both upper and lower airway to prevent entry of microorganism into the lung.[2] Nasal mucosa is the first line of prevention. Nasal cavity, paranasal sinuses and trachea are lined by pseudostratified columnar ciliated epithelial cells with a layer of mucus. Particulate materials get trapped in the mucus layer and by effective ciliary movement, they are pushed towards pharynx to be thrown out with cough or get swallowed to the acidic gastric milieu. Along with mucociliary transport, epithelial cells themselves act as an important barrier preventing entry to bacteria or virus to the deeper tissue even during acute inflammation. Mucus produced by serous and mucinous glands along with goblet cells form a protective layer over the epithelium preventing it from getting injured by bacteria and its toxins. It also contains immunoglobulin (Ig) A, lysozyme, lactoferrin, different proteases and other antibacterial molecule with varied bacteriostatic and bactericidal properties. IgG production at the local site along with complements help in opsonization of microbes followed by phagocytosis by macrophages. Proinflammatory cytokines and chemokines released at the inflamed site lead to recruitment of more macrophages followed by neutrophils and lymphocytes. The pathogenic bacteria get killed by the proteolytic enzymes and cytokines—a mechanism called "respiratory burst". Cough reflex eventually removes all the end products with mucus. All these mechanisms work in association to prevent entry of pathogenic bacteria in the lower airway. Whenever the protective mechanisms fail to function as per expectation, or there is a drop in local immunity, or the local load of microbes supersede the protective capacity; bacteria get access to the lower respiratory system leading to serious infection.

Pathophysiological Challenges with Endotracheal Intubation

Putting an endotracheal tube will compromise the protective mechanisms of airway.[3] It bypasses all the mechanical barrier provided by airway and deliver the gas directly to the lower respiratory system. It compromises effectiveness of cough reflex making the patient more prone to aspiration. During hospital stay, the oropharynx of the patients gets colonized with multidrug resistant (MDR) Gram-negative bacteria replacing his normal flora. Some high-risk patients (e.g. patients with multiple hospital admissions, broad spectrum antibiotic usage, critical illness, on haemodialysis) may be already colonized with MDR bugs even at admission. Oropharyngeal secretion along with these MDR bugs get collected over ETT cuff and leads to micro-aspiration through the creases. Besides, the bacteria form a biofilm inside the ETT lumen as there is no access of antibiotics in that area. This biofilm acts as a source of infection and leads to entry of bacteria to the lower respiratory system with mechanical breaths. It may be aggravated by a drop in local immunity. Presence of orogastric or nasogastric tube compromise the patency of upper esophageal sphincter and along with supine position, may increase the risk of aspiration. Presence of nasogastric tube or ETT through the nasal cavity (uncommon practice in critical care medicine) may compromise the drainage of paranasal sinuses, leading to retention of secretion and sinusitis.

Ventilated patients are mostly sick and requiring other invasive lines like central vascular access and urinary catheter, leading to infection related to those lines. Restricted mobilization in bed, specially when fractional inspiratory oxygen (FiO_2) and positive end expiratory pressure (PEEP) requirements are high, may lead to pressure sore and subsequently skin and soft tissue infection. They usually come under hospital associated infection (HAI) and does not have direct relationship with mechanical ventilation. But an association is very commonly seen in our daily practice.

HOSPITAL-ASSOCIATED INFECTIONS (HAI)

Hospital-associated infections are the major challenge in current critical care setting. It is defined as infection acquired by the patient while they are receiving healthcare or soon after receiving healthcare (CDC definition).[4] The timeline is 48 hours after hospital admission or within 30 days of receiving healthcare service.[5] It causes significant morbidity and mortality to hospitalised patients along with cost burden to the patient and to the healthcare system. Hospital associated infection (HAI) is a more scientific term rather than hospital acquired; as most of the time patients develop infection with their own bacteria colonized inside the body (e.g. gut, nasopharynx, etc.).

In an intubated patient, the following HAIs are most important:

- Ventilator-associated pneumonia (VAP), currently termed as ventilator associated events (VAEs)
- Catheter-associated blood stream infection (CLABSI)
- Catheter-associated urinary tract infection (CAUTI)

Ventilator-Associated Events (VAEs)[6]

Ventilator-associated pneumonia (VAP) is a new onset lower respiratory tract infection while the patient is on mechanical ventilation. It is characterized by worsening respiratory function along with inflammatory, radiological and microbiological criteria.[7] It is a clinical diagnosis with lots of interobserver variability. Diagnostic criteria are not very sensitive or specific leading to significant diagnostic dilemma.[8] So, centers for Disease Control and Prevention (CDC) has modified it to a more objective surveillance definition, i.e. ventilator associated event (VAE).

VAEs[9] is diagnosed when there is a progressive deterioration of respiratory function after initial stabilization for 2 or more days on ventilator, measured in terms of FiO_2 and PEEP changes (increase compared to its baseline value). It needs to be associated with inflammatory markers, empirical escalation in antibiotics and microbiologically positive report of respiratory sample or pleural fluid. It has been divided into three categories by CDC:

1. **Ventilator-associated condition (VAC):** VAC is defined as deterioration of respiratory function (for 2 or more days) after a period of improvement or stabilization (stable for 2 or more calendar days). Worsening respiratory function is measured by increase in FiO_2 by >0.2 or increase in PEEP by 3 cm H_2O.

2. **Infection-related ventilator-associated condition (IVAC):** IVAC is considered when VAC is associated with:
   - Positive inflammatory markers (temperature >38°C or <36°C/white blood cell count >12,000 cells/mm^3 or <4,000 cells/mm^3) and
   - Antimicrobial escalation for 4 or more days

3. **Possible-ventilator-associated pneumonia (PVAP):** PVAP will be diagnosed if IVAC is present along with:
   - Positive microbiological culture (by quantitative or semiqualitative method) from appropriate respiratory sample (tracheobronchial secretion or lung tissue) **(Table 16.1)**
   - Purulent respiratory sample with insufficient microbiological growth
   - Organism identified from pleural fluid or lung histopathology
   - Organism identified by non-culture-based tests (PCR based method)

Table 16.1: Microbiological cut-off for qualitative culture method from different respiratory sample

Type of sample	Microbiological cut-off
Endotracheal aspirate	$\geq 10^5$ CFU/ml
Bronchoalveolar lavage (bronchoscopy guided or blind)	$\geq 10^4$ CFU/ml
Protected specimen brushing (bronchoscopy guided or blind)	$\geq 10^3$ CFU/ml
Lung tissue	$\geq 10^4$ CFU/gm

CFU = Colony forming unit

Adopted from: Ventilator associated event (VAE), National healthcare safety network, CDC

Catheter Associated Blood-Stream Infection

Mechanically ventilated patients usually have invasive lines for giving multiple medications, like central venous line (CVL), for organ support like haemodialysis (HD) line and also for monitoring purpose like pulmonary arterial catheter (PAC) and arterial line. Although these invasive lines have important role to play in patient management; they put the patient at increased risk of infection. CVL is most common among the lot and nearly all ventilated ICU patients have CVL. Some long-standing patients may have peripherally inserted central line (PICC). Haemato-oncology and transplant patients have long term catheters like Hickman catheter or permcath. Infection to any of these invasive lines cause substantial morbidity to the patients, in terms of removal of line, sending laboratory work up, insertion of new line along with complications related to sepsis. It prolongs ICU stay, hospital stay, cost of therapy and can also cause death.[10]

Central line (CL), by definition, is an access that terminates at, or closer to heart in a great vessel (e.g. aorta, pulmonary artery, superior or inferior vena cava, internal jugular and subclavian vein, femoral and iliac vein, etc.) and used for infusion or transfusion of product, blood sampling and haemodynamic monitoring.[11] Routine arterial line and intra-aortic balloon pump are not considered as CL.

- **Primary blood-stream infection (Primary BSI):** It is laboratory confirmed bloodstream infection (LCBI) not secondary to infection to any specific organ/body site.
- **Secondary BSI:** LCBI due to infection to another body site/any specific organ (e.g. pneumonia, urosepsis, surgical site infection).
- **Central line associated BSI (CLABSI):** LCBI where an 'eligible' organism has been identified, and an 'eligible central line' (>2 days old) present on the positive culture day or before, without any evidence of secondary site of infection (LCBI 1).
- The 'eligible' organism must not be a commensal. If it is commensal, it should be clearly present in two or more blood samples sent separately, without any secondary source along with clinical symptoms (e.g. fever, chill, hypotension) (LCBI 2).
- **Mucosal barrier injury laboratory confirmed blood-stream infection (MBI – LCBI):** LCBI in an immunocompromised patient (post-transplant, neutropenic) where intestine is the source of infection and organisms are mostly enterobacteriaceae. Occasionally Viridans group of *Streptococcus* or *Rothia* sp. can cause can also be the causative agent (LCBI 2). Patient's factors are allogenic hematopoietic stem cell

transplant less than one year with Grade 3 or 4 gut Graft vs Host Disease (GVHD) or diarrhoea >1 lit/day within 7 days of positive culture, or neutropenic (absolute neutrophil count <500/mm^3 for two consecutive days) within 7 days of positive culture.

Catheter-associate Urinary Tract Infection (CAUTI)

Urinary catheter is another important semi-invasive line present routinely in critically ill patients. Urine output monitoring is an important component of ICU monitoring and indicates overall tissue perfusion. Besides, it is a marker of renal function and diagnostic criteria for acute renal failure. Up to 25% of hospitalized patients usually have urinary catheter sometimes during their stay. But it has its own risk. It can cause bacterial colonisation and may lead to infection to urinary system. It can be cystitis, urethritis, posterities, pyelonephritis, etc. Proximity to anal canal increase the risk of infection without strict catheter handling protocol. Up to 75% of hospital associated UTI happened in presence of a catheter.

- CAUTI: It is defined as presence of clinical features of UTI along with >10^3 CFU of ≥1 bacterial growth in single catheter urine specimen or midstream urine specimen with catheter removed within 48 hours.[12]
- Catheter associated asymptomatic bacteriuria (CA-ASB)-CA-ASB is diagnosed if >10^5 CFU of ≥1 bacterial growth present in single catheter urine sample without clinical findings suggestive of UTI.
- Clinical finding of UTI in a ventilated patients are new or worsening fever, encephalopathy (requiring higher dose of sedation to keep on ventilator), flank pain /costovertebral point tenderness, haematuria. Pyuria is not diagnostic of CAUTI or CA-ASB; but its absence most likely rules out CAUTI and suggest clinicians to look for other diagnosis.

PREVENTIVE STRATEGIES AGAINST HAI

HAIs are preventable to a great extent.[13] Its incidence varies significantly from institution to institution and from country to country.[14] It mostly depends on infection prevention and control (IPC) practices of the unit and quality of nursing care. Regular training and education of the clinical team involved in patient care (e.g. doctors, nurses, housekeeping personnel, data entry officers) along with close monitoring and regular audit for the protocol compliance and hospital associated infection rate are of paramount importance. These patient centric interventions are called 'bundle'. Bundles are a group of evidence-based interventions targeting a specific clinical condition and together they shown to improve clinical outcome. There are different care bundles to ensure certain level of care, compared to an international standard. Outcome of these care bundles in before-after implementation studies are heterogenous and did not show positive outcome in all scenarios.[15,16] There can be different reasons for it. It depends on the protocol compliance of the unit along with the quality of baseline nursing and infection control practice. Besides, the basic protocol and interventions varied from study to study generating a very heterogenous kind of data.[17] All the interventions are also not supported by equal weightage of evidence. It is advisable to have written policies and check lists to prevent or minimize HAI in every clinical unit as per local challenges.

FAST HUG BIDS

This is a basic care protocol for critically ill patients in intensive care unit **(Table 16.2)**. Even in developed countries, medical errors are not uncommon along with variation in medical management. Implementing different standard protocols in patient management and following them up with varied auditable checklist can really streamline clinical practice. Daily clinical assessment is an important component of patient's care. It is advisable to review all the salient points of this pneumonic to optimize clinical management. It was developed for critically ill patients; but it is well applicable for mechanically ventilated patients too—both medical and surgical.[18]

Table 16.2: FAST HUGS BID components

	Components	Interventions
F	Feeding	NPO/oral/ enteral/ parenteral
A	Analgesia	VAS monitoring
S	Sedation	GCS/RASS score monitoring
T	Thromboprophylaxis	Mechanical, pharmacological
H	Head end elevation	30–45°
U	Ulcerative prophylaxis	H_2B or PPI
G	Glycemic control	Target CBG – 140–180 mg /dl
S	Spontaneous breathing trial	Pressure support or non-invasive ventilation
B	Bowel	Diarrhea, constipation, distension
I	Indwelling catheters	Remove if not required
D	Drug de-escalation	Antibiotics optimisation

VAS: Visual analog score; GCS: Glasgow Coma Score; RASS: Richmond Agitation Sedation Score; H_2B:H_2 blocker; PPI: Proton pump inhibitor

There are small modifications happened over time according to the specific need of the patients–specially for the surgical patients[19] and some components have been expanded (e.g. delirium, pressure sore, abdominal drain output, etc.) to improve patient monitoring.

Feeding: Nutrition is an important component of patient recovery. It is advisable to start enteral nutrition 'early' after the initial resuscitation phase once the haemodynamic is stable (vasopressor requirement is minimum and stable) via orogastric or nasogastric tube. It should be stepped up gradually to achieve targeted calorie and protein within 7–10 days. If not possible, at least tropic feed (500 ml/day) should be given for immunological benefit, to maintain gut mucosa integrity and prevention of bacterial translocation. Gastric regurgitation and aspiration can increase incidence of VAP. Some studies have suggested in favour of post pyloric feeding; but the data is very heterogenous and not recommended presently.

Sedation and analgesia: Analgo-sedation is now a standard of care for all mechanically ventilated patients. Sedation practice has been moved away towards non-benzodiazepine (non-BZD) group of drugs (e.g. propofol, dexmedetomidine) due to longer weaning time and delirium with BZD.[20] Opioids like fentanyl, though short acting, can have prolong action while given as infusion. In that case, ramifentanyl would be a better choice for weaning purpose. Sedation needs to be titrated as per RASS score to fasten the weaning process; it can be stopped once a day to assess neurological status of the patient (e.g. to assess GCS). Multimodal analgesia is currently recommended including paracetamol and other non-opioid drugs. Short acting sedatives like dexmedetomidine are more suitable for early weaning process.

Deep vein thrombosis (DVT) prophylaxis: DVT and pulmonary embolism (PE) are important preventable complications in critical care. ICU patients are at high risk of DVT and PE due to multiple reasons like sepsis, restricted mobility, underlying comorbidities (caner), etc. Mechanically ventilated patients probably has a higher risk, though the data is very limited.[21] So DVT prophylaxis is a standard of care as per recent Surviving sepsis guideline.[22] Pharmacological prophylaxis is recommended as first line. If contraindicated, mechanical thromboprophylaxis (e.g. DVT pump) is advisable.

Head end elevation: Keeping head end elevated by 30–45° has shown to decrease gastro-oesophageal reflux, and subsequently risk of aspiration in critically ill patients including those on ventilator.[23] Similar finding was observed in favour of semi-recumbent position even in Cochrane review.[24] For neurological patients, it can be 45–60° degree with neck in neutral position for better drainage of cerebral venous system and decrease of intra cranial pressure. Lateral Trendelenburg position has also been tried against semi-recumbent position to minimize VAP due to its physiological benefit. It has showed to decrease microbiologically proven VAP study;[25] but more data is needed to recommend its widespread usage.

Stress ulcer prophylaxis: Using H_2B or PPI in a mechanically ventilated patient was a standard of care to decrease stress ulcer and upper gastrointestinal (GI) bleeding. PPI has been shown to be more effective than H_2B for prevention of upper GI bleeding without any difference in mortality.[26] Currently the routine use of PPI are not recommended[27] due to increased risk of bacterial colonisation in stomach with higher probability of ventilator associated pneumonia (VAP). Current recommendation for use of PPI against stress ulcer prophylaxis are shock, thrombocytopenia and coagulopathy and patient on mechanical ventilator.[28] PPI can be stopped after 48 hours once enteral feed has been started.

Glycemic control: Targeting capillary blood glucose between 140–180 mg% is a reasonable practice in critical care setting.[29] Strict glycemic control may be helpful in certain limited subspeciality ICU (neuro, cardiothoracic, surgical ICU) by decreasing risk of infection; but at the risk of increase in hypoglycemic episodes.[30] Glycemic fluctuation has been identified to have more harmful effect rather than absolute glucose value. So, glycemic variability index is the new target for intensivist.

Spontaneous breathing trial: Daily stoppage of sedation (spontaneous awakening trial) and evaluation of the patient for liberation from ventilator (spontaneous breathing trial) is strongly recommended and a part of VAP bundle too.

Bowel movement: Maintaining optimal bladder bowel functions are important part of routine care. Diarrhea can complicate ICU care by compromising enteral feeding and increasing risk of incontinence associated dermatitis with increase in nursing workload. Constipation, though apparently benign, may cause bacterial overgrowth in gut and has shown to increase ICU morbidities by increasing ventilator days, ICU stay, hospital stay and even by increasing mortality. So optimal dietary practice along with ensuring regular bowel habit is an integral part of ventilated patient management.

Indwelling catheters: Indwelling catheters like central vascular access, peripherally inserted central catheter, arterial line, haemodialysis catheter, urinary catheter, etc. can be source of infection. Although there are guidelines and protocols for insertion and maintenance of these line; best option to minimize infection is to remove it once it is not necessary.

De-escalation: De-escalation of antibiotics is of paramount importance. So, antibiotic prescriptions need to be reviewed by antibiotic stewardship team and to be discuss with the treating doctor for its optimisation. The basic principles are use narrow spectrum antibiotics (rather than broad spectrum) once culture reports are available, change to oral medication is feasible and cut down the duration of antibiotics to 7–10 days. It can decrease antibiotic pressure in the unit and prevent an increase in MDR organism.

There are some specific preventive measures recommended against some definitive HAI.

PREVENTION OF VENTILATOR-ASSOCIATED PNEUMONIA (VAP BUNDLE)

VAP bundle[31] was launched in 2007 as a part of "Saving Lives, reducing infection, delivering clean and safe care" campaign with focusing on five high impact interventions. It had been updated in 2010 to incorporate interventions like chlorhexidine mouth wash and subglottic suction depending on the contemporary evidences.

- **Avoid invasive ventilation:** If possible, use non-invasive ventilation (NIV) in selected cases.[33] There are some Grade 1 recommendations where initial NIV trial should be given. These are—acute exacerbation of chronic obstructive pulmonary disease (COPD) with pH 7.25 – 7.35, Acute decompensated heart failure with haemodynamic stability, post organ transplant/immunocompromised patients, palliative care, and end of life care patients and in weaning of COPD patients after extubation. But it should be done in an objective manner without delaying the actual need for intubation, as that may cause poor outcome.
- **Head end elevation:** Keep head end up by 30–45°
- **Sedation vacation:** Having a patient fully conscious and obeying basic commands is an important prerequisite for liberation from ventilator. It ensures that the patient will be able to maintain his/her airway, will try to generate adequate cough to clear secretion and will follow basic commands related to physiotherapy after extubation. Daily interruption of sedation (sedation vacation) till the patient is fully awake can minimize the sedative usage and can decrease mechanical ventilator days, ICU and hospital stay.[34] Besides, nursing implemented protocolized approach[35] has also shown better outcome in terms of ventilatory days, ICU and hospital stay compared to an individualistic approach, including reduction in tracheostomy rate.

- **Daily assessment for readiness to wean:** It was done by daily implementation of spontaneous breathing trail after stoppage of sedation. It can be done either by t-piece trail or by CPAP–PS (Continuous positive airway pressure–pressure support) mode. Both are of equal efficacy and 30 minutes of spontaneous breathing trial is recommended (equally good as longer trial like 2 hours) before proceeding for extubation.
- **Chlorhexidine based oral care:** Selective decontamination of oropharynx is probably the most controversial component of VAP bundle. Thorough cleaning of oral cavity along with brushing in a ventilated patient is getting more and more importance in regular practice. Chlorhexidine is a good antibacterial molecule against Gram-positive bacteria; but ventilated patients in our country usually got colonized with MDR Gram-negative bacteria during their ICU stay. Chlorhexidine may kill normal commensals of oral cavity and select out the pathogenic bacteria to grow. Till date, evidence is still in favour of chlorhexidine. A recent meta-analysis has shown that daily chlorhexidine oral care in ventilated patients can reduce the incidence of VAP and they have recommended to use 0.02 – 0.2% solution for safe oral care.[36] Another meta-analysis involving 18 randomized control study (RCT) has shown similar result in favour of chlorhexidine.[37]
- **Selective digestive decontamination:** It constitutes of usage of oral non-absorbable antibiotics to eliminate MDR organism from gut of the patient as eventually bowel acts as an important source of infection. It has shown good result in terms of decrease mortality in center with low MDR organism rate and good infection control practice.[38] It is not recommended presently due to the risk of *Clostridium difficile* and emergence of resistant organisms due to antibiotic selection.
- **Hand hygiene:** Basic infection control policies like hand hygiene should be followed strictly to prevent HAI. '5 Point of hand hygiene' needs to be followed regularly in all patient management areas. It is recommended to use alcohol-based gel to have longer skin contact time.
- **ETT modifications:** ETT, being the conduit for the entry of the microbes, has drawn significant attention in recent days. Different focused modifications have been tried with variable clinical outcome.
    1. Cuff pressure monitoring: Micro-aspiration surrounding the ETT cuff is one of the pathophysiology for development of VAP. So, strict monitoring of cuff pressure can minimize aspiration risk and reduce complications.[39] Keeping cuff pressure within 20–30 cm H_2O is currently advisable. Lower pressure will increase risk of aspiration and higher pressure may cause tracheal mucosal ischemia and tracheal stenosis in long run. Different cuff pressure monitoring tools are routinely used in our practice, and it is usually measured once in each nursing shift.
    2. Subglottic suction: Subglottic suction system consists of a narrow tube that runs along the side of ETT and opens just above ETT cuff; so that when ETT is within trachea, this opening is placed below the vocal cords. Oropharyngeal secretions collected above the inflated cuff and cause micro-aspiration along the creases of ETT cuff. Continuous or intermittent aspiration of the secretion via this tubing system have shown to reduce the risk of aspiration, incidence of VAP, duration of mechanical ventilation and ICU stay.[40]

3. ETT cuff design: Conventional ETT cuff is high volume low pressure, made from polyvinyl chloride and on inflation, there are creases on its outer wall leading to potential channel for aspiration. Newly designed tapered shaped ultra-thin polyurethane cuff can minimize this crease formation leading to lesser chance of aspiration and VAP.[41]
4. Coated ETT: Biofilm formation on the inner side of ETT followed by bacterial colonisation is another important mechanism for development of VAP. Inner wall coating with materials with antimicrobial property (e.g. silver, chlorhexidine, titanium oxide) have been tried. Silver coated ETT has shown to have lesser VAP rate along with delayed initiation of VAP compared to conventional ETT.[42]
5. Closed suction system: Closed suction can be beneficial due to less frequent disconnection of the circuit along with less chance of contamination of the patient's airway. But routine change in ventilatory circuit is not recommended.

PREVENTION OF CENTRAL LINE ASSOCIATED BLOOD STREAM INFECTION (CLABSI)

The goal is to eliminate CLABSI to nil in that clinical area, or to minimize it as low as possible. This needs written protocol including central line insertion and maintenance prerequisites (in the form of checklist) along with regular training of the involved healthcare personal (doctors and nurses) followed by regular audit (compliance and outcome audit).[43]

CL Insertion Protocol

- Proper and periodic training of doctor about the indications, technique of insertion and associated infection control protocol for CL (Insertion checklist).
- For non-tunneled CL, subclavian line is suggested over jugular and femoral line due to lesser chance of infection. Right internal jugular cannulation is still the most common site of CL due to ease of access and scope to use ultrasound (USG). USG guided vascular canulation is strongly recommended due to safety issue. Subclavian vein should be avoided for HD catheter due to high risk of subclavian stenosis. Arterio-venous fistula is recommended for long term HD to avoid vascular access related complications.
- Minimum number of ports in CL is advisable and it should be promptly removed when not needed. CL utilisation rate of a unit can be monitored on regular basis to understand the trend.
- Strict aseptic technique for CL insertion is recommended. Proper hand hygiene and maximum sterile barrier precautions (cap, mask, sterile whole-body gown, sterile gloves, sterile full body drape) are strongly recommended for CL insertion.
- >0.5% chlorhexidine preparation with alcohol should be used for insertion site preparation. Alternative option is povidone–iodine in alcohol or 70% alcohol preparation. Antiseptic solution should be given enough time to dry up before puncturing the skin.
- Antiseptic/antibiotic impregnated catheter can be considered if the unit is having higher rate of CLABSI than expected and the catheter is expected to remain for long duration (>5 days). Two types of catheters are available–chlorhexidine/silver sulfadiazine and minocycline/rifampicin impregnated.

- Routine replacement of CL is not recommended; clinical judgement should be used to remove CL in view of source of infection. Exchange of CL over the guidewire is not recommended.

CL Maintenance Protocol

- Regular training of nursing team for aseptic CL handling, periodic audit to assess knowledge, compliance with protocol and outcome (maintenance checklist).
- Strict aseptic infection control protocol to be followed during handing the lines (hub and insertion site).
- Use sterile transparent semi-permeable dressing over CL insertion site; change it every 7 days.
- Use gauze dressing as second option or if there is bleeding from puncture site (as a part of pressure dressing); change it every 24–48 hours or as needed (damp, loosen or visibly soiled).
- Regular visual checking of CL puncture side; no topical antibiotic ointment due to risk of MDR bacterial and fungal breakthrough infection. Induration, erythema, and tenderness on palpation of the puncture side warrant detail assessment and decision regarding further course (CL removal). 'Suture less fixation' of CL may be beneficial in terms of reduced infection.[44]
- Chlorhexidine impregnated sponge dressing[45] can be considered if high CLABSI rate is a concern even after all IPC measures.
- No systemic or local antimicrobial prophylaxis, antimicrobial lock, or catheter flush, or anticoagulant are recommended.
- Administration set and tubing involved in blood/blood product or fat emulsion should be changed every 24 hours; rest can be changed between 4–7 days.
- Implementation of 'CLABSI prevention bundle' for ease of implementation of protocol.[46]

Prevention of Catheter-Associated Urinary Tract Infection (CAUTI)

Like other HAIs, CAUTI is also a preventable complication[47], with a target to minimize it to as low as possible. Just like monitoring any other device utilisation, urinary catheter days need to be monitored in any clinical area and audit to be done to look at the trend.

Urinary Catheter Insertion Protocol

- Use urinary catheter only with definitive indication and remove it once there is no clinical need. Higher threshold for catheterisation should be there for high-risk patients like elderly, female, immunocompromised patients where risk of CAUTI is more. Urinary incontinence is not a definitive indication.
- Routine catherization in surgical patients is not needed. If urinary catheterisation is done during surgery (prolong surgery, strict input output measurement is required, urological/genitourinary interventions); need for the catheter should be reviewed postoperatively and advisable to remove within 24 hours if not needed.
- Patient with bladder emptying dysfunction, intermittent catheterisation is preferred over indwelling catheter.
- Proper hand hygiene and adequate training is mandatory for medical staffs involved in urinary catheter insertion.

- In hospital setting, catheterisation should be done by aseptic technique with sterile equipment (sterile gloves, drape, sponge forceps, sterile gauge, povidone iodine solution, lubricant jelly). Routine use of antiseptic jelly is not recommended. Antiseptic solution (povidone iodine) is used for periurethral cleaning before insertion; sterile water or normal solution are reasonable option.
- Minimum bore catheter should be preferred for insertion followed by secure fixation to prevent catheter movement and urethral stretching.
- For intermittent catheterisation in non-acute set up, clean technique is reasonable at regular interval for urinary retention.
- Hydrophilic catheter is preferred for intermittent catheterisation and silicon catheter is preferred for long term catheterisation.
- Antibiotic/antiseptic impregnated (e.g. silver alloy) catheter can be considered if CAUTI rate is persistently high even after implementation of ICP protocols.

Urinary Catheter Maintenance Protocol

- Maintain a closed drainage system with properly connected and sealed catheter tubing junction. Close monitoring needed to identify breach in aseptic technique, any leak, block, or accidental disconnection. In such case, catheter and collecting system may need to be changed.
- The collecting bag needs to be kept hanging below the level of bladder (not on the floor). Avoid kinking of the tubing. Empty the urinary bag to a container without contamination of the surrounding. Standard precautions to be followed all the time.
- Urinary catheter and collecting system should be changed as per clinical indication and not on routine basis. No role of systemic antibiotic prophylaxis to prevent CAUTI in patients with short- or long-term catheter.
- Routine cleaning of catheter area during bathing is sufficient without any antibiotics. Bladder irrigation or installation of antibiotics/antiseptics are not recommended routinely. Close continuous irrigation is advised in case of obstruction (e.g. clot due to bleeding).
- Routine clamping of catheter to check for bladder sensation before removal of catheter is not recommended.
- Urinary sample to be collected from needleless sampling port of the collection system without disconnecting the closed system.
- It should be removed once it is not clinically necessary. Nurse-based or electronic daily reminder system to the physician to review the need for catheter can be an important intervention to reduce device utilisation rate.
- Routine screening of catheterized urine to diagnose CAUTI or CA- ASB followed by treatment are not recommended.

MANAGEMENT OF HOSPITAL-ASSOCIATED INFECTIONS (HAIS)

Ventilator-Associated Pneumonia

Diagnosis: Microbiological diagnostic criteria (Surveillance definition of VAP) has been already discussed. It has good sensitivity and positive predictive value; but poor specificity has limited its clinical usage. There are different scoring systems that have been used in practice; like The Clinical Pulmonary Infection Score (CPIS), Johannson criteria, HELICS criteria, etc.

The Clinical Pulmonary Infection Score (CPIS) has been developed by Pugin and his team.[48] It consists of six clinic-radio-laboratory findings (six criteria) with grading system for severity (0 to 3). The criteria are temperature, leucocyte count, PaO_2/FiO_2 ratio, Chest X-ray, quality of tracheal secretion and microbiological culture of tracheal aspirate. Value more than 6 is suggestive of VAP. Some parameters of CPIS are subjective (chest X-ray and quality of tracheal aspirate) and have interobserver variability. Johannsan criteria[49] have some overlapping assessment points with CPIS and also has poor sensitivity and specificity when compared with postmortem microbiology finding. HELICS criteria[50] is also a surveillance diagnostic criterion which classify PVAP into five categories (PN1 TO PN5) depending on type and representativeness of the respiratory sample. Lack of radiological findings was the significant drawback of this scoring system.

In 2016, Infectious Disease Society of America and American thoracic Society has jointly published guideline for management of ventilator-associated pneumonia in adults.[51] Non-invasive sampling (ETT aspirate) with semiquantitative culture rather than invasive technique (bronchoalveolar lavage) for diagnostic workup was advocated. Biomarkers like procalcitonin (PCT), sTREM-1, C-reactive protein (CRP) or any scoring system are unlikely to contribute more than clinical findings in diagnosis.

Treatment: Empirical choice of antibiotics should be guided by hospital/local epidemiology of bacteria and antibiogram against them. Enterobacteriaceae like *E. coli*, Klebsiella and non-lactose fermenters like Pseudomonas and Acinetobactor with methicillin resistant *Staphylococcus aureus* (MRSA) are the main concern. Empirical MRSA cover (linezolid or vancomycin) is advocated if the incidence of MRSA is >10–20%. Risk for multi-drug resistant pathogen as causative factor needs to be evaluated, e.g. intravenous antibiotics within 90 days, hospital admission >5 days, acute respiratory distress syndrome (ARDS) or septic shock on admission, patient on haemodialysis, etc. Combination therapy can be considered for MDR Pseudomonas, specially if the patient is in septic shock with high risk of mortality. For bacteria with limited therapeutic option, inhalational antibiotics (colistin or tobramycin) can be combined with systemic therapy. Vibrating mesh nebulizer is strongly recommended for delivery of inhalational antibiotics. For MDR acinetobactor, polymyxin B based therapy is recommended along with sulbactam. Carbapenem resistant Enterobacteriaceae should receive Polymyxin-based therapy or ceftazidime avibactam-based therapy. Duration of antibiotics of 7 days is mostly adequate and should be prolong only on case-to-case basis (neutropenic, slow clinical response, inadequate source control). PCT can play an important role to in escalation of antibiotics along with clinical finding.

Central Line Associated Blood Stream Infection[52]

Diagnosis: Microbiologically confirmed blood culture is required for diagnosis of CLABSI. Clinical diagnostic criteria are little different from surveillance definition by CDC. Paired blood culture should be sent from the suspected catheter and from peripheral vein at the same time, preferably before first dose of antibiotic. If peripheral venous sample is not available; then two or more blood sample should be sent from different lumens of the suspected catheter. On removal of the suspected catheter, the tip should be sent for microbiological culture. Any pus or discharge from catheter hub or puncture site should be cultured. Catheter colonisation is diagnosed if >15

CFU growth is observed from 5 cm catheter tip by semi-quantitative roll-plate culture method or >10^2 CFU by quantitative broth culture method. Alcoholic chlorhexidine (>0.5%) solution should be preferred for skin preparation and cleaning of catheter hub followed by adequate time for dryness.

If the peripheral blood culture is positive with the same organism from the catheter tip or catheter blood sample (meeting quantitative criteria or differential time of positivity criteria); it is 'Definite CLABSI'. If blood sample from one lumen of suspected catheter shows 3 times CFU growth of bacteria compared to the other one, is called 'Possible CLABSI'. Microbiologically meeting criteria consists of 3-fold greater CFU growth of bacteria from suspected catheter compared to peripheral sample, or 2 hours earlier microbial growth from catheter hub sample compared to peripheral venous sample. Microbiological instruction regarding the volume of blood for each culture bottle should be followed.

Treatment: Basic principle of treatment of CALBSI incorporates broad-spectrum empirical antibiotics (+/– antifungal) along with removal of the suspected catheter (if possible). Empirical antibiotics should be according to hospital epidemiology and local antibiogram. Gram-negative bacterial sepsis is most prevalent and as a result piperacillin tazobactam or meropenem with/without combination therapy is the initial choice. Combination therapy is justified against suspected MDR bacteria (e.g. Pseudomonas) with high-risk host factors (neutropenia, critically ill with high APCHE 4 score, septic shock, on mechanical ventilation, already colonized with MDR bacteria). Empirical MRSA cover can be considered as per hospital policy, specially after removal of femoral CL.

Empirical treatment against Candida should be considered with specific risk factors like prolong broad-spectrum antibiotic usage, haematological malignancy, bone marrow or solid organ transplant, neutropenia, femoral CL, total parenteral nutrition (TPN), etc. Echinocandin is the drug of choice specially if the patient is sick, received fluconazole therapy/prophylaxis in last 3 month or if *C. glabrata* or *C. krusei* are of concern. Persistent bacteremia or fungaemia warrants ruling out of infective endocarditis.

Removing long-term catheter in the background of CLABSI, can be really challenging specially in presence of thrombocytopenia and coagulopathy. Persistently positive blood culture even after 72 hours of appropriate antibiotics may need removal of catheter. There are other indications for removal of long-term catheter like severe sepsis, suppurative thrombophlebitis, endocarditis, bacteria like *S. aureus*, *Pseudomonas*, fungi, or mycobacteria. In uncomplicated CLABSI, long term catheter can be kept, and appropriate antibiotics can be continued—sometimes through the infected catheter. Lock therapy can be used too in certain cases.

Single positive blood culture with coagulase negative *Staphylococcus sp.* does not warrant treatment. Repeat culture should be sent from the catheter and peripheral vein and treatment should be considered only if multiple cultures are positive.

Catheter-Associated Urinary Tract Infection[12]

Diagnosis: CAUTI needs to be differentiated from catheter associated asymptomatic bacteriuria (CA-ASB) to decide about treatment beyond change of catheter. In case of MDR bugs, it can be a challenging decision to choose antibiotics. So, CA-ASB can be kept under monitoring for clinical progression rather than giving antibiotics.

A urine sample should be collected from the catheter/tubing (not from the collecting bag) for routine microscopy and culture before starting empirical antibiotics. Removal of the catheter would be clinical judgement depending on the strength of clinical suspicion of CAUTI. If the catheter is >2weeks old, it is advisable to replace it and send urine sample from the new catheter. Lower abdominal radiological work up (e.g. USG kidney ureter bladder) should be considered if upper urinary tract infection (pyelonephritis) is suspected. A blood culture should be sent along with urine sample to diagnose secondary BSI.

Treatment: Empirical antibiotics should be started as per institutional/local epidemiology and antibiotic protocol. Most common causative organisms are Enterobacteriaceae (*E. coli* most common) followed by Pseudomonas, enterococci, other non-fermenters like acinetobactor, etc. frequently Enterobacteriaceae are extended spectrum beta lactamase (ESBL) and carbapenemase producers; so empirical antibiotics need to be select accordingly.[53] Usually, 7 days of therapy are sufficient if the patient responded promptly with treatment. Shorter duration can be considered in female, <65 years with minimum symptoms and when catheter has been removed promptly. On the contrary, 10–14 days of therapy can be needed in case of poor/delayed clinical response. Source control is an important step if there is any obstruction in routine urinary drainage (e.g. stone). Identification of atypical bacteria (e.g. myroides) in catheterized urine sometimes only need change in catheter and no antibiotic is needed.

There are other hospital associated infections of clinical significance in mechanically ventilated patients like surgical site infection (SSI), *Clostridium difficile* infection, skin soft tissue infection on pressure sore, etc. These can happen in mechanically ventilated patients also, without much direct relationship.

Conclusion

HAIs in mechanically ventilated patient poses significant challenges to the intensivists. Mostly it creates a new onset clinical deterioration over the primary medical event. New onset organ failure along with current respiratory failure will definitely increase morbidity in terms of increase ICU and hospital stay, increase ventilatory days and eventually there is increase mortality too. In this era of MDR bacteria, empirical choice of antibiotics is very challenging, and we are forced to use broad-spectrum antibiotics empirically with significant clinical failure. So, prevention is the only way forward. Strict implementation of IPC measures along with education of medical personnel can minimize these HAIs to a significant level.

References

1. Wunsch H. The outbreak that invented intensive care. Nature. 2020 Apr 3. doi: 10.1038/d41586-020-01019-y. Epub ahead of print. PMID: 32246120.
2. Fokkens WJ, Scheeren RA. Upper airway defence mechanisms. Paediatr Respir Rev. 2000 Dec;1(4):336-41. doi: 10.1053/prrv.2000.0073. PMID: 16263461.
3. Gunasekera, P. and Gratrix, A. Ventilator-associated pneumonia. BJA Education 2016; 16(6), 198–202. doi:10.1093/bjaed/mkv046
4. https://arpsp.cdc.gov/profile/infections?tab=nhsn

5. Revelas A. Healthcare - associated infections: A public health problem. Niger Med J. 2012 Apr;53(2):59–64. doi: 10.4103/0300-1652.103543. PMID: 23271847; PMCID: PMC3530249.
6. Peña-López Y, Ramírez-Estrada S, Rello J. Ventilator-Associated Events: Definitions and Uses. Encyclopedia of Respiratory Medicine. 2022:523–9. doi: 10.1016/B978-0-12-801238-3.11482-5. Epub 2021 Sep 17. PMCID: PMC7157436.
7. Novosel TJ, Hodge LA, Weireter LJ, *et al.* Ventilator-associated pneumonia: depends on your definition. Am Surg 2012;78(8): 851–54.
8. Tejerina E, Esteban A, Fernandez-Segoviano P, *et al.* Accuracy of clinical definitions of ventilator-associated pneumonia: com- parison with autopsy findings. J Crit Care 2010;25(1):62–68.
9. National Healthcare Safety Network, Centers for Disease Control and Prevention. The National Healthcare Safety Network (NHSN) Manual: Patient Safety Component Protocol. July 2013. https://www.cdc.gov/nhsn/pdfs/pscmanual/10-vae_final.pdf
10. Mishra SB, Misra R, Azim A, Baronia AK, Prasad KN, Dhole TN, Gurjar M, Singh RK, Poddar B. Incidence, risk factors and associated mortality of central line-associated bloodstream infections at an intensive care unit in northern India. Int J Qual Healthcare. 2017 Feb 1;29(1):63-67. doi: 10.1093/intqhc/mzw144. PMID: 27940521.
11. National Healthcare Safety Network, Centers for Disease Control and Prevention. The National Healthcare Safety Network (NHSN) Manual: Patient Safety Component Protocol. July 2013. http://www.cdc.gov/nhsn/PDFs/pscManual/4PSC_CLABScurrent.pdf. Accessed September 28, 2013.
12. Hooton TM, Bradley SF, Cardenas DD, Colgan R, Geerlings SE, Rice JC, *et al.* Infectious Diseases Society of America. Diagnosis, prevention, and treatment of catheter-associated urinary tract infection in adults: 2009 International Clinical Practice Guidelines from the Infectious Diseases Society of America. Clin Infect Dis. 2010 Mar 1;50(5):625-63. doi: 10.1086/650482. PMID: 20175247.
13. Schreiber PW, Sax H, Wolfensberger A, Clack L, Kuster SP; Swissnoso. The preventable proportion of healthcare-associated infections 2005-2016: Systematic review and meta-analysis. Infect Control Hosp Epidemiol. 2018 Nov;39(11):1277-1295. doi: 10.1017/ice.2018.183. Epub 2018 Sep 20. PMID: 30234463.
14. Haque M, Sartelli M, McKimm J, Abu Bakar M. Healthcare-associated infections - an overview. Infect Drug Resist. 2018 Nov 15;11:2321-2333. doi: 10.2147/IDR.S177247. PMID: 30532565; PMCID: PMC6245375.
15. Rello J, Afonso E, Lisboa T, Ricart M, Balsera B, Rovira A, Valles J, Diaz E; FADO Project Investigators. A care bundle approach for prevention of ventilator-associated pneumonia. Clin Microbiol Infect. 2013 Apr;19(4):363-9. doi: 10.1111/j.1469-0691.2012.03808.x. Epub 2012 Mar 22. PMID: 22439889.
16. Morris AC, Hay AW, Swann DG, Everingham K, McCulloch C, McNulty J, *et al.* Reducing ventilator-associated pneumonia in intensive care: impact of implementing a care bundle. Crit Care Med. 2011 Oct;39(10):2218-24. doi: 10.1097/CCM.0b013e3182227d52. PMID: 21666444.
17. Zilberberg MD, Shorr AF, Kollef MH. Implementing quality improvements in the intensive care unit: ventilator bundle as an example. Crit Care Med. 2009 Jan;37(1):305-9. doi: 10.1097/CCM.0b013e3181926623. PMID: 19050626.
18. Vincent JL. Give your patient a fast hug (at least) once a day. Crit Care Med. 2005 Jun;33(6):1225-9. doi: 10.1097/01.ccm.0000165962.16682.46. PMID: 15942334.
19. Nair AS, Naik VM, Rayani BK. FAST HUGS BID: Modified Mnemonic for Surgical Patient. Indian J Crit Care Med. 2017 Oct;21(10):713-714. doi: 10.4103/ijccm.IJCCM_289_17. PMID: 29142387; PMCID: PMC5672681.

20. Barr J, Fraser GL, Puntillo K, Ely EW, Gélinas C, Dasta JF, *et al.* American College of Critical Care Medicine. Clinical practice guidelines for the management of pain, agitation, and delirium in adult patients in the intensive care unit. Crit Care Med. 2013 Jan;41(1):263–306. doi: 10.1097/CCM.0b013e3182783b72. PMID: 23269131.
21. Minet C, Lugosi M, Savoye PY, Menez C, Ruckly S, Bonadona A, Schwebel C, Hamidfar-Roy R, Dumanoir P, Ara-Somohano C, Ferretti GR, Timsit JF. Pulmonary embolism in mechanically ventilated patients requiring computed tomography: Prevalence, risk factors, and outcome. Crit Care Med. 2012 Dec;40(12):3202–8. doi: 10.1097/CCM.0b013e318265e461. PMID: 23164766.
22. Evans L, Rhodes A, Alhazzani W, Antonelli M, Coopersmith CM, French C, *et al.* Surviving sepsis campaign: international guidelines for management of sepsis and septic shock 2021. Intensive Care Med. 2021 Nov;47(11):1181–1247. doi: 10.1007/s00134-021-06506-y. Epub 2021 Oct 2. PMID: 34599691; PMCID: PMC8486643.
23. Drakulovic MB, Torres A, Bauer TT, Nicolas JM, Nogué S, Ferrer M. Supine body position as a risk factor for nosocomial pneumonia in mechanically ventilated patients: a randomised trial. Lancet. 1999 Nov 27;354(9193):1851-8. doi: 10.1016/S0140-6736(98)12251-1. PMID: 10584721.
24. Wang L, Li X, Yang Z, Tang X, Yuan Q, Deng L, *et al.* Semi-recumbent position versus supine position for the prevention of ventilator-associated pneumonia in adults requiring mechanical ventilation. Cochrane Database Syst Rev. 2016 Jan 8;2016(1):CD009946. doi: 10.1002/14651858.CD009946.pub2. PMID: 26743945; PMCID: PMC7016937.
25. Li Bassi G, Panigada M, Ranzani OT, Zanella A, Berra L, Cressoni M, *et al.*; Gravity-VAP Network. Randomized, multicenter trial of lateral Trendelenburg versus semirecumbent body position for the prevention of ventilator-associated pneumonia. Intensive Care Med. 2017 Nov;43(11):1572–84. doi: 10.1007/s00134-017-4858-1. Epub 2017 Jun 20. PMID: 29149418.
26. PEPTIC Investigators for the Australian and New Zealand Intensive Care Society Clinical Trials Group, Alberta Health Services Critical Care Strategic Clinical Network, and the Irish Critical Care Trials Group; Young PJ, Bagshaw SM, Forbes AB, Nichol AD, Wright SE, Bailey M, *et al.* Effect of Stress Ulcer Prophylaxis With Proton Pump Inhibitors vs Histamine-2 Receptor Blockers on In-Hospital Mortality Among ICU Patients Receiving Invasive Mechanical Ventilation: The PEPTIC Randomized Clinical Trial. JAMA. 2020 Feb 18;323(7):616–26. doi: 10.1001/jama.2019.22190. PMID: 31950977; PMCID: PMC7029750.
27. Alhazzani W, Guyatt G, Alshahrani M, Deane AM, Marshall JC, Hall R, *et al.* Canadian Critical Care Trials Group. Withholding Pantoprazole for Stress Ulcer Prophylaxis in Critically Ill Patients: A Pilot Randomized Clinical Trial and Meta-Analysis. Crit Care Med. 2017 Jul;45(7):1121-1129. doi: 10.1097/CCM.0000000000002461. PMID: 28459708.
28. Buendgens L, Koch A, Tacke F. Prevention of stress-related ulcer bleeding at the intensive care unit: Risks and benefits of stress ulcer prophylaxis. World J Crit Care Med. 2016 Feb 4;5(1):57-64. doi: 10.5492/wjccm.v5.i1.57. PMID: 26855894; PMCID: PMC4733456.
29. NICE-SUGAR Study Investigators; Finfer S, Chittock DR, Su SY, Blair D, Foster D, Dhingra V, *et al.* Intensive versus conventional glucose control in critically ill patients. N Engl J Med. 2009 Mar 26;360(13):1283–97. doi: 10.1056/NEJMoa0810625. Epub 2009 Mar 24. PMID: 19318384.
30. Ling Y, Li X, Gao X. Intensive versus conventional glucose control in critically ill patients: a meta-analysis of randomized controlled trials. Eur J Intern Med. 2012 Sep;23(6):564–74. doi: 10.1016/j.ejim.2012.02.013. Epub 2012 Mar 24. PMID: 22863436.
31. Klompas M, Branson R, Eichenwald EC, Greene LR, Howell MD, Lee G, *et al.* Society for Healthcare Epidemiology of America (SHEA). Strategies to prevent ventilator-associated

pneumonia in acute care hospitals: 2014 update. Infect Control Hosp Epidemiol. 2014 Aug;35(8):915-36. doi: 10.1086/677144. PMID: 25026607.

32. Morris AC, Hay AW, Swann DG, Everingham K, McCulloch C, McNulty J, Brooks O, Laurenson IF, Cook B, Walsh TS. Reducing ventilator-associated pneumonia in intensive care: impact of implementing a care bundle. Crit Care Med. 2011 Oct;39(10):2218-24. doi: 10.1097/CCM.0b013e3182227d52. PMID: 21666444.
33. Aboussouan LS, Ricaurte B. Non-invasive positive pressure ventilation: Increasing use in acute care. Cleve Clin J Med. 2010 May;77(5):307-16. doi: 10.3949/ccjm.77a.09145. PMID: 20439563.
34. Kress JP, Pohlman AS, O'Connor MF, Hall JB. Daily interruption of sedative infusions in critically ill patients undergoing mechanical ventilation. N Engl J Med. 2000 May 18;342(20):1471-7. doi: 10.1056/NEJM200005183422002. PMID: 10816184.
35. Brook AD, Ahrens TS, Schaiff R, Prentice D, Sherman G, Shannon W, Kollef MH. Effect of a nursing-implemented sedation protocol on the duration of mechanical ventilation. Crit Care Med. 1999 Dec;27(12):2609-15. doi: 10.1097/00003246-199912000-00001. PMID: 10628598.
36. Dai W, Lin Y, Yang X, Huang P, Xia L, Ma J. Meta-Analysis of the Efficacy and Safety of Chlorhexidine for Ventilator-Associated Pneumonia Prevention in Mechanically Ventilated Patients. Evid Based Complement Alternat Med. 2022 Jul 30;2022:5311034. doi: 10.1155/2022/5311034. PMID: 35942379; PMCID: PMC9356777.
37. Veitz-Keenan A, Ferraiolo DM. Oral care with chlorhexidine seems effective for reducing the incidence of ventilator-associated pneumonia. Evid Based Dent. 2017 Dec 22;18(4):113–114. doi: 10.1038/sj.ebd.6401272. PMID: 29269816.
38. de Smet AM, Kluytmans JA, Cooper BS, Mascini EM, Benus RF, van der Werf TS, *et al.* Decontamination of the digestive tract and oropharynx in ICU patients. N Engl J Med. 2009 Jan 1;360(1):20-31. doi: 10.1056/NEJMoa0800394. PMID: 19118302.
39. Nseir S, Zerimech F, Fournier C, Lubret R, Ramon P, Durocher A, Balduyck M. Continuous control of tracheal cuff pressure and microaspiration of gastric contents in critically ill patients. Am J Respir Crit Care Med. 2011 Nov 1;184(9):1041-7. doi: 10.1164/rccm.201104-0630OC. PMID: 21836137.
40. Muscedere J, Rewa O, McKechnie K, Jiang X, Laporta D, Heyland DK. Subglottic secretion drainage for the prevention of ventilator-associated pneumonia: a systematic review and meta-analysis. Crit Care Med. 2011 Aug;39(8):1985-91. doi: 10.1097/CCM.0b013e318218a4d9. PMID: 21478738.
41. Coppadoro A, Bittner E, Berra L. Novel preventive strategies for ventilator-associated pneumonia. Crit Care. 2012 Dec 12;16(2):210. doi: 10.1186/cc11225. PMID: 22429668; PMCID: PMC3681356.
42. Kollef MH, Afessa B, Anzueto A, Veremakis C, Kerr KM, Margolis BD, Craven DE, Roberts PR, Arroliga AC, Hubmayr RD, Restrepo MI, Auger WR, Schinner R; NASCENT Investigation Group. Silver-coated endotracheal tubes and incidence of ventilator-associated pneumonia: the NASCENT randomized trial. JAMA. 2008 Aug 20;300(7):805-13. doi: 10.1001/jama.300.7.805. PMID: 18714060.
43. National Healthcare Safety Network, Centers for Disease Control and Prevention. The National Healthcare Safety Network (NHSN) Manual: Patient Safety Component Protocol. July 2013. https://www.cdc.gov/infectioncontrol/pdf/guidelines/bsi-guidelines-H.pdf
44. Yamamoto AJ, Solomon JA, Soulen MC, Tang J, Parkinson K, Lin R, *et al.* Sutureless securement device reduces complications of peripherally inserted central venous catheters. J Vasc Interv Radiol. 2002 Jan;13(1):77-81. doi: 10.1016/s1051-0443(07)60012-8. PMID: 11788698.

45. National Healthcare Safety Network, Centers for Disease Control and Prevention. The National Healthcare Safety Network (NHSN) Manual: Patient Safety Component Protocol. July 2013. https://www.cdc.gov/infectioncontrol/guidelines/bsi/c-i-dressings/considerations.html
46. National Healthcare Safety Network, Centers for Disease Control and Prevention. The National Healthcare Safety Network (NHSN) Manual: Patient Safety Component Protocol. July 2013. https://www.cdc.gov/hai/pdfs/bsi/checklist-for-CLABSI.pdf
47. National Healthcare Safety Network, Centers for Disease Control and Prevention. The National Healthcare Safety Network (NHSN) Manual: Patient Safety Component Protocol. July 2013. https://www.cdc.gov/infectioncontrol/pdf/guidelines/cauti-guidelines-H.pdf
48. Pugin J, Auckenthaler R, Mili N, Janssens JP, Lew PD, Suter PM. Diagnosis of ventilator-associated pneumonia by bacteriologic analysis of bronchoscopic and nonbronchoscopic "blind" bronchoalveolar lavage fluid. Am Rev Respir Dis. 1991 May;143(5 Pt 1):1121-9. doi: 10.1164/ajrccm/143.5_Pt_1.1121. PMID: 2024824.
49. Fàbregas N, Ewig S, Torres A, El-Ebiary M, Ramirez J, de La Bellacasa JP, *et al.* Clinical diagnosis of ventilator associated pneumonia revisited: comparative validation using immediate post-mortem lung biopsies. Thorax. 1999 Oct;54(10):867-73. doi: 10.1136/thx.54.10.867. PMID: 10491448; PMCID: PMC1745365.
50. Pugh R, Harrison W, Harris S, Roberts H, Scholey G, Szakmany T; WICSARG Investigators and WHAIP. Is HELICS the Right Way? Lack of Chest Radiography Limits Ventilator-Associated Pneumonia Surveillance in Wales. Front Microbiol. 2016 Aug 18;7:1271. doi: 10.3389/fmicb.2016.01271. PMID: 27588017; PMCID: PMC4988982.
51. Kalil AC, Metersky ML, Klompas M, Muscedere J, Sweeney DA, Palmer LB, *et al.* Management of Adults With Hospital-acquired and Ventilator-associated Pneumonia: 2016 Clinical Practice Guidelines by the Infectious Diseases Society of America and the American Thoracic Society. Clin Infect Dis. 2016 Sep 1;63(5):e61-e111. doi: 10.1093/cid/ciw353. Epub 2016 Jul 14. Erratum in: Clin Infect Dis. 2017 May 1;64(9):1298. Erratum in: Clin Infect Dis. 2017 Oct 15;65(8):1435. Erratum in: Clin Infect Dis. 2017 Nov 29;65(12):2161. PMID: 27418577; PMCID: PMC4981759.
52. Leonard A. Mermel and others, Clinical Practice Guidelines for the Diagnosis and Management of Intravascular Catheter-Related Infection: 2009 Update by the Infectious Diseases Society of America, Clinical Infectious Diseases, Volume 49, Issue 1, 1 July 2009, Pages 1 - 45, https://doi.org/10.1086/599376
53. Nicolle LE. Catheter associated urinary tract infections. Antimicrob Resist Infect Control. 2014 Jul 25;3:23. doi: 10.1186/2047-2994-3-23. PMID: 25075308; PMCID: PMC4114799.

CHAPTER 17

The Role of Respiratory Therapist in the Management of Mechanical Ventilation

❒ Jithin K Sreedharan

Keywords: Mechanical ventilation, respiratory therapy, scope of practice.

ABSTRACT

The need for ventilator assistance is one of the most conventional cause of patient admission to the intensive care units. In numerous circumstances, mechanical ventilation settings should be tailored to the individual, and warrants careful attention because improper ventilation can induce damage to the lungs or respiratory muscles and aggravate morbidity and mortality. Respiratory Therapists (RTs) are projected to be the specialists or consultants of the mechanical ventilator and all traits of its utilization in the clinical practice. In the recent past, the role of the RT evolved together with the advancement of medicine, particularly critical care. The evolution of the profession of respiratory care can be invariably linked with the development of the advanced ventilators and the generic changes in the nature of disease progression and pathophysiological background. This chapter is outlining inevitable role of RTs as front liners in the management of patients requiring ventilator support over a broad-range of practice areas and its implications in the patient outcome.

INTRODUCTION

Respiratory therapy emerged as a known profession in the 1940s and 1950s. By tradition, the scope of the Respiratory Therapists (RTs) practice comprises performing diagnostic and therapeutic interventions for patients with cardiopulmonary disease.[1] The COVID-19 pandemic has highlighted the importance of interprofessional collaborative practice and spotlighted the contributions of Respiratory Therapist (RT) to the healthcare team. RTs can serve an essential role in the multidisciplinary team by providing diagnostic testing (e.g. pulmonary function, cardiopulmonary exercise testing, 6-min-walk tests), medication administration and education, airway clearance, sleep therapy, smoking cessation, and dyspnea management. The RT profession is moving toward expanding the role of the RT across the continuum of care including prevention and health promotion, acute care, out-patient clinics, and physician offices. A good bit of required interventions are carried out by RTs, the connoisseurs on the application of mechanical ventilation. Rapid and efficient decisions are required to prepare for patients requiring mechanical ventilation. As the physician workforce within the specialization of pulmonary and critical care medicine continues to decline,

RTs can help fill a well-needed demand of specialized providers to care for patients with chronic pulmonary disease. Moreover, farther group of healthcare professionals have little insight to support ventilated patients, only the respiratory therapist has the depth of knowledge and expert ability required to blend technical skills with patient specific clinical requirements.[2] RTs possess the knowledge, skill, and ability to deliver the whole range of diagnostic and therapeutic procedures to patients who necessitate basic, advanced, and prolonged cardiopulmonary and associated services. The ventilator is an intricate machine with diverse modes, settings, and alarms that RTs have gone through firm training in a university for two or four-year to master the skill. Moreover, RTs are most constructive in mending patient outcomes and thus curtailing morbidities. It is witnessed, that ICUs around the world are realizing the importance of standard guidelines and protocols and implementing them for managing mechanical ventilation, and this empowers RTs to be involved actively in the ventilator management. That includes the selection of ventilator mode, determining the ventilation strategy, and participating in the decision to wean and liberate. Numerous randomized controlled studies have concluded that RT-driven mechanical ventilation protocols result in shorter weaning times, augmented successful extubation rate, and ventilator-free days, as well as a decrease in overall morbidities.[3]

The competencies of a Respiratory Therapist to Manage Mechanical Ventilation

Competency is the talent of a practitioner to integrate the professional attributes such as knowledge, skill, judgment, attitudes, values, and beliefs required to perform in a given role, situation, or practice setting. It is imperious that each clinician prove competency before partaking in the initiation and management of mechanical ventilation. Over recent years the role of the RT advanced correspondingly with the development of medicine, in particular critical care practice. Precisely, the maturing of the respiratory care profession can be associated to the development of the mechanical ventilator and the application of mechanical ventilation. The refinement and continual development in conjunction with the expanded clinical application of the mechanical ventilator have been prominent factors in the development and growth of the respiratory care profession and critical care medicine. Indeed, the expansion and increased sophistication of the mechanical ventilator parallels similar developments in the respiratory therapy profession. RTs possess the ability to comprehend in detail, the operational intricacies of the contemporary features of the new generation ventilators. They are clever to determine when one feature is indicated over the other. RTs are highly competent to be certain that the ventilator is accurately doing what it is anticipated to do and that the patient is responding as likely to the intervention.[4]

RT education is primarily focused on the over-all understanding of research techniques and statistical methodology, which is making them proficient and critiquing the growing body of evidence published regarding mechanical ventilation. As a result, during rounds it is commonly observed the RTs are discussing the nuances of recently published literature regarding mechanical ventilation. In the multidisciplinary team RTs are believed to be the specialists in mechanical ventilation and it is desirable to seek their opinion on how to manage the ventilatory aspects of patient care, and what is best suitable care plan. RTs are well able to powerfully argue for an explicit approach to ventilatory support and constantly function as a patient advocate in the management of the mechanically ventilated patient, that basically lies on the essential communication skill every RT possess. A survey of respiratory therapy educational programs acknowledged that 99.71% of all respiratory therapy programs included competencies on the application of invasive and non-invasive mechanical ventilation, 97.98% comprised competencies on the application of all ventilation modes, and 97.96% encompassed the competencies on the interpretation of ventilator data.[5] The essential competency of a respiratory therapist with regards to mechanical ventilation covers every technical properties of mechanical ventilators **(Table 17.1)**.

Table 17.1: Competencies required of respiratory therapists to manage MV

Bedside monitoring	Modes of mechanical ventilation
Complications of mechanical ventilation	Monitoring MV
Effective communication	Non-invasive ventilation
Evidence-based application of MV	Pathophysiology of lung disorders that require MV
Independent application of MV	Patient-ventilator interactions
Indications for mechanical ventilation	Pharmacology of critical care
Initiating ventilation	Protocols and guidelines
Management of the airway	Respiratory physiology
Mechanical ventilation adjuncts	Weaning and extubation

MV: Mechanical Ventilation, RT: Respiratory Therapist

Initiation of Mechanical Ventilation; The RT Approach

Initiating and maintaining both invasive and non-invasive mechanical ventilation is a multifaceted procedure, and there large quantity of data showing the strong association between initial ventilator adjustments and clinical outcomes, as well as the high safety and favourable risk-benefit profile. Ventilatory physiology is significantly changed when positive pressure is applied to the respiratory tract. Initial ventilator settings should provide maximal support for the patient in whom mechanical ventilation, and not mere airway protection, is necessary. Typically, the patient is fatigued, agitated, hypoxic and possibly hypercarbic, and unable to ventilate effectively on his own. Hence, the patient's entire ventilatory requirements must be met. The RT must discriminate amongst different manufacturers, ventilator models, offered modes, and breath types to decide which is suitable for each individual patient. Particularly because there is a lack of standardized terminology, which leads to ambiguity and confusion regarding mechanical ventilation. Once initiated, the RT must be able to fine-tune the ventilatory support for the patient attributed to the physiologic response as measured by invasive and non-invasive monitoring.[6]

Inspiratory flow rates are often set by the respiratory therapist, but it may need to increase for the patients with severe air hunger or airways obstruction who require prolonged expiratory times, or reduce it for patients generating high peak airway pressures. On some machines, inspiratory flow rates are controlled by setting the inspiratory time or I:E ratio. It is noteworthy to appreciate that breathing through the ventilator circuit spontaneously or even assisting is linked with a workload that may equal or exceed that of unassisted ventilation. Therefore, total support with MV should guarantee maximum rest of fatigued ventilatory muscles in the early management.[7]

A ventilator pre-use check must be performed to affirm the function and reliability of the ventilator circuit, internal components, and the type (active or passive) humidifier system. This procedure is generally performed by an RT during the circuit or humidifier setup, and usually repeated anytime the circuit is replaced or modified. The initial settings are generally done based on specific lung protective strategies by meticulously understanding the patient history, reason for ventilatory assistance, anatomy and goal for mechanical ventilation, which will help to mitigate the risk of ventilator induced lung injury.[8] It is equally important to adjust both informative and protective alarms, predominantly the volume and pressure limits, rate, etc.

Managing Mechanical Ventilation in the Emergency Department; Role of a Respiratory Therapist

Since the emergency department is the entry point to the ICU for hundreds of thousands of mechanically ventilated patients, a lung-protective ventilation strategy instituted from the emergency department demonstrated to have benefits concerned with the prevention of volutrauma, setting appropriate positive end-expiratory pressure setting, prevention of hyperoxia, aspiration precautions. Studies also have proven the repercussions of having RTs in the supervision of mechanically ventilated patients during their stay in the emergency department. The issues commonly faced in the emergency department while managing the ventilated patients are multifaceted, as there are many elements to take into consideration. First, for patients supported with invasive mechanical ventilation, the need to put high standards of care into action early are associated with the prevention of complications such as barotrauma, volutrauma, and ventilator-associated pneumonia.[9] RTs knowledgeable to provide the basic care such as 30–45 head-of-bed elevation and oral hygiene with chlorhexidine, etc. and they hold competence regarding the delivery of safe tidal volumes and airway plateau pressure targeted for protective ventilation strategies and management of patient-ventilator dyssynchronies. The initial ventilator settings done by the RTs in the emergency departments are frequently continued on ICU admission, these early ventilator adjustments are vital for continued high quality care (**Fig. 17.1**).[10, 11]

Monitoring the Mechanically Ventilated Patient

Respiratory therapists are the front-line care providers for patients requiring mechanical ventilation, especially those in intensive care units or other chronic ventilator units. Along with the clinical assessment of vital signs, mental status, and respiratory effort, pulse oximetry, End-tidal CO_2, Airway cuff pressure, RTs are responsible to ensure the patient is interacting seamlessly with the ventilator by simultaneously assessing the patient and the ventilator waveforms. It is also imperative to identify air trapping by looking at the expiratory portion of the flow vs. time graphic on the ventilator.[12] If the flow is not returning to zero or at least plateauing, some degree of air trapping is likely present. Air trapping can be assessed by adjusting the respiratory rate and monitoring the effects on airway pressure or tidal volume. Tidal volumes (VT) are a simple parameter to monitor, it is the duty of the RT to monitor and ensure that patients receive low tidal volumes (4–8 cc/kg of ideal body weight). If patients consistently receive tidal volumes beyond the acceptable range (high or low), RTs and physicians must work together to delineate an acceptable plan for the patient. Monitoring the plateau pressure by applying inspiratory hold manoeuvre is an essential component of the lung protective strategy. Increasing plateau pressure at a steady tidal volume and PEEP is an indication of worsening lung compliance (Fig. 17.1).[13]

Relatively, low levels of Driving Pressure (DP) were found to be significantly associated with survival in ARDS patients, whereas VT and PEEP were not independently

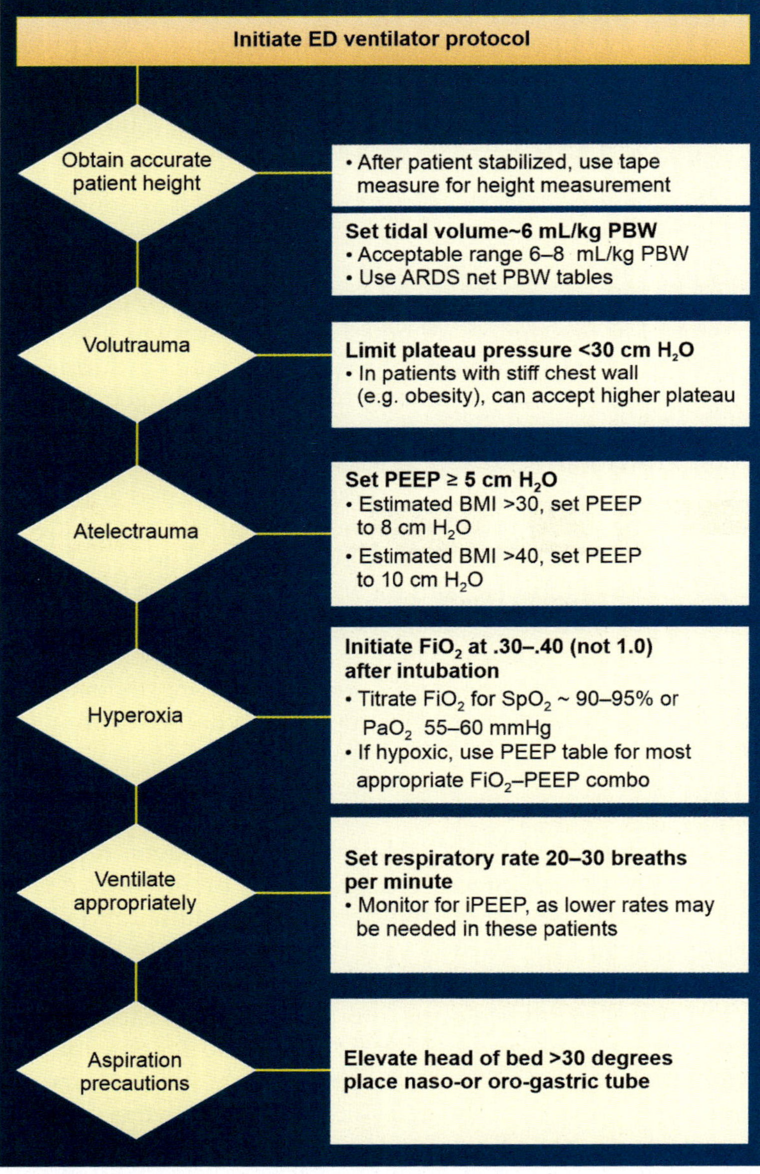

Fig. 17.1: Emergency department protocol for mechanical ventilation in the immediate post intubation period[11]

associated with survival. Studies pointed out that curtailing the DP by regulating the ventilator parameters has significant correlation with the associated clinical outcome and survival; adjustments in VT, VT calculated by PBW, P-plat, or PEEP is influencing the outcome only when there is a change in DP.[14] RT should routinely monitor to ensure patients are not being ventilated with excessively high driving pressures, especially in those with severely injured lungs. Mechanical ventilation is a prevalent class of life support used worldwide to support patients with respiratory failure. Unfortunately, while potentially life-saving, it carries with it the potential for significant harm even when provided for only short periods. Hence, it is a demanding fact that patients receiving mechanical ventilation should be monitored closely to minimize the risk of lung injury. This exercise involves a skilled respiratory therapist checking both non-ventilator- and ventilator-specific parameters (**Fig. 17.2**).

Troubleshooting the Ventilator

After ventilator support has been initiated, it is essential to be conscious of latent complications that may manifest immediately or early in the patient's course of treatment. When ventilator alarms repetitively signal that the high airway pressure threshold is exceeded at the Vt set, RT should investigate the patient's respiratory system compliance. If there is an upsurge in peak pressure, the first step to take is to do an inspiratory hold and check the plateau. If there is an elevation in peak pressure and normal plateau pressure that means there is a high airway resistance and normal

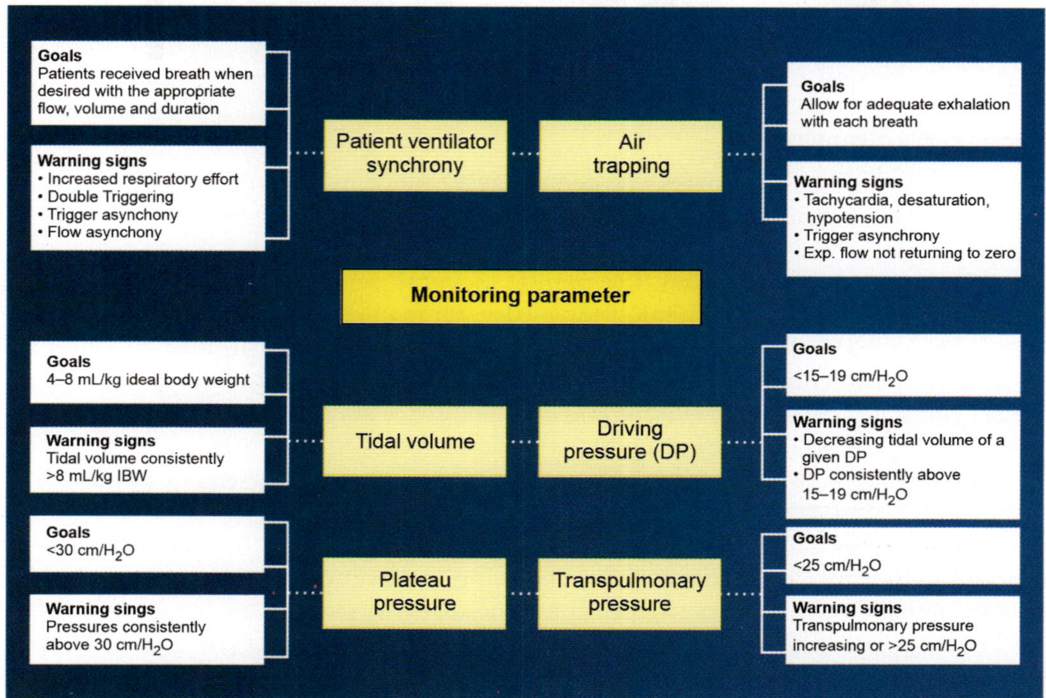

Fig. 17.2: Monitoring parameters of mechanically ventilated patient

compliance. Possible causes are, (1) distorted endotracheal tube—to resolve this issue; unkink the tube or insert a bite block if the patient is biting on the tube, (2) if there is a mucus plug, suction the patient, (3) If there is bronchospasm administer bronchodilators. Whereas, if there is an elevation in both peak airway pressure and plateau, that is compliance problem. The possible causes include; (1) Mainstem intubation—the solution is to retract the endotracheal tube, (2) Pneumothorax—the solution is placing a chest tube, (3) Atelectasis—chest physiotherapy and recruitment manoeuvres, (4) Pulmonary edema—the solution is diuresis, inotropes and apply high PEEP, (5) ARDS—the solution could be using low tidal volume, high PEEP titration.[15]

The initial step in managing a patient in respiratory distress on the ventilator is to disconnect the machine from the endotracheal tube, and begin to ventilate manually by hand with 100% oxygen. This allows the RT attending the emergency to investigate the ventilator function and breathing circuit while gaining a sense of the patient's lung compliance with hand ventilation. Sedation and anti-anxiolytics are required to control the reflexes and reduce the discomfort, particularly caused by the intense irritation to the tracheal and laryngeal mucosa as a consequence of the endotracheal tube. In the worse scenario, neuromuscular blockade is appropriate to reduce muscle fatigue and myocardial oxygen demand. Using these pharmacological agents may be particularly useful when patient "bucking" or fighting the ventilator contributes to unacceptably high airway pressures. Nurses are typically the first in recognising those types of issues while delivering care mechanically ventilated patients. In-depth knowledge about the pathophysiology and managing the patient and the mechanical ventilation in concurrence with that is fundamental for successful outcome. The nurses and other care providers must be vigilant and alert the RTs managing the case immediately if there are any issues with ventilator use. This sort of interprofessional partnership will impart greater results in handling patients on ventilators.[16]

Weaning from Ventilator

Weaning is defined as a progressive decline in the amount of ventilatory support that a patient receives from a ventilator. The course of weaning take account of decreasing ventilator support, evaluating the patient's responsiveness, and conceivably liberating from the support or extubating the patient. Several patients who are mechanically ventilated every so often extubated long after being clinically prepared to breath by own.[17] Stretched and superfluous mechanical ventilation time can lead to a number of deleterious outcomes, such as increased risk of infection, ventilator-induced lung injury, ventilator-associated events, and extra length of stay. Generally, the reasons for delayed extubations (after meeting the criteria for weaning and extubation) are many; resident physician hesitancy, lack of attending physician's presence, or proximity to end of shift remains top in the practice.

Exceptional knowledge and skills coupled with the care of patients on mechanical ventilation (e.g. airway management, suctioning, mechanical ventilator modes, blood gas interpretation) are indispensable capabilities of every single clinician for instigating the weaning process. The respiratory therapist remains with the patient, especially at the start of the weaning trial; ensure frequent assessment of breathing characteristics and prognosis during the trial; train the patient about the synchronous breath; underpins the objectives on ventilator support and desired outcomes; and moreover they reminds the patient that successful weaning and extubation enable speaking, eating, self-care activities, and mobilization. Weaning indices are mostly used to evaluate the patient's willingness to wean by evaluating the breathing pattern, respiratory muscle strength etc. these indices are commonly measured and applied by RTs. Implementing an RT driven weaning and extubation procedure will benefit greatly to facilitate and expedite extubation. Using well-defined criteria and with an established care plan, the RT can efficaciously evaluate, and execute extubation without direct physician supervision.[18] While weaning, respiratory therapists, working in association with the healthcare team, are vital for implementation of evidenced based practices that improve patient safety. An example of this is the daily evaluation for readiness for extubation component of the VAP bundle. Implementing an RT driven protocol for weaning results better patient outcomes, increased safety, and cost savings, however these changes does not assure its immediate acceptance, even within an institution where the RT department has wide acceptance of diverse group of healthcare professionals and specialists. Suboptimal compliance with protocol implementation itself may not improve over all outcome as well, however, through diligence and the passage of time, an ongoing change of culture can be achieved that allows protocol implementation and appropriate amendment of bedside practice.[19]

Role of Respiratory Therapists in the Management of Ventilated Patients in the Alternative Care Settings

The cost savings and patient welfare and fringe benefits concomitant with the home care and other non-acute care settings were recognized well in the literature. Numerous sub-acute facilities, rehabilitation facilities, and long term nursing facilities, provide respiratory care to patients especially those who require long term mechanical ventilator support. They are very popular in the recent times, since they offer the benefit of lower costs and superior patient comfort when compared with acute care facilities. However, inappropriate or untimely discharging of patients to alternative care settings and poor patient care plan implementation can wipe away these benefits and result in short-term readmission. Even though physicians are generally initiating the process of discharging a ventilated patient to an alternative site, many other healthcare professionals are also involved in the discharge process, including RTs.[20] Prompt communication and mutual respect for the talents and abilities of every single team member are the two key elements in making patient care in the alternative care setting to work successfully. The primary factors defining the suitable site for discharge are the objectives and wishes of the patient. These goals and needs should be met in an optimal and economical way using the resources available at the suggested location. The team of the designated capacity, essentially the RTs must have all the basic competencies required to manage ventilated patients, provide airway care and other respiratory needs at the alternative setting. Furthermore, the RTs must remain proficient in providing the other desirable healthcare services such as pulmonary rehabilitation, chest physical therapy and provide adequate 24-hour coverage. If the plan is to discharge the patient to the home, it is essential that the ability of caregivers to absorb and perform the required care be evaluated before transfer. RTs are responsible to train the caregivers, prepare them to clearly demonstrate the essential competencies to care for the specific patient. To confirm that a nonprofessional caregiver can perform a particular skill, the critical role of the RT is to go beyond to for the demonstration and verbal confirmation of the caregiver's understanding.[21] The RT must observe a return demonstration, whereby the caregiver properly performs the same procedural steps the RT demonstrated. In addition, providing the caregiver with written information relating to the procedural sets and equipment setup, maintenance, and basic troubleshooting can help reinforce key areas and ensure caregiver mastery of the competency before the transfer. RTs are often among the final healthcare professional in contact with a terminally ill patient MV, and much of the support not only pertains to physical comfort, but also to psychosocial management. How to recognize the symptoms of psychosocial distress in the final stages of a patient's life and how to make a referral to the most responsible physician is the talent of the RT in-charge.

Role of Respiratory Therapist in the Transport of Mechanically Ventilated Patients

Inter- or intra-hospital transport of mechanically ventilated patient (adult, paediatric or neonate) is always linked with a degree of risk. Careful preparation ahead of moving, good hand-off communication amongst all parties involved, continuous monitoring throughout the transport, and assurance of patient stability with final hand-off are essential to minimize these risk factors. Take advantage of using the right transport equipment that has the potentiality to function from a battery source in case if there is power failure and personnel appropriately trained to deal with unpredictable situation is also important.[22] Transport of a mechanically ventilated patient should be performed by an expert team consisting of an RT and a registered nurse with critical care experience, with ACLS certification. The RT assures endotracheal or tracheostomy tube is intact and patent, and confirms the proper connection between ventilator and artificial airway, preparing the air-bag-mask, check the amount of oxygen in the tank for transportation to assure that the oxygen will be sufficient during the transportation. RT holds the responsibility to check the functions of transport ventilator to assure its normal functions and alarm settings, and confirms the power charge is sufficient during the transportation, especially for the returning to the ICU. Prior to the transport the in-charge RT can perform trial of mechanical ventilation by using the planned transport MV device to appraise the patient tolerance and stability before proceeding with the transport when possible.[23]

Respiratory Therapist as the Custodian of Ventilators in the Hospital

Mechanical ventilators, used in critical care settings, are complex microprocessor-driven devices designed to support wide-ranging medical conditions, acuteness, ventilation modes, flow rates, and pressure settings. The high cost of procuring and maintaining such machines makes stockpiling these devices economically impractical. Extensive training and competency requirements are compulsory to manoeuvre these sophisticated devices safely and effectively. Ramping up ventilator capacity, founded on any capacity building initiative, will likewise require progressive elevation of human resources such as hiring RTs for the treatment of patients requiring mechanical ventilation. It is a key element in ventilator selection in the procurement process, of no less importance than the ventilator itself. RTs play an integral part in the hospital management and public health agencies regarding the procurement of mechanical ventilators by providing rapid reviews and evidence-based recommendations. The multi-criteria decision-making (MCDM) technique, usually by TOPSIS (Technique for Order Preference by Similarity to an Ideal Solution) and PROMETHEE II (preference ranking organization method for enrichment evaluation) techniques to select the best ventilator prior to their purchase by the Respiratory Therapists proved to be very advantageous in decision making. TOPSIS and PROMETHEE II are powerful techniques used to support decisions and handle evaluation of some of the alternative basis of numerous criteria, with the aim of classifying the negatives and positives of alternatives and obtaining the order of alternatives and then tracking down the best alternative.[29] Typically, for the same reason the purchase of mechanical ventilators has been with the Respiratory Care Departments in many countries. Since these departments in the past have been classified among the revenue-generating departments of the acute care hospital, it was fairly easy to rationalise capital equipment budgets to substitute old equipment or expand the ventilator army.[24]

Ventilator designs are demanded to undergo verification before manufacturing and, ultimately, testing of a prototype possibly will take place. Therefore, it is essential to have the presence of someone with expertise in mechanical ventilation in the designing phase itself, and that is necessary to be a respiratory therapist. This kind of a prompt association with the RTs, who serves as a liaisons between technical and clinical workforce of research and development teams will help to minimize the time from design to testing a prototype mechanical ventilator capable of providing advanced ventilator support for patients.

Performing proper preventative maintenance of mechanical ventilators are essential to ensure the patients receive the critical care they need to make a full recovery in the shortest time possible **(Table 17.2).** Improperly maintained or the use of malfunctioned lifesaving equipment such as ventilators can spell disaster for patients in vulnerable situations.

RTs are committed to carry out a regular visual inspection for anything erroneous in the wiring, console, or screens of the ventilator in every duty shift. It also involves running a performance check to verify all the modes of the ventilator and the various alarms are working correctly. Never overlook, or neglect any damages; no matter how tiny and insignificant it may seem. Usually ventilator batteries required to change once a year. Still, it is important to periodically check the ventilator's battery life, especially for ventilators in the ICUs that experience a high volume of patients. This can be exercised by freeing the electricity and checking to see if the ventilator still operating. RTs are responsible to do this every so often, and, as much as possible, they should make sure the ventilators are not functioning in the battery mode unless it is required.[25]

Table 17.2: Preventive maintenance of mechanical ventilator

Simple steps to follow when performing preventative maintenance of a ventilator
1. Perform a visual inspection and make sure there is no physical damages.
2. Clean and sanitize the ventilator unit.
3. Examine all air and oxygen filters and make sure they are clean.
4. Inspect for any electrical damage, ground, etc.
5. Connect the simulator/test-lung and permit it to run according to the manufacturer's suggested settings.
6. Change any components per the manufacturer's recommendation.

Guarantee the ventilator filters are clean, and change them as stated by the manufacturer's directives. A filter shields the patient from breathing hazardous materials and guards the machine and those tending to the patient from encountering anything detrimental that may be on the patient's breath. RTs should be familiar with the manufacturer guidelines of how often they need to change different ventilator filters and whether the frequency differ depending on patient volume. Disinfecting the medical equipment is a standard infection control procedure in any hospital settings, but to keep ventilators running accurately, disinfecting should not end with the cleaning of console and changing the circuit. If the ventilators use water or moist collector vials, it should be removed and clean them regularly, sometimes even daily, when high use is experienced. These aspects of the preventative maintenance process that can help prevent healthcare-acquired infections.[8] It is worth if frequently perform maintenance of the ventilators in the hospital facility, because the well-being of patients and delivering extraordinary care is the priority of all healthcare professionals.

Prevention of Infection; Strategies of a Respiratory Therapist

Ventilator associated pneumonia (VAP) is one of the most common hospital acquired infection among patients in the ICU, with an estimated incidence of 10–20% in some institutions. Notwithstanding the foregoing research, the application of VAP prevention measures or "bundles" in acute care hospitals, approaches of vigorous surveillance and early recognition, developments in antimicrobial therapy and stewardship, and multiple centralized tracking methods, VAP remains to be significantly related with patient morbidity and mortality.[26] Numerous healthcare facilities implemented a VAP "bundle" for prevention, with the most prevalent elements being head of the bed elevation, oral hygiene, daily sedation interval, spontaneous breathing trials, gastrointestinal prophylaxis, and thrombotic disease prevention; but with all these bundle components, full devotion to all the elements is a main barrier. Recent studies recommend a multidisciplinary team approach is paramount to safeguard adherence to evidence-based practices of a VAP bundle. Consecutively, a decrease in the prevalence of VAP is stated. In a retrospective cohort study conducted in a single-center setting, VAP bundle adherence was assessed with RT participation. Conventionally, the oral care component of the bundle had been done by the nurses, with hydrogen peroxide solution in a 4-hour interval. However, poor adherence to oral care was reported (33%), and the responsibility was reallocated to the RTs. Around the same time of this shift in responsibility, they also substituted hydrogen peroxide with chlorhexidine 2% solution every 12 hours.[27] Significant drop-in antibiotic days were also noted. Even though this study could not conclusively establish causality in the decrease of VAP rates, the RTs' assumption of oral care and the improved bundle adherence (along with a chlorhexidine solution change) accomplished a modest reduction in VAP rates. The distinct impact of the improved adherence under RT care, or of the transformation to chlorhexidine from hydrogen peroxide, is mysterious; nonetheless the effect on VAP rates was considerable and that highlights the role of multidisciplinary team in prevention of VAP in mechanically ventilated patients. Arroliga, *et al.* pointed out the importance of a multidisciplinary task force to carry out best practices, with the duty and accountability is shared among nurses and RTs. This study also highlighted the role RT can play in VAP prevention outside of ventilator management and faster initiation of spontaneous breathing trial. Their work can expand to the bedside team further and that will directly influence VAP rates.[28]

Role of Respiratory Therapists in Training Mechanical Ventilation

RT's role has been integral in the management and treatment of mechanically ventilated patients, and the ventilator is considered a property of the RT department. Any trouble or alarm of the ventilator activates an alert signal to the RT to troubleshoot a problem. Nevertheless, some of that alarm or issues could be so emergent that there is no sufficient time to call an RT particularly when they are not directly available in the ICU or they are stuck with a different procedure. The nurses and the multidisciplinary team members concerning their own inevitable roles at the ICU, and many of them are not practically taught on the ventilator, and their clinical experience and capacity might differ. Training this multi-disciplinary team members on the basics of a ventilator can meaningfully help the patients (**Fig. 17.3**). RTs have a pivotal role in educating them about the basic operation of a ventilator (e.g. what are the type of alarm mean and how to troubleshoot, etc.) are not proposed to overstrain the already busy nursing fraternity, and other healthcare professionals but to empower them to take on a more diligent role in the patients' welfare. It might support their patients wean off and get liberated off the ventilator quicker and safer. RTs' clinical and academic experience allows them to share and critique mechanical ventilation and critical care related empirical literature experienced clinicians in the medical community.[20]

To prevent hazardous occurrences or events, RTs play a decisive role in educating patients and training the family members or care givers in the safe use of oxygen therapy equipment, monitoring and caring the mechanically ventilated patient at home, and medications. It takes a comprehensive understanding of respiratory therapy to expedite a smooth change between hospital care to that of their management in the home. Occupied in the home care setting entails solid patient assessment skills and proficient knowledge in the management and trouble shooting of all respiratory care equipment. Critical care skills are truly applied in a home environment where limited availability of equipment, skilled personnel assistance and less-invasive monitors are available. RTs can also

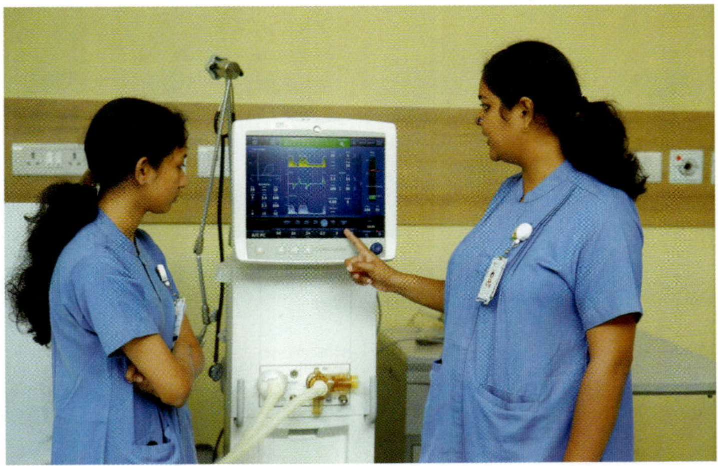

Fig. 17.3: Hands on session on mechanical ventilation by an RT educator

advice the patients on how their illness may affect them, what they can assume, and how to be mindful of any significant or acute changes. Early intervention still remains key.[21] Once again, teaching and training is vital and RTs can cover a broad range of topics. Dedicated and passionate RTs are enthusiastic to undertake the task of being involved in the training and community awareness to combat spreading of infections like COVID-19. For them supporting the heart and pulmonary health of patients with respiratory disease and ensuring cardiorespiratory stability is highly gratifying. RTs working in the community can prove what RTs can bring to the healthcare rapport by stepping outside the box and engaging with practitioners from other disciplines.

Conclusion

Although the COVID-19 pandemic has emphasised the status of the respiratory therapist in an interprofessional healthcare line-up, it has also added to an already mounting patient population demanding multifaceted cardiopulmonary care. The RT brings value to the team of providers necessary to meet expanding practice needs. Because of their incomparable combination of education and experience, RTs are inimitably equipped to deliver abrupt contributions to a cardiopulmonary specialty care and practice. Further, as RT educators assure the advanced curriculum and training address the expanding roles in a variety of complex situations, the one and only professional who is enormously suited to manage, adjust, and document the ventilator is the respiratory therapist.[30] Furthermore, to offer safe care to ventilated patients, the number of healthcare professionals who are permitted to make alterations to the ventilator should be restricted. All respiratory therapists, by their training and day-to-day experience, have remarkably greater exposure and clinical competence than most healthcare professionals when it comes to the ventilator. Whenever an adjustment is made on the ventilator, the respiratory therapist must be informed so that the alarm settings can be reviewed and attuned as desired for the safety of the patient. Any healthcare worker who makes changes to the ventilator settings must be brave enough to demonstrate the same degree of competency and training as that of a qualified respiratory therapist.

Key Points

- Respiratory therapists involved in taking care of ventilated patients should participate in regular educational roundtables on mechanical ventilation.
- Respiratory therapists should be instructed to take continuing medical education programs on mechanical ventilation safety at least once in every 2 years.
- Whenever a new machine, or a new technique is introduced the competency of the RTs involved in the care of ventilated patients must be assessed or otherwise an annual assessment is recommended.
- Respiratory therapists should make it as a custom practice to document ventilator settings, or any changes including the alarm range. Such changes must be evidence based, and communicated to oncoming staff and the whole healthcare team taking care of the patient.
- A statutory board ought to be formed to create and update policies and procedures on mechanical ventilators. There should be directives as to who can change or modify the settings should explicitly be stated, and it must clearly state the time required to respond to a ventilator alarm.
- The primary person in charge of the ventilator must be a respiratory therapist.
- All healthcare establishments must confirm that a respiratory therapist is available at all times to anage interventions pertaining to mechanical ventilation.

References

1. American Association for Respiratory Care Advanced practice respiratory therapist. Available from : https://www.aarc.org/careers/advanced-practice-respiratory-therapist/. [Last Accessed on 18th September 2022].
2. Rickards, T. and Kitts, E., 2018. The roles, they are a changing: Respiratory Therapists as part of the multidisciplinary, community, primary healthcare team. Canadian Journal of Respiratory Therapy, 54(4), pp.83–85.
3. Stoller JK. Respiratory therapist-driven protocols. Rationale and efficacy. West J Med. 1997 Dec;167(6):408-10.
4. Barnes TA, Gale DD, Kacmarek RM, Kageler WV. Competencies needed by graduate respiratory therapists in 2015 and beyond. Respir Care. 2010 May;55(5):601–16.
5. Kacmarek RM, Barnes TA, Durbin CG. Survey of directors of respiratory therapy departments regarding the future education and credentialing of respiratory care students and staff. Respir Care 2012;57(5):710–20.
6. Hajdukovic, D. and Spasojevic, I., 2016. Initiation and deescalation of mechanical ventilation. Acta chirurgica Iugoslavica, 63(2), pp.65–70.
7. Wilcox SR, Richards JB, Fisher DF, Sankoff J, Seigel TA. Initial mechanical ventilator settings and lung protective ventilation in the ED. Am J Emerg Med. 2016 Aug;34(8):1446–51.
8. Williams LM, Sharma S. Ventilator Safety. [Updated 2022 Jun 13]. In: StatPearls [Internet]. Treasure Island (FL): StatPearls Publishing; 2022 Jan. Available from: https://www.ncbi.nlm.nih.gov/books/NBK526044/. [Last Accessed : 20th September 2022].
9. Weingart SD. Managing Initial Mechanical Ventilation in the Emergency Department. Ann Emerg Med. 2016 Nov;68(5):614–17.
10. Miller AG, Gentile MA, Coyle JP. Respiratory Therapist Endotracheal Intubation Practices. Respir Care. 2020 Jul;65(7):954–60.
11. Fuller BM, Ferguson I, Mohr NM, *et al*. Lung-protective ventilation initiated in the emergency department (LOV-ED): a study protocol for a quasi-experimental, before-after trial aimed at reducing pulmonary complications. BMJ Open 2016;6:e010991. doi: 10.1136/bmjopen-2015-010991.
12. Sanborn WG. Monitoring respiratory mechanics during mechanical ventilation: where do the signals come from? Respir Care. 2005 Jan;50(1):28–52.
13. Hess DR. Respiratory mechanics in mechanically ventilated patients. Respir Care. 2014 Nov;59(11):1773–94.
14. Sreedharan, J and Alqahtani, J 2018. Driving pressure: Clinical applications and implications in the intensive care units. Indian Journal of Respiratory Care, 7(2), p.62.
15. Cairo, J.M. (2020). Chapter 18: Troubleshooting and problem solving. In Pilbeam's mechanical ventilation: Physiological and clinical applications (7th ed., pp. 334-354). St. Louis: Elsevier.
16. Wilcox, S.R., Aydin, A., Marcolini, E.G. (2019). Troubleshooting the Ventilated Patient. In: Mechanical Ventilation in Emergency Medicine. Springer, Cham. https://doi.org/10.1007/978-3-319-98410-0_11.
17. Ely EW, Bennett PA, Bowton DL, Murphy SM, Florance AM, Haponik EF. Large scale implementation of a respiratory therapist-driven protocol for ventilator weaning. Am J Respir Crit Care Med. 1999 Feb;159(2):439–46.
18. Dries DJ, McGonigal MD, Malian MS, Bor BJ, Sullivan C. Protocol-driven ventilator weaning reduces use of mechanical ventilation, rate of early reintubation, and ventilator-associated pneumonia. J Trauma. 2004 May;56(5):943–51.

19. Krawiec, C, Carl, D, Stetter, C, Kong, L, Ceneviva, G and Thomas, N, 2017. Challenges With Implementation of a Respiratory Therapist–Driven Protocol of Spontaneous Breathing Trials in the Pediatric ICU. Respiratory Care, 62(10), pp.1233–40.
20. Glass C, Grap MJ, Battle G. Preparing the patient and family for home mechanical ventilation. Medsurg Nurs. 1999 Apr;8(2):99-101, 104–7.
21. Smith CE, Mayer LS, Perkins SB, Gerald K, Pingleton SK. Caregiver learning needs and reactions to managing home mechanical ventilation. Heart Lung. 1994 Mar-Apr;23(2):157–63.
22. Stephens RJ, Siegler JE, Fuller BM. Mechanical Ventilation in the Prehospital and Emergency Department Environment. Respir Care. 2019 May;64(5):595–603.
23. Bowen SL. Transport of the mechanically ventilated neonate. Respir Care Clin N Am. 2002 Mar;8(1):67–82.
24. Pham T, Brochard LJ, Slutsky AS. Mechanical Ventilation: State of the Art. Mayo Clin Proc. 2017 Sep;92(9):1382–1400.
25. Grace K. The ventilator: selection of mechanical ventilators. Crit Care Clin. 1998 Oct;14(4):563–80.
26. Oliveira J, Zagalo C, Cavaco-Silva P. Prevention of ventilator-associated pneumonia. Rev Port Pneumol. 2014 May-Jun;20(3):152–61.
27. Chacko R, Rajan A, Lionel P, Thilagavathi M, Yadav B, Premkumar J. Oral decontamination techniques and ventilator-associated pneumonia. Br J Nurs. 2017 Jun 8;26(11):594–99.
28. Alecrim RX, Taminato M, Belasco A, Longo MCB, Kusahara DM, Fram D. Strategies for preventing ventilator-associated pneumonia: an integrative review. Rev Bras Enferm. 2019 Mar-Apr;72(2):521–30.
29. Alyazji, Q and Asiksoy, G, 2021. Evaluating Mechanical Ventilators Using Multi-Criteria Decision-Making Techniques. International Journal of Online and Biomedical Engineering (iJOE), 17(07), p.4.
30. Kollef, M., 2017. Evaluating the Value of the Respiratory Therapist: Where Is the Evidence? Focus on the Barnes-Jewish Hospital Experience. Respiratory Care, 62(12), pp.1602–10.

Abbreviations:

ACLS	Advanced Cardiac Life Support
ARDS	Acute Respiratory Distress Syndrome
COPD	Chronic Obstructive Pulmonary Disease
DP	Driving Pressure
I:E ratio	Inspiratory Expiratory Ratio
MCDM	Multi-criteria decision-making
PBW	Predicted Body Weight
PROMETHEE II	Preference ranking organization method for enrichment evaluation
RT	Respiratory Therapist
TOPSIS	Technique for Order Preference by Similarity to an Ideal Solution
VAP	Ventilator associated pneumonia
VT	Tidal Volume

CHAPTER 18

Mechanical Ventilation in Clinical Scenarios

I. CHRONIC OBSTRUCTIVE PULMONARY DISEASE (COPD)

❒ Lisha PV ❒ Vijay Deshpande

Patients with chronic obstructive pulmonary disease (COPD) admitted to an intensive care unit (ICU) due to an acute exacerbation are still confronted with a substantial hospital mortality rate of 24% and worse clinical outcomes, respectively.[1] About 10% of COPD patients are at high risk for prolonged mechanical ventilation and mortality ranges 55–78%.[2] Non-invasive Positive Pressure Ventilation (NIPPV) is the modality of choice for managing respiratory failure in COPD exacerbations. However, invasive mechanical ventilation may become necessary in a case of clinical worsening on NIPPV or if there are contraindications to NIPPV.

PATHOPHYSIOLOGY OF COPD

It is imperative that we have a clear understanding of the pathophysiology of COPD before initiating mechanical ventilation. COPD is defined by a persistent reduction in FEV_1/FVC.

1. Airflow Obstruction

COPD differs from asthma in that the low FEV_1 and FVC are not reversible fully. FEV_1 demonstrates the relation between the elastic recoil of lung which promotes expiratory airflow and the airway resistance which limits flow during a forced vital capacity manoeuvre. In COPD, the maximal expiratory flow diminishes as the lung volume decreases. This is because of two reasons—the low elastic recoil of the lung parenchyma at low lung volumes and the increased airway resistance due to decreased cross-sectional area of airways secondary to small airway disease. In advanced COPD, this airflow limitation occurs throughout expiration. The airways are also unable to remain open at the end of expiration due to the parenchymal destruction leading to air trapping and emphysema. This leads to incomplete expiration, higher residual volumes, hyperinflation and auto-positive end expiratory pressure or auto-PEEP.

The most important pathophysiology of COPD that is expiratory airflow limitation, is compensated by an increased inspiratory flow and lung volume. But when this is combined with an increased respiratory drive as occurs in COPD exacerbations associated alone or along with pneumonia, cardiac failure or pulmonary embolism, inspiratory muscle fatigue sets in. Adding to this is the short expiratory time, which leads to air trapping, auto-PEEP and dynamic hyperinflation. The Work of Breathing WOB increases as a conz equence of DHI and the subsequent generation of Auto-PEEP.[3,4]

2. Abnormal Distribution of Ventilation and Ventilation Perfusion (V/Q) Mismatch

VQ mismatch due to the non-homogenous involvement of the pathogenic process of COPD in the airways and lung parenchyma is the cause of hypoxia in COPD. In acute exacerbations and other infective and non-infective complications like pneumonia, cardiac failure or pulmonary embolism, this mismatch can be augmented. If the hypoxemia is difficult to correct with oxygen alone, then an additional shunt pathology should be considered.[3]

3. Hyperinflation

The expiratory airflow limitation is overcome by increasing the lung elastic recoil and decreasing the airway resistance by increasing the cross-sectional area of airways. This is achieved by the chronic hyperinflation which develops in COPD. There is increase in Functional Residual Capacity (FRC), Residual Volume (RV), Total Lung Capacity (TLC) and RV/TLC ratio. The problem with hyperinflation is that it pushes the diaphragm down and flattens it, which leads to:

- Decrease in the zone of apposition between diaphragm and abdominal wall
- Shortening of the muscle fibre length, thus decreasing the force of contraction
- Increases radius of curvature of diaphragm and thus decrease the transpulmonary pressure generated
- Changes the direction of diaphragmatic muscle fibres medially, thereby impairing their action.

4. Gas Exchange Abnormalities in COPD

$PaCO_2$ usually does not rise above normal unless the FEV_1 is less than one fourth of its predicted normal values. Increase in physiological dead space is an important factor in COPD. The increase in dead space ventilation and increase in alveolar arterial oxygen gradient causes abnormalities in gas exchange for O_2 and CO_2. Therefore, more than normal ventilation is required to maintain eucapnia in COPD. In severe COPD and in exacerbations the minute ventilation required is typically two to three times the normal. The increased airway resistance and hyperinflation leads to increased intrathoracic pressure swings to generate the required tidal volume and airflow rates. This greatly increases the respiratory muscle oxygen uptake to even greater than 50% of the total oxygen uptake by the body. The hyperinflation also causes mechanical disadvantage, and decreases the capacity of inspiratory muscles to generate Pmax. This is compounded by advanced age, and malnutrition in patients with COPD. The consequent inspiratory muscle fatigue plays an important role in weaning a COPD patient from mechanical ventilation.[3]

Hypoxemia in COPD is generally due to VQ mismatch and corrected easily by oxygen therapy. But during exacerbations other factors which lead to lung failure like pneumonia, atelectasis, embolism pulmonary oedema should be looked for and corrected. Hypoxemia is rarely refractory to supplemental oxygen in patients with exacerbations of COPD. Unless if a shunt physiology is at play like a coexisting ARDS.

Indication for Invasive Mechanical Ventilation in COPD

Non-Invasive Positive Pressure Ventilation (NIPPV) is the preferred choice when a COPD patient presents in respiratory failure. But in many situations like a comatose patient who is unable to control his airway or patient who is having vomiting or facial trauma, we may have to go for invasive mechanical ventilation upfront. The indications for initiation of invasive mechanical ventilation in COPD are as follows:[5,6]

Major criteria (any one of the following)

- Respiratory arrest
- Loss of consciousness
- Psychomotor agitation requiring sedation
- Hemodynamic instability
- Heart rate less than 50 beats/min with loss of alertness
- Gasping for air

Minor criteria (any two of the following)

- Respiratory rate >35 breath/min
- Worsening acidemia or pH <7.25
- PaO_2 less than 40 mm Hg or PaO_2/FiO_2 less than 200 mm Hg despite oxygen
- Decreasing level of consciousness

Interaction between Ventilator and Lung in COPD and Monitoring

The primary goals of invasive mechanical ventilation in patients with chronic obstructive pulmonary disease (COPD) are the following:[7]

- Correct derangements in oxygenation and ventilation
- Reduce the work of breathing
- Prevent dynamic hyperinflation (DHI)

It is important to assess the pre-ventilator status while taking control of the intubated COPD lung. Dynamic hyperinflation and intrinsic PEEP may be the most common problem you may have to face in the initial periods.

1. Selection of Initial Mode

The initial mode can be an Assist Control mode, Synchronised Intermittent Mandatory Ventilation mode or Pressure support mode depending on the ability of the patient to trigger and cycle his own breaths. In the fully obtunded or comatose patient always choose an Assist Control mode till he is conscious enough to trigger his own breaths. If the patient is fully conscious, even an initial pressure support mode can be selected, however, SIMV to be preferred initially in the conscious patient. Pressure or volume targets may be chosen according to the expertise available to monitor the patient.[8]

2. How to Detect Dynamic Hyper Inflation (DHI) and auto-PEEP

In the presence of increased expiratory airflow resistance, the time available to empty the inspired volume may not be sufficient. Thus, the respiratory system is unable to return to its normal relaxation volume at the end of expiration. This results in a new resting state where the FRC is greater than the Vrel. This condition of air trapping is otherwise called DHI. The DHI results in positive alveolar pressure at the end of expiration also referred to as auto-PEEP (positive end expiratory pressure). This can be recognised by the following:

- Clinically a patient with DHI and significant auto-PEEP will develop tachypnoea, tachycardia, hypertension, or hypotension; decrease in arterial oxygen saturation; use of accessory muscles of breathing; reduction or absence of breath sounds over a region of the lung, wheezing, rib-cage abdominal asynchrony, paradoxical movement of the abdominal wall during inspiration, cyanosis, inability to trigger the ventilator, and apnea. All these point to the need for urgent interventions or ventilator adjustments.[9]
- When the manual bag is connected to the ventilator a slow filling of the bag will be noted.
- Auto-PEEP can also be detected on ventilator graphic waveform monitoring. Although not readily quantifiable, auto-PEEP is easily recognized on the expiratory portion of the flow waveform. If expiratory flow does not return to zero before the next inspiration, auto-PEEP is present as shown in **Figs 18.1 and 18.2**.

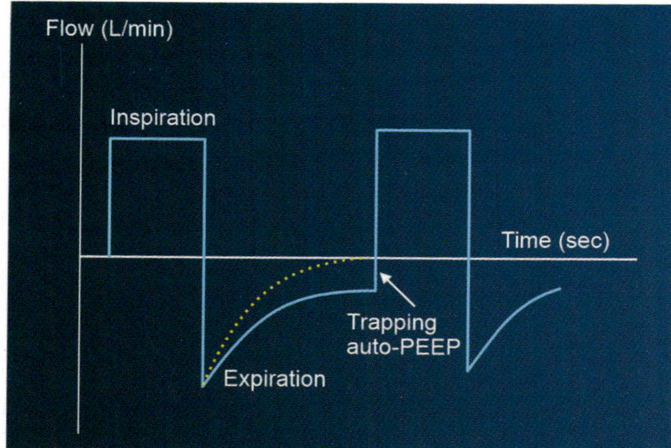

Fig.18.1: Auto-PEEP in a flow time scalar (*Courtesy:* Rajiv Dhand. Ventilator Graphics and Respiratory Mechanics in the Patient With Obstructive Lung Disease;Respir Care 2005;50(2):246–259.)

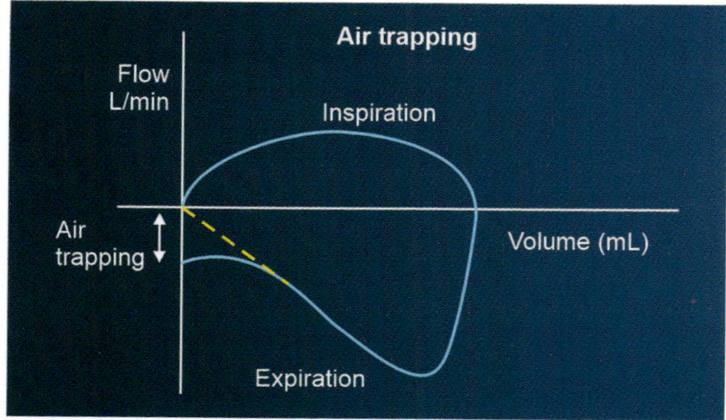

Fig. 18.2: Air trapping in a flow volume loop (*Courtesy:* Rajiv Dhand. Ventilator Graphics and Respiratory Mechanics in the Patient With Obstructive Lung Disease; Respir Care 2005;50(2):246–259.)

- Observing the ventilator waveforms for a missed breath or cycle will also give an idea that the patient's effort is ineffective in overcoming the intrinsic PEEP to trigger a breath.
- Some ventilators allow a breath hold for 2 seconds during expiration which will allow in detecting the total PEEP which is the sum of the applied PEEP plus the intrinsic PEEP. But this method is not applicable in a patient a patient with spontaneous breathing efforts. The patient should be fully sedated and paralysed for this method to measure auto-PEEP.
- If there is active respiratory effort from the patient, dynamic PEEP can be measured using a simultaneous recording of oesophageal pressure and airflow tracings. It is measured at end expiration as the negative deflection of oesophageal pressure to the point of zero flow.
- For patients who are making spontaneous efforts to breathe, observing their respiratory efforts and the ventilators response is another useful technique, provided the ventilators sensitivity is set correctly (at 1 cm H_2O or on flow triggering). Because auto-PEEP increases the pressure gradient required to inhale, the patient's effort may not be able to trigger the ventilator; the result is a missed breath or cycle.

3. *Disadvantages of Auto-PEEP*

- **Increased work of breathing:** During an exacerbation, tidal breathing occurs towards the total lung capacity in an effort to improve the flow rates. In this situation the respiratory system is acting on the flatter part of the pressure volume curve where increase in pressure generates only small changes in volume (**Figs 18.3 and 18.4**). In the presence of auto-PEEP, the intrapleural pressure generated must be more than the amount of auto-PEEP for airflow to begin which imposes a substantial inspiratory burden on the respiratory muscles.[10,11]
- **Compromise in cardiac function:** Increased intrathoracic pressure can lead to decreased venous return which in turn decreases left ventricular preload. DHI can increase pulmonary vascular resistance by compressing alveolar capillaries leading to increased right ventricular afterload. These changes can lead to hypotension especially soon after intubation when other factors like sedatives and hypovolemia

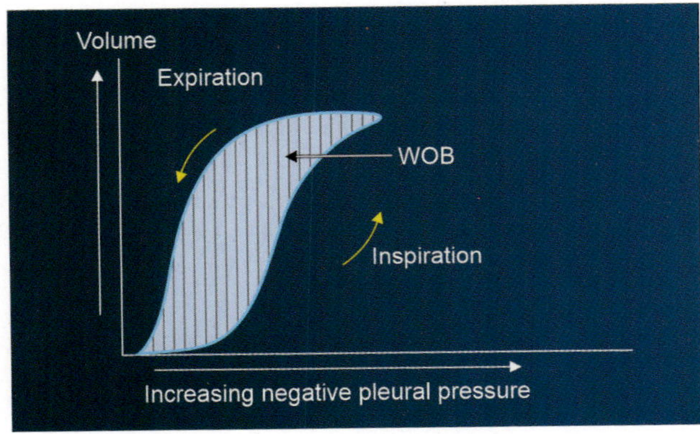

Fig. 18.3: WOB representing the relation between pressure and volume

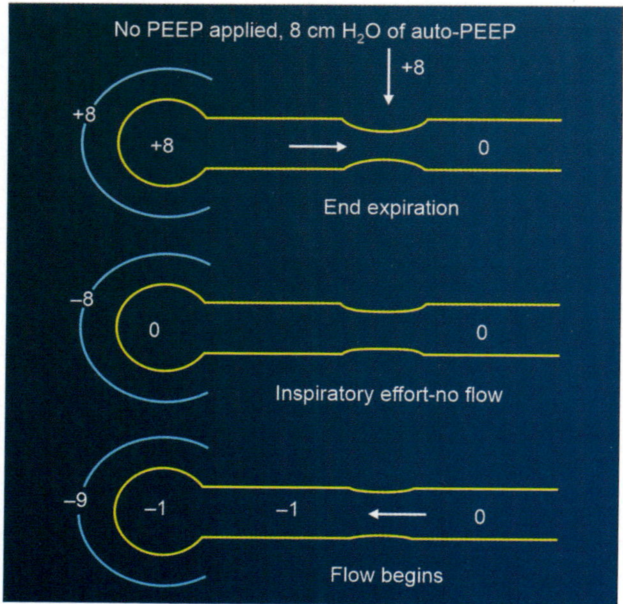

Fig. 18.4: Effect of Auto-PEEP on Work of breathing

may be coexisting. Sometimes this combination of reduced cardiac output, high filling pressures and hypotension may be mistaken the dynamic hyperinflation continues it will cause Pulse less Electrical Activity and cardiac arrest.[12–16]

- **Barotrauma:** Excessive PEEP can lead to barotrauma related adverse effects like pneumothorax and pneumomediastinum. Barotrauma correlates better with the plateau pressures than the peak inspiratory pressures. Therefore, it is advisable to maintain a plateau

4. Strategies to overcome Auto-PEEP and Decrease DHI

Auto-PEEP depends on three factors:

- Minute ventilation
- Inspiratory expiratory ratio
- Expiratory time constants

So, the strategy to decrease auto-PEEP should be aimed primarily at decreasing minute ventilation and allowing more time to expiration which may be done by a low tidal volume, lower respiratory rates, higher inspiratory flow rates and a longer expiratory time. This strategy should be targeted to normalise the PH with some permissive hypercapnia. Minute ventilation should be adjusted to the pH and target to attain normal pH and prevent overventilation rather than trying to normalise the $PaCO_2$ levels.[4]

The initial settings after intubation of the patient should be targeted to prevent or mitigate DHI and auto-PEEP. Therefore, the tendency to increase respiratory rates and thus increase minute ventilation and correct acidosis is to be curbed. Instead, the rates should be set around 10 to 14 breaths, tidal volume at 6 to 8 ml per kg ideal body weight, high inspiratory flow rates of 80 to 100 L per minute, a square wave form and a flow trigger. I:E ratio should be kept at 1:3 or above. The idea is to improve respiratory acidosis by giving more time for expiration and allowing the intrinsic PEEP to come down. This should be accompanied by pharmacological measures to decrease airway resistance like bronchodilators and anti-inflammatory therapy.

5. Effects of Expiratory Time, Minute Ventilation and Expiratory Flow Rates on DHI

The important determinants of DHI are minute ventilation, tidal volume, time for expiration (TE), and severity of airway obstruction. Reduction in end expiratory volume which indicates air trapping is achieved by decreasing the respiratory rate which increases the time for expiration, while increasing the tidal volume to keep the minute ventilation constant. Simply altering the I:E ratio will not bring about the change in expiratory time.[17] Correctable factors causing increased work of breathing should be targeted in the ventilated patient with COPD. This includes airway resistance due to bronchospasm, decreased parenchymal compliance due to pulmonary oedema, pneumonia or atelectasis, and decreased chest wall compliance due to pleural effusion or ascites. Respiratory muscle weakness caused by sedatives, electrolyte abnormalities or nutritional wasting can also increase work of breathing. Ventilator-associated factors like a narrow endotracheal tube, external PEEP increased trigger threshold of the ventilator should also be considered as causing increased work of breathing.[4]

6. Effect of Peak and Plateau Pressure

Peak pressure threshold of 50 cm of H_2O has been suggested to decrease chance of barotrauma. But rather than peak pressure, coincides risk of barotrauma with plateau pressure and is advisable to keep plateau pressures less than 30 cm of H_2O. Low minute ventilation, low tidal volume and correction of auto-PEEP helps to achieve this target.[18,19]

7. PEEP as a Strategy to Counter auto-PEEP

Presence of auto-PEEP increases the work of breathing by making it difficult for the patient to generate the pressures needed to trigger a breath. Applying an external PEEP to counter auto-PEEP is a strategy which can be used. This is explained in the following figure. The external PEEP should be kept below 75 to 80% of auto-PEEP to avoid worsening of DHI (**Fig. 18.5**).[20,21]

8. Setting the Trigger in COPD

A high trigger will make it difficult for the patient to initiate a breath whereas a low trigger will lead to initiation of unwanted breaths leading to DHI. The trigger sensitivity is usually set at –1 to –2 cm H_2O when pressure triggering is used. This means that ventilator-assisted breaths will be triggered when the airway pressure decreases to 1 to 2 cm H_2O below atmospheric pressure. The trigger sensitivity is usually set at 2 L/min when flow triggering is used. This means that ventilator-assisted breaths will be triggered once the patient's inspiratory effort generates a flow of 2 L/min above the bias flow running through the circuit.

Adjust inspiratory trigger sensitivity to reduce ineffective triggering and lower the degree of wasted work of breathing.[22]

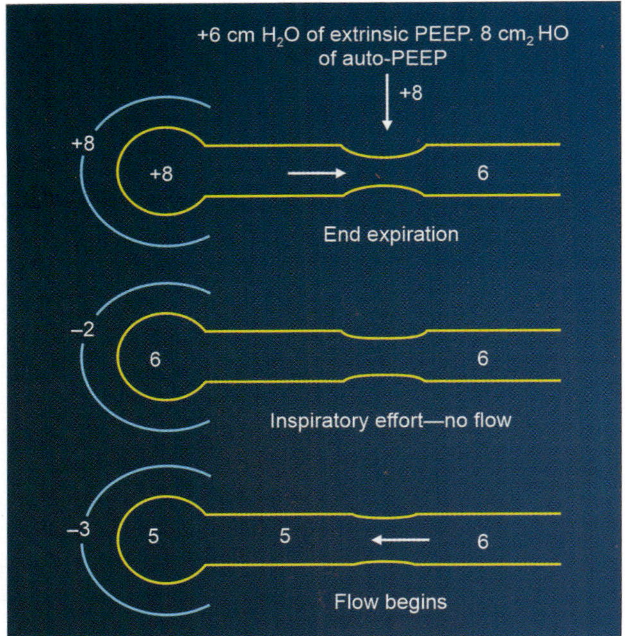

Fig. 18.5: Application of external PEEP to counter auto-PEEP

Medical Management of COPD Exacerbation

Medical management of COPD targeted to the pathophysiology is essential and should go hand in hand with the ventilatory adjustments.[23]

Bronchodilators

Inhaled short acting beta agonists with or without short acting anticholinergics administered through nebulisers is the preferred choice. They help in reducing airway resistance.

Corticosteroids

At a dose of 40 mg of prednisolone equivalents for 5 days corticosteroids are used in severe exacerbations and decrease airway inflammation and resistance.

Antibiotics

Antibiotics targeting bacterial infection according to the local resistance pattern is indicated in COPD patients requiring invasive mechanical ventilation. The duration of antibiotic therapy is usually five days.

Other important aspects of management are adequate secretion clearance, preventing the complications of immobility and adequate nutrition.

Complications of Mechanical Ventilation in COPD

- Worsening of DHI and auto-PEEP is the most important complication that can occur in COPD patients. Prompt recognition and introducing the necessary changes is necessary as has been described in previous sections will be needed.

- Barotrauma causing pneumothorax and pneumomediastinum
- Mortality in ventilated COPD is increased in proportion the following factors
  - Prolonged hospital stay prior to initiation of mechanical ventilation
  - Presence of multiple organ failure and sepsis
  - Presence of cardiac failure or pulmonary embolism

Interpreting Loops and Scalars (Figs 18.6 to18.12)

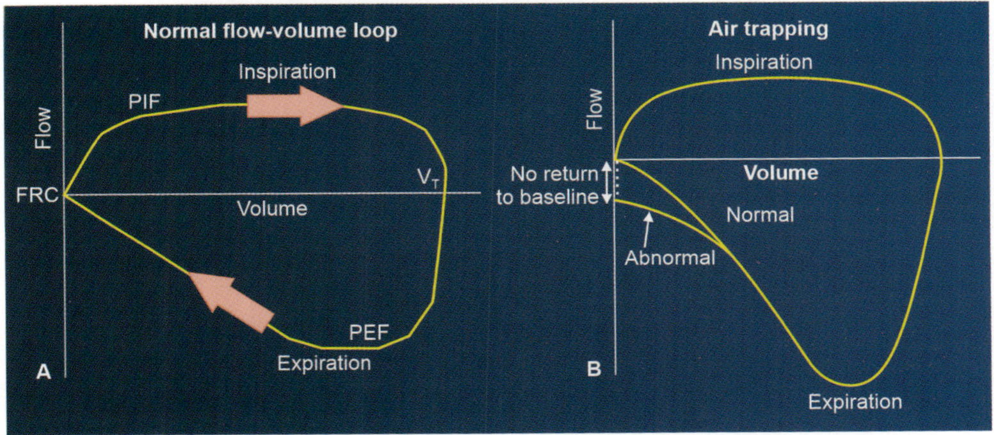

Fig. 18.6A and B: Air trapping in flow volume loop

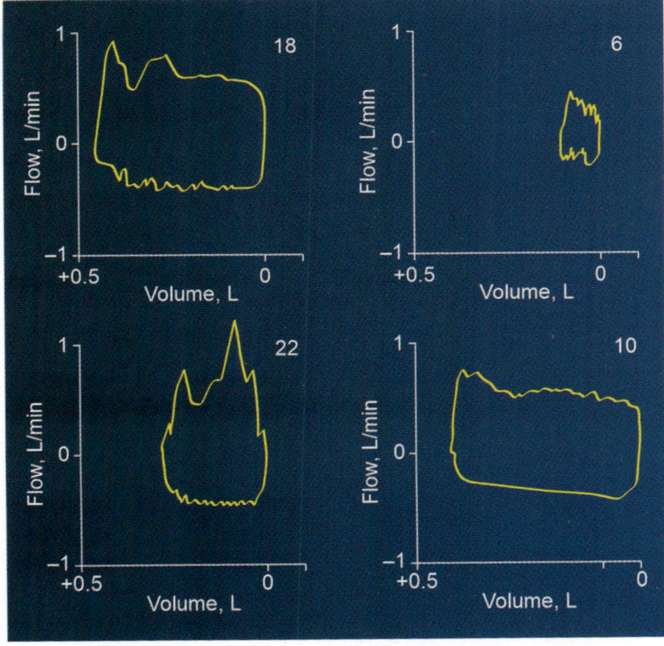

Fig. 18.7: Flow volume curve indicating secretions

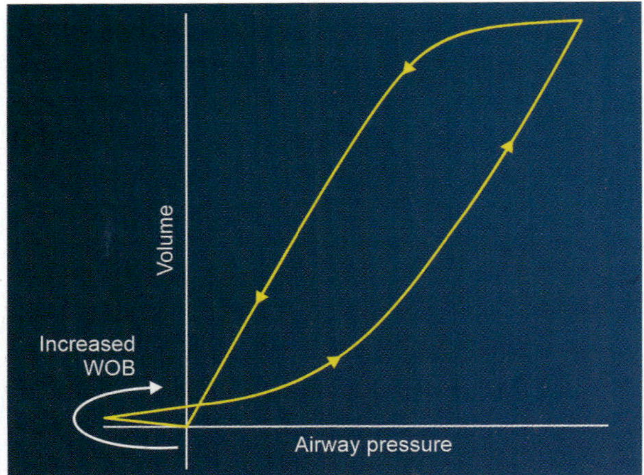

Fig. 18.8: Pressure-volume loop showing excessive patient effort due to inadequate trigger sensitivity

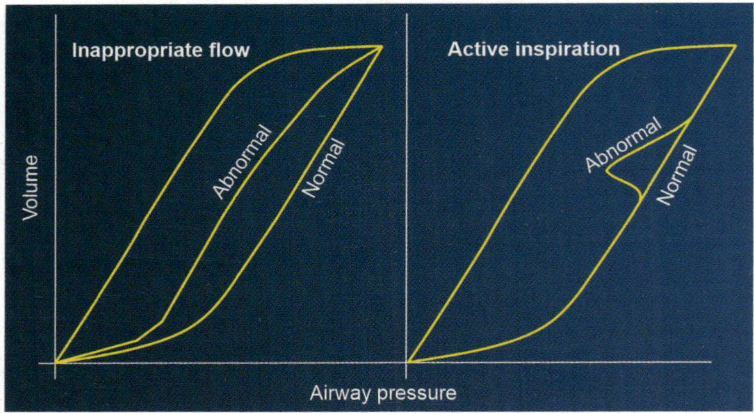

Fig. 18.9: Pressure-volume loops may also be helpful in detecting an inappropriately low inspiratory flow setting (left) and active patient efforts during inspiration (right)

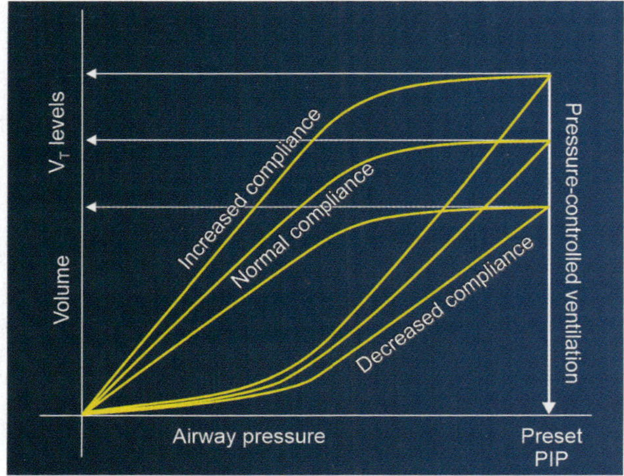

Fig. 18.10: Changes in pressure volume loop according to compliance of lung in pressure controlled modes

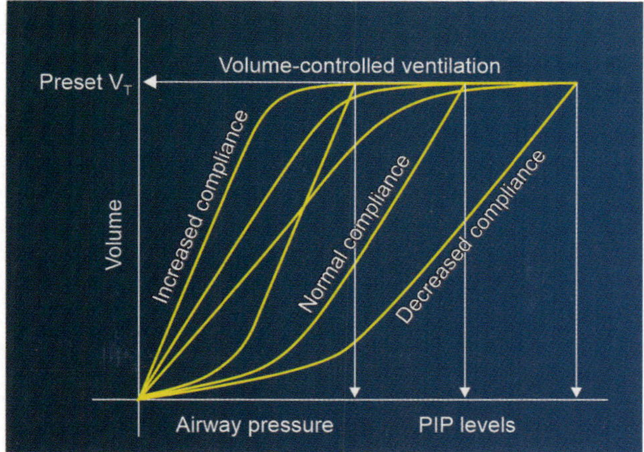

Fig. 18.11: Change in pressure volume loop according to compliance in volume controlled modes

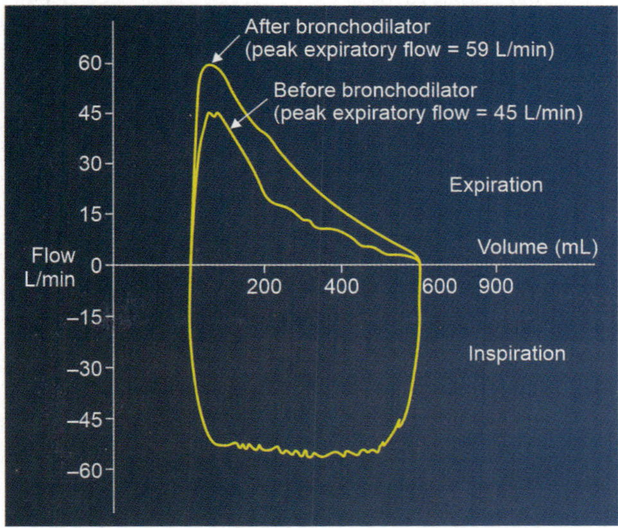

Fig. 18.12: Flow volume loop showing response to bronchodilator administration

Conclusion

Invasive mechanical ventilation at the right time is an invaluable tool in the management of COPD exacerbation. Rapid correction of physiology and early weaning is possible with careful monitoring in many of these patients. The therapeutic goals of invasive mechanical ventilation are to improve gas exchange, rest fatigued respiratory muscles, and relieve respiratory distress. Early weaning with attention to other pharmacological measures especially nutrition, will ensure the best outcome. Ventilator graphics should be used in the early detection of complications before the signs of complications set in. If not properly used mechanical ventilation itself may cause mortality in COPD.

References

1. Ward NS, Dushay KM. Clinical concise review: Mechanical ventilation of patients with chronic obstructive pulmonary disease. Crit Care Med 2008; 36: 1614–19.
2. Mohan A, Premanand R, Reddy LN, *et al.* Clinical presentation and predictors of outcome in patients with severe acute exacerbation of chronic obstructive pulmonary disease requiring admission to intensive care unit. BMC Pulm Med 2006; 6: 27.CrossRefPubMedGoogle Scholar
3. In: Grippi MA, Elias JA, Fishman JA, Kotloff RM, Pack AI, Senior RM, Siegel MD. eds. Fishman's Pulmonary Diseases and Disorders, Fifth Edition. McGraw Hill; 2015. Accessed October 02, 2023. https://accessmedicine.mhmedical.com/content.aspx?bookid=1344§ionid=79339192
4. Nathan T. Mowery, MD. Ventilator Strategies for Chronic Obstructive Pulmonary Disease and Acute Respiratory Distress SyndromeSurg Clin N Am 97 (2017) 1381–1397 http://dx.doi.org/10.1016/j.suc.2017.07.006
5. Brochard L, Mancebo J, Wysocki M, *et al.* Non-invasive ventilation for acute exacerbations of chronic obstructive pulmonary disease. N Engl J Med 1995;333(13): 817–22.
6. Brochard L, Isabey D, Piquet J, *et al.* Reversal of acute exacerbations of chronic obstructive lung disease by inspiratory assistance with a face mask. N Engl J Med 1990;323(22):1523–30
7. AU Davidson AC, Banham S, Elliott M et al, BTS Standards of Care Committee Member, British Thoracic Society/Intensive Care Society Acute Hypercapnic Respiratory Failure Guideline Development Group, On behalf of the British Thoracic Society Standards of Care Committee. BTS/ICS guideline for the ventilatory management of acute hypercapnic respiratory failure in adults.Thorax. 2016 Apr;71 Suppl 2:ii1–ii35.
8. Ozlem Ediboglu. Mechanical Ventilation for Patients with COPD. 14 July 2021DOI: 10.5772/intechopen.96633
9. Tobin MJ. Respiratory monitoring in the intensive care unit. Am Rev Respir Dis. 1988a;138:1625–42. [PubMed] [Google Scholar] [Ref list]
10. Tobin MJ. Respiratory monitoring in the intensive care unit. Am Rev Respir Dis. 1988a;138:1625–42. [PubMed] [Google Scholar] [Ref list]
11. Fluery B, Murciano D, Talamo C, *et al.* Work of breathing in patients with chronic obstructive pulmonary disease. Am Rev Respi Dis. 1985;131:822. [PubMed] [Google Scholar] [Ref list]
12. Mahler DA, Brent BN, Loke J, *et al.* Right ventricular performance and central hemodynamics during upright exercise in patients with chronic obstructive pulmonary disease. Am Rev Respir Dis. 1984;130:722–9. [PubMed] [Google Scholar] [Ref list]
13. Martens R, Vandekerhove Y, Mullie A (1993), Restoration of spontaneous circulation after cessation of cardiopulmonary resusitation. Lancet 341:1217
14. Kollef MH (1992) Lung hyperinflation caused by inappropriate ventilation resulting in electromechanical dissociation: a case report. Heart Lung21: 74-77
15. Myles PS, Madden H, Morgan EB (1995). Intraoperative cardiac arrest after unrecognized dynamic hyperinflation. Br J Anaesth 74:340–42.
16. Scharf SM, Iqbal M, Keller C, *et al.* Hemodynamic characterization of patients with severe emphysema. Am J Respir Crit Care Med. 2002;166:314–22. [PubMed] [Google Scholar] [Ref list]
17. Tuxen DV, Lane S. The effects of ventilatory pattern on hyperinflation airway pressures, circulation in mechanically ventilation of patients with severe air flow obstruction. Am Rev Respir Dis. 1987;136:872. [PubMed] [Google Scholar] [Ref list]
18. Williams TJ, Tuxen DV, Scheinkestel CD, *et al.* Risk factors for morbidity in mechanically ventilated patients with acute severe asthma. Am Rev Respir Dis. 1992;146:607. [PubMed] [Google Scholar] [Ref list].

19. Slutsky AS. Mechanical ventilation—ACCP consensus conference. Chest. 1993;104:1833. [PubMed] [Google Scholar] [Ref list].
20. Ranieri VM, Giuliani R, Cinnella G, *et al.* Physiologic effects of positive end-expiratory pressure in patients with chronic obstructive pulmonary disease during acute ventilatory failure and controlled mechanical ventilation. Am Rev Respir Dis. 1993;147:5–13. [PubMed] [Google Scholar] [Ref lis].
21. Reddy RM, Guntupalli KK. Review of ventilatory techniques to optimize mechanical ventilation in acute exacerbation of chronic obstructive pulmonary disease. Int J Chron Obstruct Pulmon Dis. 2007;2(4):441–52. PMID: 18268918; PMCID: PMC2699957.
22. Ward ME, Corbeil C, Gibbons W, Newman S, Macklem PT Optimization of respiratory muscle relaxation during mechanical ventilation. Anesthesiology. 1988;69(1):29.
23. Global Initiative for Chronic Obstructive Lung Disease 2023 Report: GOLD Executive Summary. Eur Respir J. 2023 Apr 1;61(4):2300239. doi: 10.1183/13993003.00239-2023.

II. MECHANICAL VENTILATION IN ASSHMA

❒ Nalini Nagalla

Asthma, a chronic inflammatory airway disease, can cause severe exacerbations that may require ICU admission or may turn life threatening. Improved asthma treatment plans and healthcare access have led to reduced incidence of life threatening exacerbations (LTAE). Still, about 25,000 to 50,000 of asthma patients every year require admission to an ICU in the United States.[1]

Of all the acute asthma exacerbations requiring hospital care, 10% require Intensive Care unit (ICU) admission and 2% require invasive ventilation.[2] Hence it is very important for clinicians taking care of these patients to be familiar with timely assessment and management of LTAE.

The Global Initiative for Asthma guidelines refers to severe asthma exacerbation as a patient who talks in words, sits hunched forward, is agitated, uses accessory respiratory muscles, has a respiratory rate >30/min, heart rate >120/min, O_2 saturation on air <90% and PEF 50% of their best or predicted. This can turn life threatening if there is poor response to emergency room treatment.

Though life threatening asthma events are most frequent with severe and poorly controlled asthma, they can occur in patients with mild or moderate asthma also. A multi-centre study of clinical feathers of asthma by Ramnath VR, *et al*. showed that there are two distinct clinical entities of acute severe asthma:

1. The Slow Onset Group (80 to 85%), where patients have symptoms for several days prior to the severe attack,
2. The Sudden Onset Group (6%), who present with severe attack in one to three hours of beginning of symptoms.[3,4]

Risk factors for Acute Severe Asthma (Table 18.1)

There are definite identified risk factors for acute severe asthma.

Table 18.1: Risk factors for fatal asthma exacerbations

A History of near fatal asthma requiring intubation and machanical ventilation
✦ Hospitalization or emergency care visits for asthma in the past year
✦ Currently using or having recently stopped using oral steroids
✦ Not currently using inhaled steroids
✦ SABA over-use (more than one cainster of salbutamol/month (or equivalent))
✦ History of psychiatric disease or psychosocial problems
✦ Female sex
✦ Age >40 years
✦ Smoking history
✦ Poor preception of airflow limitation
✦ Hyperinflation in chest radiograph
✦ Poor adherence with asthma medications and/or poor adherence (or lack of with a written asthma action plan
✦ Food allergy

SABA: Short acting beta agonists. (*Adapted from*: Global Initiative for Asthma (GINA), 2018)

A prior history of ICU admission or invasive ventilation should always be asked when an acute severe asthma patient comes to ED (Emergency Department) as it helps the clinician in escalating the therapy quickly in case of poor response to initial treatment.

Obesity is also a risk factor for severe exacerbations. It has been seen that in patients who have undergone bariatric surgery, the asthma attacks and hospitalization has come down.[5]

Key Areas of Acute Asthma Management

Patients with acute severe asthma are more at risk for ventilator induced dynamic hyperinflation and barotrauma. It is very important for clinicians in the ICU to prevent and manage these devastating complications.

As described by James Leatherman, MD, for successful outcome of acute severe asthma patients who require mechanical ventilation, a strategy that prioritizes avoidance of ventilator-related complications over correction of hypercapnia was first proposed 30 years ago and has become the preferred approach.[6]

Brenner *et al.* reviewed the evidence-based data regarding the indications, techniques, and complications of intubation and mechanical ventilation in the treatment of acute asthma in the emergency department (ED) and came up with strategies for intubation and practical management recommendations.[7]

Emergency Department (ED) task force had identified 7 key areas for management of acute severe asthma based on review of literature and clinical experience:[7]

1. Prevention of intubation
2. Criteria for intubation
3. Recommendations for intubation technique
4. Recommendation for appropriate ventilator settings
5. Management in the immediate post-intubation period
6. Medical management of asthma in the ventilated patient
7. Prevention and management of complications

1. Prevention of Intubation

Most patients coming to ED with acute severe asthma can be managed without intubation. As the mortality widely ranges from 6 to 20% in patients requiring intubation, preventing intubation becomes a crucial goal in the management of acute severe asthma.

1.1 Non-invasive ventilation (NIV)

Though use of NIV is asthma exacerbations did not gain much popularity in the past, observational studies and a recent analysis showed increasing success in this group of patients. A trial of NIV should be given for LTAE patients who might otherwise require intubation.[8] Altered mental status, excessive secretions, haemodynamic instability and uncooperative patient are the contraindications for NIV use.[8]

1.2 Standard therapy

Most patients with severe asthma respond to first and second line drugs like beta 2 adrenergic agonists, systemic corticosteroids, anticholinergic agents and intravenous magnesium sulphate.

1.3 Controlled oxygen therapy

In asthma exacerbation, perfusion of non-ventilated areas causes ventilation perfusion mismatch leading to hypoxemia. SPO_2 goal of >92% is enough when starting supplemental oxygen to prevent harmful effects of hyperoxia.[9] This concept of controlled oxygen therapy is very important in managing LTAE.

1.4 Non-conventional interventions

Nonconventional approache, such as administration of heliox or bronchoscopy, may be considered only in refractory patients.

a. *Heliox (helium plus oxygen):* The turbulent airflow that occurs in LTAE is converted to laminar flow by using heliox, which is a combination of helium and oxygen. This is due to the lower density and higher viscosity of helium than air. Heliox has shown to improve peak expiratory flow, however its effects in reducing intubation remain unknown.[10] A trial of heliox can be given in LTAE who do not respond to conventional treatment but therapy should be abandoned if there is no improvement within 15 minutes.[11]
b. *Bronchoscopic mucus plug removal:* In patients in whom there is persistent airflow limitation due to mucus plugging, bronchoscopic removal of mucus plugs can be considered.[1,12]

2. Criteria for Intubation

Though most patients can be managed without intubation, there are certain clinical and laboratory criteria which mandate immediate intubation. Ignoring these signs and further waiting anticipating response to drugs could pose risk to life **(Table 18.2)**.

Table 18.2: Consensus Indicators for Intubation[7]

Clinical	Laboratory
Respiratory arrest	Severe hypoxemia with maximal oxygen delivery
Cardiac arrest	Lethargy or agitation interfering with oxygen delivery or asthma therapy
Progressive exhaustion	Lethargy or agitation interfering with oxygen delivery or asthma therapy
Altered sensorium	
Silent chest	

In the past, a respiratory acidosis was considered an indication for intubation. A systematic review by Leatherman[13] showed that intubation may not be required for most asthmatic patients with hypercapnia. The exception to this are progressive hypercapnia despite treatment and altered mental status.[7]

ABGs are not routinely required for all asthma patients coming to ED. They are done for patients with refractory acute asthma. Corbridge and Hall[14] have emphasized that observing the course of clinical condition of the patient is more important than laboratory testing.

Respiratory rate >40/minute and silent chest despite respiratory effort are also ominous signs

3. Recommendations for Intubation Technique

Patients with LTAE should always be considered as having difficult airways due to potential complications that may arise in the peri-intubation period.

Intubation by experienced persons is important as multiple attempts could trigger vagal response which might lead to laryngospasm and worsening of bronchospasm.

Orotracheal intubation is the preferred choice of intubation. Orotracheal intubation also allows the use of an endotracheal tube of a larger diameter (>8 mm), facilitating secretion removal and bronchoscopy, and decreasing inspiratory airway resistance.

Delayed sequence intubation is an alternative to rapid sequence intubation that can be beneficial in LTAE. Delayed sequence intubation intends to separate the induction agent from the paralytic to resuscitate, preoxygenate and denitrogenate better.[1]

Peri-intubation resuscitation can prevent hemodynamic instability in patients who might have become hypovolemic from insensible losses.[15] The shock index is a simple bedside calculation (heart rate/systolic BP) that can help to identify occult shock and is predictive of peri-intubation cardiac arrest. If a patient has a shock index of >1, pre-emptive resuscitation with fluids or vasopressors is needed.[16]

Ketamine should be used as an induction agent because it does not cause hemodynamic instability.[1] As soon as the SpO_2 goal is achieved, paralysis with rocuronium is favoured when needed. Bag-mask ventilation should be avoided because it can worsen DHI or cause barotrauma.[1]

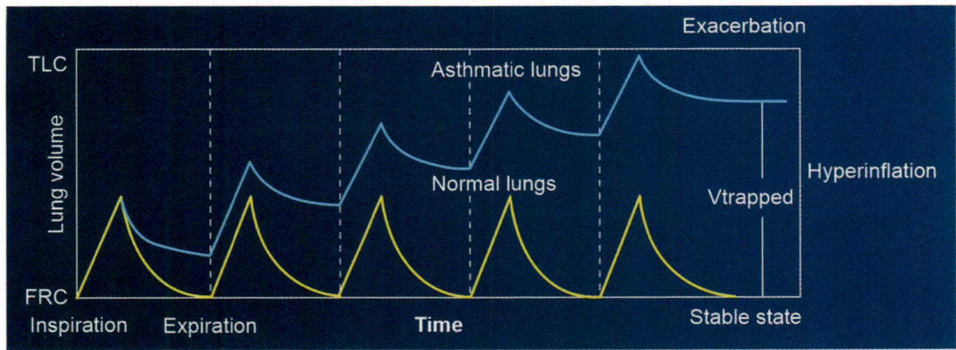

Fig. 18.13: Dynamic hyperinflation during exacerbation[18]

4. Recommendations for Appropriate Ventilator Settings

The aim of mechanical ventilation is to maintain adequate oxygenation, to reduce the work of breathing and to prevent and confront further hyperinflation without any circulatory compromise or ventilator induced lung injury.[17]

4.1 Anticipated problems due to intubation and ventilation

a. *Hyperinflation:* Ventilation of LTAE patients leads to breath stacking as expiratory time is not enough to empty the alveoli due to airflow limitation. This leads to severe dynamic hyperinflation (DH) due to prolonged expiration. DH causes generation of auto-PEEP and barotrauma which might lead to pneumothorax and pneumomediastinum.[22]

b. *Hypotension:* Hypotension, the most common complication after intubation is caused by DH and aggravated by dehydration, sedatives and neuromuscular blocking agents.

c. *Others:* Severe acidosis, arrythmia, seizers, etc.

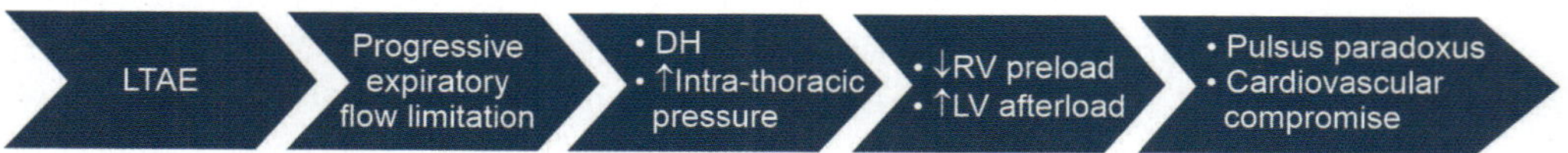

Fig. 18.14: Cardiovascular changes due to dynamic hyperinflation (DH)[18,19]

4.2 Ventilation settings

Mechanical ventilation can be initiated either with volume cycled or pressure cycled ventilation. DH and lung injury can be prevented by manipulating minute ventilation, I:E ratio and respiratory rate as shown in **Table 18.3**.

Table 18.3: Initial ventilator settings in intubated patients with acute severe asthma exacerbation

Mode	Settings
Tidal volume	6–8 ml/kg ideal body weight
Respiratory rate	8–10/min
Minute ventilation	<10 L/min
Inspiratory flow rate	60–80 L/min
Inspiratory to expiratory ratio	≥1:3
Inspiratory waveform	Decelerated waveform
Expiratory time	4–5 s
Plateau pressure	<30 cm H_2O
PEEP	0–4 cm H_2O
FiO_2	100% initially and titrate to maintain SaO_2 >90%

SaO_2: Oxygen saturation; PEEP: Positive end expiratory pressure

Response of DH to low minute ventilation can be seen in flow times scalar. The expiratory portion of this scalar should come to baseline before a new breath is initiated suggesting resolution of DH **(Fig. 18.15)**.[1]

Extrinsic PEEP should be kept below 5 cm H_2O in most intubated patients. Sometimes extrinsic PEEP might help in overcoming the auto-PEEP and improve work of breathing in spontaneously breathing patients. [1] Auto-PEEP should be measured at least 6 hours.[1]

4.3 Strategies for refractory DH

There are 3 ventilatory strategies that can be used to reduce DH and auto-PEEP in ventilated asthmatic patients.

a. Reduction of respiratory rate
b. Reduction of tidal volume
c. Increasing inspiratory flow

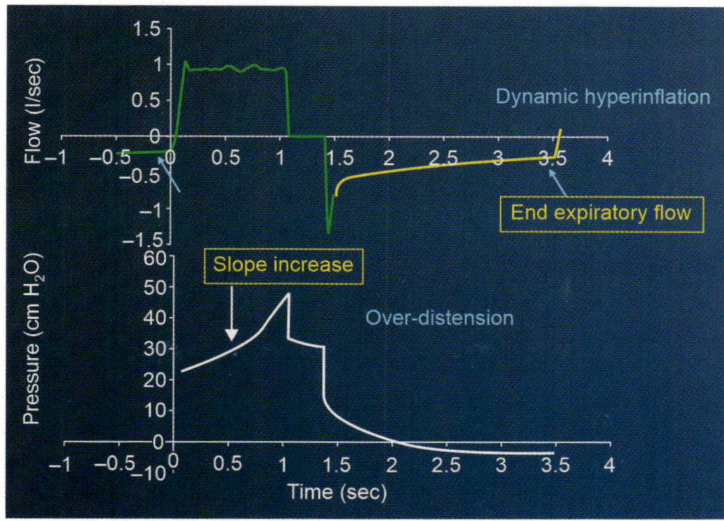

Fig. 18.15: Flowtime tracking of a patient with persistence of flow at the end of expiration which indicates dynamic hyperinflation and pressure time tracing with a slope increase indicative of over-distension[18]

Changes in respiratory rate have the greatest effect on DH and auto-PEEP.[7] Routinely, inspiratory flow with decelerating waveform configuration is used as initial setup.[7] If one is unable to reduce respiratory rate enough to reduce DH and auto-PEEP (10–15 cm water) to acceptable levels, inspiratory time can be shortened by increasing inspiratory flowrate and using square waveform configuration.[24] Sometimes this could be counter productive by increasing the respiratory rate and worsening auto-PEEP **(Table 18.4)**.[25]

Decreasing respiratory rate can cause hypercapnia. Fortunately hypercapnia is well tolerated up to $PaCO_2$ value as high as 90 mm Hg.[7] This concept of permissive hypercapnia is safer than over ventilating the patient leading to hyperinflation.[7] Anoxic brain injury and sever myocardial dysfunction are contraindications to permissive hypercapnia.[26]

If hypoxia persists, an alternative cause should be looked into.[21]

4.4 Assessment of lung hyperinflation

It is crucial to assess and monitor severity of lung hyperinflation for successful outcomes of ventilated asthmatic patients. This will help in adjusting ventilator settings when needed and prevent further lung injury.[23]

Measurement of exhaled gases and volume at end inspiration (Vei) gives an indication of lung hyperinflation (Vei >20 ml/ kg correlates with barotrauma).[27] This requires staff training and patient paralysis and is not performed in routine ICU practice.[7]

Two easy to measure pressures are used as surrogate markers of lung inflation in daily practice: Auto-PEEP and plateau pressure (P_{plat}).[7]

a. Auto-PEEP is obtained by measuring airway opening pressure during an end-expiratory hold manoeuvre. Presence of expiratory gas flow at the beginning of inspiration (on flow tracing) also suggests auto-PEEP.[7] When there is poor

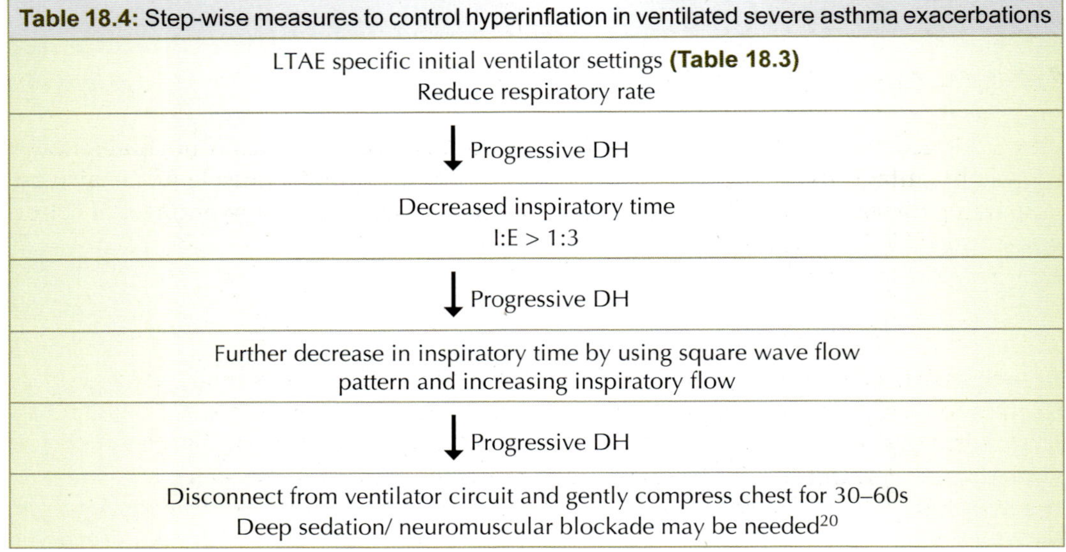

Table 18.4: Step-wise measures to control hyperinflation in ventilated severe asthma exacerbations
LTAE specific initial ventilator settings **(Table 18.3)** Reduce respiratory rate
↓ Progressive DH
Decreased inspiratory time I:E > 1:3
↓ Progressive DH
Further decrease in inspiratory time by using square wave flow pattern and increasing inspiratory flow
↓ Progressive DH
Disconnect from ventilator circuit and gently compress chest for 30–60s Deep sedation/ neuromuscular blockade may be needed[20]

communication between alveoli and airway opening, the severity of hyperinflation gets under estimated by auto-PEEP.[28]

b. P_{plat} is determined by temporarily stopping flow at end inspiration during a single delivered breath.[7]

Though both have not been validated as a predictor of complications of mechanical ventilation, it is agreed that complications are rare when P_{plat} is < 30 cm H_2O and auto-PEEP is <15 cm H_2O.[29]

5. Management in the Immediate Post-intubation Period

Adequate sedation is important to achieve the desirable patient–ventilator synchronization.[18] Sedation and analgesia will also decrease the metabolic rate, oxygen consumption and carbon dioxide production.[18]

Dexmedetominide, propofol and remifentanyl are the appropriate drugs for sedation and analgesia.[18] Their usage has been associated with shorter length of ICU stay, shorter duration of mechanical ventilation and improved long-term neurocognitive outcomes when compared to benzodiazepines.[30] It is important to use agents that accomplish deep sedation, while at the same time allow rapid awakening, should the patient improve quickly, which is common in the asthma cases.[18] Morphine should be avoided because it can cause histamine release.

Patients with severe asthma with persistently dangerous levels of hypercapnia and arterial hypoxemia, and extreme patient-ventilatory asynchrony may require paralysis in addition to sedation.[18] Paralytic agents can be administered either intermittently through bolus injections, or by continuous intravascular infusion.[18] Its duration must be as short as possible, because concomitant use of intravascular corticosteroids and paralytic neuromuscular agents increases the incidence of critical illness myopathy.[31]

6. Medical Management of Asthma in the Ventilated Patient

6.1 Inhaled short-acting beta$_2$ agonists (SABAs) and muscarinic antagonists

SABAs are the first-line treatment for acute asthma. A high-dose strategy (7.5 mg) offers no benefit over a low-dose (2.5 mg) of albuterol.[32] IV β_2 agonists should be reserved for when inhaled therapy is not feasible. Ipratropium bromide relaxes bronchial smooth muscle by antagonizing the muscarinic M_3 receptor on smooth muscle of the airway, alleviating airway obstruction.[1] Compared with SABAs, it has a slower onset of action (60–90 min).[1] When used, ipratropium bromide should be administered in combination with SABAs, and its benefit is limited to patients with severe disease.[33]

6.2 Systemic corticosteroids

Systemic corticosteroids improve outcomes in patients with acute asthma and reduce the likelihood of repeat exacerbation.[1] They should be administered as soon as possible as the clinical effects may take 6 to 12 hours to start their action.[34] IV methylprednisolone is recommended in those with severe respiratory distress who are being admitted to the hospital or ICU.[1] The potential role of inhaled corticosteroids in managing acute asthma has not been evaluated fully in large trials, although some studies in children and adults suggest a benefit.[35]

6.3 Magnesium Sulphate

Magnesium sulphate acts as a bronchodilator by inhibiting calcium channels and blocking parasympathetic tone.[1] The role of IV magnesium in the treatment of acute asthma has been studied as an adjunct therapy to SABAs, ipratropium bromide, and corticosteroids.[1] Evidence has shown that this intervention reduced hospital admissions in severe asthma and improved pulmonary function, but it has not been found to reduce mortality or need for NIV.[36]

6.4 Methylxanthines

Aminophylline is a methylxanthine that traditionally has been used as an infusion in acute asthma. It is a nonselective phosphodiesterase inhibitor.[1] However, aminophylline is an inferior bronchodilator to SABA monotherapy. Because of the safety profile of aminophylline, its use is no longer recommended in the treatment of acute asthma.[37]

6.5 Nonventilator Strategies

a. **Inhaled anaesthetics:** Inhaled anaesthetics can be used in patients with LTAE with high P_{paw}, excessive hypercarbia, and refractory bronchospasm who are receiving invasive ventilation.[1] Isoflurane or halothane can reduce bronchospasm, and evidence of improvement should be seen quickly, but only while the gases are being administered because their effect is short-lived.[1] These anaesthetics are delivered through an anaesthesia ventilator, and their use may be limited by the experience of the ICU staff. Inhaled anaesthetics can cause hemodynamic instability by reducing venous and vascular tone.[1]

b. **Extracorporeal Life Support (ECLS):** Though ECLS has shown to give excellent results in refractory acute severe asthma, it is rarely required. One scenario in which ECLS would be appropriate would be the combination of severe refractory respiratory acidosis and extreme hyperinflation that had resulted in significant barotrauma or hemodynamic instability

7. Prevention and Management of Complications

Intubation-induced bronchospasm: It is well known that tracheal intubation increases airway resistance in patients with bronchial hyperreactivity.[38] Pre-treatment with bronchodilators appears to be useful in decreasing or preventing this complication of intubation in patients with hyperreactive airways.[7]

7.1 Persistent or worsening hypoxemia could be due to severe bronchospasm.[7] However other causes of worsening hypoxemia like endotracheal tube displacement for blockage, ventilator malfunction, pneumothorax, aspiration, infection, pulmonary edema, and pulmonary embolism need to be ruled out when required.[7]

7.2 Hypotension can be caused by dehydration, sedatives, neuromuscular blocking agents and dynamic hyperinflation. A fluid bolus is the first measure to be taken in case of hypotension. In case od hypotension due to DH, respiratory rate should be reduced to allow more time for expiration.[7] In critical hypotension a trial of hypopnea (2–3 breaths/ min) or apnea in a pre-oxygenated patient for 30–60 seconds can be useful.[7]

7.3 Cardiac arrest in LTAE can occur due to severe hypoxia, tension pneumothorax, critical lung hyperinflation leading to circulatory collapse, acidosis, electrolyte abnormalities or associated acute coronary syndrome.[7]

7.4 Barotrauma: Careful clinical examination, chest X-ray and point of care ultrasound help in detecting pneumothorax and pneumomediastinum.

7.5 Myopathy: About 15% of severe asthma patients who are ventilated develop acute myopathy.[39] Acute myopathy usually does not cause delay in extubation as diaphragm is relatively spared.[6]

7.6 Cerebral injury: Cardiorespiratory arrest prior to intubation is the most common reason for permanent cerebral injury.[6]

Extubation

A spontaneous breathing trial can be given in an awake patient once $PaCO_2$ normalizes, airway resistance is less than 20 cm H_2O, auto-PEEP is less than 10 cm H_2O, and neuromuscular weakness has not been identified. After extubation, observation in an ICU is recommended for an additional 12 to 24 hours.[7]

Mortality

The reported mortality rates from four large databases range from 6 to 20%. It might range from 0.6 to 2.5% in centres with extensive experience in managing acute severe asthma patients. The cause of death could be sepsis, pulmonary embolism, myocardial infarction, tension pneumothorax, and hypotension due to dynamic hyperinflation.

Prognosis

Usually, outcomes of acute severe asthma patients who are ventilated are good, as long as they do not have a cardiac arrest before coming to the hospital. Every minute of care counts for a patient having a life threatening asthma attack.

Prior intubation has been identified as the strongest risk factor for death, these patients are at increased risk for subsequent fatal attacks. It is very important for these patients to follow a proper asthma treatment plan which includes avoidance of known triggers, regular use of controller medicines, and early use of oral corticosteroids for exacerbations (Fig. 18.16).

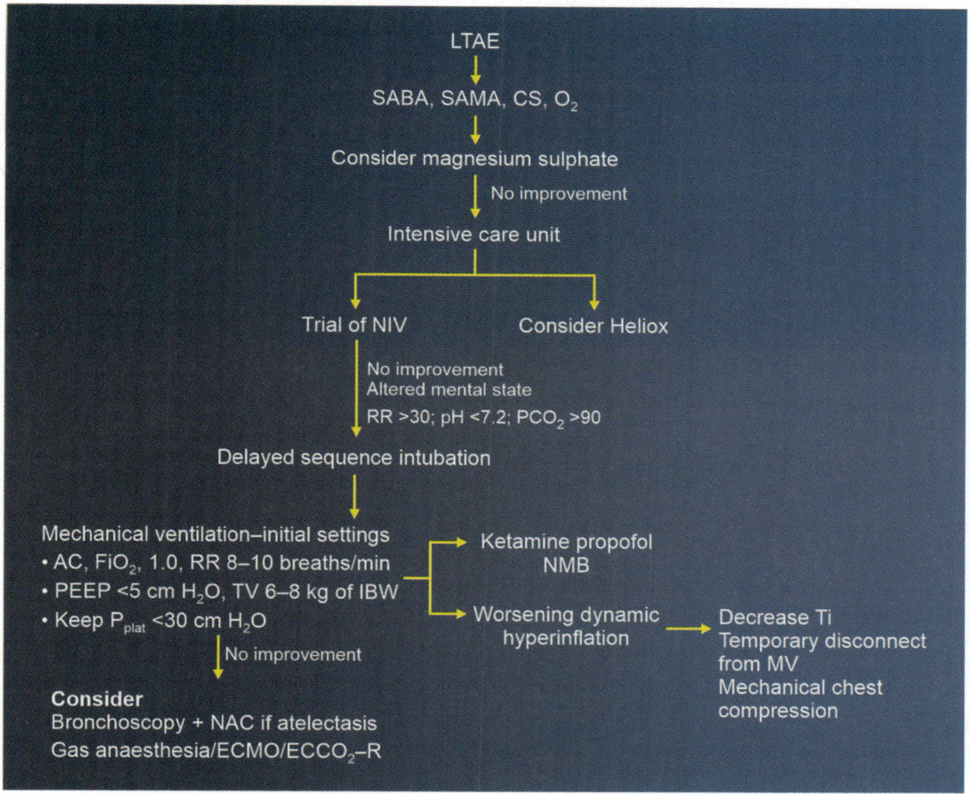

Fig. 18.16: LTAE Management algorithm[1]

AC—assist control; ECCO-R—extracorporeal carbon dioxide removal; ECMO—extracorporeal membrane oxygenation; IBW—ideal body weight; NAC—N-acetylcysteine; NMB—neuromuscular blockade; PEEP—positive end-expiratory pressure; RR—respiratory rate; SABA—short-acting β_2-agonist; SAMA—short-acting muscarinic antagonist; CS—corticosteroid; SpO_2—oxygen saturation; Ti—inspiratory time; TV—tidal volume.

Conclusion

LTAE is a rare but fatal complication of asthma and requires timely, systematic management. Immediate treatment should be started with inhaled SABAs, inhaled ipratropium, controlled oxygen (when required) and intravenous corticosteroids. If the respiratory distress progresses despite this treatment, intravenous magnesium sulphate can be considered when there are no contraindications. Patients who deteriorate despite these treatments should be admitted to the ICU. A trial of NIV can be given but intubation should be delayed if there is no response to NIV in an hour. Special ventilation strategies are required to avoid ventilator induced dynamic hyperinflation and barotrauma for successful outcome of LTAE. The ICU which focus on the strategy of permissive hypercarbia and lung protective ventilation will have very low mortality rates and should be the goal in treating such patients.

References

1. Orlando Garner, MD; James Scott Ramey, MD; and Nicola A. Hanania, MD, FCCP. Management of Life-Threatening Asthma Severe Asthma Series. j.chest.2022.02.029
2. Louie S, Morrissey BM, Kenyon NJ, Albertson TE, Avdalovic M. The critically ill asthmatic—from ICU to discharge. Clin Rev Allergy Immunol. 2012;43(1-2):30–44.
3. Barr RG, Woodruff PG, Clark S, Camargo CA. Sudden-onset asthma exacerbations: Clinical features, response to therapy, and 2-week follow-up. Eur. Respir. J. 2000;15:266–273. doi: 10.1034/j.1399-3003.2000.15b08.
4. Ramnath VR, Clark S, Camargo CAJ. Multicenter Study of Clinical Features of Sudden-Onset Versus Slower-Onset Asthma Exacerbations Requiring Hospitalization. Respir. Care. 2007;52:1013–20.
5. Peters U., Dixon A.E., Forno E. Obesity and asthma. J. Allergy Clin. Immunol. 2018;141:1169–1179. doi: 10.1016/j.jaci.2018.02.004.
6. James Leatherman, MD. Mechanical Ventilation for Severe Asthma. CHEST 2015; 147 (6): 1671–80.
7. Brenner B, Corbridge T, Kazzi A. Intubation and mechanical ventilation of the asthmatic patient in respiratory failure. Proc Am Thorac Soc. 2009;6(4):371–79.
8. Nanchal R, Kumar G, Majumdar T, *et al.* Utilization of mechanical ventilation for asthma exacerbations: analysis of a national database. Respir Care. 2014 ; 59 (5): 644–53.
9. Chien JW, Ciufo R, Novak R, *et al.* Uncontrolled oxygen administration and respiratory failure in acute asthma. Chest. 2000;117(3):728–33.
10. Rodrigo GJ, Castro-Rodriguez JA. Heliox-driven β_2-agonists nebulization for children and adults with acute asthma: a systematic review with meta-analysis. Ann Allergy Asthma Immunol. 2014;112(1):29–34.
11. Anderson M, Svartengren M, Bylin G, Philipson K, Camner P. Deposition in asthmatics of particles inhaled in air or in helium oxygen. Am Rev Respir Dis. 1993;147(3):524–28.
12. Henke CA, Hertz M, Gustafson P. Combined bronchoscopy and mucolytic therapy for patients with severe refractory status asthmaticus on mechanical ventilation: a case report and review of the literature. Crit Care Med. 1994;22(11):1880–83.
13. Leatherman J. Life – threatening asthma. Clin Chest Med 1994;15:453–79.
14. Corbridge TC, Hall JB. The assessment and management of adults with status asthmaticus. Am J Respir Crit Care Med 1995;151:1296–16.

15. Weingart SD, Trueger NS, Wong N, Scofi J, Singh N, Rudolph SS. Delayed sequence intubation: a prospective observational study. Ann Emerg Med. 2015;65(4):349–55.
16. Acker SN, Bredbeck B, Partrick DA, Kulungowski AM, Barnett CC, Bensard DD. Shock index, pediatric age-adjusted (SIPA) is more accurate than age-adjusted hypotension for trauma team activation. Surgery. 2017;161(3):803–07.
17. Williams TJ, Tuxen D, Scheinkestel CD, Czarny D, Bowes G. Risk Factors for Morbidity in Mechanically Ventilated Patients with Acute Severe Asthma 1, 2. Am. Rev. Respir. Dis. 1992;146:607–615. doi: 10.1164/ajrccm/146.3.607.
18. Eirini Kostakou,1,† Evangelos Kaniaris,1,† Effrosyni Filiou,1 Ioannis Vasileiadis,1 Paraskevi Katsaounou,2 Eleni Tzortzaki,3 Nikolaos Koulouris,1 Antonia Koutsoukou,1 and Nikoletta Rovinal. Acute Severe Asthma in Adolescent and Adult Patients: Current Perspectives on Assessment and Management J Clin Med. 2019 Sep; 8(9): 1283.
19. Pepe PE, Marini JJ. Occult Positive End-Expiratory Pressure in Mechanically Ventilated, PA tients with Airflow Obstruction. Am. Rev. Respir. Dis. 1982;126:166–170
20. Laher AE, Buchanan SK. Mechanically ventilating the severe asthmatic. J Intensive Care Med. 2018;33(9):491–501.
21. Jain S, Hanania NA, Guntupalli KK. Ventilation of patients with asthma and obstructive lung disease. Crit Care Clin. 1998;14(4): 685–705.
22. Lougheed MD, Fisher T, O'Donnell DE. Dynamic hyperinflation during bronchoconstriction in asthma: implications for symptom perception. Chest 2006;130:1072–81.
23. Reddy VG. Auto-PEEP: how to detect and how to prevent—a review. Middle East J Anaesthesiol 2005;18:293–312.
24. Mayo P, Radeos MS. The severe asthmatic: intubated and difficult to ventilate. In: Brenner B, editor. Emergency asthma. New York: Marcel-Dekker; 1999. pp. 469–87.
25. Corne S, Gillespie D, Roberts D, Younes M. Effect of inspiratory flow rate on respiratory rare in intubated patients. Am J Respir Crit Care Med 1997;156:304–08.
26. Tuxen DV. Permissive hypercapnic ventilation. Am J Respir Crit Care Med 1994;150:870–74.
27. Tuxen DV, Lane S. The effects of ventilatory pattern on hyperinflation, airway pressures, and circulation in mechanical ventilation of patients with severe air-flow obstruction. Am Rev Respir Dis 1987;136:872–79.
28. Leatherman JW, Ravenscraft SA. Low measured auto-positive end-expiratory pressure during mechanical ventilation of patients with severe asthma: hidden auto-positive end-expiratory pressure. Crit Care Med 1996;24:541–46.
29. Corbridge T, Corbridge S. Severe asthma exacerbation. In: Fink M, Abraham E, Vincent JL, Kochanek PM, editors. Textbook of critical care, 5th ed. Philadelphia: Elsevier Saunders; 2005. pp. 587–97.
30. Burburan SM, Xisto DG, Rocco PRM. Anaesthetic management in asthma. Minerva Anestesiol. 2007;73:357–65.
31. Behbehani NA, Al-Mane F, D'yachkova Y, Pare P, FitzGerald JM. Myopathy following mechanical ventilation for acute severe asthma: The role of muscle relaxants and corticosteroids. Chest. 1999;115:1627–31. doi: 10.1378/chest.115.6.1627.
32. Emerman CL, Cydulka RK, McFadden ER. Comparison of 2.5 vs 7. 5 mg of inhaled albuterol in the treatment of acute asthma. Chest. 1999;115(1):92–96.
33. Agnihotri NT, Saltoun C. Acute severe asthma (status asthmaticus). Allergy Asthma Proc. 2019;40(6):406–09.

34. Rowe BH, Edmonds ML, Spooner CH, Diner B, Camargo CA Jr. Corticosteroid therapy for acute asthma. Respir Med. 2004;98:275–84.

35. Dembla G, Mundle RP, Salkar HR, Doifoide DV. Oral versus intravenous steroids in acute exacerbation of asthma—randomized controlled study. J Assoc Physicians India. 2011;59:621–23.

36. Long B, Lentz S, Koyfman A, Gottlieb M. Evaluation and management of the critically ill adult asthmatic in the emergency department setting. Am J Emerg Med. 2021;44:44–451.

37. Maselli DJ, Peters JI. Medication regimens for managing acute asthma. Respir Care. 2018;63(6):783–96.

38. Silvanus MT, Groeben H, Peters J. Corticosteroids and inhaled salbutamol in patients with reversible airway obstruction markedly decrease the incidence of bronchospasm after tracheal intubation. Anesthesiology 2004;100:1052–57.

III. MECHANICAL VENTILATION IN TRAUMATIC BRAIN INJURY

❐ Sagar Sunka ❐ Pavan Kumar Reddy N

Severe traumatic brain injury is defined as a GCS of 8 and below, such patients usually require intubation and mechanical ventilation for prevention of aspiration pneumonitis/ pneumonia, and for preventing secondary brain injury as a consequence of hypoxemia and hypercapnia [defined as arterial PaO_2 <60 mmHg and arterial $PaCO_2$ >45 mmHg].

These patients develop ARDS secondary to aspiration of oropharyngeal or gastric contents or due to neurogenic pulmonary edema. As a general rule lung protective ventilation strategies like low tidal volume ventilation, moderate to high PEEP, inverse ratio ventilation which is normally employed in ARDS, may not be the norm in all severe brain injury patients.

Traditionally in severe brain injury patients high tidal volumes, low PEEP is employed to achieve the following goals

1. Maintaining adequate oxygenation PaO_2 (60–100 mmHg)
2. Maintaining normocapnia $PaCO_2$ (35 – 40 mmHg)
3. Maintaining cerebral perfusion pressure [CPP = MAP – ICP]
4. Minimising the intrathoracic pressure by adjusting PEEP, so that it does not translate to raised ICP (Fig. 18.17)

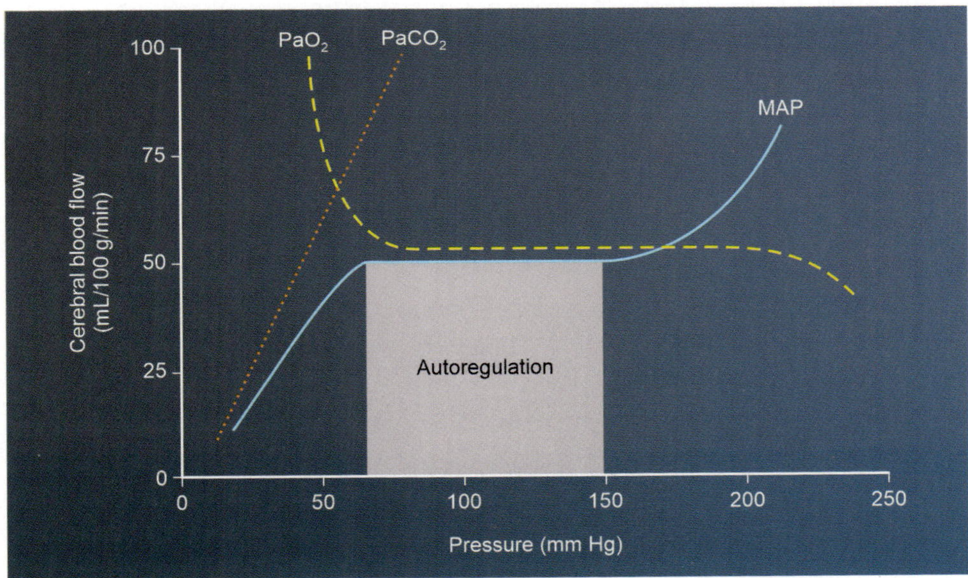

Fig. 18.17: Factors affecting cerebral blood flow and autoregulation

- Cerebral autoregulation operates in a narrow zone, despite the breach in blood–brain barrier. PaO_2, $PaCO_2$, CPP plays a vital role in maintaining the cerebral blood flow.
- PaO_2 has to be given atmost importance because, hypoxemia determines the extent of secondary brain injury. If required one should not hesitate to apply rescue ventilatory strategies [which are discussed subsequently]. At the same time hyperoxia is also

equally bad, hyperoxia leads to increase in free radical injury, especially after revascularisation in the ischemic bed.

- Other two parameters which are of importance are the $PaCO_2$ and the PEEP.
- Role of $PaCO_2$: As known hypercapnia causes cerebral vasodilatation, which leads to increased CSF production, thereby increasing the ICP, when uncontrolled may lead to brain herniation. In the ischemic zones cerebral vessels are already maximally dilated, but when hypercapnia occurs, rest of the cerebral vessels dilate, there by diverting the blood flow from the ischemic bed, and thus can aggravate the ischemic insult in penumbra region, this phenomenon is known as cerebral steal, when this is compounded by increased ICP as a result of hypercapnia, can be detrimental.[2]
- On the other hand, hypocapnia, secondary to hyperventilation causes cerebral vasoconstriction which leads to reduced ICP. This phenomenon is utilized only in emergency conditions like impending brain herniation. Prolonged hyperventilation in the absence of high ICP should be avoided as this leads to cerebral vasoconstriction and could worsen secondary brain ischemia. The degree of hypocapnia/hypercapnia is also a vital factor as values less than 25 mmHg or more than 60 mmHg is very detrimental, because the relation of CO_2 and CBF is a linear one, unlike the PaO_2 and the MAP curve which is a sigmoid curve.

Role of PEEP in Severe Brain Injury

TBI patients may require significant levels of PEEP to maintain oxygenation. Hypoxia is due to severe lung injury as a result of chest trauma, aspiration pneumonia or secondarily due to neurogenic pulmonary edema.

The effect of PEEP on ICP is predominantly determined by the compliance of the respiratory system and the hemodynamic status of the patient. In patients with low compliance, a moderate PEEP increase (up to 10–12 cmH_2O) is not associated with ICP increase; whereas in patients with normal compliance, high PEEP causes lung overdistension, reduction in cerebral venous return and increase in ICP (**Fig. 18.18**).

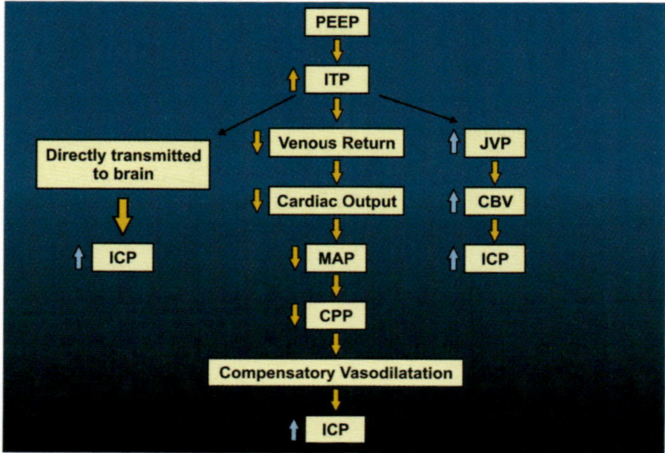

Fig. 18.18: Effect of PEEP on intracranial pressure (ICP)

How to Ventilate a Severely Brain Injured Patient?

Traditionally PAO_2, $PACO_2$ operate in a very narrow range in a patient with already raised ICP, when compared to a patient with normal ICP. It is provident to take help of neuromonitoring devices in patients with raised ICP, while titrating the ventilatory settings.

In case of severe hypoxemia with severe brain injury, importance should be given to correction of hypoxemia first, and rescue maneuvers should be employed **(Table 18.5)**.

Table 18.5: Normal ICP and raised ICP

	Normal ICP	Raised ICP
Begin with	Normocapnia Low V_T (6 ml/kg) Limit P_{plat} <30 cm H_2O	Normocapnia Low V_T (6 ml/kg) Limit P_{plat} <30 cm H_2O
Raising $PaCO_2$	✦ Moderate hypercarbia ✦ Follow ICP ✦ Remove excess dead space ✦ Sedation/Ensure synchrony ✦ Drain large effusions/ascites	✦ Consider increasing V_T Normocarbia ✦ Follow ICP ✦ Remove excess dead space ✦ Sedation/Ensure synchrony ✦ Drain large effusions/ascites
Next	Alternative modes, prioritizing lung protection (but following ICP)	Alternative modes, prioritizing CO_2 elimination

In case of severe hypoxemia with severe brain injury, impotance should be given to correction of hypoxemia first, and rescue maneuvers should be employed

Rescue maneuvers used are:

1. Use of neuromuscular blocking agents (NMBA)
2. Recruitment maneuvers
3. Prone position ventilation
4. Bronchoscopy
5. Use of ECCOR and VV-ECMO
6. Use of nitric oxide (NO)

1. NMBA: High level evidence exists for use of NMBAs. Its use is associated with good patient ventilatory synchrony and thereby improving global oxygenation. When used with sedation it also has the added advantage of reducing cerebral metabolic rate and there by aiding in reducing the secondary brain insult and thus recovery.
2. Recruitment maneuvers: Role of recruitment maneuvers is controversial, but can be used in cases of severe ARDS with p/f ratio <100 and should be used for shorter duration. New evidence do not support the use of recruitment maneuvers even in severe ARDS without brain injury. While performing recruitment maneuvers one should be cautious, and invasive monitoring of vital signs is mandatory. Additional benefit can be seen in patients with neuromonitoring like (ICP monitoring, NIRS)
3. Bronchoscopy is associated with very high rise in intrathoracic pressures approx. (80–100 mmHg) and similar rules apply, as performing recruitment maneuvers.

4. PRONE position: In patients with severe ARDS, prone position has shown to improve oxygenation, but in those with signs of raised ICP, proning may cause further increase in ICP, despite the improvement in oxygenation.[4] In all the prone ventilation trials, patients with brain injury are generally excluded. Hence evidence is lacking. But if mandatory, it should be done with caution and preferrable with ICP monitoring and invasive hemodynamic monitoring.

   Off note employing bolsters while proning, taking care to keep the head in centre, employing reverse Trendelenburg position, with a slight head up position, and trying to minimise the duration of prone position once P/F ratios improve is logical.
5. ECCOR: In patients in whom increase in intrathoracic pressures translate to increase in ICP (where high TVs and high PEEP cannot be applied) or in those patients where hypercapnia cannot be managed with conventional ventilatory strategies, extracorporeal CO_2 removal (ECCOR) can be considered. Though the usage of anticoagulation is not as high as in ECMO, one should consider the possibility of worsening intracranial bleed, and should be employed as a rescue measure only after multidisciplinary discussion.[3]
6. VV-ECMO: Veno-venous extracorporeal membrane oxygenation is generally used in severe ARDS patients in whom prone position in not helping, and can be considered in severe TBI only if there is no evidence of intracranial bleed, as patients with diffuse axonal injury, or in patients with only cerebral edema.[5] It should be considered only if above rescue measures fail.
7. Niric oxide: Even in patients without brain injury patients nitric oxide (NO) has shown no proven benefits. In severe brain injured patients, probably vasodilatory effects of NO cause more harm than improvement in oxygenation, and evidence is against the use of NO.

Weaning: Once goals of oxygenation are achieved and the patient is stable for >48 hr, one should consider early tracheostomy (within 7 days), weaning and early neurorehabilitation.

- Tracheostomy should be considered early in all severe brain injured patients in whom neuro recovery is expected to be delayed. It has the added advantage of good tracheal toileting, faster weaning and reduced sedation requirements.[6]

Conclusion

A. Hypoxia is detrimental for the penumbra zone, hence intensivist should not be reluctant in:
   1. Early intubation and ventilation of the patient.
   2. To apply moderate to high PEEP where required, for correction of hypoxia.
   3. Should not be reluctant to use rescue measures for optimising oxygenation and ventilation.
   4. Where available one should use neuromonitoring devices like ICP monitoring and NIRS, in whom there is deviation from normal ventilatory settings and to understand the effects of PaO_2, $PaCO_2$ and PEEP on the CBF.
   5. Prolonged hyperventilation must be avoided if ICP is not high and hyperventilation for short period can be used only if ICP is very high with high risk of herniation. Brain oxygenation should be monitored if hyperventilation is used.

6. Lung compliance can change rapidly in patients with severe brain injury, when they develop neurogenic pulmonary edema, new onset ventilatory associated pneumonias, hence close monitoring is warranted.

B. Early tracheostomy, early weaning, and early neurorehabilitation translates to better outcomes.

References

1. Papazian L, Forel JM, Gacouin A, Penot-Ragon C, Perrin G, Loundou A, *et al.* Neuromuscular blockers in early acute respiratory distress syndrome. N Engl J Med. 2010;363(12):1107–16. 29.
2. WarnerDS Hansen TD, Vust L, *et.al*. Distribution of cerebral blood flow during deep isoflurane vs pentobarbital anesthesia with middle cerebral occlusion J Neuro anesthesia 2005,1,219.
3. Combes A, Fanelli V, Pham T, Ranieri VM. European Society of Intensive Care Medicine Trials Group and the "strategy of ultra-protective lung ventilation with extracorporeal CO_2 removal for new-onset moderate to severe ARDS " (SUPERNOVA) investigators. Feasibility and safety of extracorporeal CO_2 removal to enhance protective ventilation in acute respiratory distress syndrome: the SUPERNOVA study. Intensive Care Med. 2019;45(5):592–600.
4. Reinprecht A, Greher M, Wolfsberger S, Dietrich W, Illievich UM, Gruber A. Prone position in subarachnoid hemorrhage patients with acute respiratory distress syndrome: effects on cerebral tissue oxygenation and intracranial pressure. Crit Care Med. 2003;31(6):1831–8.
5. Della Torre V, Robba C, Pelosi P, Bilotta F. Extracorporeal membrane oxygenation in the critical trauma patient. Curr Opin Anaesthesiol. 2019; 32(2):234 –41.
6. de Franca, Sabrina Araujo BaSN1; Tavares, Wagner M. MD, PhD1,2; Salinet, Angela S. M. MSc, PhD1,3; Paiva, Wellingson S. MD, PhD_2; Teixeira, Manoel J. MD.

IV. MECHANICAL VENTILATION IN CHEST TRAUMA

❒ Pavan Kumar Reddy N ❒ Shweta Ram Chandankhede

Hypoxia and hypoventilation are the two major causes of mortality and morbidity following chest trauma in a traumatized patient. Chest trauma accounts for around 10 % hospital admissions globally with a mortality ranging from 5 to 8% for isolated chest injuries. The mortality differs if chest trauma is presented in combination with other major injuries. Management of chest trauma is challenging to its complexity and thus needs an individual approach depending on the type and location of the chest trauma, associated injuries and the severity. It is very important to optimize the oxygenation and hemodynamics by improving the cardiac output in chest trauma keeping in mind to avoid any further injury due to ventilation (**Fig. 18.19**).

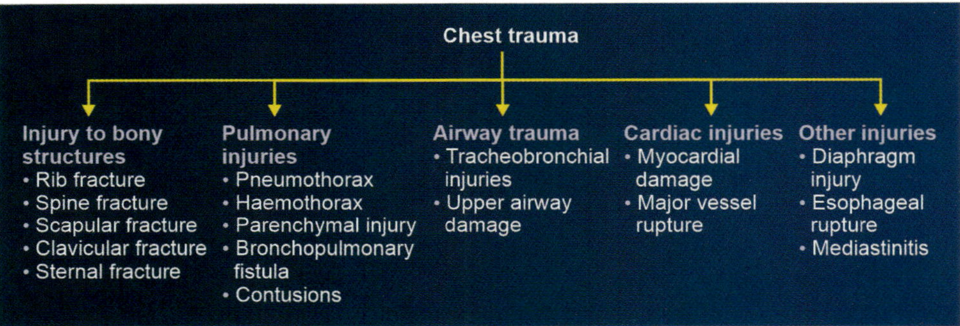

Fig. 18.19: Various injuries in chest trauma

Chest trauma involving various pulmonary and associated injuries are depicted in **Fig. 18.20**. Broadly chest trauma is classified into either blunt trauma which often has no exterior signs or symptoms of injury to the chest or penetrating chest injury. Blunt chest trauma carries more mortality than penetrating trauma as it is often associated with more systemic injuries which can be missed during early resuscitation hour.

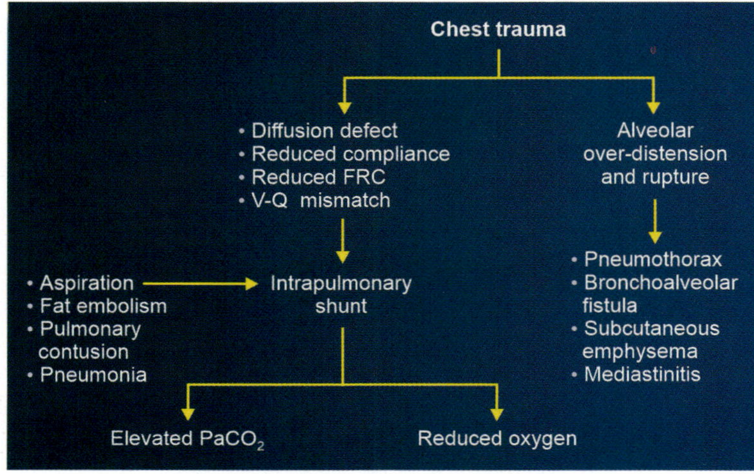

Fig. 18.20: Pathophysiology of chest trauma

General Approach to Chest Trauma

Resuscitation of the patient by securing the airway, breathing and circulation followed detailed history, physical examination and bedside imaging using ultrasound is utmost important to rule out severe chest trauma **(Table 18.6)** and carry out immediate interventions. In case of hemodynamic instability due to pneumothorax or hemopneumothorax, putting a chest drain may at times unnecessitate the need of intubation and mechanical ventilation. Complexity of chest trauma makes it difficult to generalize the indication of intubation and optimal ventilatory strategy for all patients.

Direct and indirect injuries like sepsis, massive transfusion and multiorgan dysfunction have potential for development of ARDS. Thus, it is prudent to understand the pathophysiology of individual patient and optimize the oxygenation, utilize open lung ventilation with lung protective ventilation, lung toilet and minimize or prevent further ventilator-associated lung injury (VALI). Apart from this supportive care **(Table 18.9)** plays vital role in early recovery and prevention of complications.

Table 18.6: Clinical signs of severe trauma

Clinical signs of severe chest trauma
✦ Haemorrhagic shock
✦ Instability of thorax
✦ Diaphragmatic rupture

Non-invasive Ventilation (NIV)

Recently more emphasis is being given to the use of non-invasive ventilation in early phase to trauma patients who are conscious, cooperative and hemodynamically stable. NIV improves hypoxemia, prevents atelectasis, decreases work of breathing and thus reduces the incidence of intubation, mechanical ventilation and its associated complications thereby, reducing the number of days in ICU. It is contraindicated in patients who are unconscious, high risk for aspiration and facial trauma.

Invasive Mechanical Ventilation

In the event of contraindications, noncompliance or failure of non-invasive ventilation, intubation and initiation of invasive positive pressure ventilation is required. The other indications of invasive mechanical intubation are given in **Table 18.7**. The application of PEEP prevents alveolar collapse, atelectasis, maintains the respiratory compliance and augments cardiac output. Good analgesia can help in providing adequate ventilation with support mode. Aim is to optimize gas exchange with lowest inspiratory pressure keeping in mind the patient's comfort. When using control mode aim should be to prevent barotrauma by minimizing airway pressure, allowing permissive hypercapnia (except in associated head injury where normocapnia is desirable) and avoiding collapse or over-distension of the lung.

Table 18.7: Indications of mechanical ventilation in chest trauma

✦ GCS< 8
✦ Failed Non-invasive ventilation
✦ Severe hypoxemia (PaO_2 <60 mmHg on 100% FiO_2)
✦ Pulmonary contusion
✦ Large narcotic doses for pain management causing respiratory compromise
✦ Flail chest with severe pain, dyspnoea, hypoxemia and underlying lung parenchymal injury
✦ Hemodynamic and metabolic instability
✦ Deteriorating respiratory status
✦ Emergency surgery
✦ Postoperatively after surgical repair

Table 18.8: Supportive care

✦ Pain management
✦ Physiotherapy to prevent atelectasis
✦ Bronchoscopy for removal of secretions and blood clots
✦ VAP bundle
✦ Nutritional care
✦ Early rehabilitation

Table 18.9: Ventilatory strategy

Calculate predicted body weight	✦ Men = [50+0.91 • (body height in cm – 152.4)] ✦ Women = [45.5+0.91 • (body height in cm – 152.4)]
FiO_2	✦ Set at 1, and then titrate to the desired level of PaO_2 (60–80 mmHg) and SpO_2 (90%)
Mode	✦ PCV or VCV
PEEP	✦ Start with 5 cm H_2O, titrate to oxygenation and hemodynamic stability, avoid overdistension of alveoli ✦ Avoid high peep in associated tramatic brain injury. ✦ In cases of subcutaneous emhysema, pneumothorax and air leak from chest tube, set peep as low as 0 cm H_2O ✦ High PEEP in pulmonary shunt
Tidal volume	✦ 6 to 8 mL/kg of predicated body weight
Plateau pressure	✦ <30 cm H_2O
Respiratory rate	✦ Start with 15/min and titrate to desired $PaCO_2$ ✦ Permissive hypercapnia accepted with exception to associated traumatic brain injury
Inspiratory time	✦ <1 second

Flail Chest

Flail chest is a painful traumatic condition caused by fracture of 3 or more ribs in at least 2 places causing loss of stability of the rib cage often associated with an underlying pulmonary parenchymal injury and can be fatal. It results in significant ventilatory disturbances such as hypoventilation due to pain, paradoxical movement of thorax resulting in inadequate expansion and underlying lung parenchymal damage. The paradoxical floating segment of chest wall and soft results in pain, dyspnoea, atelectasis, elevated respiratory effort and hypoxemia. Flail chest can be managed adequately with oxygenation, good analgesia and non-invasive ventilation with a very few patients requiring invasive mechanical ventilation. Continuous monitoring and reassessing the need for invasive mechanical ventilation frequently is must (Fig. 18.21).

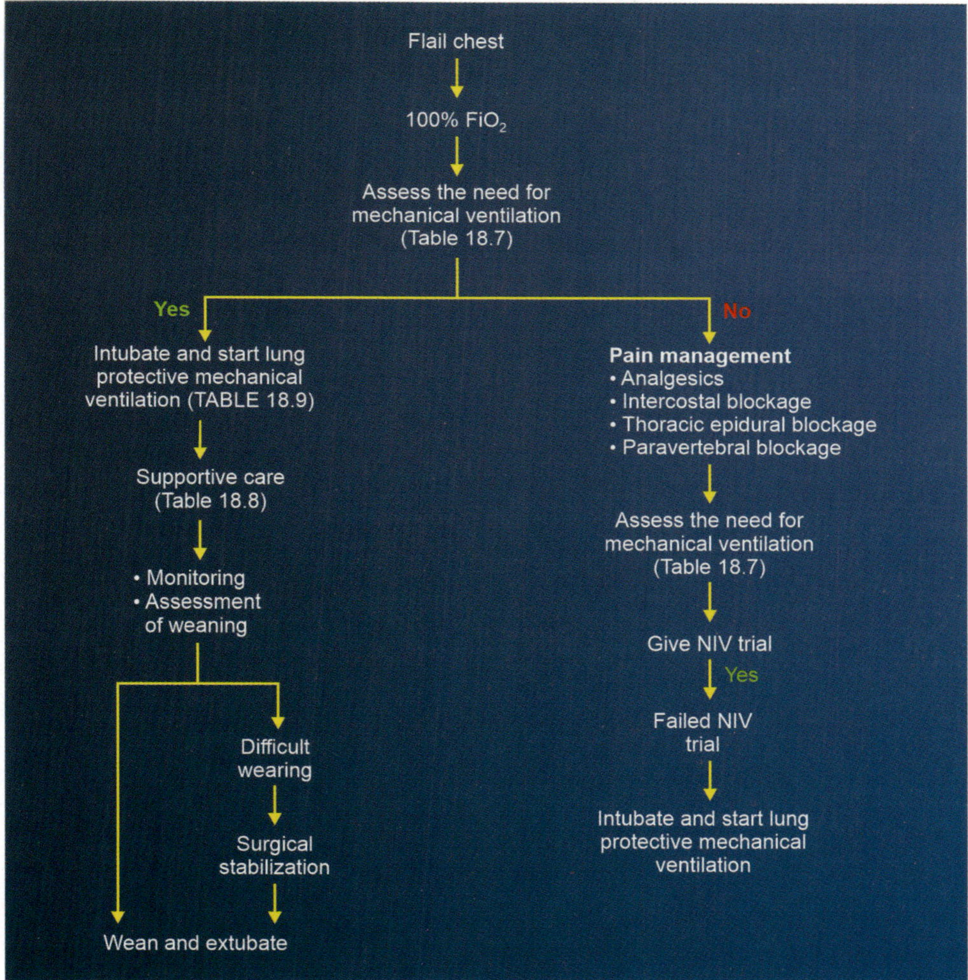

Fig. 18.21: Management of flail chest

Pulmonary Contusion

Pulmonary contusion is intrathoracic injury resulting from high impact blunt chest trauma leading to leakage of blood and protein from the vascular to the interstitial and alveolar space of the lungs over a period of 24 hours. This causes poor gas exchange, increased pulmonary vascular resistance and reduced lung compliance as well as development of ARDS. CT thorax and blood gas analysis is important to assess the severity of lung contusion.

Management of hypoxemia is the mainstay of the treatment along with supportive care **(Table 18.3)**. Mild to moderate forms of pulmonary contusion can be satisfactorily treated oxygen supplementation and non-invasive ventilation. In cases with severe form of pulmonary contusions, intubation and initiation of lung protective mechanical ventilation are required. If complication like acute respiratory distress syndrome (ARDS) develops it is always better to go for surgical repair of related injuries (diaphragmatic rupture, long bone fracture) to facilitate ARDS ventilation and proning.

Pneumothorax, Haemothorax and Hemopneumothorax

Injury to the pleura due to blunt and penetrating chest trauma can lead to pneumothorax or haemothorax associated with a collapse of the lung. Chest radiograph, CT scan and ultrasound are useful in the diagnosis of pneumothorax and haemothorax. Patient on mechanical ventilation should be treated urgently with tube thoracostomy of size 28 or 32 French for thoracic drainage to prevent the development of tension pneumothorax and decrease the air leakage due to bronchopleural fistula. The application of negative pressure to the drainage system can improve lung expansion with a risk of increased fistula flow and delayed closure.

Practice of intermittent thoracostomy tube closure during mechanical inhalation and a release during exhalation under continuous monitoring of ventilator setting such as peak, plateau and end expiratory pressure can be useful.

Bronchopleural Fistula

Bronchopleural fistula is a sinus tract formed between mainstem, lobar or segmental bronchus and pleural cavity due to either traumatic chest injury or after thoracocentesis. bpf offers a path of least resistance to air movement and thus leads to volume loss, inadequate lung expansion disturbing the gas exchange resulting in hypoxemia and hypercarbia. Conventional mechanical ventilation can be very challenging in bpf and needs specialize care **(Table 18.10)**. The disproportionate ventilation of both the lungs may necessitate independent lung ventilation with double lumen tube. This can help in differential ventilation of the affected and the normal lung with two ventilators set as per the lung requirement. Simultaneous high frequency jet ventilation for affected lung and lung protective ventilation for normal lung can be thus be established for optimal oxygenation and hemodynamic stability.

Table 18.10: Goals of mechanical ventilation in BPF
✦ Lowest effective tidal volume
✦ Short inspiratory time
✦ Lower respiratory rate
✦ Low PEEP
✦ Low mean airway pressure

Key Points

- Chest trauma either blunt or penetrating can be lethal
- Hypoxia and hypoventilation are the major causes of mortality
- Complexity of chest trauma leads to ventilatory challenges
- Generalized approach to chest trauma is difficult
- Individualized ventilatory approach according to the type, site and magnitude of trauma is a prudent approach
- Pain management and supportive care plays a vital role in early recovery
- Ventilatory setting should aim for prevention of further lung injury and enhance the oxygenation
- Monitoring and reassessment of the ventilatory setting is must

References

1. Richter T, Ragaller M. Ventilation in chest trauma. J Emerg Trauma Shock. 2011 Apr;4(2):251–9. doi: 10.4103/0974-2700.82215. PMID: 21769213; PMCID: PMC3132366.
2. Razi E. Mechanical ventilation in chest trauma. Arch Trauma Res. 2014 Nov 28;3(4):e25446. doi: 10.5812/atr.25446. PMID: 25821753; PMCID: PMC4360598.
3. Rico FR, Cheng JD, Gestring ML, Piotrowski ES. Mechanical ventilation strategies in massive chest trauma. Crit Care Clin. 2007 Apr;23(2):299-315, xi. doi: 10.1016/j.ccc.2006.12.007. PMID: 17368173.

V. MECHANICAL VENTILATION IN NEUROMUSCULAR DISORDERS

❒ Saurabh Biswal ❒ Pavan Kumar Reddy N

Neuromuscular diseases that affect the respiratory system are a major cause of morbidity and mortality in both acute and long-term settings. Long standing congenital and acquired neurological disease can cause respiratory failure requiring ventilator support. Neuromuscular diseases include a wide variety of disorders where the defect or disease could be at the upper motor neuron or lower motor neuron level.

Causes of neuromuscular diseases frequently referred to the ICU:

Table 18.11: Neuromuscular disorders referred to ICU[2]

Level of Lesion	Disease
Cortex	✦ Stroke (bilateral MCA)
Brainstem	✦ Infarction or hemorrhage in lower pons
Spinal Cord	✦ Trauma, tumour, abscess
	✦ Mulitiple sclerosis
	✦ Transverse myelitis.
Motor neuron	✦ Motor neuron disesase
	✦ Poliomyelitis
Peripheral nerve	✦ Guillain-Barré syndrome
	✦ Critical illness neuropathy
Neuromuscular junction	✦ Myasthenia gravis
	✦ Organophosphate poisoning
	✦ Botulism
Skeletal muscles	✦ Critical illness myopathy
	✦ Muscular dystrophy
	✦ Steroid induced myopathy
	✦ Alcohol induced myopathy
	✦ Electrolyte disturbances—hypokalemia, hypophosphatemia, hypomagnesemia.
	✦ Necrotising myopathy
	✦ Toxins

Patients with NMD usually have normal respiratory drive and normal lungs. The main problem with these type of patients is respiratory muscle weakness.

ICU-acquired Weakness (ICU-AW)

ICU-acquired weakness (ICU-AW) is recognized as a major complication of critical illness. Both functional and structural abnormalities in muscle and nerve causing critical illness polyneuropathy and myopathy (CIP and CIM), have been implicated in the development and maintenance of the generalized progressive muscle weakness and atrophy seen in ICU-AW. Neuromuscular weakness typically becomes apparent when an attempt is made to wean the patient from the ventilator, although there are earlier clues, which include grimacing without movement with noxious stimuli before recovery of consciousness, relative lack of movement after regaining consciousness and (not inevitably) loss of deep tendon reflexes that had been present earlier(seen with neuropathy than myopathy). The presence of severe muscle abnormalities that cannot be fully explained by disuse atrophy or compressive neuropathies suggests that ICUAW may be a primary myogenic problem. Electrophysiological studies and histology show axonal degeneration in neuropathy and muscle necrosis in myopathy. It is associated with longer time on ventilator, increased length of stay and increased morbidity and mortality.

Diagnosis

Experts advocate physical examination as the primary determinant of ICU-AW. In cooperative patients daily grading of muscle strength as per Medical Research Council (MRC) score is a good practice. Symmetric weakness and facial sparing are classical findings, along with difficult to wean and profound weakness despite return of sensorium that causes quadriplegia gives a clue that the patient has developed ICU-acquired weakness (ICU-AW).Patients develop these symptoms in a background of sepsis with multi organ dysfunction or an acute severe illness requiring extended periods of mechanical ventilation Patients demonstrating the characteristic examination combined with any evidence of recovery on serial examination usually require no further investigation. Patients with a protracted altered sensorium or fixed motor deficit should undergo further testing for CNS pathology. When a reliable motor examination is not possible muscle biopsy and electrophysiological studies may be warranted.

Risk factors associated with increased incidence for ICU-acquired weakness, are severe systemic inflammation, medications (specifically, corticosteroids and neuromuscular blocking agents, sedatives), glycemic control and immobility.

Management Protocol for ICU-acquired Weakness (ICU-AW) (Fig. 18.22)

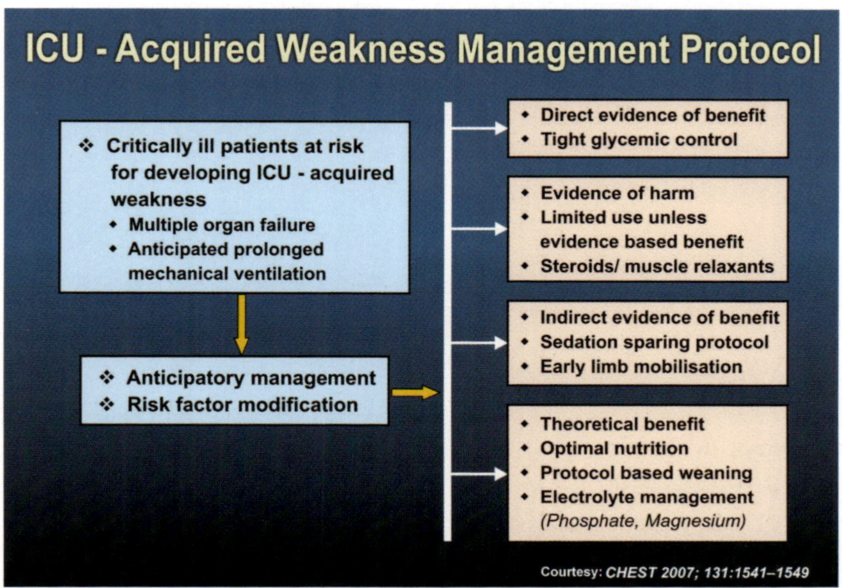

Fig. 18.22: Management protocol for ICU-acquired weakness (ICU-AW)

The most common pre-existing NMD referred to ICU are Guillain-Barré syndrome (GBS) and myasthenia gravis (MG).

Guillain-Barré syndrome (GB syndrome)

Neuromuscular respiratory failure requiring mechanical ventilation occurs in 20 to 30% of GBS patients. The clinician must monitor for clinical signs of impending respiratory failure, including tachypnea, use of accessory muscles of respiration, asynchronous movements of the chest and abdomen and tachycardia. Vital capacity has to be regularly monitored to detect any worsening in respiratory failure. A vital capacity below 20 ml/kg or less than 30% of the predicted VC, maximal inspiratory pressure (PImax) less than 30 cm H_2O, or maximal expiratory pressure (PEmax) less than 40 cm H_2O or a increasing PCO_2 level on arterial blood gas predicts imminent respiratory arrest. Time from onset to admission of less than 1 week, facial weakness, inability to cough, inability to lift head off the pillow, dyspnea and atelectasis on chest radiograph are other factors associated with respiratory failure and need for mechanical ventilation. Point of care scoring systems like the Erasmus GBS Respiratory Insufficiency score (EGRIS) can be used to predict the chances of respiratory failure in these patients BTS guidelines have advocated the use of NPPV in GBS patients if there are no contraindications. Invasive mechanical ventilation with lung protective strategies is warranted when used. The mean duration of mechanical ventilation for GBS is 2 to 6 weeks. Weaning from the ventilator should follow improvement in serial pulmonary function tests and strength. Plan for tracheostomy should be based on the status of the individual in the context keeping in mind the advantages of the procedure **(Table. 18.12)**.

Table 18.12: Erasmus GBS respiratory insufficiency Score

Measure	Categories	Score
Days between onset of weakness and hospital admission	>7days	0
	4–7 days	1
	≤3days	2
Facial and/or bulbar weakness at hospital admission	Absence	0
	Presence	1
MRC sum score at hospital admission	60–51	0
	50–41	1
	40–31	2
	30–21	3
	≤20	4
EGRIS		**0–7**

Myasthenia gravis (MG)

Complaints of shortness of breath and bulbar dysfunction, especially dysphagia, in patients with MG, especially if they are of recent onset, along with other clinical signs of respiratory failure must be taken very seriously. When accurate measures are possible, patients with a peak negative inspiratory force (NIF) of less than 20 cm (absolute value) H_2O or positive expiratory force (PEF) of <40 cm H_2O often require tracheal intubation. In general, a low forced vital capacity (especially <25–30 ml/kg) is worrisome and carefully following FVC in a closely monitored setting is important. Patients with marked bulbar dysfunction that compromises airway protection should be admitted to the intensive care unit even in the absence of overt respiratory failure. It is important to note that endotracheal intubation may be necessary to maintain airway patency in such patients who are having difficulty handling oral secretions even in the absence of overt respiratory failure. Earlier elective intubation may avert the likelihood of requiring emergency intubation and its inherent risks. Use of Non-invasive Positive Pressure Ventilation (NPPV), ventilator setting, weaning and tracheostomy principles are same as discussed in GB syndrome section.

Of late NPPV has become a cost effective alternative to IPPV in scenarios where there is mild respiratory insufficiency, during weaning from IPPV and in patients with inadequate pharmacological control.

Recent evidence has shown NPPV use in select myasthenia gravis patirnts has been effective in decreasing ICU and hospiatal length of stay, lessening incidence of intubation and pulmonary complications. For better outcomes with NPPV patient selection has to be appropriate, with better results seen in patients with lesser severity of illness (APACHE II<6) and higher failure rates among patient with PCO_2 >45 mmHg at the time of NIV initiation.

Spinal Cord Injuries

Higher the level of the cord injury higher is the mortality and morbidity, due to an increasing risk of respiratory muscle weakness.

Cervical cord lesions (C3–C8) predominantly affects inspiratory muscles (diaphragm and accessory muscles).These patients may need IPPV and are usually difficult to wean needing tracheostomy and rehabilitation. Thoracic cord lesions (T1–T11) affect the intercostal muscles hampering mainly inspiration and to some extent expiration. Thoracolumbar cord lesions (T6–T11) mainly involve the abdominal muscles affecting expiration. Thoracic and lumbar cord lesions have poor cough effect.

APPLICATION OF NPPV

Patient selection should be appropriate for NPPV to be effective. NPPV is contraindicated if there is hemodynamic instability, bulbar palsy causing inability to manage oral cavity secretions, comatose patients, facial injury or abnormality causing inability to fix an interface, copious secretions and life threatening hypoxemia.

Steps to apply NPPV

- Patient needs to be explained the process to ensure compliance.
- An appropriate interface, e.g. oronasal, nasal needs to be chosen.
- Approriate mode, Pressure support or pressure control needs to be selected.
- Start with low pressure settings of pressure support of 5–6 cm H_2O and PEEP of 4 cm H_2O. It can be increased in increments of 2–4 cm H_2O till adequate minute ventilation is achieved. Usually a pressure support of more than 10–12 cm H_2O and PEEP of 4–6 cm H_2O is not required as lung parenchyma is not affected.

- At the beginning of ventilation interface needs to be held with hand against the patients face and once the patient synchronises then the NPPV mask needs to be fixed with straps minimising air leaks.

Once the patient is on NPPV close monitoring regularly to look for any signs of worsening in the form of worsening respiratory distress, patient non-compliance, worsening sensorium, worsening PH, PCO_2, PO_2. Immediate transition to IPPV if the need arises needs to be available from the point of initiating NPPV.

Initial Ventilator Settings for IPPV:

- Tidal volume–6–8 ml/kg IBW
- Respiratory rate–12–20 breaths/min
- PEEP 4–5 cmH_2O
- I:E 1:2
- Plateau pressure <30 cm H_2O
- FiO_2 1.0 to begin with and then titrate to the lower FiO_2 as per oxygenation levels.

Goals of mechanical ventilation in chronic neuromuscular disease:

- Maintain pulmonary compliance
- Support muscles of respiration to maintain normal alveolar ventilation

These goals can be achieved with respiratory muscle training with frequent spontaneous breathing trails, cough assist techniques, when respiratory failure ensues, patients may require NPPV and intubation with mechanical ventilation if contraindications to NPPV are present. Ventilator support in chronic NMD patients can be provided with NPPV.

The indications for NPPV are symptoms of fatigue, dyspnea, orthopnea, and early morning headache with either $PaCO_2$ of more than 45 mm Hg or nocturnal desaturation with SpO_2 of less than 88% for 5 consecutive times. The advantage of NPPV includes respiratory muscle rest, improves alveolar ventilation, lung compliance, ventilation/perfusion matching and also avoidance of complications associated with intubation and complications of long term IPPV.

Selection of settings for NPPV in patients with neuromuscular disease is often done based on symptoms of the patient. Initially the NPPV settings are selected based on short-term symptoms such as chest expansion, accessory muscle use, and patients comfort and adjusted later for long term goals. Initially started with low settings and gradually titrated to the patients requirements.

Lung protective ventilator protocols should be implemented when they have acute deterioration in lung status. The ultimate goal in these patients on NPPV is to improve symptoms of morning headache, fatigue and daytime sleepiness.

Conclusion

Many patients with NMD require mechanical ventilation for a short duration till the acute cause is resolved. In some chronic conditions mechanical ventilation may be instituted in the ICU if there is an acute deterioration in the respiratory status with lung protective settings. NPPV and airway clearance in properly selected patients can be life prolonging. Cough and secretions are important determinates of extubation success.

References

1. Non-invasive Ventilation in Neuromuscular Disease. Dean R Hess. Respiratory care: August 2006 vol 51 no 8.
2. Neuromuscular Disease in Respiratory and Critical Care. Nicholas S Hill: Respir Care 2006; 51 (9): 1065–1071.
3. Principles and Practice of Mechanical Ventilation. 2nd edition. Martin.J.Tobin.
4. ICU-Acquired Weakness. William D. Schweickert and Jesse Hall. Chest 2007; 131:1541–49.
5. Rabinstein A, WijdicksEF.BiPAP in acute respiratory failure due to myasthenic crisis may prevent intubation. Neurology.2002;59(10):1647–49.
6. Senevratne J, Mandrekar J, Wijdicks EFM, Rabinstein AA. Non-invasive ventilation in myasthenic crisis.Arch Neurol. 2008;65[1]:54–8.
7. Agarwal R, Reddy C, Gupta D. Non-invasive ventilation in acute neuromuscular respiratory failure due to myasthenic crisis: case report and review of literature. Emerg Med J. 2006:23[1]:e6.
8. Wu JY, Kuo PH, Fan PC, Wu HD, Shih FY, Yang PC. The role of non-invasive ventilation and factors predicting extubation outcome in myasthenic crisis. Neurocrit Care. 2009;10[1]:35–42.

VI. ACUTE RESPIRATORY DISTRESS SYNDROME (ARDS)

❒ Srinivas Samavedam

INTRODUCTION

Acute respiratory distress syndrome (ARDS), initially referred to, as "Shock Lung" is one among the most commonly encountered life-threatening emergency faced by an intensivist, associated with high mortality and morbidity. The recent COVID 19 pandemic witnessed the burden of mortality and morbidity due to severe ARDS. In spite of more than 5 decades of research, ARDS carries a high mortality and only a few effective therapeutic modalities exist to combat it.

DEFINITION

Based on his study published on a case series of 12 patients treated in a civilian environment in the USA, Ashbaugh was the first to describe ARDS in 1967. Later, in 1988 Murray and co expanded the definition to incorporate the risk factors, acute nature of the disease process and measures of severity. Followed by the initial description, many others definitions have been used by various physicians involved in the care of ARDS patients, until the joint American European Consensus Conference (AECC) met and redefined the definition of ARDS, in the year 1994. Following this the definition by AECC was widely used to clinically identify patients with ARDS and for patient enrollment in various trials, but has many limitations due to its simplicity. Since the recognition of ARDS as a distinct clinical entity there has been a huge publications addressing various pathogenic mechanisms responsible for the development of ARDS, with a focus on the therapeutic strategies. Due to the inconsistent definitions used by various physicians across different ICUs and also the drawbacks of the AECC definition, the published prevalence of ARDS ranged from 10–90%, associated with a high mortality of around 35–55%. The current definition is the Berlin definition, clinically in practice since the year 2013, which was created by a consensus panel of experts convened in 2011.

Ashbaugh described a clinical entity associated with:

1. Severe dyspnea, tachypnea
2. Cyanosis refractory to oxygen therapy
3. Associated with loss of lung compliance
4. Diffuse alveolar infiltrates on CXR
5. Hyperaemia, atelectasis, interstitial and alveolar edema and hemorrhages with hyaline membrane at autopsy.

   This was the first description of "The ARDS " more than 50 years ago.

Following this, definition of ARDS was refined by the AECC in 1994, which has subsequently gained wide popularity and was widely employed in clinical practice. The key components include:

1. The presentation should be acute
2. Hypoxia, measured by PF ratio, PF <300 consistent with ALI and PF ratio <200 is ARDS

3. Bilateral infiltrates on a frontal CXR
4. Absence of left atrial hypertension, PCWP<18 mmHg, no clinical signs of CHF.

This definition was widely used due to its simplicity, was incorporated in various papers and also defined the entry criteria for patients into various trials for over a period of 20 years until the Berlin definition has been proposed. Due to its pitfalls, the AECC definition has faced criticism.

The limitations of AECC definition are:

A. Time limit has not been clearly defined
B. The term ALI was used inconsistently leading to confusion
C. CXR interpretation is unreliable
D. PF ratios can be manipulated by adjusting PEEP
E. PCWP may be elevated for reasons other than heart failure.

All these pitfalls led to the development of the Berlin definition, which is in practice currently.

Berlin definition of ARDS: It is a form of acute diffuse lung injury in patients with predisposing risk factors. The key components are:

1. Timing: Acute onset, i.e. onset with in 1 week of a known clinical insult or new/worsening respiratory symptoms.
2. Presence of bilateral opacities on the chest radiographs, not fully explained by effusions, lobar/lung collapse or nodules
3. Respiratory failure not fully explained by cardiac failure or fluid overload, with the need for objective assessment (echo) to exclude hydrostatic edema
4. Presence of hypoxemia, defined by a PaO_2/FiO_2 ratio measured with a minimal PEEP of > 5 cm H_2O, and defines 3 mutually exclusive categories of severity
   a. Mild: PaO_2/FiO_2 between 200 and 300
   b. Moderate: PaO_2/FiO_2 between 100 and 200
   c. Severe: PaO_2/FiO_2 less than 100

This new definition has addressed several important issues:

- Clear timing of the insult was mentioned.
- Radiological criteria were specified
- PCWP criteria was removed
- PEEP was added and the term ALI was removed

With in a very short span even the Berlin definition has faced criticism. The main pointers being that it does not allow early identification of patients before ARDS becomes established, lacks direct measure of lung injury, diagnosis still includes CXR, which when compared to a CT scan has a poor correlation and in particular measurement of PF ratio after 24 hr using predefined ventilator settings might improve the class of severity of ARDS and it is unclear how the diagnosis and management in the real world have changed, and also its ability to predict mortality is still poor. In the real world especially in the resource limited settings application of the Berlin criteria has faced challenges and hence a slight modification was done to this in the year 2014, " the Kigali modification", according to which ARDS is defined without the need of PEEP and the cut off for SpO_2/FiO_2 is less than or equal to 315. Before its application, validity and reliability of the Kigali modification has to be further studies. The LUNG SAFE study which was a multicenter, prospective study done across 50 ICUs looking at the ICU incidence of ARDS and the ability of the clinician to recognize ARDS, also supports and the strengthens the rationale of Kigali modification to the 2012 Berlin definition of ARDS.

Though several efforts have been made constantly to better define ARDS, major drawback of the current Berlin definition is that it defines ARDS as all or none phenomenon, and many clinical entities are often confused with ARDS, e.g. a cute cardiogenic pulmonary edema. These clinical entities can be grouped under one category as "ARDS Mimics". It is important to clearly differentiate the ARDS mimics so that treatment strategy can be optimized.

Patients with true ARDS compared to the mimics usually:

- Have prolonged and severe hypoxia which may need several recruitment techniques
- Lung compliance is impaired
- Aerated lung volume is decreased
- Dead space is increased leading to ineffective CO_2 clearance
- Recovery usually takes several days to weeks and often-residual fibrosis is seen.

PATHOPHYSIOLOGY, TYPES AND CAUSES OF ARDS

The pathophysiology of ARDS is a complex process and not fully understood to date in health, for the gaseous exchange to happen it requires dry lungs with a patent alveoli and an intact pulmonary capillary endothelium.in ARDS there occurs a diffuse alveolar damage (DAD), releasing pro-inflammatory cytokines like tumor necrosis factor, IL 6, il8, that are ultimately responsible for the pulmonary alveolar–capillary endothelial damage. This results in increased permeability leading to pulmonary edema, loss of surfactant and alveolar collapse. As a consequence the physiological dead space increases, gaseous exchange is impaired, lung compliance decreases, and pulmonary arterial hypertension develops. In ARDS the acute lung injury is an evolving process and tends to progress through three relatively distinct and overlapping pathologic phases.

The exudative phase: Lasts for 5–7 days, due to epithelial and endothelial injury fluid exudates

The proliferative phase: Lasts from 7–14 days, repair of the damaged endothelium and epithelium begins along with proliferation of fibroblasts.

The fibrotic phase: Begins after 2 weeks, fibrosis occurs only in some patients due to chronic inflammatory process **(Fig. 18.23)**.

It was previously assumed that the lung passes through all these 3 phases over a specified time period, i.e. it was usually thought that exudative phase occurs in the 1st week of insult, proliferative during the 2nd week and fibrotic phase begins after 10 days after the insult, but as we better understand the pathology, there seems to be an overlap of the inflammatory and the fibro proliferative phases in contrast to the what was previously imagined and this may begin as early as 24 hr after the insult. The ventilator strategies used in the management of ARDS can also exacerbate the acute lung injury.

The underlying causes for ARDS are multiple. Based on the insult ARDS can be classified as pulmonary and extrapulmonary ARDS.

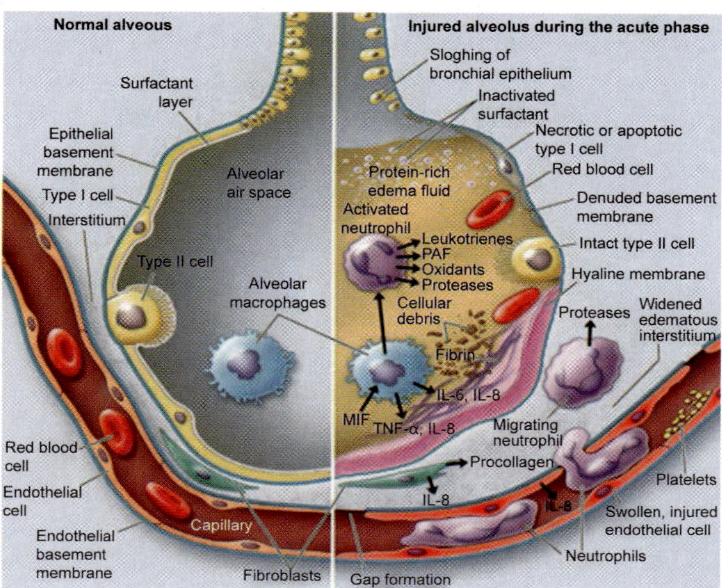

Fig. 18.23: Pathophysiology of ARDS

Table 18.13

Pulmonary ARDS/direct injury	Extrapulmonary ARDS/indirect injury
Pneumonia	Sepsis
Aspiration	Pancreatitis
Smoking/toxic gas inhalation	Blood transfusion
Lung contusion/Trauma	Burns
Drowning	Neurogenic pulmonary edema
VILI	Cardiopulmonary bypass

THE " BABY LUNG " IN ARDS

Until mid 1980s the injured lung in ARDS was considered to be homogenous and stiff. On contrary to our belief, the use of CT in ARDS showed that, we were actually dealing with an heterogeneous lung, and the amount of normally aerated lung was around 20 % of the normal size, which weighed to around 200–500 g at end expiration in severe ARDS, and this was roughly equal to the size of a healthy lung in a 5–6 year old. From this our concept of ARDS lung has changed from it being a "homogenous and stiff " lung to our current concept of a "heterogeneous baby lung" (**Fig. 18.24**).

The compliance of the respiratory system strongly correlated well with this small-aerated lung tissue, which had a near normal elasticity as measured by the specific tissue compliance. With this it was assumed that the Baby lung was an anatomical structure in the non-dependent areas of the lung and hence the concept of prone ventilation was introduced. With prone ventilation, oxygenation has improved, but when a CT was done in prone, they observed a shift in the position of the baby lung to dorsal zones. This observation led to the understanding that the baby lung is not an anatomical structure but a functional structure that is a diseased but aerated part of the lung and another

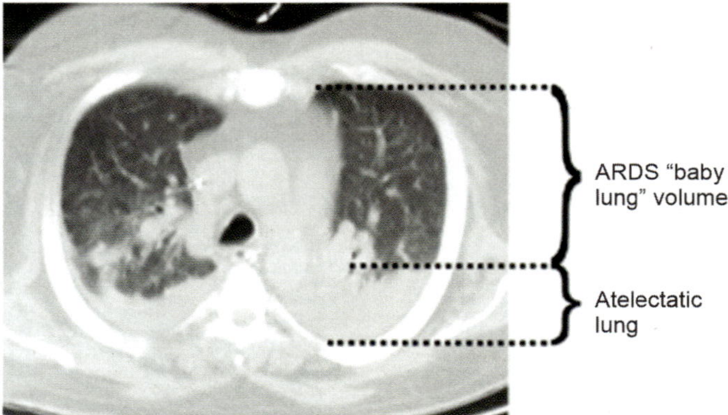

Fig. 18.24: An HRCT of ARDS Lung. Note the heterogeneity and the relatively small (baby) normal lung

interesting finding was that the edema in the injured lung was evenly distributed, due to which the weight of the lung increases, and there occurs loss of alveolar gas as a result of the compressive gravitational force including the weight of the heart, which are off loaded in the prone position, resulting in improvement this lead to the so called concept of "Sponge lung" (Fig. 18.25).

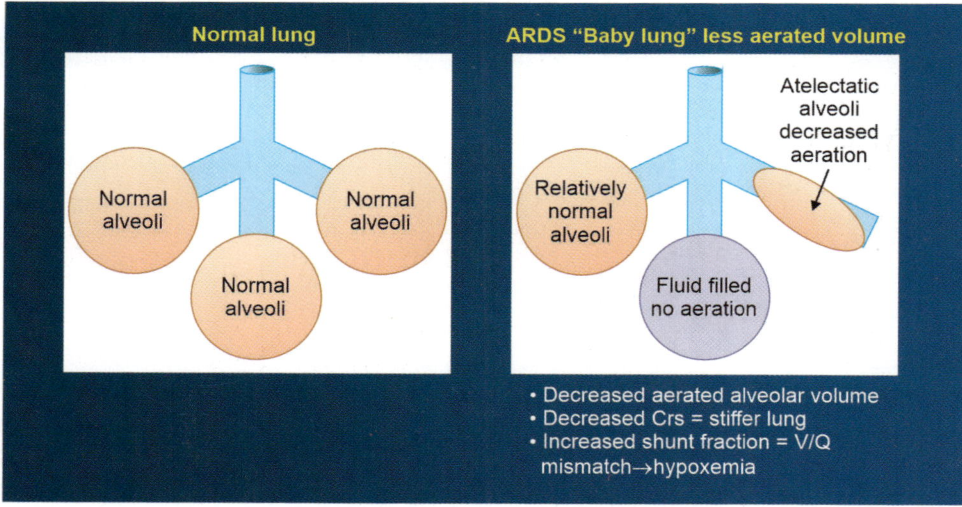

Fig. 18.25: Three alveoli model of the lung

This concept held reasonably good until the recent COVID 19 pandemic. COVID 19 represented an atypical form of ARDS, and the CT performed in initial stages of the disease in patients who met the ARDS criteria showed that they still had an adult lung with normal specific compliance. But over a period of time either due to the disease progression or due to inappropriate treatment strategies the adult lung shrinked to a baby lung. The cause of hypoxemia in COVID patients was mainly due to the VQ mismatch, and to combat hypoxia respiratory drive is activated leading to high tidal volume breaths ultimately leading to a high transpulmonary pressure, resulting in Stress and Strain, imitating the changes similar to VILI. Due to this the dependent regions of the lung collapse, resulting in reduction in the compliance and transitioning the lung from an adult to baby lung. If these changes are not a interrupted, the vicious cycle of events continue causing the baby lung to shrink, which is a result of a dynamic lung injury (**Fig. 18.26**).

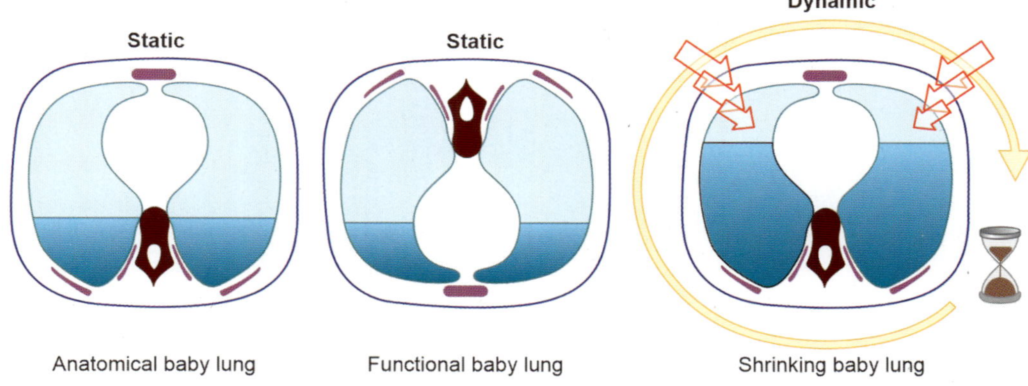

Fig. 18.26: Development of the baby lung concept

MANAGEMENT OF ARDS

ARDS is a complex disease with multifactorial causes and poorly understood pathophysiology. Treatment is directed at optimizing the oxygenation and ventilation. The main lines of management include:

1. Identifying the underlying cause and treating it
2. Supportive therapy
3. Rest to the lung, so as to provide time for the injured lung to repair
4. Preventing further insults to the injured lung.

Treatment categories can be broadly divided as:

1. Ventilatory and non-ventilatory strategies **(Table 18.14)**
2. Pharmacological and non-pharmacological interventions

Table 18.14

Ventilatory strategies	Non-ventilatory strategies
Lung protective ventilation	Prone ventilation
Inverse ratio ventilation	Sedation and paralysis
HFOV	Fluids, Steroids
	ECMO

Ventilator Management

Providing supplemental oxygen is the basic and the most crucial step in the management of ARDS patients. In the past, most of the clinicians managed ARDS by putting patients on Invasive mechanical ventilation, which was presumed to be a better way of management, but off late as we better understand the etio-pathogenesis of ARDS today NIV, HFNC has been used with successful outcomes especially in patients with mild ARDS and with careful vigilance in patients with moderate ARDS, keeping in view the advantages and disadvantages of each.

NIV and HFNC in ARDS

For more than two decades NIV has been used by clinicians in patients with mild to moderate ADRS, though we do not have a strict guideline driven protocol except in immunocompromised patients where use of NIV has a strong level of recommendation. By providing positive pressure, NIV reduces the inspiratory effort, work of breathing, improves the gaseous exchange. Thus has a strong rationale from physiological perspective, but to date various studies published on the use of NIV in ARDS patient's shows inconclusive data. The recently published LUNG SAFE study has shown that in patients with a PF ratio <150, mortality was higher with use of NIV compared to IMV and also the failure of NIV co-related with the severity of ARDS. Apart from the severity of ARDS, patient compliance and attaining a proper seal also determine the success. In a recent single center trial published by Patel *et al.* the interface with helmet compared to face mask, showed the intubation rates to be lower in the helmet group, and this translated into more ventilator free days and lower mortality rates. The main disadvantage of the use of NIV is that in spontaneously breathing, patients tend to hyperventilate due to the higher respiratory drive resulting in significantly increased incidence of VILI.

HFNC is one of the recent technique and currently widely being used the physiological effects of HFNC differ from NIV in that, with HFNC constant flow rate of gas generated variable pressure according to the patients effort and dynamic thoracic compliance compared to NIV where in the gas flow rate varies to maintain a preset PS and PEEP. HFNC also generates PEEP that is proportional to the gas flow that is not constant due to air leakage. Most studies also reported a better comfort with HFNC compared to NIV resulting in better compliance. In the FLORALI trial, HFNC was shown to be non-inferior to NIV and also intubation rates were significantly reduced, with a statistically significant higher ventilator free days in the HFNC group.

Though there are multiple studies published on the use of NIV and HFNC in patients with mild to moderate ARDS, till date we do not have clear guidelines driven protocol for their application in real world and the success tends to lie in careful patient selection, with careful vigilance and monitoring, and recognizing failures with low threshold for intubation in such seems to be the key for successful outcomes. Lately, HFNC has been the initial choice by many clinicians as it consistently proved to be non-inferior to NIV and also the fact that patients showed better tolerate it. In the subset of patients where HFNC fails, there is no practical advantage of switching over to NIV and vice versa, rather in such delaying IMV may increase the mortality.

INVASIVE MECHANICAL VENTILATION (IMV)

1. Mode of Ventilation

IMV has been the main stay of treatment for patients with ARDS and over the last few decades various ventilator strategies have been tried with variable outcomes. Today we also clearly understand and agree to the fact that IMV per se can worsen the ALI, referred to as ventilator induced lung injury (VILI).

Clinicians have used both VCV and PCV in the management of ARDS. To date many RCTs done comparing both these modes have not shown a major benefit of one over the other. It is important for the treating physician to have a basic understanding of each mode of ventilation with its advantages and disadvantages.

In VCV, a fixed tidal volume is delivered, that produces stable minute ventilation, but the pressure is not controlled. As it delivers a guaranteed tidal volume VCV favors the control of ventilation. The main disadvantage is that the mean airway pressures are lower and hence recruitment may be poor in a lung with poor compliance. But ADRS net have used VCV in ARDS, as it seemed to be practically easy to practice the low tidal volume ventilation.

On contrary in PCV the inspiratory pressure is a controlled variable and flows are variable. Tidal volume is variable and is dependent on the compliance of the lung. As the PCV increases the mean airway pressure, it helps in alveolar recruitment and hence favors the control of oxygenation. Because pressure is a control variable, it protects from barotrauma, but as volume is uncontrolled, volutrauma is a possible side effect.

Either mode of ventilation has not shown any mortality or morbidity benefit of one over the other, the important point to be remembered and practiced is that irrespective of the mode used, the main principle is to follow the lung protective ventilation (LPV) which is now the well-established and accepted method of ventilating an ARDS lung. It is achieved by:

A. Using a low tidal volume of approximately 4–6 ml/kg PBW
B. Targeting a plateau pressure of 25–30 cm of H_2O
C. Optimal PEEP

2. Tidal Volume

Traditional approach in managing hypoxic ARDS lung was to use high tidal volumes, as high as 10–15 ml/kg. As the use of mechanical ventilator as supportive therapy became widespread out of OT in the ICUs, many clinicians also had a concern that mechanical ventilation per se has the ability to inflict lung injury. To further clarify this, Webb and Tierney published a landmark paper in 1974. In their study, they ventilated rats with normal lungs with varying peak inspiratory pressure (PIP) with and without PEEP. The key observations from this study was that ventilation with lower PIP of 14 cm of H_2O does not cause significant injury, high PIP and high TV without PEEP lead to severe lung injury due to worsening pulmonary edema and addition of PEEP has shown beneficial. This aptly holds good for our current understanding that in ARDS, we are ventilating the baby lung, trying to avoid secondary insults to it and helping the injured lung rest so as to heal over a time period. Following this. Dreyfuss, *et al.* has done a experimental study to better answer whether it is the high pressure or the high tidal volume that is responsible for the VILI. They have subjected rats to 5 different ventilator strategies:

a. Low PIP and TV (7 cm H_2O/13 ml/kg)
b. High PIP and TV (45 cm H_2O/40 ml/kg)
c. High PIP with addition of PEEP
d. High PIP with restricted TV by using thoracoabdominal binders

e. Using negative inspiratory pressure with high TV. The key observations were that PEEP had a protective effect, low TV irrespective of PIP had beneficial effects and high TV irrespective of PIP was harmful. Similar findings from multiple small trials led to the landmark trial published by the ARDS network in the year 2000. This study clearly showed a mortality benefit in patients being ventilated with low TV (6 ml/kg with P_{plat} <30 cm H_2O) compared to those ventilated with high TV (12 ml/kg with P_{plat} <50 cm H_2O). This trial has changed our practice of ventilating ARDS patients with high TV to the low TV ventilation followed currently. But this practice comes with accepting the side effect of low TV, so called "permissive hypercapnia" and auto-PEEP (**Fig. 18.27**).

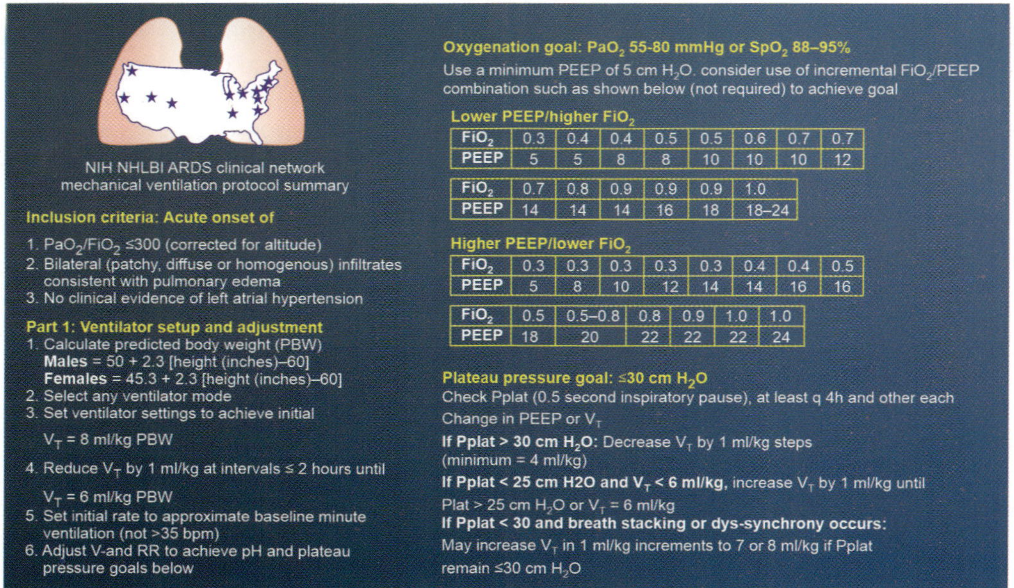

NIH NHLBI ARDS clinical network mechanical ventilation protocol summary

Inclusion criteria: Acute onset of

1. PaO_2/FiO_2 ≤300 (corrected for altitude)
2. Bilateral (patchy, diffuse or homogenous) infiltrates consistent with pulmonary edema
3. No clinical evidence of left atrial hypertension

Part 1: Ventilator setup and adjustment

1. Calculate predicted body weight (PBW)
   Males = 50 + 2.3 [height (inches)–60]
   Females = 45.3 + 2.3 [height (inches)–60]
2. Select any ventilator mode
3. Set ventilator settings to achieve initial
   V_T = 8 ml/kg PBW
4. Reduce V_T by 1 ml/kg at intervals ≤ 2 hours until
   V_T = 6 ml/kg PBW
5. Set initial rate to approximate baseline minute ventilation (not >35 bpm)
6. Adjust V-and RR to achieve pH and plateau pressure goals below

Oxygenation goal: PaO_2 55-80 mmHg or SpO_2 88–95%

Use a minimum PEEP of 5 cm H_2O. consider use of incremental FiO_2/PEEP combination such as shown below (not required) to achieve goal

Lower PEEP/higher FiO_2

FiO_2	0.3	0.4	0.4	0.5	0.5	0.6	0.7	0.7
PEEP	5	5	8	8	10	10	10	12

FiO_2	0.7	0.8	0.9	0.9	0.9	1.0
PEEP	14	14	14	16	18	18–24

Higher PEEP/lower FiO_2

FiO_2	0.3	0.3	0.3	0.3	0.3	0.4	0.4	0.5
PEEP	5	8	10	12	14	14	16	16

FiO_2	0.5	0.5–0.8	0.8	0.9	1.0	1.0
PEEP	18	20	22	22	22	24

Plateau pressure goal: ≤30 cm H_2O

Check Pplat (0.5 second inspiratory pause), at least q 4h and other each Change in PEEP or V_T

If Pplat > 30 cm H_2O: Decrease V_T by 1 ml/kg steps (minimum = 4 ml/kg)

If Pplat < 25 cm H2O and V_T < 6 ml/kg, increase V_T by 1 ml/kg until Plat > 25 cm H_2O or V_T = 6 ml/kg

If Pplat < 30 and breath stacking or dys-synchrony occurs: May increase V_T in 1 ml/kg increments to 7 or 8 ml/kg if Pplat remain ≤30 cm H_2O

Fig. 18.27: The PEEP-FiO_2 table

3. PEEP

Setting an optimal PEEP is the most challenging aspect of ventilator settings in ARDS. PEEP was traditionally used to improve oxygenation but today we have enough evidence that it also prevents VILI by preventing alveolar collapse and the stress caused by repeated collapse and re-opening of the alveoli. On the other hand PEEP can also cause alveolar over distension, increase dead space and reduce the RV afterload and LV preload resulting in reduced biventricular compliance and decreased cardiac output. The main consequence of applying PEEP is that it increases the end expiratory lung volume (EELV), so it opens the previously collapsed alveoli but may over distend the already open alveoli. Rather it is a double-edged sword, with both beneficial and harmful effects. Hence there has been lot of research to determine the ideal PEEP and many methods proposed for setting the ideal PEEP. When applying PEEP one thing to be remembered is that every ARDS lung should be assessed for recruitability to determine the optimal PEEP for that lung and this has to be repeated frequently over a time frame, rather PEEP should be individualized.

To date 3 major trials published on high vs low PEEP, the ALVEOLI, LOV and EXPRESS, did not show any mortality benefit of high PEEP over low PEEP, but high PEEP did result in better oxygenation, more ventilator free days. Practically a very low PEEP of <6 cm H_2O seems to be ineffective and a high PEEP of >15 cm H_2O can lead to alveolar over distension and hence may be harmful. In any individual an optimal PEEP is that PEEP where

A. Oxygenation is maximized
B. There is minimal end expiratory atelectasis
C. There is minimal end inspiratory over distension.

Today PEEP is considered to protect the injured lung.

Numerous methods for setting this optimal PEEP have been described in literature, but none were comparatively superior to the other.

A. ARDS Net Table

The most commonly used method for setting PEEP by beginners is to use the ARDS net table, comparatively an easy method of selecting PEEP, but may not be an ideal method for selecting optimal PEEP as it has no evidence and they are based on expert opinion. A combination of PEEP and FIO_2 are used to achieve a target SPO_2 of 88–95% or PAO_2 of 555–80 mmHg **(Table 18.15)**.

Table 18.15: Two examples of PEEP/FiO_2 tables used by the ARDS Network

Conservative approach																
FiO_2	.30	.40	.40	.50	.50	.60	.70	.70	.70	.80	.90	.90	.90	1.0	1.0	1.0	1.0
PEEP	5	5	8	8	10	10	10	10	12	14	14	14	16	18	18	20	22
Aggressive approach																	
FiO_2	.30	.30	.40	.40	.50	.50	.60	.60	.70	.80	.80	.90	1.0	1.0			
PEEP	12	14	14	16	16	18	18	20	20	20	22	22	22	24			

B. By using PV Loops

Using PV loop to determine the upper inflection point (UIP) and lower inflection point (LIP) was a popular method in setting PEEP **(Fig. 18.28)**.

The LIP is the point where alveolar recruitment starts and below this there occurs atelectasis. The UIP is the point where recruitment ends and pressure above this leads to over distension. It is recommended to set PEEP 2 cm above the LIP. Bedside estimation of the PV loop is cumbersome, it requires deeper sedation and paralysis for the correct loops and identification of the LIP may also be difficult.

c. Stress Index (SI)

The shape of the Pressure Time scalar with constant inspiratory flow in VCV helps to determine the stress index that corresponds to the elastance of the respiratory system. The stress index is determined from the shape of the Pressure time scalar.

Which can take 3 different shapes, that are: Linear, concavity upwards or concavity downwards. To measure the stress index we need dedicated software that limits its use **(Fig. 18.29)**.

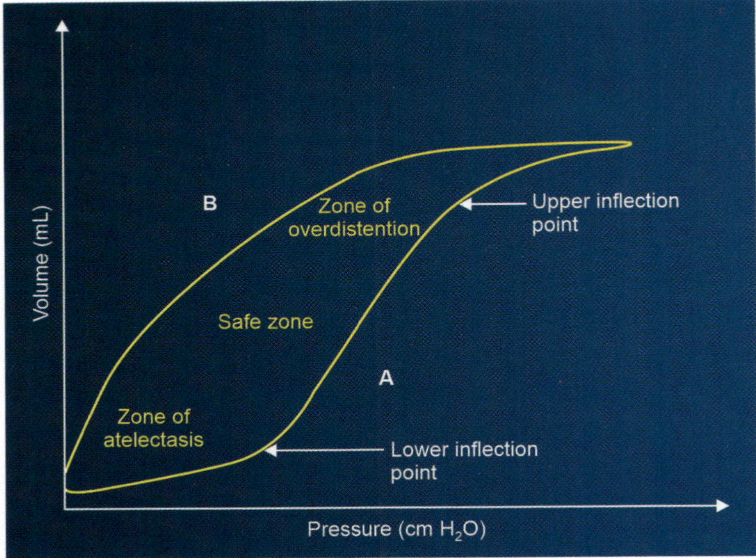

Fig. 18.28: The conceptual lower inflection point

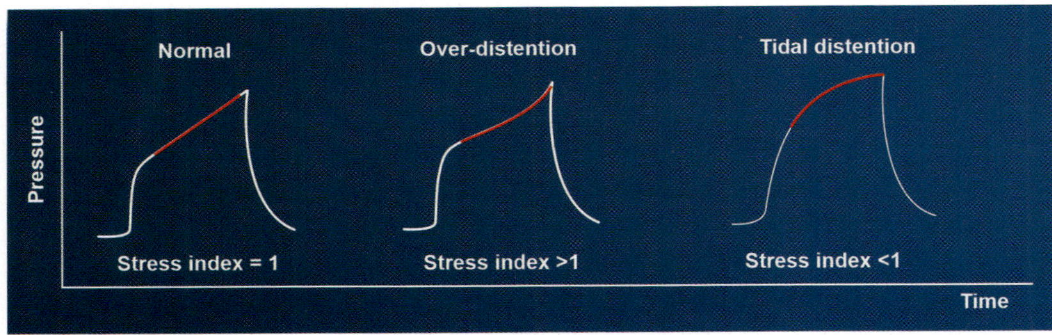

Fig. 18.29: Patterns of the pressure time scalar according to the stress index

A linear curve, SI = 1, suggest recruitment without over distension
Upward concavity, SI >1 suggests over distension
Downward concavity, SI <1 suggests potential for recruitment.

D. Imaging

Imaging has been one of the reasonable methods of setting PEEP; many clinicians have used CT and CXR to assess the alveolar recruitment. But practically transporting to imaging is difficult and needs expertise in measuring the density changes that occur with change in PEEP. Off late USG nag Electrical impedance tomography have been used. USG due to its of availability, reliability and ease of performance has gained wide popularity. EIT though may be a more reliable method needs expertise and also not available at many centers making its use limited.

E. Best Compliance

In this method the level of PEEP that coincides with best static compliance is determined to determine the ideal PEEP either by applying incremental or decremental PEEP.

F. Lung Volume

In ARDS, FRC is severely compromised. FRC plus PEEP induced increase in the lung volume together is the End Expiratory Lung Volume (EELV). A modified nitrogen wash out technique is used to measure the EELV at various levels of PEEP. EELV combined with compliance helps to determine the response to PEEP, there by its titration.

G. Esophageal Manometry

Esophageal pressure is measured using balloon manometry, as a surrogate to pleural pressure and the transpulmonary pressure (TPP) is calculated by subtracting it from the P_{plat}. PEEP is adjusted so as to maintain a TPP between 0 and 10 cm H_2O at end expiration. This method may be beneficial in patients with morbid obesity.

4. P_{plat}, Driving Pressure

Low TV ventilation is a strategy employed to reduce the P_{plat}, with a target to maintain P_{plat}< 30 CM H_2O in ARDS, a value that roughly corresponds to the Total lung capacity. Since the publication of the ARMA trial, most of the clinicians have used a P_{plat} target of <30 cm H_2O in the management of ARDS, by adjusting the TV between 4–8 ml/kg PBW. Bedside measurement of P_{plat} can be done by putting the patient in VCV, with either deep sedation or paralysis and performing an inspiratory hold **(Fig. 18.30)**.

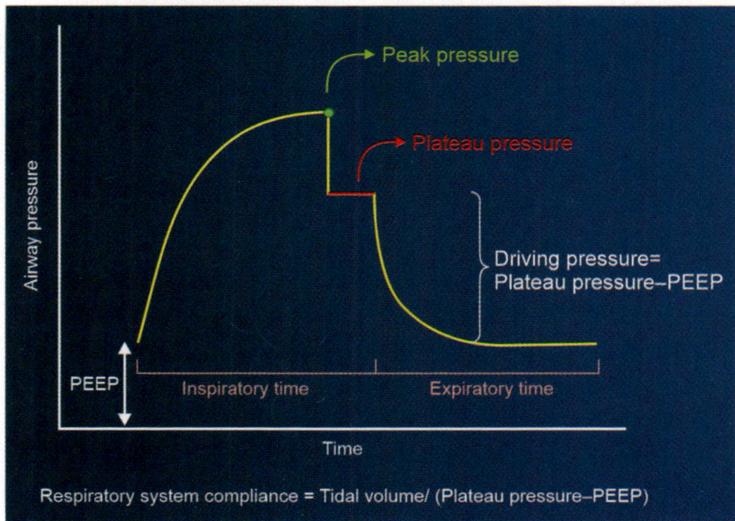

Fig. 18.30: The concept of driving pressure

The main aim of LPV is to protect the lungs; the low TV as per ARDS net does not take into account the concept of ventilating "baby lung "in ARDS. Normalizing the TV to compliance of the respiratory system that indicates the functional lung, may be a better predictor and this ratio VT/CRS, is called the DRIVING PRESSURE, which can be calculated as the difference of the PLAT and PEEP. In 2015, Amato *et al.* in his study demonstrated that by increasing the PEEP, if Pplat decreases or remains same, the driving pressure decreases and the mortality improves and vice versa. In a multi level mediation analysis in the LUNG SAFE study it has been shown that a driving pressure of < 14 cm H_2O was associated with a lower hospital mortality, making it a reasonable target of ventilation.

5. Neuromuscular Blockers

There are very few indications for the use of NMB agents in the ICU, ADRS being top on the list. In spite of using LPV, ARDS patients can hyper inflate due to spontaneous respiratory effort during CMV even when sedated leading to asynchrony. The ACURASYS trial was the first trial that evaluated the role of NMBs in ARDS patients. In this trial patients with moderate to severe ARDS as defined with a PF ratio <150 with a PEEP of > 5 cm H_2O during the first 2 days after the diagnosis of ARDS received cis atracurium or placebo for 48 hr. This study clearly showed mortality benefit with higher ventilator free days in the patients who were paralyzed. This benefit was mainly attributed to the elimination of asynchrony. After this paralysis in ARDS was widely used by many clinicians though the results of the trials were criticized. After nearly a decade another trial was published in 2019, ROSE PETAL trial, reevaluating the role of NMBs. The results of this study did not show significant 90 day mortality benefit in contrary to the ACURASYS, questioning the routine the recommendation for the use of NMBs in moderate to severe ARDS. But most of the clinicians do agree that the use of NMBs have a strong physiological basis and may be considered in management after ensuring adequate sedation.

6. Permissive Hypercapnia

Permissive hypercapnia is an accepted side effect of LPV, which was well tolerated by most of the patients without any significant side effects. The usual accepted range of $PACO_2$ is 65–85 mmHg with an acceptable PH of 7.2–7.25. There are no clinical trials so far that examined the effect of hypercapnic acidosis independent from other ventilator parameters. Data from experimental animal models suggest beneficial effects of hypercapnic acidosis. In these experimental models hypercapnic acidosis has shown to attenuate VILI, improve oxygenation, reduction in the level of inflammatory markers. Except in patients with co-existing neurological injury and pregnants hypercapnic acidosis need no particular attention.

7. Recruitment Maneuvers (RMs)

RMs are simple, dynamic process where in the atelectatic alveoli are opened by transiently intentional increase of transpulmonary pressure with the aim to improve EELV and there by oxygenation. By applying RMs a potentially aerated alveoli that requires high opening pressure than the tidal ventilation are opened, and the success of RMs depends on the magnitude of pressure rather than the duration of time frame during which the maneuver is performed. The benefit may be seen when applied early in the disease process rather than in late stages where application may result in more harm than benefit especially when the lung has undergone a fibrotic change. Based on the methods of intervention RMs are:

a. Pressure based
b. Position based
c. Based on mode of ventilation
d. Based on chest wall modification

Of the different techniques, airway pressure based recruitment maneuvers were most frequently used in clinical settings, followed by the current day prone ventilation. Several RCTs that have looked at RMs also used high PEEP as co-intervention in the management, making it difficult to evaluate the effect of RMs alone on the outcomes. To date, evidence is not strong enough to recommend the routine use of RMs as standard practice, and rather have to be applied on case-to-case basis in patients with severe ARDS as a life saving procedure keeping in view the potential side effects. It is important to emphasize on the fact that ARDS lung can easily be derecruited and interventions that cause derecruitment should be avoided.

8. Prone Ventilation

In patients with moderate to severe ARDS, prone ventilation has been used as a means of improving oxygenation since early 1970s. Prone positioning has multiple physiological effects that improve the oxygenation and decrease VILI. Being a relatively simple cost effective, easily applicable bedside technique with fewer side effects and proven beneficial effects, prone ventilation today is a part of the treatment algorithm followed in the moderate to severe ARDS patients. In cooperative patients with mild to moderate ARDS, awake prone position when applied early has shown to reduce the intubation rates. Prone ventilation has many physiological advantages.

It improves oxygenation by improving the respiratory mechanics, optimizes the VQ match, causes a more homogeneous distribution of transpulmonary and plateau pressure, increases the FRC, helps in better secretion clearance and off loads the weight of the heart from the lungs, all of them contributing to an improvement in oxygenation. Prone position can be practically applied in all patients exception being those with head injury and unstable spine, rest all being relative contraindications **(Table 18.16)**. The PROSEVA trial has shown that early and prolonged prone ventilation has reduced all cause mortality and improved survival compared to supine ventilation in patients with moderate to severe ARDS. This was the practice changing trial after which prone ventilation has been widely used in clinical practice with a very few maneuver related complications (**Fig. 18.31**).

Contraindications of prone ventilation:

Table 18.16: Contraindications for prone ventilation

Absolute contraindications	Relative contraindications
Spine instability	Pregnancy
Pelvic fractures	Facial trauma
Severe arrhythmias	BPF
Intracranial hypertension	Ophthalmic surgery
Recent cardiac surgery	Mild hemodynamic instability

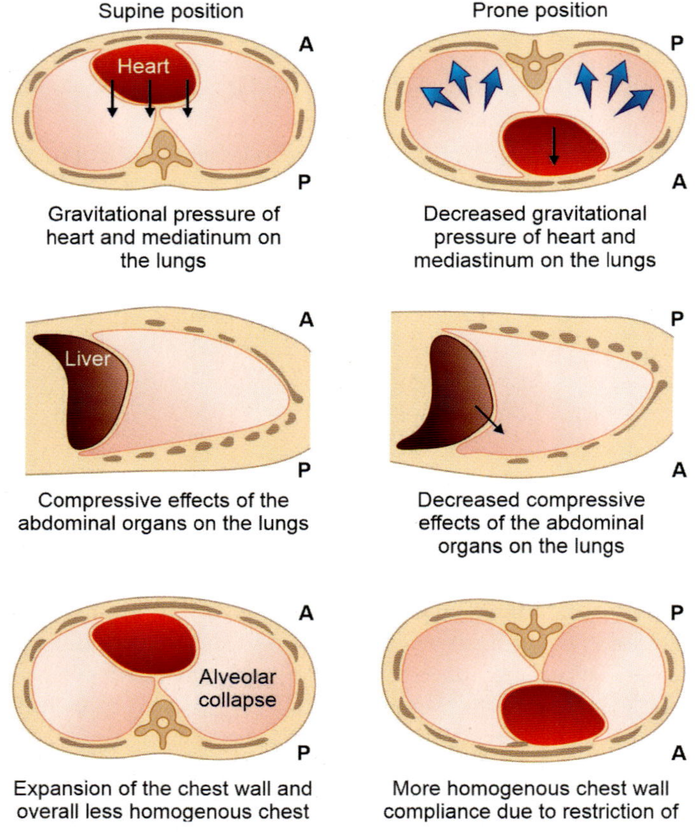

Fig. 18.31: Physiological impact of prone ventilation

9. Fluids in ARDS

Fluids should be used judiciously in ARDS patients. The alveolar edema of ARDS can be worsened by injudicious use of IV fluids. Choosing the optimal fluid strategy is one of the greatest challenges. The functional barrier, the glycocalyx can be damaged by several factors such as hypervolemia, rapid crystalloid administration, etc. When compared to liberal fluid strategies, conservative fluid replacement strategies have shown to prevent lung edema, and there by associated with less invasive mechanical ventilation, less organ dysfunction and a trend towards less renal replacement. There is also enough evidence in favor of deresuscitation compared to liberal fluid strategy. But to date, there is no ideal method for monitoring the response to fluid replacement in ARDS.

10. Steroids

Steroids have been one of the adjuvant drugs used widely in ARDS patients.

There is no clear-cut benefit with corticosteroids in mild ARDS management. In moderate to severe ARDS (PF ratio <200) steroid accelerates weaning, reduces ICU length of stay. This benefit is seen if following conditions are met

PF ratio < 200 despite optimization of ventilation strategies for 24 hr

Started early in course of illness, <14 days

Etiology of ARDS—pneumonia or sepsis

In other ARDS patients (trauma, pancreatitis, etc.), late ARDS, >14 days the role of steroids is doubtful. Recommended dose is dexamethasone 20 mg IV or equivalent for 5 days and tapered.

11. ECMO in ARDS

ECMO is a prolong cardiopulmonary support. Between 2 types of ECMO, VV ECMO is offered in acute respiratory failure. The indications for ECMO in ARDS include-Hypoxemic respiratory failure with PF ratio <100 despite optimization of ventilator settings, peep, I: E ratio. In severe ARDS patient should be transferred early to ECMO center. The benefit with ECMO is more if started early in course of illness (<7 days) when conventional strategies fail. The survival rates in patients who require ECMO are in range of 60–70%. The CESAR trial in 2009 showed improved survival with ECMO in patients with Murray lung injury score >3. But the ventilation strategies in control group were not uniform. Another trial EOLIA in 2018 also showed that survival is higher in those who received early. The complications seen in VV ECMO include bleeding manifestations, thrombocytopenia, thrombotic events, and neurological injury.

TO SUMMARIZE

ARDS a potentially fatal condition, and one of the commonest form of acute severe hypoxic respiratory failure has been a challenge to the clinicians despite considerable advances in our knowledge about the pathophysiology, diagnosis, ventilatory management, supportive care. In spite of research of more than 50 years there still seems to be lacuna in our understanding and management of severe ARDS resulting in significant mortality and morbidity. Probably the current emerging therapies focusing on modulating the immune response, vascular endothelial barrier, may enhance ARDS resolution and improve long term survival.

CHAPTER 19

Patient–Ventilator Asynchrony

❒ Hillary Vaughan ❒ Dharani Narendra ❒ Kalpalatha K Guntupalli

INTRODUCTION

Mechanical ventilation is a crucial component of caring for the critically ill patient with respiratory failure. The goal of mechanical ventilation is to support the patient by unloading respiratory muscles, matching metabolic demands, and enhancing patient comfort during acute respiratory failure. Patient–ventilator interaction involves a harmonious balance between the patient's demand and the level of support delivered by the ventilator. An interactive breaths can be described as assisted (patient-triggered and time- or volume-cycled breaths) or supported (patient-triggered and flow-cycled breaths). Assisted or supported ventilator breaths interact with patient efforts during all three breath phases: Trigger (initiation of breath), target (gas delivery), and cycling (termination of breath). The patient–ventilator interaction during all three phases of breath delivery supports respiratory requirements while protecting the lungs and muscles of respiration from potential ventilator-induced lung injury. The scalars commonly reviewed are the pressure-, flow- and volume-time. Others include the flow- volume loop, volume-pressure loop. Ventilator waveforms provide a wealth of insight into the physiology of the respiratory system.

DEFINITIONS

Patient–ventilator asynchrony (PVA) occurs when there is an absence of patient effort or absence of ventilator response during the breath initiation phase (trigger). Patient ventilator dyssynchrony (PVD) results from a mismatch between patient's demand and the amount of ventilator response delivered.[3] However, PVA and PVD are used interchangeably, for the purpose of this chapter, we will use the term PVA for both. PVA is often under-recognized despite affecting one third of patients on mechanical ventilation.[1] PVA events can be classified according to which phase the PVA event is occurring, with target dyssynchrony occurring during the gas delivery phase, and cycling dyssynchrony occurring during the termination phase (**Fig. 19.1**). Identifying the phase in which these events occur may help clinicians to recognize contributing factors and intervene appropriately.

Deleterious Effects of PVA

Recognizing patient–ventilator mismatch is important as PVA events impart significant mechanical and biochemical stress resulting in increased work of breathing,

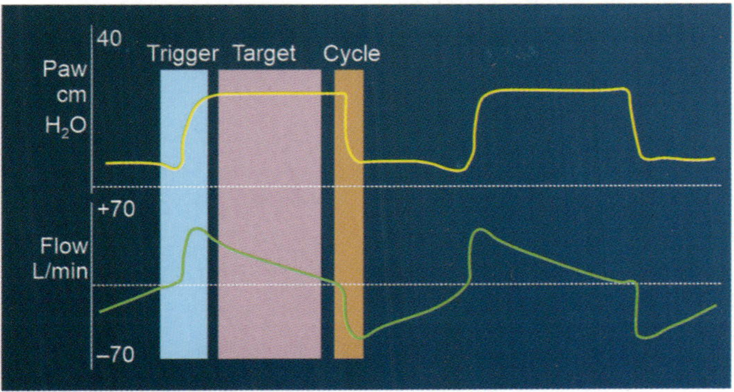

Fig. 19.1: Identifying PVA events by phase

diaphragmatic injury, and over-distention of the alveoli **(Table 19.1)**.[4] They have been associated with excessive tidal volumes up to 15 ml/kg increasing the risk of ventilator-induced lung injury and diaphragmatic dysfunction.[1] PVA events contribute to patient discomfort, anxiety, and dyspnea.[4] In addition to direct injury, adverse effects include over-sedation, increased ventilator days, and prolonged intensive care unit (ICU) stay.[1] The quantification of PVA events is best expressed as a percentage and is termed the asynchrony index (ASI). The asynchrony index equals the number of PVA events divided by the total respiratory rate (number of ventilator cycles + ineffective efforts) multiplied by 100.[11] Data suggests that an asynchrony Index more than 10% is associated with increased ventilator days, increased need for tracheostomy, and increased mortality.[1] Notably, common conditions in the ICU such as acute respiratory distress syndrome (ARDS), Chronic obstructive pulmonary disease (COPD), and asthma predispose patients to experiencing PVA during mechanical ventilation **(Fig. 19.2)**.[4]

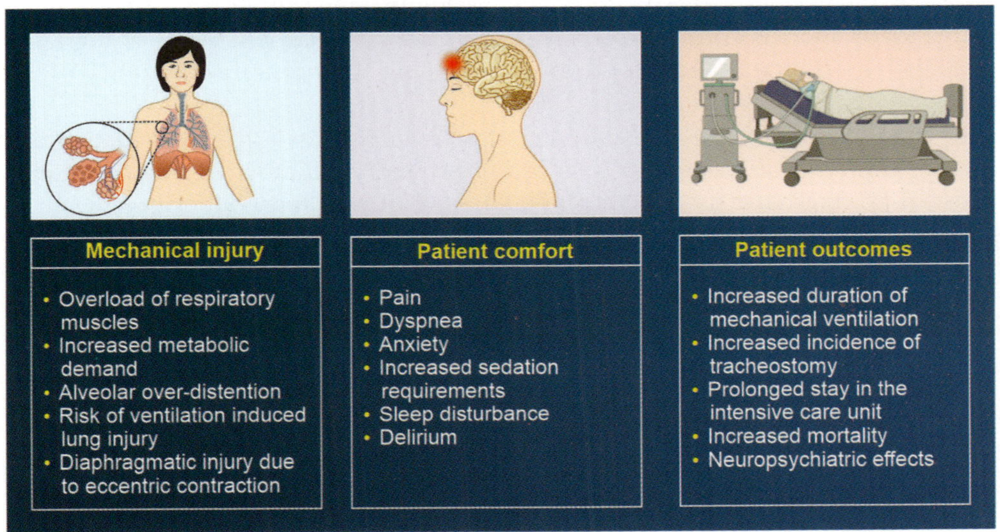

Fig. 19.2: Deleterious effects of patient–ventilator dyssynchrony

Respiratory Physiology

The initiation of spontaneous breath results from the neuroventilatory coupling of the ventilatory control center with the muscles of respiration, resulting in the generation of a respiratory rhythm and tidal volume optimized to facilitate efficient gas exchange while minimizing the load on respiratory muscles.[4] Chemoreceptors in the brainstem detect local changes in pH, PO_2, and PCO_2, influencing the timing and intensity of phrenic nerve signaling upon mechanoreceptors in the musculature in order to coordinate optimized minute ventilation. In the critically ill patient, the ventilatory control center must respond to increased metabolic demands in the setting of acidosis, hypoxemia, discomfort, anxiety, and stress. Conversely, certain conditions such as sedation, central nervous system injury, and sleep result in depressed ventilatory drive. Mechanical ventilatory support must be ideally programmed to support the ventilatory requirements of the patient.

In a spontaneously breathing patient, contraction of the respiratory muscles provides force sufficient to overcome intrinsic PEEP and generate flow against the resistive and elastic recoil properties of the respiratory system. The efficiency of the spontaneous ventilatory system to generate flow and volume is therefore dependent upon the contractile properties of the respiratory muscles and the impedance of the respiratory system.[4] Respiratory failure occurs when inspiratory efforts fail to generate volume and flow sufficient to meet ventilatory requirements.

A variety of factors contribute to respiratory muscle failure during critical illness. Though the diaphragm is primarily responsible for generating contractile force and initiating inspiration, physiologic stress during critical illness causes recruitment of external intercostal and accessory muscles to assist in maintaining minute ventilation. Increased ventilatory demands and supine positioning increase the load on the respiratory muscles, while systemic inflammation and high metabolic states (such as sepsis) increase oxygen requirements and decrease oxygen delivery, further weakening the respiratory muscles.[8] Airway impedance is compromised in disease states with high resistive loads such as chronic obstructive pulmonary disease (COPD) or high elastic loads such as pulmonary edema, further increasing the pressure required to initiate spontaneous breath.

Respiratory muscle failure may also manifest as an inability to wean patients from the ventilator despite resolution of illness and improved ventilatory demand. Ventilator-induced diaphragmatic dysfunction (VIDD) is a known consequence of mechanical ventilation and describes the phenomenon of diaphragmatic atrophy and muscle fiber injury that develops within hours of initiating mechanical ventilation and results in decreased diaphragmatic contractility.[7] Supine positioning, dyssynchronous breath delivery, and oxidative stress are all associated with VIDD and prolonged mechanical ventilation.[4]

Patient–Ventilator Interactions

In positive pressure ventilation, extrinsic pressure is supplied from the mechanical ventilator to assist in meeting patient demands. This extrinsic pressure is added to the intrinsic pressure generated by spontaneously contracting respiratory muscles in order to overcome resistive forces of the airways. The introduction of extrinsic pressure has the potential to uncouple the relationship between ventilatory effort and output, decreasing the efficiency of the system and increasing the risk of mechanical injury.[4] The delivery of dyssynchronous positive pressure breaths imparts stressful loads onto respiratory muscles and alveoli resulting in over distention, which the patient experiences as dyspnea and discomfort. The intrinsic ventilatory control center may respond to this stress by increasing the respiratory rate, decreasing the tidal volume, shortening the neural inspiratory time, or may ultimately suppress spontaneous ventilatory effort.[4] An optimized Patient–ventilator interaction facilitates minute ventilatory requirements and unloading of respiratory muscles while imposing the least amount of extrinsic stress to the system. The chosen ventilator mode determines the level of pressure support introduced to the Patient–ventilator system.

During controlled ventilation, the total pressure required to overcome the resistive and elastic forces of the respiratory system is provided by the mechanical ventilator, resulting in constant flow and pressure delivery to the patient independent of muscle activity or respiratory drive, and effectively uncoupling the intrinsic neuroventilatory system.[4] Except in cases of neuromuscular disease, sedation is often required to reduce patient–ventilator dyssynchrony.

Detecting Patient–Ventilator Asynchrony

Detecting PVA at the bedside is possible by interpreting ventilator waveforms without the need of invasive methods such as esophageal pressures or measuring the electrical activity of the diaphragm.[11] PVA events are classified according to the phase of breath cycle affected (**Fig. 19.1**). Some PVA are more frequently associated with either insufficient or excessive ventilatory support compared to patient demand due to patient-related factors as seen in **Fig. 19.3**.[2] Patient–ventilator mismatch may occur because of patient-related factors, ventilator-related factors (**Table 19.1**), or a combination of both. Interventions are aimed at minimizing the mismatch between ventilatory demand and support delivered improve Patient–ventilator interaction and comfort.[9] These measures could be as simple as adjusting ventilator settings, changing mode of ventilator or managing sedation and paralytics.

Table 19.1: Ventilator-related factors contributing to Patient–ventilator mismatch
1. Trigger sensitivity (flow/pressure) ✦ Trigger sensitivity too low → Auto-triggering ✦ Trigger sensitivity too high → Ineffective trigger
2. System leak or water in the tubing → Auto-triggering, ineffective triggering, doulbe triggering Ventilator misinterprets change in pressure or flow and provides a breath unrelated to patient effort
3. Insufficient Flow → Flow Starvation Gas delivery fails to meet patient demand
4. Ventilator inspiratory time: ***Machine Ti > Neural Ti → Delayed Cycling*** Mechanical breath delivery persists after inspiratory effort is complete. ***Neural Ti > Machine Ti → Premature cycling*** Patient inspiratory effort continues during mechanical exhalation

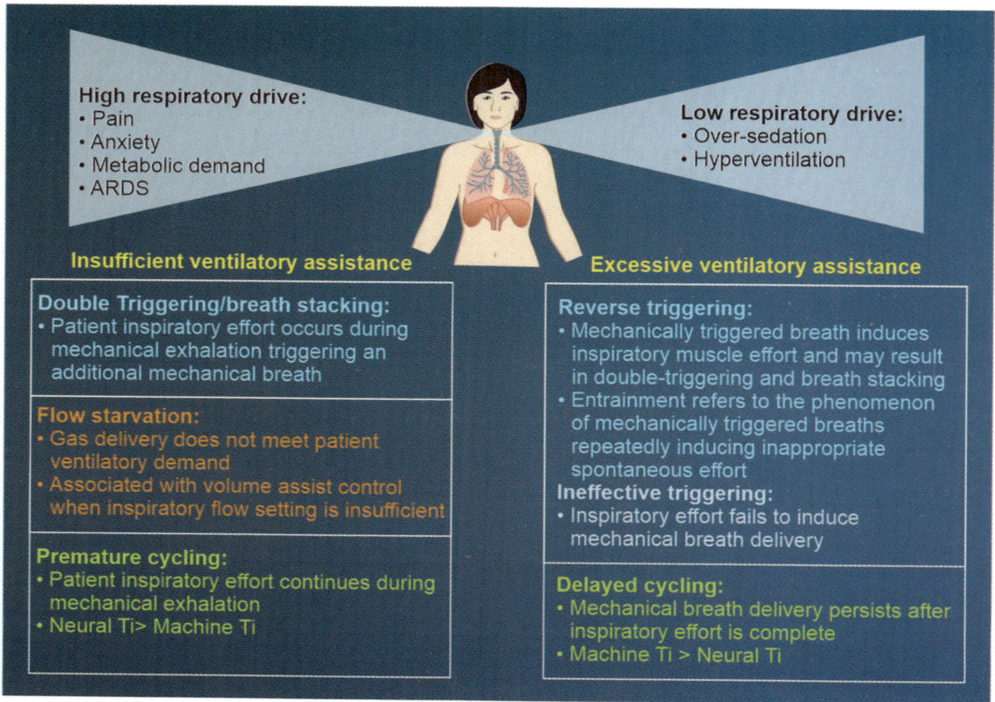

Fig. 19.3: Patient-related factors contributing to patient–ventilator mismatch

A. Trigger Asynchrony

Occurs during trigger or breath initiation phase of the ventilatory cycle **(Fig. 19.7)**. These are the most common form of PVA.

Ineffective Triggering or Missed Triggering

Ineffective triggering manifests as an inspiratory effort that is not followed by a mechanical breath **(Fig. 19.4)**.[10] Ineffective efforts may be due to incorrectly programmed trigger sensitivity or malfunctioning sensitivity on the ventilator. Patients with low respiratory drive in conditions such as deep sedation, central nervous system disease, weak inspiratory muscles (critically ill and myasthenia gravis) have poor respiratory effect leading to ineffective trigger.

Ineffective triggering may also be seen when auto-PEEP resulting from dynamic hyperinflation (DHI) in obstructive airway diseases, as these patient have to overcome the auto-PEEP and the applied PEEP to initiate a breath.[9] Ineffective efforts are sometimes associated with excessive ventilation, particularly in patients with high tidal volumes, alkalemia, and COPD in which excessive ventilation decreases the respiratory drive resulting in ineffective inspiratory efforts.[11] The ventilator waveform will show an abrupt drop in airway pressure (≥0.5 cmH_2O) associated with a decrease in flow, not followed by an assisted breath as shown in **Fig. 19.4**. Interventions are aimed at optimizing trigger sensitivity or addressing patient-related factors such as decreasing sedation or neuromuscular blockers. In DHI, bronchodilators remain mainstay therapy,

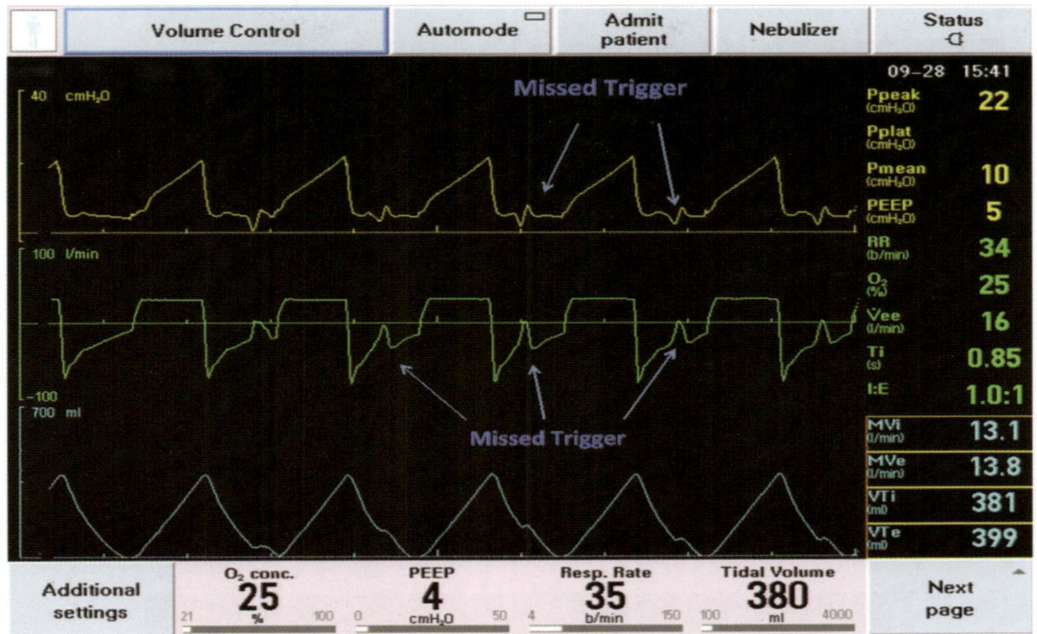

Fig. 19.4: Missed or ineffective trigger; patient inspiratory effort is not sufficient to trigger a mechanical breath, shown by blue arrows in pressure-, flow-time scalar. (*Courtesy:* Felix Khusid, RRT, New York-Presbyterian Brooklyn Methodist Hospital)

as they take time, minimize hyperinflation by reducing minute ventilation and or increase extrinsic PEEP slightly lower to the intrinsic PEEP to facilitate the initiation of breath.

Double Triggering

Double triggering occurs when the patient initiates inspiration while the ventilator is still in mechanical expiration and this inspiratory trigger results in a second mechanically delivered breath before exhalation is complete **(Fig. 19.5A and B)**. The consequence of this extra "stacked" breath is delivery of double the set tidal volume, increased load on respiratory muscles, diaphragmatic dysfunction, and decreased venous return to the heart.[1] Breath stacking is particularly deleterious in patients with ARDS, as the additional tidal volume hyperinflates the compliant (baby) lung via the pendelluft effect thus increasing the risk of ventilator-associated lung injury.[13]

Factors associated with double triggering include use of volume control ventilation (VCV) mode with low tidal volumes, and short inspiratory time in all modes.[11] Management of double triggering dyssynchrony should address ventilator settings to better match patient respiratory drive by increasing machine inspiratory time to match neural inspiratory time in VCV or PCV mode, increase tidal volume in VCV mode and consideration of pressure-targeted rather than volume-controlled ventilation. Decrease cycling threshold percentage of peak flow in pressure support mode. Additionally, the clinician should address reversible factors of increased respiratory drive such as pain, anxiety, acidosis, and high metabolic states.[8]

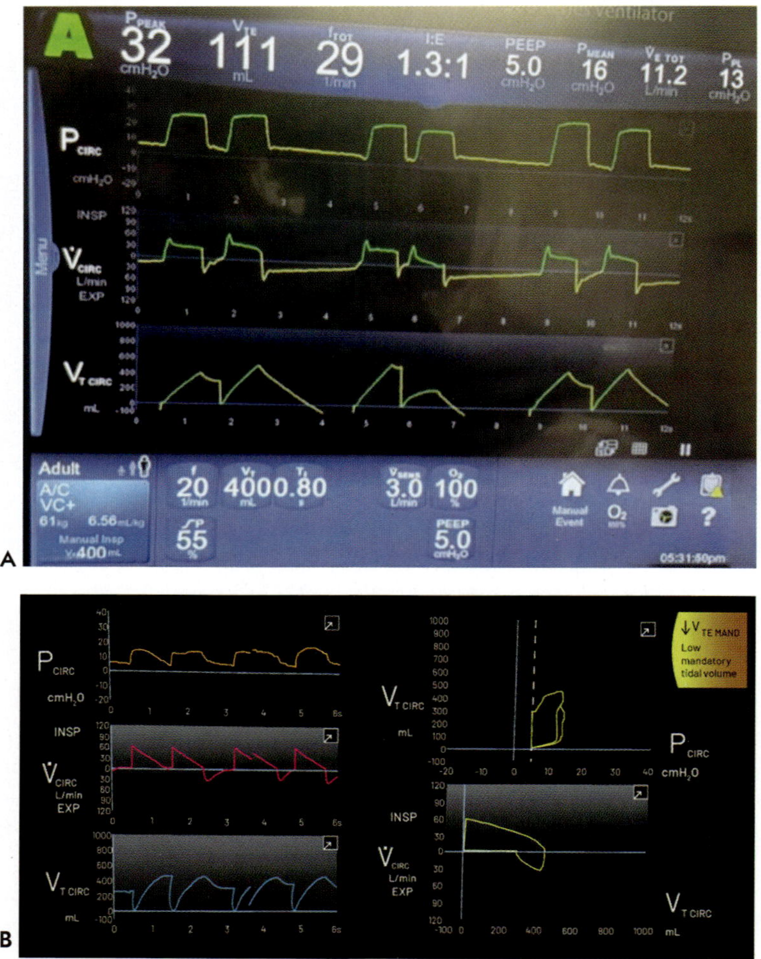

Fig. 19.5A and B: Double trigger due to air leak in VC mode and decreased inspiratory time

Reverse Triggering

Reverse triggering occurs when a mechanically delivered breath induces a reflex inspiratory muscle effort. If the inspiratory muscle effort is sufficient, a second breath will be delivered by the ventilator leading to a double triggering (**Fig. 19.6**) resulting in excessive tidal volumes and breath stacking. If the inspiratory muscle effort is not sufficient to trigger a second full breath (**Fig. 19.7**). In reverse triggering, the first breath is always machine triggered whereas in double triggering the first breath is patient triggered. Reverse triggering is typically seen in low respiratory drive states such as deep sedation or those on neuromuscular blocking agents.[9] Persistent episodes of reverse triggering in which each mechanically delivered breath prompts an inspiratory muscle effort is known as entrainment and is attributed to a reflexive muscular response to repetitive lung distention mediated by mechanoreceptors in the inspiratory muscles and chest wall, rather than vagal stimuli.[9] The management involves decreasing sedation and neuromuscular blockade.

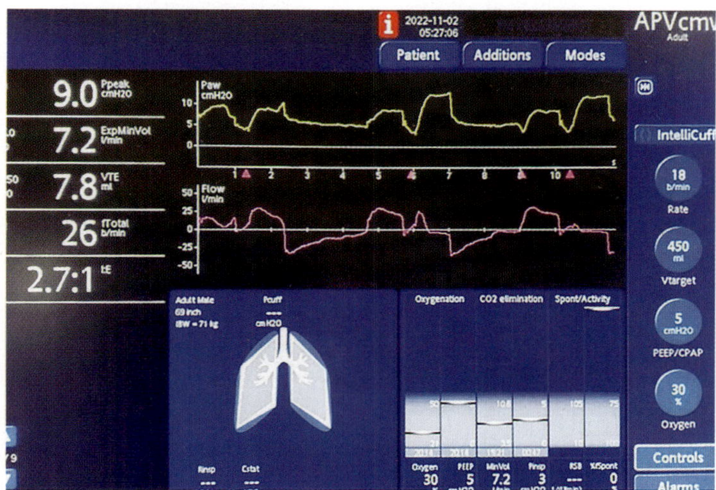

Fig. 19.6: Reverse Triggering. A mechanical breath is delivered first and causes a reflexive inspiratory effort (pink arrows) resulting in elevated airway pressures. The reflexive inspiratory effort occurs after the mechanical breath triggering a second breath

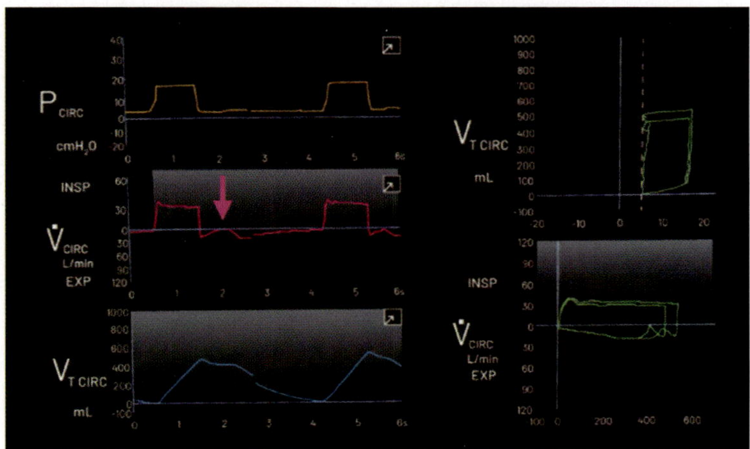

Fig. 19.7: Incomplete reverse triggering in a deeply sedated patient. Mechanical breath causes a reflexive inspiratory effort (Pink arrow: positive deflection in flow wave after breath is delivered) that is not sufficient to trigger a second full breath

Auto-triggering

Auto-triggering occurs when the ventilator delivers a breath that is unrelated to patient inspiratory effort. Air leaks, cardiac oscillations, condensation in the ventilator tubing, or vibrations from equipment such as renal replacement therapy may inappropriately trigger the ventilator and result in hyperventilation.[3] Auto-triggering due to air leak is shown in **Fig. 19.8**. Managing auto-triggering involves addressing the underlying cause (fix air leaks, remove condensation in the tubing) and increasing the trigger sensitivity threshold.

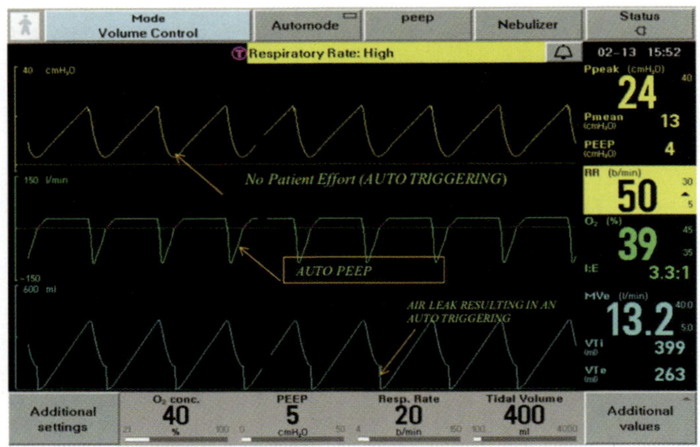

Fig. 19.8: Auto-triggering (*Courtesy:* Felix Khusid, RRT New York-Presbyterian Brooklyn Methodist Hospital)

B. Target Dyssynchrony: Flow dyssynchrony is the only type of target dyssynchrony

Flow Starvation

Flow starvation occurs when a preset fixed flow during volume control ventilation is insufficient to meet patient ventilatory demands. Flow starvation prompts the patient to generate an inspiratory effort during mid-flow which is visualized on the pressure waveform as a negative deflection or "suck down" during mid inspiratory flow corresponding to the additional effort as shown in **Fig. 19.9A.**[4] The inspiratory effort during mechanical insufflation is in addition to patient effort during triggering resulting in increased load on respiratory muscles and excess energy expenditure.[9] Recognition of flow starvation should prompt the clinician to adjust ventilator settings to meet ventilatory demands, increase patient comfort, and decrease excessive load on muscles of respiration. Proposed interventions include increasing flow rates on volume controlled mode **(Fig. 19.9B)** or utilizing pressure-controlled, or pressure supported modes of ventilation in which the flow varies to meet patient demand.[8]

C. Cycling Dyssynchrony: Occurs during the Cycling Phase (Exhalation) of the Breath

Premature Cycling

Premature or short cycling is another example of PVA associated with insufficient ventilatory support seen in patients with high respiratory drive. Premature cycling refers to continued inspiratory effort by the patient during mechanical exhalation where neural time is more than machine time indicating the preset cycle time in volume-controlled ventilation is too short to meet patient demand as shown in **Fig. 19.10.**[4] If the inspiratory effort is sufficiently vigorous, double triggering may occur resulting in excessive tidal volumes.[9] In patients with ARDS or other high respiratory drive states, the mismatch between neural Ti and machine Ti may be primarily contributed to patient discomfort.[4] Premature cycling can also manifest in patients with normal inspiratory time if fixed cycle time set by the clinician is inappropriately low resulting in hypoventilation.[4] Premature cycling is also seen in pressure support ventilation in which cycle time is determined by decelerating inspiratory flow. Attempting to address

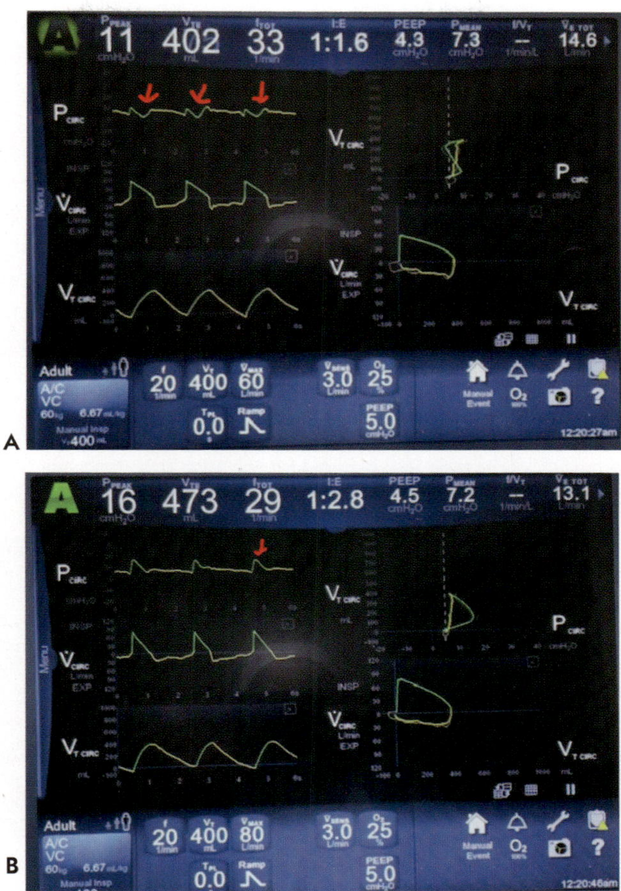

Fig. 19.9: (A) Flow dyssynchrony: Insufficient flow causing negative deflection in pressure-time scalar; (B) Increasing flow rates from 60 L/min to 80 L/min in VCV mode, flow starvation resolved

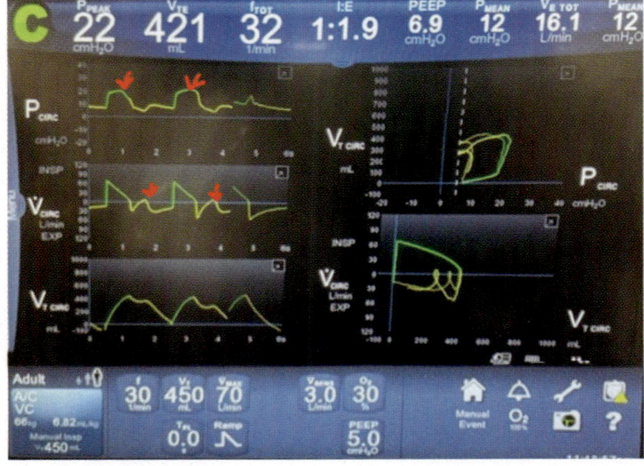

Fig. 19.10: Premature cycling with neural Ti > Ventilator Ti. Note the upward notch on the pressure wave at the termination of the cycle signaling persistent patient inspiratory effort. The expiratory flow is decreased (upward deflection) as patient continues to exert inspiratory effort

this PVA is by increasing inspiratory time in VCV or PCV mode, increase tidal volume in VCV or decrease inspiratory flow.

Delayed Cycling

Delayed cycling occurs when the ventilator inspiratory time exceeds the neural inspiratory time and causes the patient to exert effort in attempt to exhale as shown in **Fig. 19.11**. This causes an abrupt increase in airway pressure late in the breath cycle, increasing the risk of barotrauma.[3] Delayed cycling may be the result of inappropriately long machine Ti or pathological respiratory mechanics in the patient. For example, in patients with obstructive airway diseases, the prolonged inspiratory time with short expiratory time may contribute to dynamic hyperinflation.[6] This is addressed by decreasing machine time by increase inspiratory flow or decrease tidal volume.

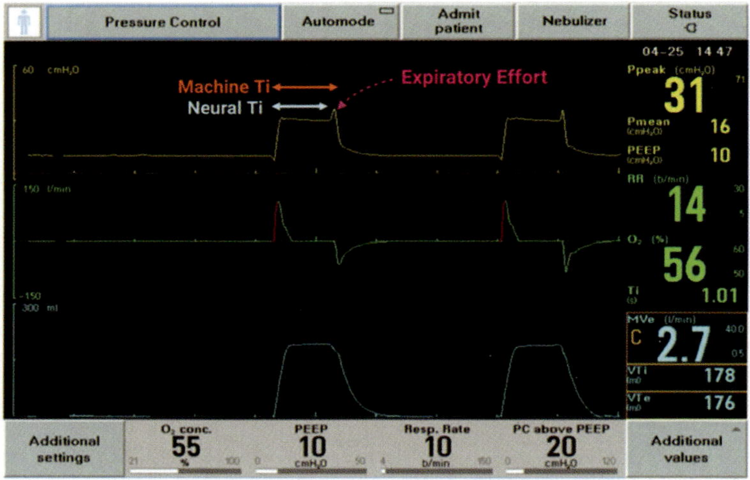

Fig. 19.11: Delayed Cycling in which machine Ti > neural Ti. Note the upward deflection at the end of the pressure tracing which indicates patient effort to exhale despite mechanical inflation. (*Courtesy:* RRT New York-Presbyterian Brooklyn Methodist Hospital)

Conclusion

PVA events are common but often go undiagnosed until a patient is in respiratory distress. Missed triggers and other seemingly harmless PVA events go entirely unnoticed. However, the data shows that the frequency of the events during mechanical ventilation, calculated as the asynchrony index, have a direct impact on ICU length of stay, ventilator days, and mortality.[9] New ventilator technologies such as neurally adjusted ventilatory assist have emerged that aim to decrease Patient–ventilator mismatch, but they are not yet widely adopted.[12] Close evaluation of scalars and loops at the bedside will aid the trained clinicians in detecting and evaluating PVA events without the need for invasive monitoring or advanced equipment. **Tables 19.2 and 19.3** summarize the asynchrony type, causes, waveform and strategies to correct the patient ventilator asynchrony. It is imperative for intensivist to adopt a systematic approach in evaluating ventilator waveforms and determine whether a dyssynchrony is occurring in trigger, target or cycling to initiate appropriate interventions.

Table 19.2: Waveform: (A) Ineffective Triggering; note missed triggers illustrated by diaphragmatic contractions (yellow) that fail to trigger a mechanical breath; (B) Patient inspiratory effort during mechanical exhalation triggers an additional breath, results in elevated airway pressures;

Troubleshooting patient-ventilator mismatch			
Type	**Cause**	**Waveform**	**Intervention**
✦ **Ineffective triggering** Inspiratory effort fails to trigger breath delivery	✦ Incorrectly programmed trigger senseitivy ✦ Low respiratory drive (sedation, CNS disease) ✦ Weak inspiratory muscles (critical illness myopathy, myasthenia) ✦ Dynamic hyperinflation in obstructive airway disease; patient cannot overcome auto-PEEP	**(A)** Paw cm H_2O 20 10 0 −10 −20; Pmus Flow L/min 100 0	✦ Decrease trigger threshold (flow trigger is more sensitive than pressure trigger) ✦ Decrease sedation ✦ Discontinue neuromuscular blockers ✦ DHI: Minimize hyperinflation via bronchodilators, add extrinsic PEEP to a value 80% of auto-PEEP ✦ Decrease pressure support in PSV mode
✦ **Double triggering:** Patient inspiratory effort occurs during mechanical exhalation, triggering an additional breath	Machine inspiratory time is too short compared to neural Ti Tidal volume set too low in VCV	**(B)** Paw 20 10 0 −10 −20 Flow L/min 100 50 0 −50 −100	✦ VCV of PCV mode: Increase Machine Ti ✦ PSV mode: Decrease cycling threshold percentage of peak flow. ✦ VCV: Increase tidal volume ✦ Switch to PCV for variable tidal volume mode ✦ Increase sedation +/– neuromuscular blockade

Contd.

Table 19.2: Waveform: (C) Mechanical breath is delivere first and causes a feflexive inspiratory effort (negative inflection on green esophageal pressure waveform); (D) Auto-triggering due to air leak in volume-controlled (VC) ventilation mode (Contd.)

Troubleshooting patient-ventilator mismatch			
Type	**Cause**	**Waveform**	**Intervention**
✦ **Reverse triggering:** Mechanically triggered breath induces inspiratory muscle effort	✦ Reflexive inspiratory effort caused by machine-triggered breath in deeply sedated and/or paralyzed patients	**(C)**	✦ Reduce sedation ✦ Reduce neuromuscular blockade
✦ **Auto-triggering:** Ventilator provides a breath in response to a stimulus unrelated to patient effort	✦ Triggering threshold set too low ✦ Air leak ✦ Cardiac oscillations, condensation in ventilator tubing ✦ External vibrations (Renal replacement therapy, chest tube, gastric tube)	**(D)**	✦ Increase trigger theshold to account for external vibrations ✦ Fix air leaks ✦ Remove condensation

Abbreviations: P musc: Diaphragmatic muscle pressure, PEEP (Positive end expiratory pressure), VCV: Volume controlled ventilation, PCV: Pressure controlled ventilation, PSV: Pressure support ventilation

Table 19.3: PVD types by waveform: (A) Flow starvation is a target dyssynchrony: Flow does not meet patient demand; patient inspiratory effort results in "sucked down" appearance of pressure waveform in VC mode; (B) Premature cycling in VC and pressure controlled (PC) modes. Neural Ti is greater than machine Ti; persistent inspiratory effort triggers a second breath (C) Delayed cycling; Mechanical inhalation persists in opposition to patient expiratory effort. Machine Ti is greater than neural Ti

Troubleshooting patient-ventilator misamatch			
Type	**Cause**	**Waveform**	**Intervention**
✦ **Target/Flow dyssynchrony: flow** insufficient to meet patient demand	✦ Fixed flow in VCV is insufficient to meet patient demand	(A) Paw 20 10 0 −10 −20; Flow L/min 100 50 0 −50 −100; Vol mL 1000 500 0	✦ Increase flow in VCV mode ✦ Change to PCV or PSV modes where flow is variable
✦ **Premature cycling**: Neural Ti > Machine Ti	✦ Machine Ti in VCV or PCV is too short and insufficient	(B) cm H_2O 10; Volume control; Pressure-Time; Pressure contract; Ventilator Ti; 0; L/min 70; Flow-Time; Neural Ti; 0; −70; 1.0; Volume-Time; 0	✦ VCV or PCV: Increase machine Ti ✦ VCV: Increase tidal volume or decrease flow
✦ **Delayed cycling:** Machine Ti > Neural Ti	✦ Machine Ti is too long and provides excessive support ✦ Obstructive respiratory mechanics (COPD)	C cm H_2O 10; Pressure-Time; 0; 6; L/min 70; Flow-Time; 0; 6; −70; 1.0; Volume-Time; 0; 6	✦ VCV or PCV: Decrease machine Ti ✦ VCV: Decrease tidal volume or Increase flow

References

1. De Haro, C, *et al.* (2019). "Patient–ventilator asynchronies during mechanical ventilation: current knowledge and research priorities." Intensive Care Med Exp 7(Suppl 1): 43.
2. De Oliveira, B, *et al.* Patient–ventilator Dyssynchrony in Critically Ill Patients. J Clin Med, 2021. 10(19).
3. Flynn, BC, *et al.* Stepwise Ventilator Waveform Assessment to Diagnose Pulmonary Pathophysiology. Anesthesiology, 2022. 137(1): p. 85–92.
4. Gilstrap, D. and N. MacIntyre (2013). "Patient–ventilator interactions. Implications for clinical management." Am J Respir Crit Care Med 188(9): 1058–68.
5. Hess, D. R. (2005). "Ventilator waveforms and the physiology of pressure support ventilation." Respir Care 50(2): 166-186; discussion 183–166.
6. Holanda, MA, *et al.* Patient–ventilator asynchrony. J Bras Pneumol, 2018. 44(4): p. 321–33.
7. Jaber, S, *et al.* Rapidly progressive diaphragmatic weakness and injury during mechanical ventilation in humans. Am J Respir Crit Care Med, 2011. 183(3): p. 364–71.
8. MacIntyre, N. (2021). "Managing Patient–ventilator Dyssynchrony." Crit Care Med 49(12): 2149–51.
9. Pham, T, *et al.* (2018). "Asynchrony Consequences and Management." Crit Care Clin 34(3): 325–341.
10. Sottile, PD, *et al.* Ventilator dyssynchrony-Detection, pathophysiology, and clinical relevance: A Narrative review. Ann Thorac Med, 2020. 15(4): p. 190–98.
11. Thille, AW, *et al.* (2006). "Patient–ventilator asynchrony during assisted mechanical ventilation." Intensive Care Med 32(10): 1515–22.
12. Unroe, M and N MacIntyre. Evolving approaches to assessing and monitoring Patient–ventilator interactions. Curr Opin Crit Care, 2010. 16(3): p. 261–8.
13. Yoshida, T, *et al.* (2018). "Understanding spontaneous vs. ventilator breaths: impact and monitoring." Intensive Care Med 44(12): 2235–38.

CHAPTER 20

Fluid and Electrolytes

❐ Srinivas Samavedam

Fluid management in ventilated patients is an important aspect of critical care. There are studies showing adverse outcome with positive fluid balance in ventilated patients. And patients who are hypovolemic will not tolerate positive pressure ventilation. Hence maintaining appropriate fluid balance according to clinical situation plays an important role in management of critically ill patients. This chapter will deal with fluid management followed by electrolyte disturbances and their management.

PHYSIOLOGY

Body fluids in human body include blood, lymph, saliva, mucous secretions, milk, csf, pleural fluid, synovial fluid, etc. These fluids are mainly composed of water with some contribution from electrolytes, proteins (albumin, globulins, coagulation factors, hormones) and metabolites (urea, glucose, etc.). In a healthy adult male total body water equals 60% of body weight, of which 65% is intracellular, 35% extracellular. This extracellular fluid can be further compartmentalized into interstitial (75%) and plasma volume (25%) (**Fig. 20.1** and **Table 20.1**).

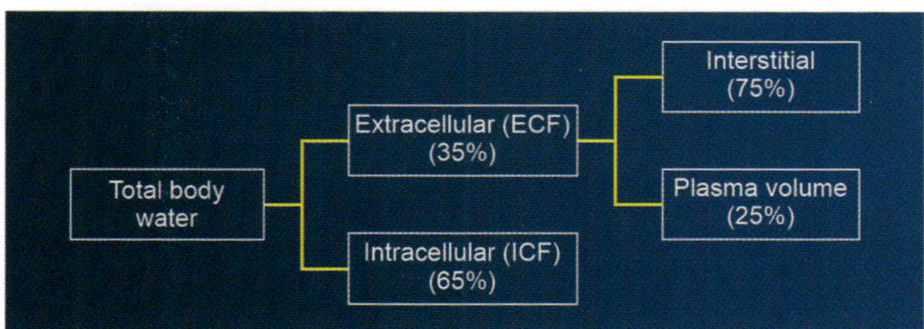

Fig. 20.1

Table 20.1: Body fluid composition percentage

Adult male	60% of body weight
Adult female	50%
Elderly male/female	50%
Child	65%
Infant	70%

Example: In a 70 kg healthy adult male total body water equals to 42 L of which 27 L is intracellular and 15 L is extracellular (11 L is interstitial fluid, 4 L is plasma volume).

Factors Controlling Distribution of Total Body Water

Several factors control the distribution of fluid between compartments which is tightly regulated.

1. Serum osmolarity—in order to maintain steady state, the body fluids will redistribute itself from low osmolarity to high osmolarity. This causes fluid to move between intracellular and extracellular compartments. And high osmolarity triggers ADH secretion
2. Starling forces–distribution of water within ECF (between interstitial and intravascular space) is determined by starling forces which include capillary hydrostatic and oncotic pressure, interstitial space hydrostatic and oncotic pressure (**Fig. 20.2**).

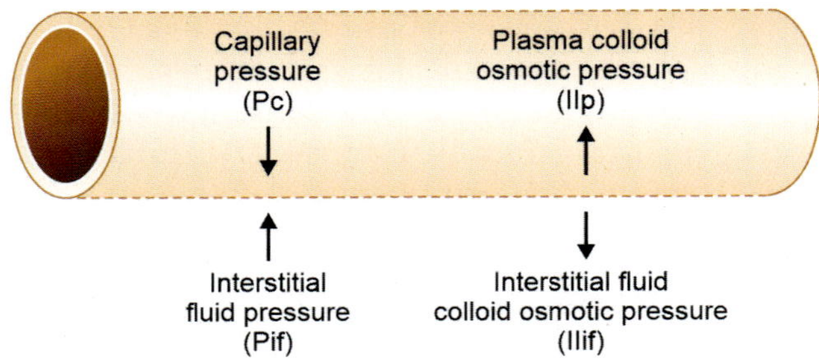

Fig. 20.2

Starling forces determine the movement of fluid across vessels. At arteriolar end fluid moves out of vessel due to high hydrostatic pressure and at venule end there is reabsorption of fluid. Any fluid accumulated in interstitium is removed by lymphatics. The alveolar tight epithelial junctions prevents movement of fluid. So any inciting event causing rise in hydrostatic pressure or increase in capillary permeability will lead to alveolar or interstitial edema in lungs.

In lungs where gas exchange is already compromised due to ARDS, pulmonary edema can further worsen it. The fluid therapy is one of the intervention in ARDS management.

Assessment of Fluid Requirement in ARDS Patients

Fluid management in ARDS is complicated. Fluid overload can lead to pulmonary edema impairing gas exchange and hypotension decreases pulmonary blood flow thereby increasing dead space. Clinically it is difficult to determine volume status of patient based on heart rate, blood pressure, urine output. A CXR has limited value in this. So balancing tissue perfusion and tissue oxygenation is challenging aspect.

A large prospective RCT compared conservative fluid strategy (maximum +400 ml) with liberal fluid strategy (approximately +7 Litres) in first 7 days and found that conservative fluid strategy group did well in terms of oxygenation index, ventilator free days, lung injury score. There is no difference in shock, 60 day mortality between 2 groups. Overall conservative fluid strategy is recommended in ARDS management.

Parameters to Assess Volume Responsiveness

Table 20.2	
Static parameters	✦ Volume parameters–global end diastolic volume, left ventricular end diastolic volume, IVC diameter, IVC collapsibility/distensibility ✦ Pressure parameters – CVP, PAOP
Dynamic parameters	✦ Stroke volume variation, pulse pressure variation, passive leg raise, fluid challenge, end expiratory occlusion, Tidal volume challenge

Fluid responsiveness is termed when 500 ml of crystalloid administered over 15 min increases stroke volume by 15%. A fluid responsiveness does not mean fluid is indicated, fluid should be given only when indicated (shock). Among various parameters, static parameters are less sensitive and specific in predicting fluid responsiveness. In practice dynamic parameters do well in predicting but they too have limitations.

Table 20.3

Parameter	Comments
CVP/PAWP	✦ Traditionally used to guide fluid therapy. Using pressure to estimate volume indirectly. CVP used as surrogate for RV preload and PAWP for LV preload. But there is poor relationship between blood volume and CVP. And also it is affected by RV function, tricuspid valve function. ✦ Same as above IVC diameter also is poor predictor of fluid responsiveness
✦ IVC distensibility index	✦ During mechanical ventilation changes in intrathoracic pressure leads to changes in IVC diameter which can be used to estimate fluid responsiveness. ✦ IVCd = [max diameter (inspiration)–min diameter (expiration)]/min diameter(expiration. ✦ Value >18% indicates fluid responsiveness. ✦ Not reliable in spontaneously breathing patients and low tidal volume ventilation.
✦ Pulse pressure variation(PPV)/stroke volume variation (SVV)	✦ Pulse pressure was used to estimate stroke volume in mechanically ventilated patients ✦ PPV = PPmax – PPmin/PPmean * 100 during single breath ✦ Value >12% predicted fluid responsiveness with 88% sensitivity and 89% specificity. PPV is extensively studied marker. ✦ Pulse pressure monitoring requires invasive arterial line monitoring whereas stroke volume can be measured invasively by pulse contour analysis or non-invasively by velocity time integral in echocardiography, aortic blood flow from esophageal Doppler. ✦ Limitations – not reliable in spontaneously breathing patients, ards patients ventilated with low tidal volume, patients with arrhythmias. ✦ SVV – SVmax – SVmin/SVmean *100 ✦ Value >12% indicates fluid responsiveness ✦ Just like IVC distensibility PPV and SVV are also based on cyclic variations in intrathoracic pressure and changes in blood volume ✦ Limitations – not reliable in spontaneously breathing patients, ards patients ventilated with low tidal volume, patients with arrhythmias.

Contd.

Table 20.3 (Contd.)

Parameter	Comments
✦ Extra Vascular Lung Water (EVLW)	✦ Used to estimate fluid in interstitial space of lung. It can result from both cardiogenic and non-cardiogenic edema. ✦ EVLW estimated by thermodilution technique and pulse contour analysis (>7ml/kg) indicated fluid in interstitial space ✦ Another method to estimate EVLW is using lung ultrasonography. The presence of B lines with B profile indicates edema. Absence of B lines and A profile indicates PAWP is <18 mmHg.

In ARDS patients the above mentioned parameters including PPV, SVV are not reliable for assessing fluid responsiveness because one prerequisite for applying this parameter is patient should be ventilated with minimum 8 ml/kg tidal volume for cyclic changes in intrathoracic pressure to happen during positive pressure ventilation. In ARDS lung protective strategy is employed where tidal volume is <8 ml/kg, so false negative results are expected.

Following parameters can be used in ARDS patients for fluid responsiveness assessment

Table 20.4

Parameter	Comments
Fluid challenge	✦ Conventional fluid challenge requires administration of 500 ml of crystalloid over 15 min and measuring cardiac output. If cardiac output >15% is termed fluid responder. Alternatively a MAP target >65 mmHg can be targeted. But main disadvantage of fluid challenge for each episode of hypotension 500ml of fluid is administered which can cause fluid overload. To overcome this mini fluid challenge is practiced. ✦ In mini fluid challenge 100 ml of colloid is given over 1 min and a change in Velocity Time Integral >10% predicts fluid responsiveness. ✦ Another approach is to give 4 ml/kg of crystalloid instead
End expiratory occlusion test	✦ In mechanical ventilation during inspiration venous return decreases thereby preload. If this cycle is interrupted for few seconds preload transiently increases. If cardiac output(measured by pulse contour analysis) increases >5% in response to end expiratory occlusion (EEO) for 15s, it indicates fluid responsiveness. This test is valid at any peep 5–15 cm.
Tidal volume challenge	✦ In this test tidal volume is transiently increased from 6 ml/kg to 8 ml/kg for 1min and observe change in PPV (delta PPV 6–8), if >3.5% indicates fluid responder with 94% sensitivity and 100% specificity. For SVV cutoff is 2.5%. A delta SVV6-8 >2.5% predicts fluid responsiveness.

ELECTROLYTES

The electrolytes exist in every fluid compartment. Water can move freely across cell membrane, not electrolytes so some of the electrolytes are predominantly confined to ECF and some to ICF but osmolarity remains same in both ECF and ICF. The composition and concentration of these electrolytes vary from one another as depicted in **Table 20.5**.

Table 20.5: Electrolyte composition of various body fluid compartment

	ICF (mmol/L)	Plasma (mmol/L)	Interstitial (mmol/L)
Na	10	140	145
K	155	3.7	3.8
CL	3	102	115
HCO_3	10	28	30
Ca (ionized)	<0.01	1.2	1.2
Magnesium	10	0.8	0.8
Phosphorus	105	1.1	1

Major ECF electrolytes include sodium, chloride and bicarbonate. So these 3 are main determinants of ECF osmolarity. Similarly potassium, phosphorus are main determinants of intracellular osmolarity.

SODIUM DISORDERS

Sodium is the major cation in ECF and accounts for 85% of osmolarity in ECF. Regulation of plasma sodium concentration depends on water intake and excretion, not by changes in sodium. When there is excess water in the body development of hyponatremia is prevented by suppression of ADH release. Similarly, excess water loss and development of hypernatremia is controlled by thirst. In mechanically ventilated patients, in depressed sensorium protective thirst mechanism is impaired. Another factor contributing to sodium and water balance is effective arterial blood volume. When there is volume expansion due to high salt intake, natriuretic peptides are released to promote renal excretion of sodium. In volume contraction low effective blood volume activates renin angiotensin aldosterone and sympathetic nervous system causing sodium and water retention.

The four basic disorders of water and sodium balance include intake of water that cannot be excreted (hyponatremia), loss of water that has not been replaced (hypernatremia), loss of sodium and water (hypovolemia), retention of sodium and water (edema).

HYPONATREMIA

Normal serum sodium concentration is 135–145 mmol/L. The term "Hyponatremia" is labelled when sodium concentration falls below 135 mmol/L. It is due to excess water intake in relation to sodium, induced by polydipsia and or impaired water excretion.

Hyponatremia is further categorized as follows

Mild	130–134 mmol/L
Moderate	125–129 mmol/L
Severe	<125 mmol/L

Acute hyponatremia	Developing in <48 hr duration
Chronic hyponatremia	>48 hr duration

Hyponatremia can be further classified based on serum osmolarity into isotonic, hypertonic, hypotonic. A true hyponatremia is always hypotonic. **Table 20.6** depicts causes for each type.

Table 20.6

Clinical classification	Etiology
Isotonic hyponatremia	Hyperlipidemia,hyperprotenemia
Hypertonic hyponatremia	Hyperglycemia,elevated mannitol, sucrose, maltose(immunoglobulin preperations), glycine (post urologic)
Hypotonic hyponatremia 1. Euvolemic 2. Hypervolemic 3. Hypovolemic	SIADH Cirrhosis, CHF, nephrotic syndrome Cerebral salt wasting, renal salt wasting,diuretics, GI losses

Symptoms

The individual may present with symptoms related to underlying illness or hyponatremia itself. The symptoms are predominantly neurological and depends on how rapid serum sodium has dropped, degree to which it dropped. A gradual drop in sodium is well tolerated because of CNS adaptation.

Mild to moderate hyponatremia/chronic hyponatremia	Nausea, vomiting, fatigue, dizziness, headache, confusion
Severe hyponatremia	Lethargy, seizures, coma

Workup for Hyponatremia

Initial workup requires serum osmolarity, urine osmolarity, urine sodium levels. Serum osmolarity helps to differentiate true hyponatremia from pseudohyponatremia. In true hyponatremia serum osmolarity is <280 mosm/kg. Urine osmolarity helps to understand ADH activity. A urine osmolarity >100 mosm/kg indicates ADH activity and inability of kidneys to dilute urine. Finally urine sodium helps differentiate hyponatremia secondary to SIADH, hypovolemia, salt wasting syndromes **(Fig. 20.3)**.

Management of Hyponatremia

In hypertonic and isotonic hyponatremia correcting cause will reverse hyponatremia. Management of hypotonic hyponatremia is based on severity of symptoms, duration of hyponatremia (acute or chronic) and volume status. Aim in acute hyponatremia is to raise serum sodium as rapid as possible by 4–6 mmol/L to prevent herniation from cerebral edema. This can be achieved by giving boluses of hypertonic saline. The recommended serum sodium correction in acute hyponatremia is 8–10 mmol/L in 24 hr. In chronic hyponatremia correction should be even slower 4–6 mmol/L in 24 hr. Over correction of serum sodium in chronic hyponatremia carries risk of osmotic demyelination syndrome (ODS). Certain individuals are at high risk for ODS such as significant hypokalemia, alcoholism, liver disease, malnutrition, baseline serum sodium <105 mmol/L. In this individuals correction should be even slow.

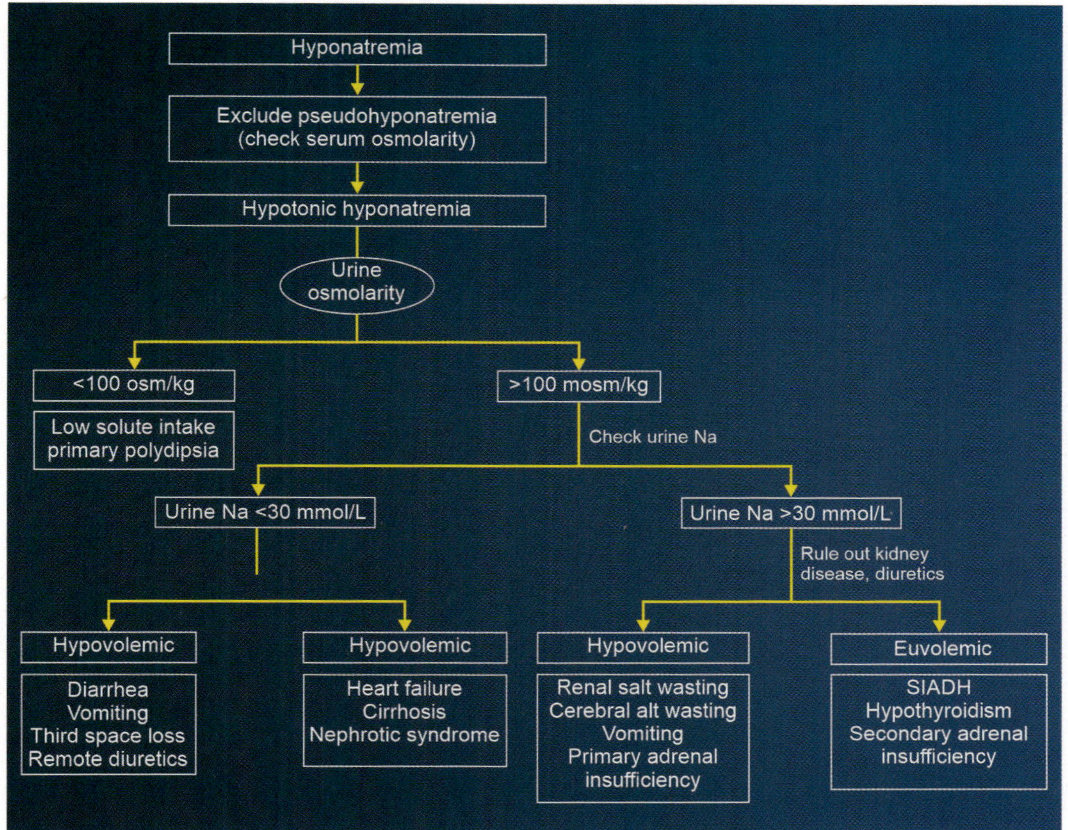

Fig. 20.3: Workup algorithm for hyponatremia

Sodium deficit can be calculated by following formula:

Sodium deficit = (desired Na – current Na) * TBW

Algorithm for hypotonic hyponatremia management (**Fig. 20.4**)

HYPERNATREMIA

Hypernatremia is coined when serum sodium is >145 mmol/L. It is always associated with high serum osmolarity. It occurs due to loss of both free water and sodium where free water loss is more than sodium. Due to osmotic shift fluid moves from cell to intravascular space causing cell shrinkage and neurological manifestations. Since this is hyperosmolar condition osmoreceptors are stimulated and leads to thirst and ADH release as compensation. So hypernatremia is seen when thirst is impaired **(Table 20.7)**.

Symptoms

- Nausea, vomiting
- Lethargy, irritability
- Seizures
- Coma

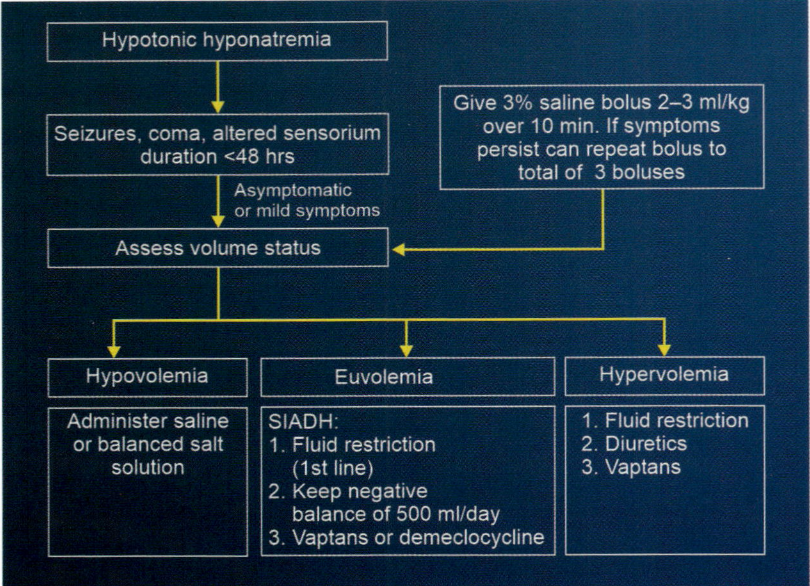

Fig. 20.4

Table 20.7: Etiology of hypernatremia

Pure water deficit	1. Insensible loss through respiratory system 2. Renal water loss 3. Impaired thirst or no access to water Intubation,immobilization, altered mental status, dementia, hypothalamic lesions 4. Diabetes insipidus
Loss of water and electrolytes (water > sodium)	1. Loop and thiazide diuretic 2. Osmotic diuresis 3. Post-obstruction diuresis 4. ATN diuretic phase
Gain of sodium	1. $NaHCO_3$ administration, hypertonic feeds 2. Excess saline administration

Management

It is by supplementing free water and correcting the etiology. In acute hypernatremia (<48 hr) rapid correction is required. For first 24 hr restrict correction to <10 mmol/L. Free water deficit is calculated as follows:

Free water deficit = TBW *(current Na – desired Na/desired Na)

Change in sodium with infusate solution can be known with below formula

Change in S.Na = (infusate Na + infusate K – serum Na/TBW+1)

The calculated water deficit is administered as pure water enterally. If IV administration is required give 5% dextrose or 0.45% saline. Pure water should not be administered intravenously due to risk of hemolysis.

Management of diabetes insipidus involves correcting cause, administration of desmopressin spray once or twice daily. Monitor SNa and avoid overcorrection. Second option include – administration of chlorpropamide 500 mg/day orally. In nephrogenic diabetes insipidus giving thiazide diuretic can help sometimes.

POTASSIUM

Total body potassium is 50 mmol/kg in adult male. It is the principal intracellular cation. About 90% of body potassium is intracellular, 95% of body potassium is exchangeable. It determines the resting membrane potential as cell membrane is 20 times more permeable to potassium than sodium. Other functions of potassium include:

1. Role in carbohydrate metabolism and glycogen synthesis
2. Role in protein synthesis

Potassium metabolism depends on activity of Na/K ATPase activity, renal excretion (aldosterone activity). When Na/K ATP pump is activated it drives potassium into cell and sodium out of cell. It happens in sympathetic stimulation, stimulation of beta receptors by salbutamol nebulization, insulin administration.

Normal serum potassium is between 3.5 to 5 mmol/L. There is no difference between serum and plasma potassium, but in thrombocytosis serum potassium is slightly higher than plasma.

HYPOKALEMIA

It is defined as serum potassium <3.5 mmol/L. It can be further graded into Mild (3–3.5mmol/L), Moderate (2.5–3 mmol/L), Severe <2.5 mmol/L. Hypokalemia is due to one of the following:

Table 20.8

Mechanism	Causes
Decreased intake of potassium	Starvation,alcoholism,anorexia,potassium poor TPN
Increased loss	1. Renal-osmotic diuresis, mineralocorticoid excess, hyperreninism, Barter syndrome, Gitelman syndrome, drugs (diuretics,amphotericin b,cisplatin) 2. Gastrointestinal—vomiting, diarrhea,colostomy, laxative 3. Skin—burns, diaphoresis 4. Dialysis
Transcellular shift	Insulin, beta agonist, barium toxicity, TPN, metabolic alkalosis

Symptoms

Mild hypokalemia is asymptomatic most of the times. Symptoms are related to muscle weakness or cardiac dysfunction. Most common symptoms fatigue,weakness. Other symptoms include muscle cramps, abdominal distension (paralytic ileus), paraperesis ECG changes in hypokalemia include –VPCs, loss of T wave, appearance of U wave, prolong QTc interval, atrial and ventricular arrhythmias.

Workup

Transtubular potassium gradient (TTKG): It is indirect measure of aldosterone activity. Normal value is 6–12 and is calculated as follows

(Urine K/serum K) * (serum Osm/urine Osm)

Expected TTKG in hypokalemia is <3. If it is more than 4 indicates renal potassium loss due to distal secretion.

Spot urine potassium—measuring 24 hr urine potassium is best method. But since it is not possible practically, measuring spot urine potassium can guide physician. In presence of hypokalemia urine potassium excretion is in range of 5–15 mmol/L. So a urine K >40 favors urinary potassium wasting and urine k <15 mmol/L favors extra renal loss. But the urine volume is variable throughout the day so measuring urine potassium to creatinine ratio is appropriate

Urine potassium to creatinine ratio—because creatinine is excreted at constant rate, measuring this ratio corrects for variations in urine volume. Ratio >13 mEq/g of creatinine is in favor of renal loss (**Fig. 20.5**).

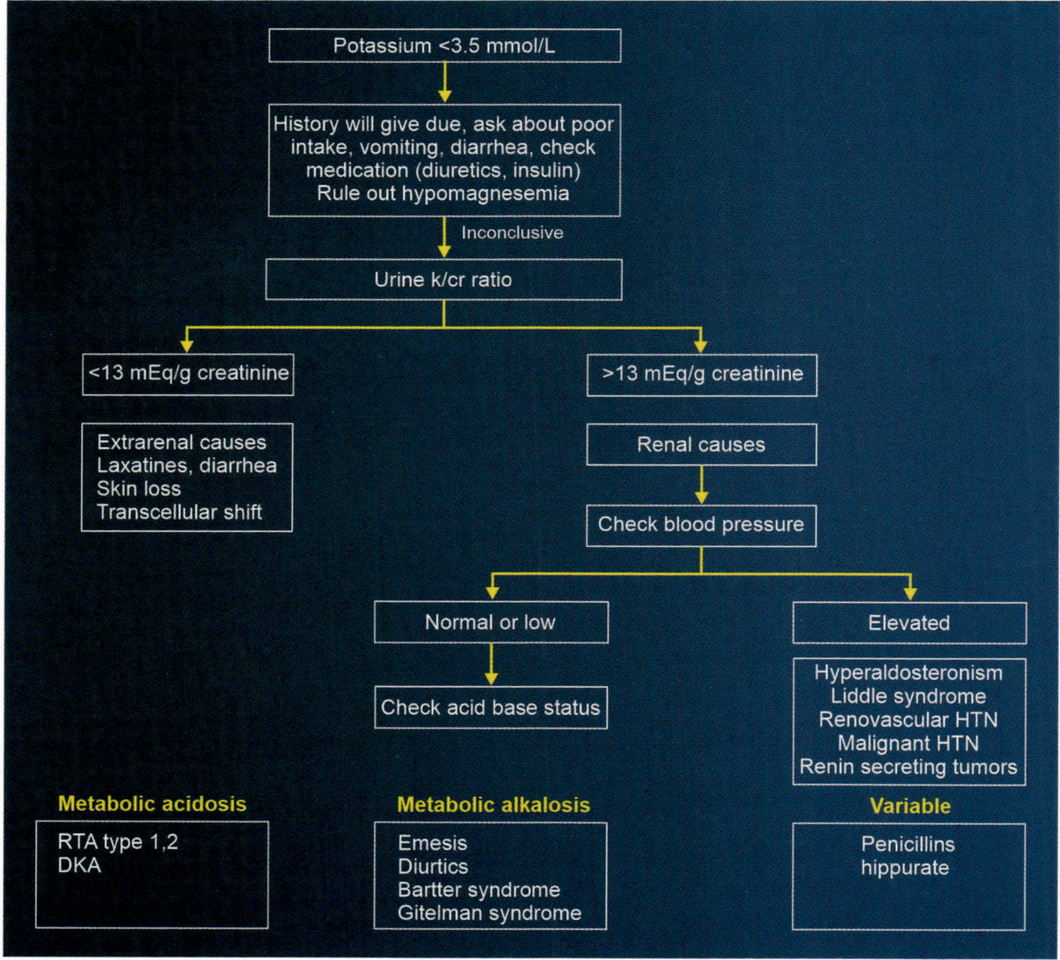

Fig. 20.5

Treatment

a. **Replacing potassium:** Potassium can be supplemented enterally or intravenous administration.In mild to moderate hypokalemia without symptoms oral supplementation is sufficient whereas in severe hypokalemia or in presence of serious symptoms—arrhythmias it has to be administered intravenously. In presence of paralytic ileus enteral supplementation will not be sufficient.

   Potassium administered IV is an irritant so it can lead to phlebitis, pain along injection site hence it should be administered in dilute concentration (<20 mEq/h) via peripheral line. The higher concentrations can be given through CVC line.

   Note: Do not overcorrect potassium in hypokalemic periodic paralysis

b. **Correct the cause:** Along with supplementation of potassium, cause of hypokalemia has to taken care of. First thing rule out hypomagnesemia, withhold diuretics, correct hyperglycemia.

HYPERKALEMIA

It is defined as serum potassium >5.5 mmol/L. It can be classified as Mild (5.5–6.4 mmol/L), Moderate (6.5 – 7.4 mmol/L), Severe (>7.5 mmol/L). Hyperkalemia should be differentiated from pseudohyperkalemia which occurs due to release of potassium during venipuncture, increase in cellular elements (Thrombocytosis, leukocytosis) are given in **Table 20.9**.

Table 20.9

Mechanism	Cause
Inadequate excretion	Renal insufficiency, hypoaldosteronism, adrenal insufficiency, heart failure, drugs (ACE inhibitors, ARBs, potassium sparing diuretics)
Transcellular shift	Acidosis,beta antagonist, digoxin, neuromuscular injury, succinylcholine, tumor lysis
Excess intake	Diet rich in potassium (banana, oranges, coconut water, dry fruits)
Pseudohyperkalemia	Thrombocytosis, leukocytosis, erythrocytosis

Clinical Features

Most of them are asymptomatic in mild cases. Patients who have chronic renal insufficiency will tolerate slightly higher potassium compared to others. Most common symptoms are weakness and fatigue. They can experience muscle paralysis, arrhythmias, chest pain, paraesthesia, nausea,vomiting.

ECG changes noted in hyperkalemia include–tall T waves, sinus bradycardia, loss of P wave, QRS widening, short QTc interval, PR prolongation, sine wave pattern, ventricular arrhythmias.

Workup

Initial step is to rule out pseudohyperkalemia. Assess for warning signs (ECG changes) which require immediate management

History and medication list will give clue to etiology in some cases. If the etiology is still not clear and once emergency management is done workup requires measurement of urine potassium, sodium and urine osmolarity. A spot urine potassium <20 mmol/L suggests impaired renal excretion and >40 mmol/L suggest non renal etiology. But in presence of high urine osmolarity >700 mosm/kg absolute urine potassium is misleading. To address this TTKG is calculated.

A TTKG <3 in hyperkalemia implies reduced renal excretion of potassium. There are certain conditions only when TTKG can be applied – urine osmolarity should be more than serum osmolarity, urine sodium >20 mmol/L.

Treatment

In presence of warning signs like ECG changes hyperkalemia should be treated immediately irrespective of serum levels. Immediate therapy requires administration of intravenous calcium 10 ml of 10% calcium gluconate to stabilize myocardium.It is administered over 2–3 min, can be repeated if ECG changes persist or recur.

a. **Rapid shifting of potassium into cells:** Insulin shifts potassium into cells. 10 units of regular insulin along with 50 ml of 50% dextrose when given shifts potassium intracellularly. The effect begins in 10 min, peaks at 60 min and lasts for 4–6 hr with close of glucose levels. If the intitial plasma glucose is >200 mg/dL then glucose/dextrose administration can be skipped.

   Beta 2 agents like albuterol nebulizations also cause intracellular shifting of potassium. Dose recommended is 10–20 mg of albuterol. It can cause tachycardia so should be used with caution in patients with cardiac disease

b. **Enhancing elimination of potassium:** Cation exchange resins–they increase gastrointestinal elimination of potassium. These resins contain sodium polystyrene sulfonate (SPS) which exchange Na with K and eliminated in fecus. Recommended dose is 15–30 gm suspended in 33% sorbitol every 4–6 hr. It acts slowly and make take upto 24 hr for full effect. It is not recommended therapy in emergent reduction of potassium. When administered to patients with reduced intestinal motility it can cause intestinal necrosis.

   Novel intestinal potassium binders—Patiromer which exchanges K with Ca^{2+} in intestine.

   Diuretics—to enhance renal excretion of potassium. Loop or thiazide diuretics are used for elimination.

   Hemodialysis—most effective method to reduce plasma potassium. Amount of potassium removed depends on blood flow rate, dialysate flow rate, duration of dialysis and potassium gradient between plasma and dialysate.

CALCIUM

Calcium plays an important role in cell signaling, neuromuscular signaling, cardiac contractility, hormone secretion, blood coagulation. The calcium concentration is tightly regulated in serum by 2 feedback mechanisms from parathyroid hormone and 1,25 hydroxy vitamin D. Normal serum calcium is in range of 9–11 mg/dL in presence of normal albumin levels.

HYPERCALCEMIA

It is coined when serum calcium concentration >11 mg/dL. Further graded as Mild (11–11.9 mg/dL), Moderate (12–13.9 mg/dL), Severe (>14 mg/dL). Hypercalcemia is due to increased bone resorption,decreased renal excretion or excess gastrointestinal absorption.

Etiology

Parathyroid mediated	Primary hyperparathyroidism, MEN syndrome, familial hyperparathyroidism, renal failure
Non-parathyroid mediated	Hypercalcemia of malignancy, vitamin D intoxication,chronic granulomatous disease
Medications	Thiazide diuretics, lithium, Excess vitamin A,teriparatide, theophylline toxicity
Miscellaneous	Hyperthyroidism, pheochromocytoma, adrenal insufficiency, immobilization, parenteral nutrition

Clinical Features

Hypercalcemia causes wide variety of symptoms. Mild hypercalcemia can be asymptomatic. CNS, renal and GI tract are commonly affected.

- CNS—irritability, seizures, coma
- Renal—polyuria, dehydration,renal calculi, renal failure
- GI tract—constipation, anorexia, pancreatitis, gastric ulcerations.

Workup

The first step in evaluation of hypercalcemia is check corrected calcium levels (correction for low albumin). A detailed history provides important clues about medications, neck surgery. Second step is check levels of PTH. If PTH is normal or elevated in presence of high serum calcium, low phosphorus then primary hyperparathyroidism is likely etiology. A calcium/creatinine clearance ratio helps in differentiating primary hyperparathyroidism from familial hypocalciuric hypercalcemia (FHH). If PTH levels are low in presence of hypercalcemia likely etiology is non-parathyroid related. Further workup needs parathyroid hormone related peptide (PTHrP) to rule out malignancy, 1,25 dihydroxy vit D to rule out granulomatous disease.

Treatment

Mild, asymptomatic hypercalcemia does not require immediate therapy. But severe hypercalcemia requires immediate intervention irrespective of etiology.

1. **Hydration:** Hypercalcemia leads to dehydration. Hence adequate hydration with crystalloids should be given, they may require 4–6 L of fluid in 24 hr. Further fluid therapy is guided by urine output. In patients with compromised cardiac function fluid should be given cautiously.
2. **Loop diuretics:** They should be given only after adequate hydration. Loop diuretics will enhance calcium excretion in urine.
3. **Calcitonin:** When given in dose of 4 u/kg subcutaneously or intramuscularly will reduce calcium in 4–6 hr by enhancing renal excretion, decreasing bone resorption.

Dose can be repeated after 12 hr. The disadvantage is development of tachyphylaxis after 48 hr. So it is used in initial management along with hydration.

4. **Bisphosphonates:** More potent agents for reducing calcium levels but onset of action is delayed by 24 hr which makes them not suitable for initial/emergent therapy. Mechanism is by inhibiting bone resorption.
5. **Glucocorticoids:** They are used in hypercalcemia due to granulomatous disease. Reduction in serum calcium is by decreasing intestinal absorption of calcium, decrease 1,25-dihydroxy vitamin D production.
6. **Other options:** Calcimimetics, denosumab, dialysis

HYPOCALCEMIA

In hypocalcemia serum calcium will be < 9 mg/dL. The presentation varies widely from asymptomatic to life threatening.

Etiology

Low PTH (hypoparathyroidism)	Digeorge syndrome,parathyroid destruction(thyroid surgery, radiation), reduced parathyroid function (hypomagnesemia)
High PTH levels	Vitamin D deficiency,hungry bone pseudohypoparathyroidism,drugs (bisphosphonates,ketoconazole,phenytoin),acute pancreatitis,rhabdomyolysis

Clinical Manifestations

Perioral tingling, numbness, wheeze, muscle cramps, dysphagia, irritability, seizures ECG shows prolong QTc interval.

Treatment

- Before labelling hypocalcemia check corrected calcium for hypoalbuminemia.
- Calcium supplementation – IV calcium gluconate 10% diluted in 100 ml saline and given over 5 min. If hypocalcemia is persistent may require continuous infusion over 24 hr (10 ampoules diluted in 1 L of 5% dextrose or saline). Simultaneously correct hypomagnesemia.
- In chronic hypocalcemia oral calcium supplementation is given 1000–1500 mg of elemental calcium per day in divided doses. In vitamin D deficiency give 60000 units of vitamin D orally or IM repeated weekly once for 6 weeks. Target is to maintain serum calcium on lower side of normal to avoid nephrolithiasis.

MAGNESIUM

It is mainly intracellular ion involved as coenzyme in numerous phosphate transfer reactions. Normal serum magnesium is 0.85 – 1.1 mmol/L (1.7–2.2 mg/dL).

HYPOMAGNESEMIA

Due to decreased intake or increased losses. Manifests as confusion, delirium, irritability, convulsions, tachyarrhythmias. It also leads to resistant hypokalemia, hypocalcemia.

Etiology

Gastrointestinal	Malabsorption, short bowel, fistulas, diarrhea, pancreatitis
Endocrine	Diabetes mellitus, hyperparathyroidism, hyperthyroidism, Conn's syndrome
Renal diseases	Renal tubular acidosis, diuretic phase of ATN
Alcoholism	
Drugs	Diuretics, amphotericin B, aminoglycosides, cisplatin, cyclosporine

Treatment

Magnesium sulphate administered IV 20–60 mmol/day. Oral supplementation can be given in mild or chronic cases. In high doses oral magnesium can cause diarrhea.

HYPERMAGNESEMIA

- It is most often due to excess administration of $MgSO_4$ in presence of renal failure. It is characterized by hyporeflexia, paralysis, hypotension, drowsiness.
- ECG demonstrates heart block at SA or AV node.
- Initial management involves administration of IV calcium to antagonize effects of magnesium. In patients with impaired excretion dialysis has to be offered.

CHAPTER 21

Weaning and Extubation

❒ Anand Vinaykumar Joshi ❒ R Vijai Kumar

INTRODUCTION

Invasive mechanical ventilation (MV) is a life-saving intervention used in intensive care units (ICU) and emergency rooms (ER) worldwide. However, it is increasingly recognized that this intervention comes with potential costs, including harmful cointerventions (e.g. sedation and paralysis), MV-related complications, increased morbidity and mortality, and financial costs to healthcare systems.[1] It is estimated that approximately 40–50% of total mechanical ventilation time is spent on the weaning process.[2–4] Thus, minimizing MV use and liberating patients from it as soon as possible has become essential.

While we have gained significant knowledge about safely initiating mechanical ventilation, less is understood about the process of liberating patients from it.

Liberation from the ventilator involves two key steps:

1. Weaning the patient from the ventilator.
2. Tracheal extubation from an endotracheal or tracheostomy tube.

Both steps are part of a continuum, with weaning typically culminating in tracheal extubation. The exception is weaning with a tracheostomy tube, where the tracheostomy can be removed later based on its indication (described elsewhere).

This chapter outlines the process of weaning and endotracheal extubation, while tracheostomy and related topics are discussed separately.

DEFINITION

Weaning from mechanical ventilation is the gradual and systematic process of reducing ventilatory support, transitioning the patient from ventilator-assisted breathing to spontaneous breathing. Some societies accept this as a definition[5], but it lacks clarity to classify all patients and introduces ambiguity in research settings.

In 2005, during the Budapest conference, Tobin proposed that weaning consists of six stages.[6] He emphasized evaluating the patient for weaning after the resolution of acute respiratory failure, which triggered the initiation of MV. Each stage was defined, with a successful endotracheal extubation or reintubation before discharge as the ultimate outcome (**Fig. 21.1** and **Table 21.1**).

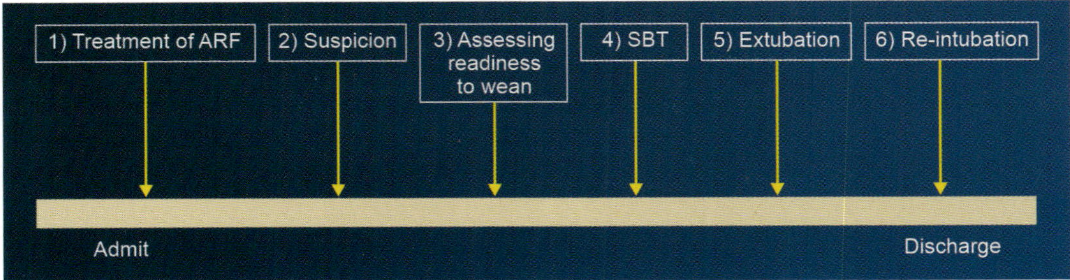

Fig. 21.1: Schematic representation of the different stages occurring in a mechanically ventilated patient. ARF: Acute respiratory failure, SBT: Spontaneous breathing test[6]

Table 21.1: Definition of the different stages, from initation to mechanical ventilation to weaning

Stages	Definitaions
Treatment of ARF	Period of care and resolution of the disorder that caused respiratory failure and prompted mechanical ventilation
Suspicion	The point at which the clinician suspects the patient may be ready to begin the weaning process
Assessing readiness to wean	Daily testing of physiological measures of readiness for weaning (MP/R/VT) to determine probability of weaning success
Spontaneous breathing trial	Assessment of the patient's ability to breathe spontaneously
Extubation	Removal of the endotracheal tube
Reintubation	Replacement of endotracheal tube for patients who are unable to sustain spontaneous ventilation

Based on this, various international societies met in 2007 to form a consensus definition of weaning from mechanical ventilation.

International consensus conference (ICC) definition: In 2007, the International Consensus Conference on Weaning from Mechanical Ventilation[3] classified patients into three different groups (ICC groups) based on the number, timing, and outcomes of spontaneous breathing trials (SBTs), as well as extubation results. SBTs were defined as either a T-piece trial or a low-level pressure support of <8 cm H_2O for 30 to 120 minutes.

The groups were:

1. **Simple weaning (ICC Group 1):** Successful extubation after the first SBT.
2. **Difficult weaning (ICC Group 2):** Successful extubation after two to three SBTs within 7 days.
3. **Prolonged weaning (ICC Group 3):** Successful extubation after more than three SBTs or after more than 7 days.

Drawbacks of ICC definition:

- This definition only considers patients who were ultimately weaned, not those who failed.
- SBTs, as defined, are not universally practiced, with significant variations in practice.[7]

- Some patients who are extubated without SBTs were not included in this definition.
- This definition, though simple, cannot be extrapolated for prognostication.

Weaning according to New Definition (WIND definition):[8] The "WIND Definition," proposed by Beduneau G, et al. defined weaning based on the initiation of any separation attempt, the duration of the weaning process, and prognosis **(Table 21.2)**.

1. **For intubated patients:**
   - Separation attempt: An SBT with or without extubation, or an extubation performed without a prior identified SBT (planned or unplanned).
   - Successful weaning or separation: Extubation without death or reintubation within 7 days, or ICU discharge without invasive mechanical ventilation within 7 days, whichever comes first.
2. **For tracheostomized patients:**
   - Separation attempt: 24 hours or more of spontaneous ventilation through the tracheostomy without mechanical ventilation.
   - Successful weaning or separation: Spontaneous ventilation through the tracheostomy without mechanical ventilation for 7 consecutive days or until discharge, whichever comes first.

Table 21.2: Compares the classification of patients based on two definition[9]

Classification	ICC	Wind
Group 1	Simple weaning: successful extubation after one SBTs	Short weaning: Successful separation from MV or death within 24 h
Group 2	Difficult weaning: Successful extubation after up to three SBTs in less than 7 days	Difficult weaning: Successful separation from MV or death in 1 to 7 day
Group 3	Prolonged weaning: Successful extubation after more than three SBTs or more than 7 days	Prolonged weaning: Unsuccessful separation 7 days after the first attempt. Subgroup A: Eventually separated from MV; B: Not separated from MV
Group "no weaning"	–	No separation attempt from MV

Extubation: Extubation is the process of removing the artificial airway from the trachea, allowing the patient to return to their natural airway or transition to a tracheostomy. It is a desired outcome after a successful SBT. Besides meeting the criteria for successful weaning, additional factors must be considered before tracheal extubation.

Some patients may require prolonged mechanical ventilation, which is defined as requiring at least 21 consecutive days of MV for at least 6 hours per day. These patients are not to be confused with those requiring prolonged weaning.[10]

IS YOUR PATIENT READY FOR WEANING

The decision to begin weaning a patient from mechanical ventilation should be considered as early as the initiation of MV to prevent MV-associated complications and premature ventilator disconnection. This requires careful planning and preparation before taking the actual steps. Inadequate preparation or improper assessment can lead to weaning and/or extubation failure.

Mechanical ventilation (MV) can cause a range of complications, and premature disconnection from MV increases the risk of adverse events. Here is a summary of some potential issues **(Table 21.3)**:

Table 21.3: Complications of MV and premature MV disconnect[11]

MV complications	Premature MV disconnect
VILI	Loss of airway protection
VAP	Respiratory fatigue
Airway trauma due to ETT	Respiratory arrest
Prolong sedation and paralysis, critical illness neuromyopathy	Compromised gas exchange

Weaning period can be considered staged approach.

1. Preparing patient for assessment
2. Assessment of readiness to wean:
3. Spontaneous breathing trials as a objective tool to determine likelihood of successful extubation.

Preparing the Patient for Weaning

Weaning can be viewed as a staged process. The first step is to prepare the patient for assessment by optimizing certain factors. The ISCCM (Indian Society of Critical Care Medicine) recommends using the "ABCDEFGHI" mnemonic for this purpose.(5) Here's a breakdown of these factors **(Table 24.4)**:

Table 21.4: Factors to be considered before assessment of readiness to wean

A	Alert, afebrile and aim for ventilation is met.
B	Breathing indices are physiologically acceptable
C	Hemodynamics are stable, with no or minimal vasopressors
D	There should be no effect of neuromuscular blocking drugs, minimal or no sedation that can threaten airway. Weaning sedation and giving sedation holidays is one of important step in weaning process. Benzodiazepines and Opioids are notorious in having residual effect and should be looked for. Non-benzodiazepine, no or low dose opioid strategy like use of dexmedetomidine or ketamine can be considered for delirious or agitated patients.
E	Electrolyte correction of sodium, chloride, potassium, phosphate, magnesium should be done before initiation of weaning
F	Fluid overload state, positive fluid balance are to be avoided.
G	Glucose control with avoiding hypoglycemia and hyperglycemia.
H	No hallucinations or delirium
I	Impending transfers or procedures are not there.

Assessment of Readiness to Wean

Once the patient has been optimised, readiness for weaning should be evaluated using both clinical assessment and objective characteristics.

- **Clinical assessment:** Ensure resolution (complete or partial) of the condition that necessitated mechanical ventilation. Check that the patient can protect their own airway (e.g. via an adequate cough reflex) and that there are no excessive tracheal secretions.
- **Objective assessment:** Clinical evaluation should be supported by objective parameters, such as stable cardiovascular status, adequate oxygenation, and acceptable ventilatory indices **(Table 21.5)**.

Table 21.5: Objective assessment for readiness to wean

Clinical stability	Adequate oxygenation	Adequate pulmonary function	Neurological status
Stabe cardiovascular status	SO_2 >90 on FiO_2 ≤0.4 PaO_2/ FiO_2>150	F ≤35 Maximal Inspiratory pressure (MIP) ≤–20 to –25	No sedation or adequate mentation on sedation
Heart rate ≤140 Systolic blood pressure `90–160 mmHg Minimal or no vasopressor	PEEP ≤8	Vt >5 ml/kg vital Capacity >10 ml/kg fR/ Vt<105 breaths/min/L	Stable neurological patient
Stable metabolic status		No significant respiratory acidosis	

Spontaneous Breathing Trials (SBT)

As early as the 1960s, weaning a patient from a ventilator involved progressively increasing the amount of "off-ventilator" time and delivering oxygen via a T-piece attached to the endotracheal tube. With the advent of intermittent mandatory ventilation (IMV), synchronized IMV (SIMV), and pressure support ventilation (PSV) modes, gradually reducing the mandatory ventilatory rate while allowing the patient to breathe spontaneously with pressure support became a popular method of weaning.

It was not until the mid-1990s that the four popular weaning methods were compared. Two major randomized controlled trials (RCTs)[12,13] and subsequent studies[14,15] failed to conclusively support any one weaning method.

Currently, the Indian Society of Critical Care Medicine recommends two methods for spontaneous breathing trials (SBTs): An off-ventilator 'T-piece' trial or an on-ventilator low-level pressure support ventilation (PSV) mode trial. The low-level PSV mode includes a PEEP of 5 cm H_2O and pressure support above PEEP of around 6–8 cm H_2O. The duration of the SBT should be 30–120 minutes. The use of SIMV and CPAP modes is no longer routinely recommended.[5]

Studies have shown that the use of the PSV mode is associated with a shorter weaning period in patients undergoing simple weaning, but it carries the risk of underestimating the respiratory workload and oxygen consumption of the respiratory muscles.[16] On the other hand, the T-piece was more suited for patients undergoing prolonged weaning.[15,17] Daily SBTs were found to be more effective than a gradual reduction in PSV or SIMV during the weaning process.[12]

Monitoring during SBTs:[7,18]

Following parameters should be monitored during SBTs **(Table 21.6)**.

Table 21.6: Monitoring during SBTs

Respiratory distress	Heart rate-trachy/bradycardia
Diaphoresis	Blood Pressure—hyper/hypotension
Use of accessory muscle	O_2 Saturation
Paradoxical breathing	$etCO_2$
Bronchospasm	ABG after 30–120 min
Altered mental status	Weaning indices (*see* below)

WEANING INDICES

Researchers have identified several tests and scoring systems that can predict the success or failure of weaning during spontaneous breathing trials (SBTs). These are referred to as "weaning indices." The most popular and widely recommended index is the Rapid-Shallow Breathing Index (RSBI). Other indices and scoring systems are detailed in **Table 21.7**.

Rapid-Shallow Breathing Index: First proposed by Tobin and Yang in 1991, this simple bedside measurement predicted successful weaning and extubation with a sensitivity of 97% and specificity of 64%, along with strong negative predictive value (98%) and positive predictive value (78%).[19,20] It is calculated by dividing the respiratory rate (f) by the tidal volume (Vt) [f/Vt]. A cut-off value of 105 is used, where values less than 105 predict weaning success, and values greater than 105 predict weaning failure.

Other weaning indices are elaborated in **Table 2.17.**

Table 21.7: Weaning indices[5]

Index	Calculation	Desired Parameter	Comment
Ventilatory drive			
Forced vital capacity	Same as Vt	>15 ml/kg	Indicate good respiratory muscle strength Need conscious and cooperative patient
Maximum inspiratory Pressure (PImax)	Breath with ventilatory valve closed. (PImax manoeuvre)	<–30 cmH_2O	Indicate good respiratory muscle strength Need cooperative patient, Watch for arrhythmia and drop in saturation.
Airway pressure at 100 ms with airway occluded. P100 or P0.1	Some ventilator has inbuilt setting while doing PImax manoeuvre	>–0.6 cm H_2O	Good central drive. Need cooperative patient

Contd.

Table 21.7: Weaning indices[5] (Contd.)

Index	Calculation	Desired Parameter	Comment
P0.1/PImax index		>0.3	Complex calculation
P0.1/RSBI		>300	Complex calculation
Scoring system			
CROP index Compliance (dynamic), Rate, oxygenation and PImax	Cdyn × PImax × $(PaO_2/PAO_2)/f$	>13	Need complex calculation
CORE Index Compliance (dynamic), Oxygenation, rate, effort	Cdyn × (PImax/P0.1) × $(PaO_2/PAO_2)/$	>8	Complex calculation
WI: Weaning Index	SRBI × EI × VDI (EI = Preak Pessure/ Negative inspiratory pressure, VDI = Minute volume /10)	<50	Cumbersome and complex calculation
IWI: Integrated weaning index	$(CRS \times SaO_2)$/RSBI, CRS = static lung compliance	>25	Complex calculation
HACOR Heart rate, acidosis, consciousness, oxygenation, repiratory rate	Clinical signs	≥5	More validated for NIV
Ultrasound guided			
Diaphragmatic RSBI	Respiratory rate/ diaphragmatic displacement	1.767 breath/ minute/ mm	Need ultrasound skills

ULTRASONOGRAPHY IN WEANING

Diaphragmatic dysfunction plays a significant role in weaning failure. Even a short duration of mechanical ventilation (MV), the use of neuromuscular blocking agents, and prolonged deep sedation can lead to diaphragmatic atrophy. The extended use of point-of-care ultrasound to assess diaphragmatic dysfunction has become an important tool for predicting weaning failure.

When using a high-frequency probe placed in the mid-axillary line, the diaphragm appears as a dark-colored sandwich structure between the bright pleura and peritoneal reflection. Normal thickness ranges from 0.22 to 0.28 mm, while a thickness of less than 0.2 mm is considered indicative of atrophy. Using a low-frequency probe placed in the mid-clavicular line, the excursion of the diaphragm is recorded. An excursion of less than 2.5 cm is classified as severe dysfunction.[21] The diaphragmatic RSBI is one of the weaning indices used to predict the success of spontaneous breathing trials (SBTs), utilising diaphragmatic excursion or displacement as one of its parameters.

FAILURE OF SBTS OR WEANING TRIAL

Patient should be closely observed for signs of failed SBTs **(Table 21.8)**.

Table 21.8: Failure criteria during SBTS	
Anxiety and agitation	Respiratory rate >35 or increase > 50%
Depressed mental status	SO_2 <90%, PaO_2 <50 mmHg on FiO_2 > 0.5
Diaphoresis	PCO_2 >50 mmHg or increase by 8 mmHg
Cyanosis	pH <7.32 or decrease by >0.07
Increased respiratory distress	RSBI >105
Increased accessory muscle activity	Heart rate >140 b/min or increase by 20%
	Hypertension >180 mmHg or increase by 20%
	Hypotension <90 mmHg
	Cardiac arrhythmia.

There are various factors that can contribute to pathophysiology of weaning failure **(Table 21.9)**.

Table 21.9: Factors causing weaning failure					
Airway and lung dysfunction	Weaning induced cardiac dysfunction	Neurological causes	Abdominal causes	Metabolic and electrolytes	Nutrition
Bronchospasm - worsening asthma, COPD, dynamic hyperinflation	Marked intrathoracic pressure changes with hypoxia and hypercarbia, increased work of breathing may induced cardiac ischemia or left ventricular dysfunction	Delirium, Depression, Anxiety	Acute abdominal pathology,	Potassium disturbance, hypophosphatemia, Hypomagnesemia	Severe malnutrition, wasting of muscles and generalised disability
Pulmonary oedema, ARDS, pneumonia		Critical illness neuromyopathy	High intra-abdominal pressure like tense ascites, AKI	Thyroid dysfunction, adrenal insufficiency	
Pleural effusion		Cervical or thoracic spinal cord injury		Morbid obesity, metabolic syndrome	
Lung fibrosis		Uncontrolled pain of any kind			
Diaphragmatic dysfunction		Drug induced like sedation and neuroparalysis			

APPROACHING FAILED SBT

If a patient fails an SBT, they should be reventilated using a strategy that avoids fatigue. The underlying cause of the failure should be identified and addressed before another weaning attempt is made. The next SBT should not be attempted for at least 24 hours or until the cause of failure has been corrected.[5]

Based on the timeline and number of failed SBTs, the patient will be classified into one of the following groups:

- Difficult weaning (ICC Group 2)
- Prolonged weaning (ICC Group 3)
- Non-weaning category (for patients who fail multiple attempts and may require long-term ventilation).

ENDOTRACHEAL EXTUBATION

A successful SBT or a wean trial leads to tracheal extubation of the artificial airway, which is a desired outcome. While there are many overlapping factors contributing to successful tracheal extubation, several airway-related factors can lead to extubation failure despite successful weaning. Airway management in the ICU has been associated with higher morbidity and mortality compared to operating theatres and emergency rooms (ER). Commonly identified factors include poor identification of at-risk patients, inadequate planning, unskilled or insufficient staff, and equipment failures, as well as the inability to recognise critical events, such as interpreting capnography. Despite adhering to current guidelines, the extubation failure rate in high-risk areas like the ICU remains around 15%.[23]

For patients intubated for more than 24 hours, additional airway problems, alongside those causing weaning failure (described earlier), can hinder successful tracheal extubation **(Table 21.10)**.

Table 21.10: Problems for successful tracheal extubation

Exaggerated laryngeal reflexes	Breathholding, coughing, bucking, laryngospasm can lead to negative pressure pulmonary dema and hypoxic cardiac arrest
Reduced airway relexes	Reduced pharyngeal tone in obese and obstructive sleep apnea (OSA) patients compounded by opioids.
Drugs effect	Residual sedation and neuromuscular blockade may reduce laryngeal reflex leading to aspiration
Airway injury	Surgical, traumatic intubation, edema from prolong intubation, infection or burns.
Human factors	Time pressure, lack of monitoring, equipment, planing and poor communication.

INDICES FOR SUCCESSFUL TRACHEAL EXTUBATION

Most of the indices used to predict SBT success can also be applied to predict successful extubation. One specific scoring system, the STAGE score, has been proposed to predict extubation success in neurological patients. The components of the STAGE score are given in **Table 21.11**:

Table 21.11: Stage scoring for sucessful extubation in neurosurgical patients

Component	Parameter	Score
Swallowing		0/3
Strong	No visibile accumulation of saliva for either conscious or comatose patient	
Poor	Visible accumulation of saliva for either conscious or comatose patients	
Tongue Protrusion		0/2
Strong	Can protrude outside the mouth	
Poor	Cannot protrude outside the mouth	
Airway protection		
Spontaneous cough		0/2
Strong	Vigorous	
Poor	Weak or none	
Suctioning cough		0/3
Strong	Vigorous	
Poor	Weak or none	
GCS–Motor response		0/2
Strong	Can obey commands or localise to pain	
Poor	Withdrawal, flexion, extension or no response to pain	
Total score	15	0/12

In the study conducted by authors, score of 6 or less had poor productivity of successful extraction while score more than 9 showed almost 100% predictivity.[24]

Other traditional tests include:

- **5-second head-lift test:** If the patient can lift their head for 5 seconds, extubation is likely to be successful.
- **Breath-holding test:** If the patient can hold their breath for at least 5 seconds after a deep inspiration, extubation success is likely.
- **Cough peak expiratory flow and cough strength using a white card test** are additional methods to assess readiness for extubation.

Steps for Performing Tracheal Extubation

Step 1: Planning

A successful weaning trial should progress to extubation. All the clinical parameters and weaning indices should be rechecked. Airway patency using the cuff leak test should be checked. A positive cuff leak test (no air leaking past the cuff) may indicate upper airway edema, suggesting that the patient may not be suitable for extubation. Risk assessment for reintubation should be performed, considering general and specific airway risk factors. High-risk factors include pre-existing airway difficulties, obesity, OSA, risk of aspiration, and airway changes due to trauma or edema.

Step 2: Prepare for extubation and possibility of extubation failure .

For airway, consider any impediments to bag-mask ventilation, to do direct laryngoscopy or cuff leak test. Clear upper and lower airway secretions. Do gastric decompression by suctioning nasogastric tube. Consider assessment of surgical airway access in high risk' patients.

Logistics and equipment should be arranged in priori. Monitoring equipment and skilled assistance as per patient risk assessment (consider need for anesthetist, surgeon if difficulty anticipated) should be done. Anticipate what oxygen delivery method patient will be extubated to HFNC, nasal prongs or NIV. Consider NIV in selected 'at risk ' patients especially COAD, LVF, OSA, obesity. Advanced airway techniques and equipment, difficult airway trolley, surgical airway should be at bedside as per patient risk assessment. Personal protective gears like goggles, gown, gloves +/- mask, hand hygiene should be acquired. Bag mask valve device should be connected to oxygen and functioning, suction checked and functioning, with yankaeur suction catheter attached.

A reintubation plan must be communicated to all team members for all patients being extubated. This may include advanced airway techniques and clear team role delineation, equipment checked and on airway trolley and the airway trolley at bedside until deemed safe by attending consultant. The key question for the consultant is whether it is safe to remove the tube. If the answer is no then postpone extubation and consider tracheostomy.

Step 3: Perform extubation

First, optimise patient position (head up), suction oral airway and aspirate subglottic port if present to remove excess secretions. Pre-oxygenate patient with 100% oxygen. Loosen the endotracheal tube securing device and instruct patient to inhale. Attach the 10 ml syringe to the pilot tube and deflate the cuff fully. Remove the ETT when the patient starts to exhale. Suction the patients oropharynx post-extubation to again remove excess secretions. Ask the patient to cough. FiO_2 and the type of oxygen delivery will be determined according to clinical situation, e.g HFNC is common first choice. NIV for high risk patients like COPD. Dispose of contaminated material appropriately and document extubation.

Step 4: Post-extubation

Life threatening complications following extubation are not limited to the immediate post-extubation period. Staffing of 1:1 nursing until airway reflexes have returned and the patient is physiologically stable should be considered. This may take 4 hours or more. Vital monitoring like respiratory rate, heart rate, blood pressure, oxygen saturations, work of breathing, secretion clearance, level of consciousness and a post-extubation ABG at 30 minutes should be done. A capnography for high risk obese/OSA patients is useful. A difficult airway trolley at bedside should be immediately available. Stridor, obstructed pattern of breathing and agitation are early signs of airway obstruction and precede a fall in oxygen saturation. A patient who is agitated or complains of difficulty breathing should never be ignored even if objective signs are normal.

STRATEGIES FOR PROLONG MECHANICAL VENTILATION AND WEANING

Patients requiring more than 21 days of mechanical ventilation (MV) requires a structured approach for management and weaning.[9]

About 6–10% of people getting intubated will end up on prolong mechanical ventilation (MV).[25–27] The duration is dependent of underlying pathology—mostly chronic respiratory disease, neuromuscular disorder and spinal cord injuries.[28]

Following approach is suggested for weaning (Fig. 21.2).

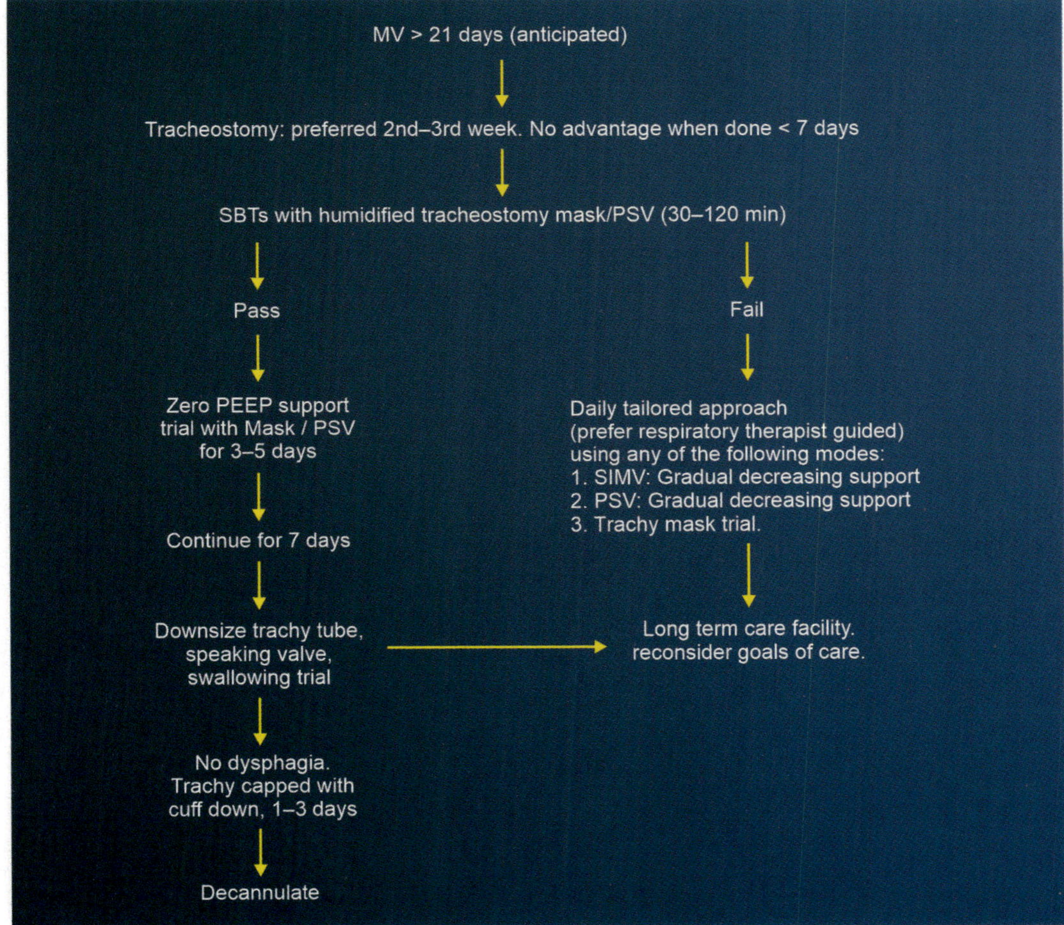

Fig. 21.2: Approach to prolong mechanical ventilation and weaning[9]

POST-EXTUBATION STRATEGIES

It is quite natural to for the ICU team to feel elated after liberating a patient from the mechanical ventilator. However, it is important to realise that the immediate phase after extubation needs utmost care and attention. The first 24 hours after extubation are difficult, and the possibility of failure or even chances of reintubation do exist. In the following section various strategies in such a situation, including the indications, outcomes and evidence will be discussed. Some of the interventions can be the use of non-invasive ventilation, high flow nasal canula and a simple venturi mask, which are targeted towards augmenting work of breathing and to maintain adequate oxygenation.

Approximately 10–20% of those patients who are extubated after a successful spontaneous breathing trial (SBT) require reintubation within 48–72 hours.[29]

Studies have shown that reintubation has several adverse effects, including prolonged ventilation, ventilator associated infections, increasing cost of healthcare and higher mortality.[30]

Post-extubation ARF can be due to several causes, including hypoxia, increased respiratory workload and ventilatory insufficiency.

High-flow nasal cannula oxygenation (HFNC) (**Fig. 21.3**), noninvasive positive-pressure ventilation (NPPV) and conventional oxygen therapy (COT) are available modalities after a residual or persisting respiratory failure post-extubation. NPPV has been shown to be effective in preventing reintubation after a planned extubation in high-risk patients.NPPV can increase the minute volume, wash out excessive CO_2, and reduce the work of breathing (WOB), however, NPPV also can cause complications, including aspiration pneumonia, mask (interface) intolerance, and in some cases patient discomfort. HFNC on the other hand can offset the complications of NPPV by delivering high concentrations of humidified oxygen via a nasal cannula. However, contradictory results from multiple studies have been shown.[31,32]

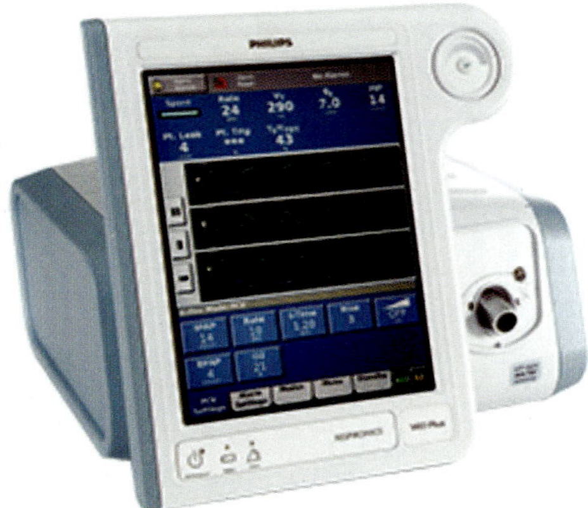

Fig. 21.3: High-flow nasal cannula (HFNC) the philips V60 plus ventilator integrates non-invasive ventilation (NIV) and high flow therapy (HFT) on one device

In this context a large network meta-analysis (NMA) by Yasuda and his colleagues[33] from Japan was to evaluate the three main strategies (NPPV/HFNC/COT) in reducing the mortality and reintubation risk. It is worth mentioning that out of the 15 studies, none had compared all the three interventions head to head. In this meta-analysis of 2600 patients, short term mortality was less in NPPV/HFNC compared to COT, reintubation again was less in both HFNC and NPPV compared to COT. There was no long term mortality benefit either in NPPV or HFNC. HFNC has shown to be superior to COT with regards to reintubation. Regarding efficacy in reducing the post-extubation respiratory failure, HFNC is better than NIV, and both these interventions are better than COT.

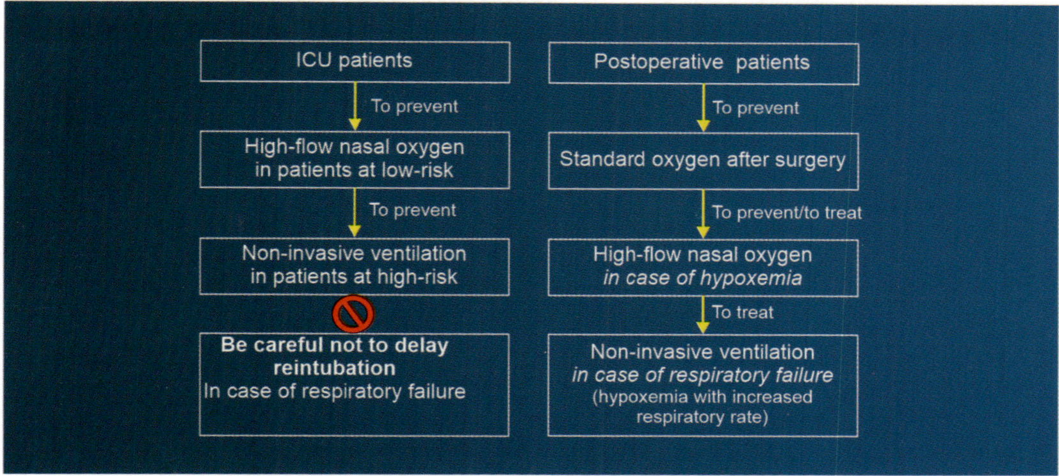

Fig. 21.4: Proposal of management of oxygenation strategies to prevent or treat respiratory failure in patients extubated in ICUs and in postoperative patients (*Courtesy:* AW Thille, et al journal of intensive medicine1 (2021) 65–70)

Yasuda et al conclude "that it is important to choose an appropriate strategy to prevent reintubation after extubation. Both NPPV and HFNC are associated with a lower reintubation rate than COT; therefore, physicians can choose a strategy according to the patient's respiratory physiology status and preference".

It is worth examining the evidence for the best strategy after post-extubation respiratory failure. In patients at low risk of extubation failure, HFNC can be an alternative strategy that may reduce the risk of reintubation as compared with standard oxygen therapy (SOT).[34,32] However in patients with high risk for reintubation, (extubation failure) several clinical trials have shown that compared with standard oxygen, NIV can reduce the post-extubation respiratory failure and eventually the need for reintubation.[35,36]

Another large scale study showed that the reintubation rates after extubation are reduced significantly when HFNC is used in an alternating fashion with NIV.[37]

Thille et al[38] have classified these patients into low risk and high risk for extubation failure.

Low risk: High flow nasal oxygen (HFNC) alone might be the most effective strategy for oxygenation **(Box 21.1)**.

High risk: HFNC can be used alternating with non invasive positive pressure ventilation (NPPV)

Thille et al also have separated those patients with post-extubation respiratory failure in postoperative situation versus those with respiratory failure in ICU after extubation **(Fig. 12.4)** since the optimal oxygenation strategy differs in these two groups. Extubations done after surgery usually have a good recovery, and may require standard oxygen therapy for a few hours before they recover completely. However those postoperative extubation patients developing respiratory failure eventually go to the ICU, and may constitute nearly 20% and may need prolonged ventilation and post-extubation respiratory failure.[39,40]

Box 21.1: High flow nasal oxygen

High Flow Nasal Oxygen

Advantages: Compact, portable and easy to use

HFNCs deliver heated and humidified 100% oxygen at a flow rate of up to 60 liters per minute. The oxygen is delivered through nasal prongs. All settings can be adjusted independently giving more control to the clinician

Mechanism High flow (60 litres per minute) provides positive pressure support, which can improve the tidal volume, and thus increase minute volume, which in turn can wash out CO_2 provides

Positive end expiratory pressure (PEEP), which increases alveolar recruitment, and thus better oxygenation

Removes the pharyngeal dead space, which can further improve gas exchange

Reduces work of breathing (WOB) as the flow rates are high, to match inspiratory flow

Reduces respiratory rate (RR) as treatment progresses, thus reducing patient distress

Since the gas mixture is heated and humidified, chances of mucosal injury are less, and patient comfort is more

Other Uses Acute respiratory failure due to COVID-19. Respiratory failure due to pulmonary fibrosis, pneumonia, COPD, cancer, and congestive heart failure.

Adverse Effects Can cause dry mouth, nasal trauma, rarely pneumothorax

Oxygen Strategies for patients extubated in ICU

Official ERS/ATS clinical practice guidelines (2017) recommend noninvasive ventilation (*see* **Fig. 21.5**) for acute respiratory failure in these patients.[41] Pooled data from various studies showed a benefit of NIV over other strategies like HFNC, including reduction in reintubations, and even risk of mortality.[42] It is important to note that unlike HFNC, NIV needs a longer learning curve to train the team.

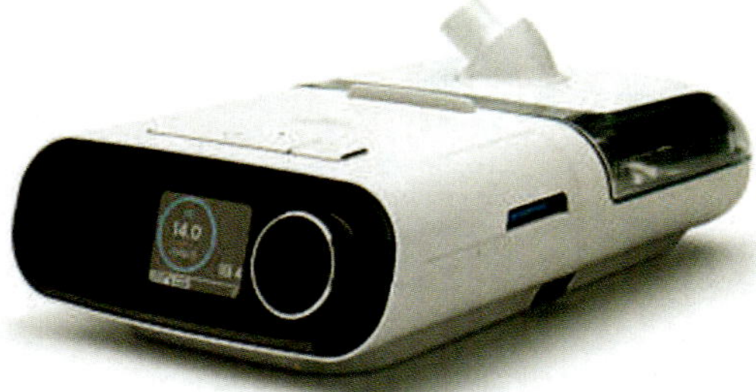

Fig. 21.5: NIV (BIPAP) dream station (Philips)

NIV can be applied for varying periods. Some studies have used it for 24 hours, 48 hours and 8 to 18 hours. NIV is particularly indicated where patient has hypercapnia ($paCO_2$ >45 mm Hg). In another large study involving 641 patients Thille[37] showed that using NIV and HFNC alternatingly gave very good results, with number of patients requiring reintubation to be much less, compared to using HFNC alone. Although NIV is very useful in cases with hypercapnia, even in those without hypercapnia, outcomes with NIV were better than HFNC (13% vs 19%). However, the ATS/ERS guidelines

(2017) has given a conditional recommendation for NIV in high-risk post-extubation respiratory failure **(Box 21.2)**. However in the last 7 years after these guidelines newer studies have demonstrated a clear advantage for the use of NIV and HFNC alternatingly than using HFNC alone.

Post-extubation respiratory failure in a low-risk setting **(Box 21.3)**: Maggiore et al[34] showed in a study of 105 patients randomised, that HFNC gave better results (reintubation rates) than delivering oxygen through venturi mask (standard oxygen therapy). Hernandez with a bigger group of 527 patients[32] of post-extubation respiratory failure, with low risk for reintubation showed that reintubation rates with HFNC better than SOT (5% vs 12%).

Box 21.2: Patients at high-risk of extubation failure

Patients at high risk of extubation failure

1. Age >65 years
2. Pre-existing heart disease
3. Pre-existing lung disease
4. Other co-morbidities
5. Prolonged ventilation
6. Hypercapnia at the time of weaning

Box 21.3: Low-risk patients for extubation

- Age <65 years
- No co-morbidities
- Ventilation <7 days
- Not obese
- Extubated after the first spontaneous breathing trial
- Normal $paCO_2$ at the time of extubation
- No laryngeal edema
- Able to clear secretions on their own

Box 21.4: Non-invasive ventilation

- Delivers pressure support along with required oxygen
- Improves tidal volume and minute volume
- Can wash out the CO_2
- It is non-invasive, uses a mask interface
- Can be used on and off to facilitate patient comfort
- Modes like average volume assured pressure support are useful in certain settings
- Needs well trained staff
- Needs close monitoring
- Pressures for inspiration and expiration need to be set (usually the EPAP is 1/3 of IPAP)

Are there any risks in using NIV for post-extubation respiratory failure?: One of the most important risk perhaps is perhaps spending too much of time on NIV, delaying intubation when needed and thus increasing the mortality.[43] Esteban et al, conducted a large clinical trial involving 221 patients of post-extubation respiratory failure, showed greater mortality than with standard oxygen therapy with venturi mask[43], although reintubation rates (48%) were similar, mortality was higher with NIV (25% vs 14%).

These end results were perhaps due to the delay in reintubation in the NIV group. This lead to the ATS/ERS guidelines to advise that NIV should not be used for post-extubation respiratory failure.

The corollary to this recommendation is those patients whose $paCO_2$ was > 45 mmHg as a result of chronic lung disease will benefit from NIV. However the fact remains that nearly 50% of patients with post-extubation respiratory failure in ICU are intubated again with a mortality of >30%

It may conclude that NIV may be used in post-extubation respiratory failure in ICU, with caution in those with underlying chronic lung disease and hypercapnia. It is important to recognize failure of NIV to improve the parameters and quickly decide to change strategy including reintubation.

Efficacy of HFNC has been reported in *de novo* respiratory failure[44], its role in post-extubation respiratory failure needs to be elucidated further.

TAKE HOME MESSAGE

1. **Weaning and Extubation Process:** Weaning involves a gradual reduction in ventilator support, transitioning the patient towards spontaneous breathing, with extubation marking the removal of the artificial airway. It is crucial to begin the weaning process early to prevent complications related to prolonged mechanical ventilation.
2. **Assessment and Readiness:** Evaluating the patient's readiness for weaning is essential, using both clinical judgment and objective parameters such as spontaneous breathing trials (SBTs). Proper assessment minimizes the risk of weaning and extubation failure.
3. **Spontaneous Breathing Trials** (SBTs): SBTs are a key tool in determining whether a patient can successfully be extubated. Daily SBTs are more effective compared to gradual reduction methods like pressure support ventilation (PSV) or synchronized intermittent mandatory ventilation (SIMV).
4. **Predictive Indices:** Weaning indices, like the rapid shallow breathing index (RSBI), are useful in predicting weaning success, guiding clinicians in their decision-making. Ultrasonography can also aid in assessing diaphragm function to predict weaning outcomes.
5. **Extubation and Post-extubation Care:** Extubation should be carefully planned and monitored, considering airway patency and potential risks for reintubation. After extubation, close observation for the first 24 hours is critical, as this period carries a significant risk of respiratory failure.
6. **Post-Extubation Strategies:** For patients at risk of post-extubation respiratory failure, interventions like high-flow nasal cannula (HFNC) or non-invasive positive pressure ventilation (NPPV) can help reduce reintubation rates. The choice between these strategies should be tailored to the patient's condition.
7. **Clinical Decision-Making:** Recognizing when to change strategies, such as opting for reintubation if non-invasive methods fail, is vital to patient outcomes. Prolonged use of NPPV without improvement can lead to worsened outcomes if it delays necessary reintubation.

In summary, successful weaning and extubation require a systematic approach, continuous evaluation, and readiness to adapt the strategy to the patient's evolving clinical status to ensure safety and minimize complications.

References

1. Tobin MJ. Mechanical ventilation. N Engl J Med. 1994 Apr 14;330(15):1056–61.
2. Esteban A, Alía I, Ibañez J, Benito S, Tobin MJ. Modes of mechanical ventilation and weaning. A national survey of Spanish hospitals. The Spanish Lung Failure Collaborative Group. Chest. 1994 Oct;106(4):1188–93.
3. Boles JM, Bion J, Connors A, Herridge M, Marsh B, Melot C, et al. Weaning from mechanical ventilation. Eur Respir J 2007;29(5): 1033–56. DOI: 10.1183/09031936.00010206.
4. Ely EW, Baker AM, Dunagan DP, Burke HL, Smith AC, Kelly PT, et al. Effect on the duration of mechanical ventilation of identifying patients capable of breathing spontaneously. N Engl J Med 1996;335(25):1864–69. DOI: 10.1056/NEJM199612193352502.
5. Clerk AM, Shah RJ, Kothari J, et al. Position Statement of ISCCM Committee on Weaning from Mechanical Ventilator. Indian J Crit Care Med. 2024;28(Suppl 2):S233-S248. doi:10.5005/jp-journals-10071–24716.
6. Tobin MJ. Role and interpretation of weaning predictors. As presented at the 5th International Consensus Conference in Intensive Care Medicine: Weaning from Mechanical Ventilation. Hosted by ERS, ATS, ESICM, SCCM and SRLF; Budapest, April 28–29, 2005. Available at www.ersnet.org/ers/lr/browse/default.aspx?id52814.
7. Burns KEA, Rizvi L, Cook DJ, et al. Ventilator Weaning and Discontinuation Practices for Critically Ill Patients. JAMA. 2021;325(12):1173-1184. doi:10.1001/jama.2021.2384
8. Béduneau G, Pham T, Schortgen F, et al. Epidemiology of Weaning Outcome according to a New Definition. The WIND Study. Am J Respir Crit Care Med. 2017;195(6):772–783. doi:10.1164/rccm.201602–0320OC.
9. Dolinay T, Hsu L, Maller A, Walsh BC, Szu cs A, Jerng,J S, Jun D. Ventilator Weaning in Prolonged Mechanical Ventilation—A Narrative Review. J. Clin. Med. **2024**, 13,1909. https://doi.org/10.3390/ jcm13071909 .
10. MacIntyre NR, Epstein SK, Carson S, et al. Management of patients requiring prolonged mechanical ventilation: report of a NAMDRC consensus conference. Chest. 2005;128(6):3937–54. doi:10.1378/chest.128.6.3937.
11. MacIntyre NR. Evidence-based ventilator weaning and discontinuation. Respir Care. 2004;49(7):830–36.
12. Esteban A, Frutos F, Tobin MJ, Alia I, Solsona JF, Valverdu I, et al. A comparison of four methods of weaning patients from mechanical ventilation. Spanish Lung Failure Collaborative Group. N Engl J Med 1995;332(6):345–50.
13. Brochard L, Rauss A, Benito S, Conti G, Mancebo J, Rekik N, et al. Comparison of three methods of gradual withdrawal from ventilatory support during weaning from mechanical ventilation. Am J Respir Crit Care Med 1994;150(4):896–903.
14. Subirà C, Hernández G, Vázquez A, Rodríguez-García R, González-Castro A, García C, et al. Effect of Pressure Support vs T-Piece Ventilation Strategies During Spontaneous Breathing Trials on Successful Extubation Among Patients Receiving Mechanical Ventilation: A Randomized Clinical Trial. JAMA. 2019 Jun 11;321(22):2175–82.
15. Thille AW, Gacouin A, Coudroy R, Ehrmann S, Quenot JP, Nay MA, et al. Spontaneous-Breathing Trials with Pressure-Support Ventilation or a T-Piece. N Engl J Med. 2022 Nov 17;387(20):1843–54.

16. Sklar MC, Burns K, Rittayamai N, Lanys A, Rauseo M, Chen L, et al. Effort to breathe with various spontaneous breathing trial techniques. A physiologic meta-analysis. Am J Respir Crit Care Med 2017;195(11):1477–85. DOI: 10.1164/rccm.201607-1338OC
17. Pellegrini JA, Moraes RB, Maccari JG, de Oliveira RP, Savi A, Ribeiro RA, et al. Spontaneous breathing trials with t-piece or pressure support ventilation. Respir Care 2016;61(12):1693–1703. DOI: 10.4187/ respcare.04816 .
18. Sklar MC, Burns K, Rittayamai N, Lanys A, Rauseo M, Chen L, et al. Effort to breathe with various spontaneous breathing trial techniques. A physiologic meta-analysis. Am J Respir Crit Care Med 2017;195(11):1477–1485. DOI: 10.1164/rccm.201607-1338OC
19. Yang KL, Tobin MJ. A prospective study of indexes predicting the outcome of trials of weaning from mechanical ventilation. N Engl J Med 1991;324(21):1445–50. DOI: 10.1056/NEJM1991052332 42101.
20. Trivedi V, Chaudhuri D, Jinah R, Piticaru J, Agarwal A, Liu K, et al. The usefulness of the rapid shallow breathing index in predicting successful extubation: A systematic review and meta-analysis. Chest 2022;161(1):97–111. DOI: 10.1016/j.chest.2021.06.030.
21. Lerolle N, Guérot E, Dimassi S, et al. Ultrasonographic diagnostic criterion for severe diaphragmatic dysfunction after cardiac surgery. Chest. 2009;135(2):401-407. doi:10.1378/chest.08–1531.
22. Akella P, Voigt LP, Chawla S. To Wean or Not to Wean: A Practical Patient Focused Guide to Ventilator Weaning. J Intensive Care Med. 2022;37(11):1417–25. doi:10.1177/08850666221095436
23. Cook TM, Woodall N, Harper J, Benger J; Fourth National Audit Project. Major complications of airway management in the UK: results of the Fourth National Audit Project of the Royal College of Anaesthetists and the Difficult Airway Society. Part 2: intensive care and emergency departments. Br J Anaesth. 2011;106(5):632–42.
24. Xu SS, Tian Y, Ma YJ, et al. Development of a Prediction Score for Evaluation of Extubation Readiness in Neurosurgical Patients with Mechanical Ventilation. Anesthesiology. 2023;139(5):614-627. doi:10.1097/ALN.0000000000004721.
25. Scheinhorn DJ, Hassenpflug MS, Votto JJ, Chao DC, Epstein SK, Doig GS, Knight EB, Petrak RA. Ventilation Outcomes Study Group. Post-ICU mechanical ventilation at 23 long-term care hospitals: A multicenter outcomes study. Chest 2007, 131, 85–93
26. Lone NI, Walsh TS. Prolonged mechanical ventilation in critically ill patients: Epidemiology, outcomes and modelling the potential cost consequences of establishing a regional weaning unit. Crit. Care 2011, 15, R102.
27. Jubran A, Grant BJB, Duffner LA, Collins EG, Lanuza DM, Hoffman LA, Tobin MJ. Long-Term Outcome after Prolonged Mechanical Ventilation. A Long-Term Acute-Care Hospital Study. Am. J. Respir. Crit. Care Med. 2019, 199, 1508–16.
28. Sahetya S, Allgood S, Gay PC, Lechtzin N. Long-Term Mechanical Ventilation. Clin. Chest Med. 2016, 37, 753–63.
29. Thille AW, Richard JC, Brochard L. The decision to extubate in the intensive care unit. Am J Respir Crit Care Med. 2013;187:1294–302.
30. Sellares J, Ferrer M, Cano E, Loureiro H, Valencia M, Torres A. Predictors of prolonged weaning and survival during ventilator weaning in a respiratory ICU. Intensive Care Med. 2011;37:775–84.
31. Fernandez R, Subira C, Frutos-Vivar F, Rialp G, Laborda C, Masclans JR,et al. High-flow nasal cannula to prevent postextubation respiratory failure in high-risk non-hypercapnic patients: a randomized multicenter trial. Ann Intensive Care. 2017;7:47.

32. Hernández G, Vaquero C, González P, Subira C, Frutos-Vivar F, Rialp G, et al. Effect of postextubation high-flow nasal cannula vs conventional oxygen therapy on reintubation in low-risk patients: a randomized clinical trial. JAMA. 2016;315:1354–61.
33. Yasuda H, Okano H, Mayumi T, et al. Post-extubation oxygenation strategies in acute respiratory failure: a systematic review and network meta-analysis. Crit Care. 2021;25(1):135. Published 2021 Apr 9. doi:10.1186/s13054-021-03550-4.
34. Maggiore SM, Idone FA, Vaschetto R, Festa R, Cataldo A, Antonicelli F, et al. Nasal high-flow versus Venturi mask oxygen therapy after extubation. Effects on oxygena- tion, comfort, and clinical outcome. Am J Respir Crit Care Med 2014;190(3):282–8. doi: 10.1164/rccm.201402-0364OC
35. Nava S, Gregoretti C, Fanfulla F, Squadrone E, Grassi M, Carlucci A, et al. Noninvasive ventilation to prevent respiratory failure after extubation in high-risk patients. Crit Care Med 2005;33(11):2465–70.
36. Ferrer M, Valencia M, Nicolas JM, Bernadich O, Badia JR, Torres A. Early noninvasive ventilation averts extubation failure in patients at risk: a randomized trial. Am J Respir Crit Care Med 2006;173(2):164–70. doi: 10.1164/rccm.200505–718OC
37. Thille AW, Muller G, Gacouin A, Coudroy R, Decavèle M, Sonneville R, et al. Effect of Postextubation High-Flow Nasal Oxygen With Noninvasive Ventilation vs High-Flow Nasal Oxygen Alone on Reintubation Among Patients at High Risk of Extubation Failure: a Randomized Clinical Trial. JAMA 2019;322(15):1465–75. doi: 10.1001/jama.2019.14901.
38. Thille AW, Wairy M, Pape SL, Frat JP. Oxygenation strategies after extubation of critically ill and postoperative patients. J Intensive Med. 2021;1(2):65–70. Published 2021 Jun 29. doi:10.1016/j.jointm.2021.05.003
39. Peñuelas O, Frutos-Vivar F, Fernández C, Anzueto A, Epstein SK, Apezteguía C, et al. Characteristics and outcomes of ventilated patients according to time to liberation from mechanical ventilation. Am J Respir Crit Care Med 2011;184(4):430–7. doi: 10.1164/rccm.201011-1887OC .
40. Esteban A, Frutos-Vivar F, Muriel A, Ferguson ND, Peñuelas O, Abraira V, et al. Evolution of mortality over time in patients receiving mechanical ventilation. Am J Respir Crit Care Med 2013;188(2):220–30. doi: 10.1164/rccm.201212–2169OC .
41. Rochwerg B, Brochard L, Elliott MW, Hess D, Hill NS, Nava S, et al. Official ERS/ATS clinical practice guidelines: noninvasive ventilation for acute respiratory failure. Eur Respir J 2017;50(2). doi: 10.1183/13993003.02426-2016 .
42. Vargas F, Clavel M, Sanchez-Verlan P, Garnier S, Boyer A, Bui HN, et al. Intermittent noninvasive ventilation after extubation in patients with chronic respiratory disorders: a multicenter randomized controlled trial (VHYPER). Intensive Care Med 2017;43(11):1626–36. doi: 10.1007/s00134-017-4785-1 .
43. Esteban A, Frutos-Vivar F, Ferguson ND, Arabi Y, Apezteguía C, González M, et al. Noninvasive positive-pressure ventilation for respiratory failure after extubation. N Engl J Med 2004;350(24):2452–60. doi: 10.1056/NEJMoa032736
44. Frat JP, Thille AW, Mercat A, Girault C, Ragot S, Perbet S, et al. High-flow oxy- gen through nasal cannula in acute hypoxemic respiratory failure. N Engl J Med 2015;372(23):2185–96. doi: 10.1056/NEJMoa1503326.

CHAPTER 22

Novel Modes of Ventilation

❐ Anand Vinaykumar Joshi ❐ Chandresh Kumar Sudani

INTRODUCTION

The discovery and application of positive pressure ventilation has resulted in the ability to manage many disease states that previously had limited treatment options, with the classic example being poliomyelitis in the 1950s.[1] There are two main goals of positive pressure mechanical ventilation:

1. To provide adequate gas exchange support
2. Minimise lung injury while doing so.

Positive pressure ventilation are only support technologies, not therapeutic technologies. They cannot be expected to "cure" disease, but only "buy time" so as other treatment act or patient has his own healing. When a patient is kept on mechanical ventilation, there is fundamental change in breathing pattern from patient's own to the one given by ventilator. Loss of patients own breathing effort (as in case of cardiac arrest or respiratory arrest) or induction of sedation and paralysis, makes this transition easier. However, difficulty arises when patient needs to be transitioned back to his own breathing and extubated. This phase requires a synchrony between patients own breathing and one delivered by mechanical ventilator. Any mismatch at this phase leads to patient-ventilator dyssynchrony. To understand the problem, it is important to know breath physiology in patient and ventilator, which are described below. In this chapter, we will overview problems of ADULT conventional modes of ventilation and newer modes that tries to address these problem.

BREATHING: PHYSIOLOGY VS MECHANICAL VENTILATORY BREATHS

The physics of normal breathing are based on pressure difference between lungs and outside atmosphere. The diaphragm contracts with its downward motion, creating a negative intrathoracic pressure. This along with ribcage expansion cause inspiration with air flowing in and expiration with air flowing out balancing the pressure. The physiological trigger comes from respiratory centres in brain, as a part of neuro-ventilatory coupling. **Figure 22.1** outlines physiological trigger leading to breath in a normal non-ventilated person. This kind of breath generated is termed as negative pressure ventilation.

Ventilator delivers breath completely in a non-breathing patient. The machine requires a signal (called trigger) to initiate breath—done by opening of inspiratory valve (and closing expiratory valve), limit the amount of air flow-done by setting volume or pressure and stopping the breath (called cycling)-done by opening expiratory valve (and closed inspiratory valve). The breath generated here induces positive pressure in thorax (as against the negative pressure in non- ventilated spontaneous breathing patient), hence it is termed as positive pressure ventilation.

In Spontaneously Breathing patient on mechanical ventilator, there need to be a synchrony between the patient and machine. With the Neuro-ventilatory signal reaching diaphragm and causing contraction, a negative pressure (in pressure trigger) or a change in flow (in flow trigger) is sensed by machine. Usually the time interval between respiratory centre signal output and the ventilator triggered inspiratory flow is around 60–80 milli second. This signals opening up inspiratory valve. The rest of the breath follows as per ventilatory breath with either flow (in volume control) or pressure (in pressure control) limit setting. Closing of inspiratory valve and opening of expiratory valve (Cycling) will again be determined by percentage fraction of flow setting or time. This will also be a positive pressure ventilation breath.

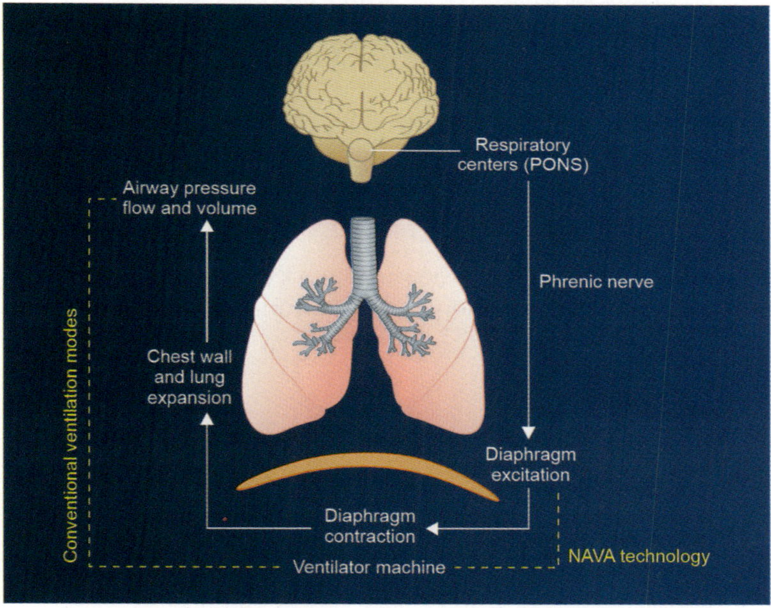

Fig. 22.1: Trigger pathway for physiological neuro-ventilatory coupling

OPEN LOOP AND CLOSE LOOP VENTILATION[2]

The previous generation ventilators had basic modes that delivered breath as per set parameters. These modes are called classic/conventional modes. Volume control, pressure control, pressure support and synchronised intermittent mandatory ventilation (SIMV) are conventional modes. These modes deliver the set parameters and take no feedback from patient's changing variables. Hence they are also called "Open loop" modes, where feedback loop is absent. In open loop system, the clinician takes feedback from patients physiological variables such as peripheral oxygen saturation (SpO_2), end-tidal CO_2 ($etCO_2$) blood gas analysis (pH, $PaCO_2$, PaO_2), etc. and sets or changes the parameters on ventilator. Thus, with clinician in between, the feedback is completed.

This makes it a labor intensive and time consuming. Clinician's presence is always required to adjust ventilator setting, especially if the patient's variables changes and there is a need to accommodate new therapeutic needs. When clinician is not there, the ventilator is unable to respond to changing patient variables and becomes insufficient to patients requirement, leading to either poorly or not protective ventilated LUNG with possible dire consequence.

With advance technologies and introduction of computer chips, newer ventilators have been able to make alterations with changing patient variables and take feedback from patient breath, thus completing feedback loop. They are called "Closed loop" modes, where feedback loop is present. All the modes included in "closed loop mode" are termed newer/non-conventional modes/novel modes of mechanical ventilators. In these modes—the control, cycle, or the limit variables undergo self—adjustment. Without limiting themselves to a single set parameters, based on feedback loop, they change from one variable to another within determined safety limits. This adjustments occur either in subsequent breath or in more advance techniques within a single breath. There can be entirely different breath delivery based on continuous feedback from patient variables. Thus, the clinicians role in open system is taken over by the computer feedback and his focus changes to choosing patient targets rather than individual parameters and regulating variables that supplement the ventilation such as hemodynamics and monitoring.

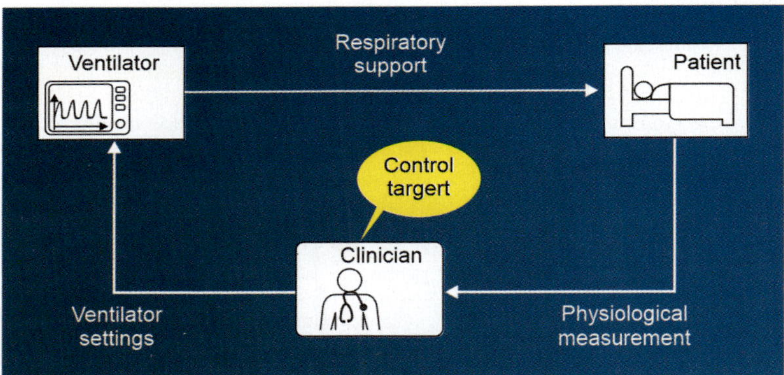

Fig. 22.2: Clinician in loop control system—open loop system

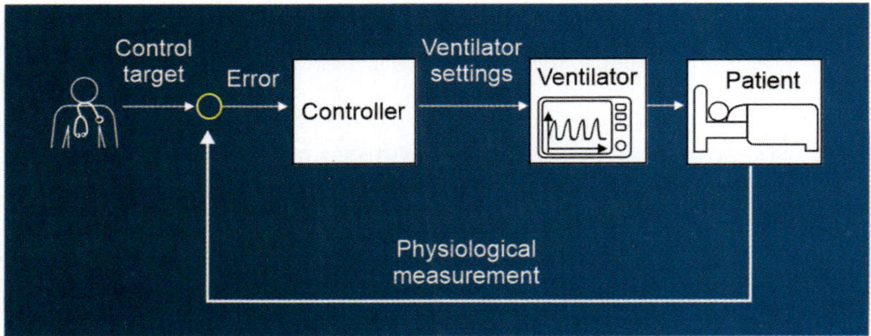

Fig. 22.3: Clinician out of loop control system—closed loop system

Disadvantages of Conventional Mode

1. Ventilator induced lung injury (VILI): A positive pressure ventilation is known to cause alveolar injury by alveolar overstretch at end of inspiration (over distension) and cyclic atelectasis - recruitment due to positive pressure breath. There are several contributing factors including repetitive insults from a fixed breath parameters and associated cytokine release and bacterial translocation.
2. Trigger delay or missed breaths, that exaggerates auto-PEEP or leak
3. Patient - ventilator dyssynchrony as ventilator parameters does not adopt to changing patient needs
4. High dose of sedation and paralysis required for control modes, leading to ventilator associated pneumonia (VAP), neuromyopathy (CINM), and ventilator induced diaphragmatic dysfunction (VIDD)
5. Hemodynamic compromise and weaning from ventilator may also get delayed due to dyssynchrony.

NEWER MODES/ NON-CONVENTIONAL MODES/NOVEL MODES[3–5]

The newer modes have solved some of the problems of conventional modes but still quest for one ideal single mode awaits. These modes are mostly patented by a particular ventilator company hence the nomenclature is associated with that ventilator. Some of the popular modes available are shown in **Table 22.1**.

Table 22.1: Newer modes of ventilator

Mode name	Ventilator company
PRVC (pressure regulated volume control)	Servo-i maquette ventilator
VAPS (volume assured pressure support)	T-Bird AVS III, Bird 8400 Ti
NeoGanesh (smart care)	Evita xl, Evita XL Neo (Drager)
(PAV+) propotional assist ventilation	Puritan Bennett 840
NAVA (neurally adjusted ventilatory assistance)	Servo-i ventilator
Adaptive support ventilation (ASV)	Hamilton medical; Galileo Drager; Evita
APRV (airway pressure release ventilation)	Drager medical Evita, Viasys Avea Bileve, Puritan Bennette 840
HFOV (high frequency oscillating ventilator)	

Novel modes can be classified based on its ability to address aspect of conventional mode disadvantage. Some of the popular modes are discussed in following script.

MODES FOR BETTER PATIENT VENTILATOR INTERACTION

Patient ventilatory synchrony is an important challenge while ventilating a lightly sedated and weaning patient. With conventional mode it is difficult to adjust the dynamic breathing pattern of the patient. Introduction of closed loop feedback seems to offer a bit of better coordination and patient comfort. *Example are:* PRVC,VAPS, SMART Care, Proportional Assist Ventilation (PAV), NAVA.

1. Pressure Regulated Volume Control (PRVC) Mode

This is a dual mode, which includes advantage of both volume control and pressure control modes. Here, Two Different Breaths, volume control breath and pressure control breath are seen. It is a control mode of ventilation (i.e Time triggered), pressure limited (decelerating flow) targeted to a set tidal volume and time cycled or flow cycled depending upon the breath. Here a set tidal volume is used as a feedback control to continuously adjust the pressure limit.

Table 22.2: Breath in PRVC

Control	Trigger	Limit	Target	Cycle
Dual: pressure and volume control	Patient or Time	Pressure (Flow in test breath)	Volume	Time

Main setting: Like in volume control tidal volume, respiratory rate, FiO_2 and PEEP are set. All alarm especially peak pressure alarm limit is set.

Breath: Ventilator gives initial couple (3–4) of volume control breath with set tidal volume as test breaths, it calculates the pressure required to reach that volume, and subsequent breaths are delivered with lowest possible pressure as a pressure control breath. Here, it is important to note that the pressure delivery will still be 5 cm H_2O less than the upper limit of pressure ALARM. The flowchart describes the continuous feedback loop under which this mode works (**Figs 22.4 and 22.5**).

Advantages

1. This mode delivers a decelerating inspiratory flow pattern with advantage of relative equal distribution in non-homogenous lungs, targeting set tidal volume.
2. Within set range, pressure automatically adjusts for changes in lung resistance and compliance

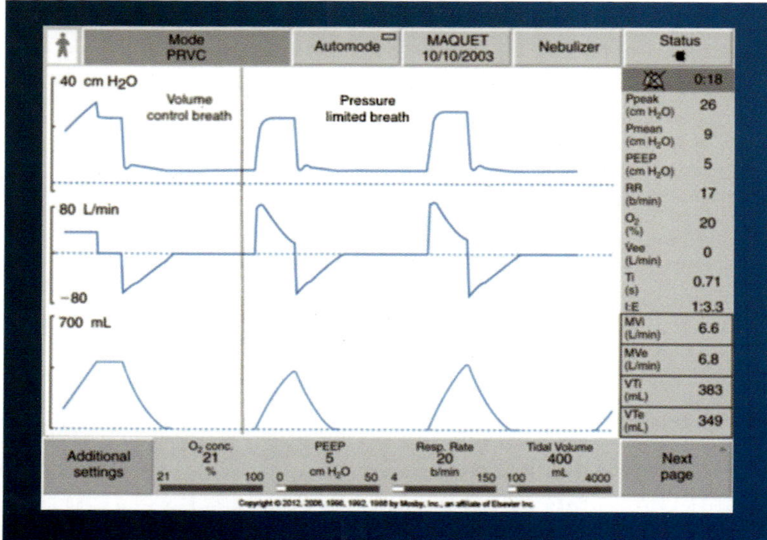

Fig. 22.4: PRVC graphics

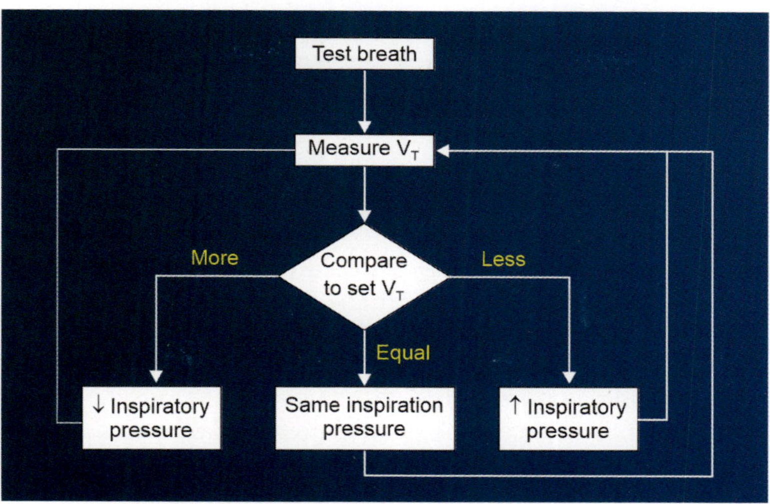

Fig 22.5: Feedback loop for PRVC mode

3. More or less, tidal volume is guaranteed
4. Prevents volutrauma by preventing excess of tidal volume delivered
5. Prevents hypoventilation by adjusting and ensuring the set tidal volume is delivered.

Disadvantages

1. Pressure delivered is dependent on tidal volume achieved on last breath. Hence with intermittent patient efforts, the tidal volume varies and confuses ventilator
2. In COPD or asthma, with dynamic pressure changes, the volume will not be delivered and feedback loop will not be effective.

Remark

Conceptually, PRVC mode seems to good mode for lung protective ventilation—setting 6–8 ml/kg of tidal volume and the ventilator would automatically adjust the applied inspiratory pressure with its synchronous variable flow feature to airway resistance. However, studies has revealed that some minority of patients got higher than targeted tidal volume. Whether this variability is an acceptable trade off needs to be seen.[6,7]

2. Volume Assured Pressure Support (VAPS)

This is also a dual mode incorporating both pressure control and volume control. However, both the pattern are seen in One Single Breath depending upon the patients lung compliance. A minimum desired tidal volume is assured. It start with pressure control breath and if at 25% of peak flow, targeted tidal volume is not reached, it switches to volume control breath and completes the tidal volume. There by increasing the inspiratory time and breaking the pressure limit. Thus a minimum volume is assured. This mode can be looked as opposite of PRVC mode. Here we set pressure limit for PC breath, but also minimum desired tidal volume, in case pressure limit does not deliver adequate tidal volume.

Table 22.3: Breath in VAPS				
Control	**Trigger**	**Limit**	**Target**	**Cycle**
Dual pressure and volume control	Patient	Pressure	Volume	Flow or Volume

Main settings: Pressure limit (as in PC mode), respiratory rate, FiO_2 and PEEP, minimum desired tidal volume.

Breath: Once triggered, ventilator give a pressure control breath, for a set pressure limit. If the delivered tidal volume is less than "set minimum tidal volume", then the breath changes to volume control to complete the "minimum set tidal volume". Here, as the breath changes from PC to VC, it breaches the peak pressure limit in order to deliver the minimum tidal volume. Thus, with this setting a minimum set tidal volume is assured. If the initial pressure control breath delivers tidal volume equal or more than set minimum tidal volume, no action occurs and a complete PC breath is delivered.

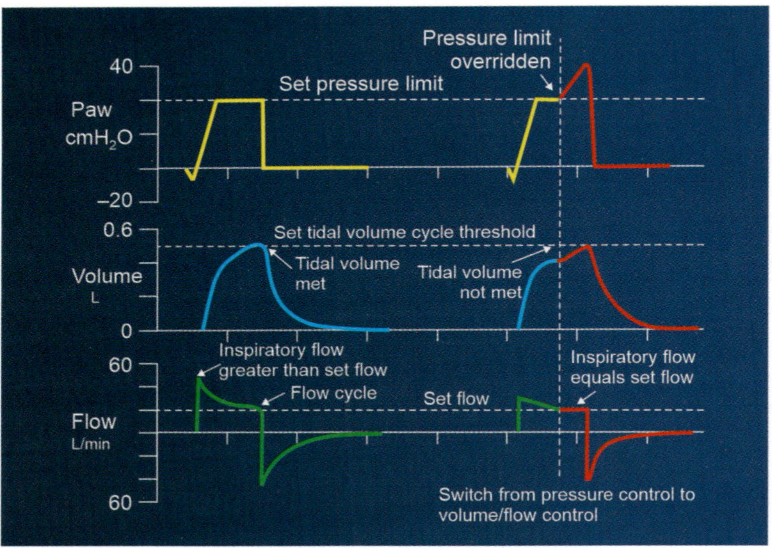

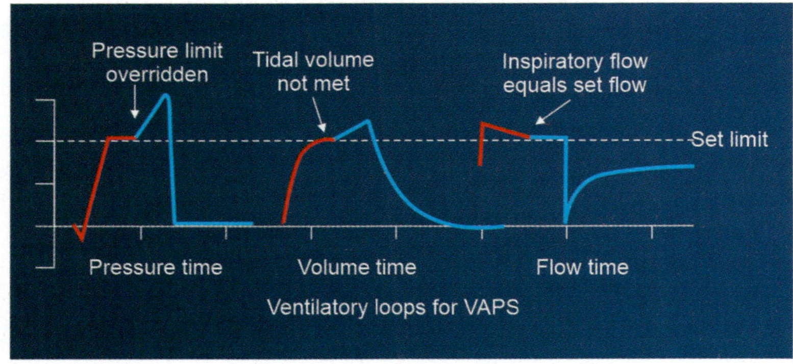

Fig. 22.6: VAPS graph

Advantage

Amato, *et al.*[8] showed that VAPS mode decreases work of breathing in dyspneic patients. There was also decrease in intrinsic PEEP and airway resistance. Overall better ventilator patient synchrony.

Disadvantage

It give same risk of barotrauma as that given by a volume control ventilation. When the delivered tidal volume is less than desired tidal volume (what ever be the reason, like change in compliance or increasing airway resistance), the ventilator changes to volume control increasing the peak airway pressure. Here setting minimum desired tidal volume is important, as that will determine the risk of barotrauma.

3. Smart Care (NeoGanesh)

This is among the first modes to have an integrated artificial intelligence. It is a closed loop modification of pressure support ventilation. Its like a clinician sitting inside ventilator and changing the settings automatically based on patients respiratory parameters. The goal is to keep patient in "safe respiratory zone" and when patients efforts are getting better, to decrease the ventilatory support and wean off the patient (of course machine cannot extubate patient).

Table 22.4: Breath in smart care (NeoGanesh)

Control	Trigger	Limit	Target	Cycle
Pressure control and patient support	Patient	Pressure	Tidal volume and end Tidal CO_2	Flow

Main setting: Patients height (to calculate ideal body weight for tidal volume), sex, End Tidal CO_2 ($etCO_2$)-usually <55 mmHg and <65 mmHg for COPD, tidal volume (>300 ml or >250 if weight is <55 kg), respiratory rate targets (between 12 and 28 breaths/min), FiO_2 and PEEP. These parameters are "safe respiratory zone" for patients to be in. The ventilator is fed with algorithm that takes inputs from patients respiratory rate, end tidal CO_2 and tidal volume, and accordingly changes pressure support for breath (*see* **Table 22.2**).

Once patient reaches and stabilise normal parameters with minimal support, it advices clinician that "patient is ready for off ventilator and extubation".

Table of Smart Care Response (Table. 22.5)

Table 22.5: Smartcare ventilator response to feedback loop

Classification	F_{spn}	VT	$etCO_2$	SC response
Normal ventilation	OK	OK	OK	↑PS by 2 or 4
Insufficient ventilation	OK	⇩	OK	↑PS by 2 or 4
	OK	OK	⇧	

Contd.

Table 22.5: Smartcare ventilator response to feedback loop (Contd.)

Classification	F_{spn}	VT	$etCO_2$	SC response
Hypoventilation	⇩	OK	⇧	↑PS by 4
Central hypoventilation	⇩	⇩	⇧	ALAEM
Tachypnea	⇧	OK	OK	↑PS by 2 or 4
	If 3 X			ALARM
Severe tachypnea	⇧⇧	OK	OK	↑PS by 4
	If 3 X			ALARM
Hyperventilation	⇩	OK	OK	↓PS by 4
Unexplained hyperventilation	⇧	OK	⇩	ALARM

Advantages

This mode seems to be replace the clinicians brain in weaning patient as it is 'decision driven' rather than 'patient driven'. It uses standard pressure support mode of ventilation to wean patient, however the support adjustment is done automatically using 3 variables from patient.

Disadvantage

While use of this mode has reduced the time to do first spontaneous breathing trial, it did not reduced the first successful spontaneous breathing trial, total duration of mechanical ventilation, time in ICU and hospital and requirement for tracheostomy.

Being a pressure support ventilation, the utility is not suitable for thoracic trauma, neuromuscular diseases or any condition where respiratory drive is affected.

Remark

Smart care is designed to support the patient's spontaneous breathing in a comfort zone of a preset defined ventilatory parameters and to automatically reduce the ventilatory support, leading to a weaning protocol. The pressure support is adjusted according to respiratory rate, tidal volume and End tidal CO_2 to meet the patient's demand. The feedback occurs every 5 minutes and there is decreases or increases the pressure support levels accordingly. Smart Care assesses and indicates if the patient is ready for extubation after a successful automatic spontaneous breathing trial.[9]

4. Proportional Assist Ventilation (PAV+)

This is another SUPPORT mode, which give support to patients breath there by decreasing its work of breathing. Simplistically, it is like pushing or pulling a person who is trying to climb a ladder. The person has to do its job, but the push or pull is going to assist in completing the job. PAV+ amplifies inspiratory efforts with the goal that patient comfortably attain whatever breathing pattern his lungs desire. The ventilator synchronises with the patients own efforts and generates pressure in proportion to patient generated flow or volume of breath. Unlike simple pressure support ventilation, where a fixed support is given to breath triggered by patient, here, pressure support changes or adapts to the patients need breath by breath.

Table 22.6: Breath in PAV+

Control	Trigger	Limit	Target	Cycle
Support mode	Patient	Pressure	Dialled percentage of whole breath (5–95%)	Flow (dialled between 1–10 L/min)

Main setting: There is no standard setting of tidal volume or respiratory rate or pressure target. Here one sets percentage of support (e.g. 5–95%). Usually it starts from higher up-say 80% means, of total breath (patients + ventilator), patient will give roughly 20% and ventilator will support 80% of breath. Other settings are FiO_2, airway type—endotracheal tube (ET) or tracheostomy tube, size of ET or tracheostomy tube, PEEP, cycling (1–10 L/min of flow) and importantly ALARM limits for pressure and tidal volume.

Mechanism for Breath: It is well known from equation of motion, that in case of a support breath from ventilnator,

$$\underset{\text{Patient effort}}{P_{mus}} + \underset{\text{support}}{P_{aw}\text{ Ventilator}} = \underset{\text{Resistive load}}{\text{Resistance} \times \text{Flow}} + \underset{\text{Elastic load load}}{\text{Elastance} \times \text{volume}}$$

Where P_{mus} is the pressure generated by respiratory muscles like diaphragm and chest wall muscles, P_{aw} is the pressure provided by ventilator (what ever pressure support is dialled by clinician). Resistance is one offered by whole of lung and respiratory tree, elastance is the distention property of lung and respiratory system along with elastic recoiling property, flow is the flow of air entering lung and volume is volume of air entering lung.

Usually in a fixed pressure support breath, if there is any change in resistive load or elastic load, patient will either get more breath or less breath for his effort. Similarly, since the ventilator breath is fixed, if patient is tired or improving, the incoming breath for a given resistive and elastic load will be more or less. In this way, the respiratory muscles will get too much offloaded causing disuse atrophy or will have to work too hard causing fatigue. This is patient-ventilator dyssynchrony.

In PAV+, the ventilator software calculates compliance or elastance of respiratory system and airway resistance using end-inspiratory occlusion performed randomly every 4–10 breaths. Every 5 milliseconds information of patients demand is collected from the flow and volume generated due to inspiratory efforts and respiratory mechanics of patient. Now once clinician adjust percentage of support, based on inspiratory effort and respiratory mechanics initiated by patient, the ventilator adjust the inspiratory pressure according to the equation of motion. If the patients demand or effort changes, the PAV+ will also change proportionally, ensuring the result is equal to airway resistance + Elastance (or compliance) as per equation of motion.

Cycling occurs with pre-set settings. With obstructive patients, it should be adjusted to high level, around 10 l/min, for restrictive patient lowest around 1 l/min, and those without any respiratory abnormalities around 3–5 l/min.

Advantages

1. Neuroventilatory coupling is very well synchronised.
2. Patient comfort as ventilator adapts to its varying demands.
3. Decreased need of paralysis or sedation.
4. Preservation of patient's own control mechanism and prevention of overuse or disuse of diaphragm.
5. Low airway pressure and decreased work of breathing.

Disadvantage

1. It will potentiate conditions with intrinsic hyperventilatory drive (like respiratory alkalosis).
2. Since its a support mode, low respiratory drive, neuromuscular weakness, bradypnea are contraindication for this mode.
3. The mode calculates compliance and resistance from a closed circuit, hence large mechanical leaks would give false results
4. External nebulisers that add flow to circuit cannot be used.
5. Pediatric patients are difficult to ventilate due to their breathing pattern.

Remark

In PAV+ mode the ventilator continuously adjust the assist pressure in a proportionate and ongoing fashion to patients respiratory efforts. This may achieve near-perfect synchrony between spontaneously breathing patient and ventilator and give relief from disease related increased work of breathing. Several studies have demonstrated favourable outcome to PAV in terms of synchronism, weaning success, sleep quality, duration of mechanical ventilation, lung and diaphragm protection and low reinutbation rates.[10–13] However, one systematic review and meta-analysis that evaluated14 randomised controlled trials with total of 931 patients showed no difference weaning time, hospital mortality, reintubation or tracheostomy.[14]

5. Neurally Adjusted Ventilatory Assistance (NAVA)

Triggering delay is one of important cause for patient ventilatory dyssynchrony, especially in pathological states like COPD, pneumonia, ARDS, etc. Conventional modes of ventilators has a time delay of around 60–80 milliseconds between neuronal respiratory centre signal output and ventilator triggering inspiratory flow. This delay is mostly due to delay in detection of change in airway pressure or flow by the ventilator (*see* **Fig. 22.1**). This delay causes air hunger and dyssynchrony especially when minute ventilation is very high.

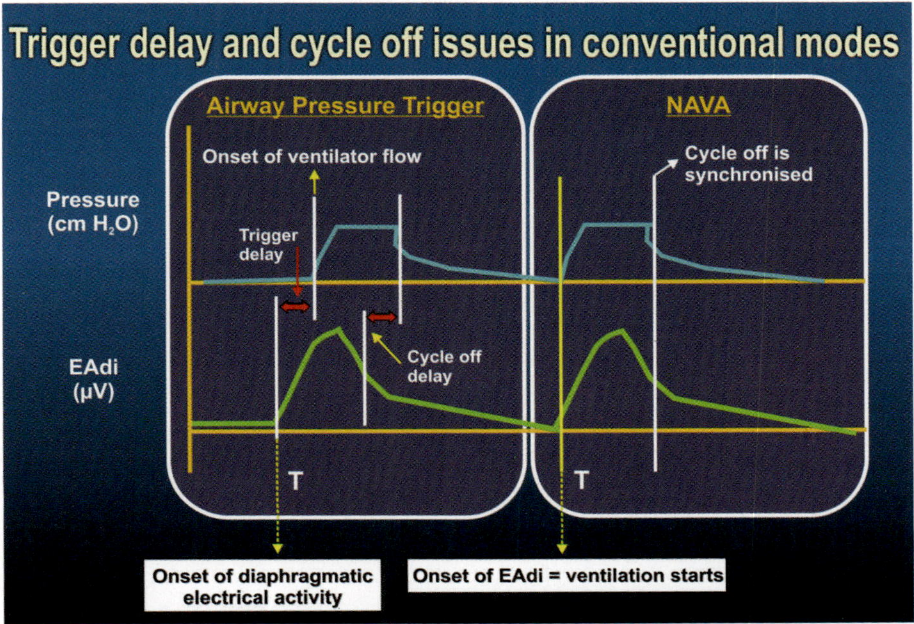

Fig. 22.7: Role of NAVA in bridging trigger delay

Neurally assisted ventilatory assistance mode bypass the mechanical triggers like pressure and flow, and senses the electrical activity of diaphragmatic contraction as a trigger. This has shown to overcome the trigger related delay and dyssynchrony.

Table 22.7: Breath in NAVA

Control	Trigger	Limit	Target	Cycle
Support mode	Patient (Electrical activity from Diaphragm: EAdi)	Peak Pressure (EAdi × NAVA level + PEEP)	Pressure calculated by EAdi × NAVA level	End of EAdi signal and drop in flow to 70–40%

Main settings: A special nasogastric tube (NG) with electrodes is inserted to position where electrical activity of crural diaphragm is noted. The size of the NG tube is determined by height and weight of patient. For reference there is also transesophageal electrocardiogram (ECG) sensed and displayed on ventilator screen. By default, the neural inspiratory trigger is set at 0.5 microvolt (uV). Below this its too sensitive and any 'noise' or ineffective muscle twitch can trigger ventilator. This is followed by setting NAVA level (no protocol, need to start with a random number usually between 0.5 and 2.0 uV/cmH_2O) that gets multiplied by EAdi to give pressure support above PEEP. Other settings include FiO_2, PEEP level. Pressure control (PC) mode is a back up mode, in case there is problem detecting the signal or apnea. Other setting are like any standard PC setting. As with other support modes, back up alarm are important.

Mechanism of Breath: Ventilator support breath starts with EAdi. As EAdi increases the assistance increases in proportion to NAVA level adjusted. Thus, NAVA trigger is a non-pneumatic trigger, unlike other modes of ventilator. Pneumatic trigger (changes in flow or pressure) is available as back up pressure control mode, in case its needed. The pressure support delivered in this case will be:

$$\text{EAdi} \times \text{NAVAL level} = \text{Inspiratory pressure (above PEEP)}$$

For example, $7\ \text{uV} \times 1.0\ \text{cm}\ H_2O = 7\ \text{cm}\ H_2O$ of PS

Also,

$$\text{Peak pressure} = \text{EAdi} \times \text{NAVA level} + \text{PEEP}$$

Cycling off occurs automatically when the EAdi signal drops down and the flow decreases to 70–40%. This cannot be set or modified by operators. If there is NO signal, and apnea is detected, it goes in PC back up mode and restarts to NAVA when the signal is again detected.

Advantages

1. NAVA works with respiratory neural signal, decreasing the trigger delay related dyssynchrony.
2. It decreases risk of hyperinflation, respiratory alkalosis and hemodynamic impairment.
3. It generates proportional assistance to patients effort, resulting in maximal unloading of his respiratory muscles.
4. Since the trigger is diaphragm electrical activity, the breath is not affected by leak, hence it is also useful in non-invasive ventilator (NAVA-NIV).
5. Since, diaphragmatic activity is monitored, appropriate depth of sedation and sedation titration can be maintained. Thus preventing development of diaphragmatic atrophy and ventilator-induced diaphragmatic dysfunction.

Disadvantage

1. NAVA depends on specialised NG tube and position of the sensors to detect diaphragmatic activity. Any movement, distort signal and ventilator going in back up mode.
2. It cannot be used where there is no diaphragmatic contraction, like muscle paralysis, neuro muscular disorder.
3. Agitation, pain, extreme respiratory distress or other causes that increase respiratory drive can result in increased EAdi and cause over assistance. This can be over come by reducing EAdi value.
4. Since the pressure support also depends on what NAVA level is set (besides patients EAdi), it takes couple of breaths before a right number is reached to get patient in comfort zone.

Remark

Large controlled studies comparing various modes with NAVA in acute respiratory failure patient did decrease the duration of mechanical ventilation but did not improve survival in ventilated patients.[15] Despite advantage, NIV NAVA also failed to improve clinical outcomes in studies.[16]

MODES TO IMPROVE GAS EXCHANGE AND DECREASE VENTILATOR INDUCED LUNG INJURY (VILI)

One of the important concept in increasing the oxygenation while on ventilator is "open lung concept". Alveoli need to be kept open and prevent collapse even during expiration by use of sustained pressure. This formed the basis of recruitment manoeuvre, inverse ratio ventilation and use of high PEEP. Advantages of keeping high airway pressure during ventilation with conventional mode has drawback of barotrauma, volutrauma, hemodynamic instability, need for deep sedation and ventilation. Also, trying to manipulate pressure 24 hr bedside is not practical. Introduction of close loop feedback has taken over this manual adjustment. Keeping intrathoracic pressure high it tends to ventilate patients and keep alveoli open within safe limits. Here we discuss some modes that uses high airway pressure and ventilate patient safely as well. For example: APRV (a Bi-Level mode), HFOV, ASV.

1. Airway Pressure Release Ventilation (APRV)[17]

APRV is a pressure-controlled mode of ventilation which can deliver prolonged high-pressure to prevent alveolar collapse, maintain recruitment and a short low level pressure to exhale carbon dioxide. The ventilator cycles between two levels, high and low, and this allows gas to move in and out of the lung. Hence the term Bi-level. The change in prolong high pressure followed by short low pressure is almost like recruitment manoeuvre, but occurring regularly as per time set by clinician. It is a unique mode where while in control mode, patient is allowed to breath spontaneously. The patient breaths his own tidal volume while in high pressure time and low pressure time. This facility intend to prevent frequent opening and closing of alveoli with each tidal volume that occurs with conventional mode and prevent stress and strain, leading to potential avoidance of VILI.

Table 22.8: Breath in APRV

Control	Trigger	Limit	Target	Cycle
Pressure control	Time	Pressure	Pressure	Time

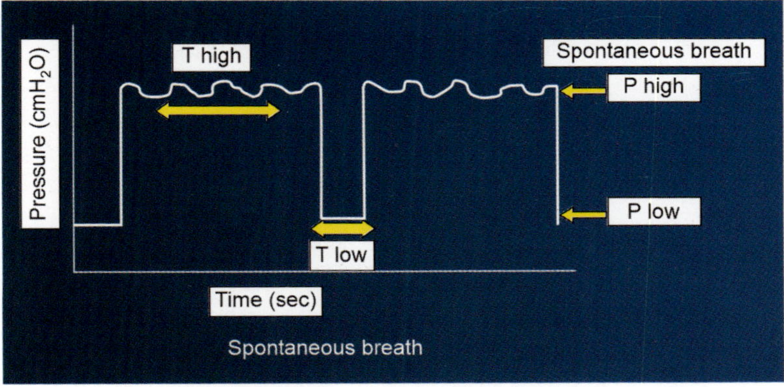

Fig. 22.8: APRV wavefrom graph

Main setting: There are two main setting, high pressure limit (P-high) and low pressure limit (P-low), and how long should be high pressure limit (T-high) and low pressure limit (T-Low). P-high is set corresponding P-plateau (up to maximum of 30 cmH_2O as per ARDSnet protocol) and P-low can be kept zero or very minimal pressure. T-high and T-low can be adjusted according to inverse ratio ventilation (For example: T-high = 4.5 to 6 sec and T-low = 0.5 to 0.8 sec). Here, T-Low has important role.It should be short enough to prevent derecruitment and it should be long enough to achieve adequate tidal volume.Other settings are FiO_2 and alarm limits.

Mechanism of breath: Once triggered, ventilator gives a pressure control breath with set high pressure (P-High), for the set time (T-High). Cycling occurs with percentage of peak flow rate, usually 25–75%. With the cycling the thoracic pressure falls to set P-low, exhaling the gas from the lung (ventilator tidal volume). This release is called 'Release breath". If tidal volume is inadequate T-low can be increased or reduced if tidal volume is high. Even though T-low is very short, CO_2 retention does not occur because patient is spontaneously breathing throughout the breathing cycle (P-high and P-low). Weaning process during APRV is called "Drop and Stretch" method where P-high is gradually decreased and T-high increased simultaneously. During weaning process one can lower P-high by 2 to 3 cm H_2O at a time and lengthen T-high by increments of 0.5 to 2.0 seconds. Once P-high is around 15 to 16 cmH_2O and T-high is at 12–15s, one can change to CPAP.

Advantages

1. A very useful mode for improving oxygenation where alveolar recruitment is indicated namely, recruitable lung, diffuse lung involvement.
2. Situations where prone position is contraindicated like morbid obesity, hemodynamic instability, trauma, burns, multiorgan dysfunction, APRV is a rescue mode.
3. Patient can be weaned off paralysis with sedation enough for patient to have spontaneous breaths.

Disadvantages

1. Increased risk of auto-PEEP and dynamic hyperinflation, if T-high or T-low are not appropriate.
2. Increased risk of volutrauma and baro-trauma, while patient is breathing spontaneously at P-high.
3. Worsening of hemodynamics in an inadequately resuscitated patients. High intrathoracic pressures will decrease venous returns and increase pulmonary afterload.
4. Not a good mode post-thoracic surgery, pneumothorax, bronchopleural fistula, restrictive lung disease, COPD and severe bronchospasm. Role in traumatic brain injury with raised intracranial tension is debated.

Remarks

This mode can be used as rescue therapy for severe ARDS to improve oxygenation where low tidal volume strategy is failing. It provides increased mean airway pressures which allow 'open-lung' ventilation. This mode can deliver CPAP with intermittent, time-cycled, short releases at a lower pressure. APRV mode can be used in spontaneously breathing patients and sedated patients as well. While theoretically APRV is attractive, there are no large multicentric trial supporting its use. Small studies showed significantly shorter stay in ICU for patients who were kept on APRV mode. It showed significantly better PF ratios and significantly better respiratory system compliance.[18] However, retrospective systematic reviews have failed to show any mortality benefits in adults.

2. High Frequency Oscillatory Ventilation (HFOV)

One of important factor for VILI is the cyclical opening and closing of alveoli along with tidal volume, causing stress and strain. HFOV works on concept of ventilating lungs with a high constant mean airway pressure that recruits alveoli and keeps them open. It needs an exclusive machine, which cannot be integrated with any other mode. The breath delivery cannot be classified in terms of control, trigger, limit and cycling. High-frequency oscillatory ventilation (HFOV) is a rescue strategy for patients with failed conventional mechanical ventilation. HFOV can be considered an alternative lung-protective ventilation strategy for patients with VILI and ARDS.

Main setting: HFOV cannot be delivered with any of conventional ventilators and need an exclusive machine (**Fig. 22.9**).

Two parameters need to be set. One is for oxygenation and another is for ventilation.

Oxygenation during HFOV is managed by two variables:

a. mPaw-mean airway pressure should be set 3–5 cm H_2O above the mPaw of conventional ventilation. Normal mPaw ranges are 25–30 cm H_2O, with a maximum of 45–60 cm H_2O.
b. FiO_2 is titrated by a blender attached to the oscillator.

Ventilation during HFOV is managed by three variables:

a. Tidal volume: It is decided by amplitude of piston. As the amplitude increases, tidal volume also increases.
b. Inspiratory time (IT%): It is a portion of the respiratory cycle that the piston spends in forward motion (similar to I:E ratio in conventional ventilator).

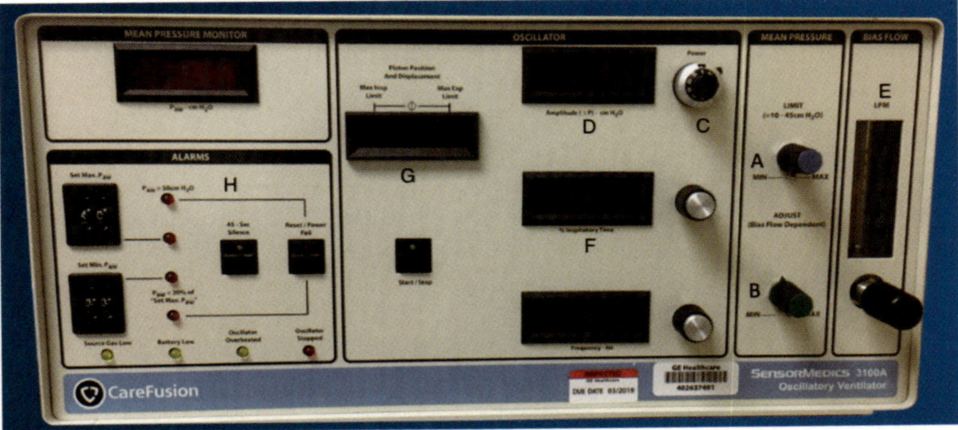

Fig. 22.9: HFOV machine: (A) Mean airway pressure limit knob; (B) Mean airway pressure adjustment; (C) Power (amplitude of piston); (D) Frequency (Hz display); (E) Bias flow; (F) Inspitatory time display; (G) Piston position; (H) ALARM settings

c. Frequency: It is derived from hertz which controls the time for piston's forward and backward movement. One hertz is 60 breaths per minute. The range is 3–15 Hz, with typical initial settings of 5–6 Hz.

HFOV Initial settings in adults:

1. BF (Bias flow) = 40 L/min (rate of continuous flow of humidified blended gas through the circuit: 0 to 60 L/min)
2. IT % (inspiratory time)= 33%
3. mPaw = 34 cm H_2O
4. FIO_2 = 1.0
5. Amplitude (delta P) = 90 cm H_2O.
6. Frequency = 4 to 7 Hz (based on ABG: pH <7.10 = 4 Hz, pH 7.10–7.19 = 5 Hz, pH 7.20–7.35 = 6 Hz, pH >7.35 = 7 Hz)

Mechanism of breath: Once switched on, HFOV builds up the airway pressure to target mPaw. It recruits collapsed alveoli and keeps them open. Ventilation is now achieved through the use of rapid (frequency), tiny oscillations (amplitude) produced by a reciprocating piston. The tidal volume are small (as low as <1 ml/kg) at extremely high frequency, around 300 bpm (120–900 bpm range). This unphysiological breaths, gas diffusion seems to occur with Taylor dispersion, coaxial flow and augmented diffusion.[19]

Advantages

Such a small tidal volume prevents cyclical opening and closing of alveoli, preventing any VILI. High mean airway pressure prevents collapse and derecruitment.

Disadvantages

HFOV delivers an unphysiological breath. Hence patient needs to be completely sedated and paralysed. Any attempt to spontaneous breathing may increase intrathoracic pressures to dangerous levels. High mean airway pressure makes patient susceptible to barotrauma - pneumothorax, pneumomediastinum, hemodynamic instability in under resuscitated patients. It requires special machine and is extremely noisy when initiated. Since its closed circuit, there is no scope of intermittent suctioning and there is likely to have mucus plugging. Stopping machine for any reason will cause derecruitement.

Remark

HFOV and APRV are the two modes that uses high mean airway pressure to prevent VILI and maintain oxygenation. Due to unconventional breath pattern, their use is more of as a rescue method in case of ARDS and hypoxemic respiratory failure due to lung issue. Despite its advantage, HFOV has failed to demonstrate any clinical outcome advantage. All the 3 major trials comparing HFOV and conventional ventilation, have shown more adverse events and high mortality with HFOV in adults.[20–22] Trials in paediatric age group has shown better outcome as compared to adults.[23] Current guidelines does not recommend HFOV to be used as rescue therapy in view of increased mortality noted in major trial.

3. Adaptive Support Ventilation (ASV)

Adaptive support ventilation mode is a highly sophisticated mode which covers whole range of control to assist modes. It can be called "3-in-1 mode", giving volume/ pressure control, intermittent mandatory breath and pressure support breath. ASV targets minute ventilation and work of breathing in a complex close loop positive and negative feedback algorithm. The mode automatically sets respiratory rate (RR) and tidal volume (TV) in different combination pattern according the patient demand and lung mechanics (compliance and resistance) to achieve set minute ventilation. Aim is to provide just enough ventilatory support for adequate gas exchange. It recognise spontaneous breathing early and switches (Adapts) from pressure control breath to pressure support. Conceptually, this minimal support should minimise the stress and strain on alveoli and hence avoid ventilator induce lung injury (VILI). ASV is assist-control, pressure-targeted and time-cycled mode which helps to provide minimal work of breathing.

Table 22.9: Breath in ASV

Control	Trigger	Limit	Target	Cycle
Pressure control	Time	Pressure and volume	Minute ventilation (respiratory rate × tidal volume)	Time

Main settings: Three important settings are—patient demographics-height in cm: Based on this it calculate Ideal body weight (IBW) and dead space 2.2 ml/kg, Gender and Percentage of minute volume (% Min Vol). Other settings are Trigger (usually Flow trigger of 2 L/min), PEEP and FiO_2 for oxygenation, tube resistance compensation (set at 100%), all alarm limit.Tidal volume and respiratory rate are not included in set parameters because, once percentage of minute volume (% min.vol) is set ventilator decides respiratory rate and tidal volume based on measurements of lung compliance and resistance. The ventilator constantly keep changing I:E ratio to avoid any autoPEEP.

Minute volume percentage is 100% or normal, based on patients ideal body weight. Once demographics are entered, ventilator calculates this percentage and that becomes basal ventilatory requirement or target minute volume. For example, if IBW is 66 kg, and basal ventilatory requirement is taken as 100 ml/kg/min (for adults - measurement differ for paediatric group), then basal minute volume becomes 6.6 L/min (=100%) for that patient. Now, based upon lung pathology this target can be increased or decreased, e.g asthma – 90%, ARDS – 120%, others – 110%, if T >101.3 F – add 20%, altitude – 5% per 500 m above sea level.

Mechanism of breath: Once triggered, ventilator give 3 test breaths to calculate resistance and compliance of lung. Based on the number generated, it calculates expiratory time constant (RCe = Resistance x compliance). This data is then inserted in formula developed by Otis, *et al.* and Mead, *et al.* to calculate frequency or respiratory rate.[24]

$$f = \frac{\sqrt{1 + 2a\text{RC}\,(V_A/V_D)} - 1}{a\text{RC}}$$

where, RC is the respiratory time constant, VA and VD are alveolar ventilation and dead space ventilation, respectively, and a is a constant that depends on the flow waveform. This data is utilised to achieve targeted minute ventilation. The data is collected breath by breath and frequency and tidal volume is adjusted accordingly to maintain that minute volume. If there is a spontaneous efforts, mandatory breaths get changed to support breath. If there are no spontaneous efforts detected, then mandatory breaths are given. This happens or changes breath by breath. The whole algorithm works in a way that patient remain in a "safe zone" avoiding any barotrauma or volutrauma.

Advantages

1. More beneficial in patients with rapid change in compliance or resistance (e.g. ARDS and Asthma)
2. Can be used as partial to full support mode during weaning process
3. Does not require constant involvement of operator
4. It is versatile and safe mode which can ventilate any patient group

Disadvantages

1. This mode is not available in all ventilators—Hamilton ventilator patented
2. We can not directly program tidal volume, respiratory rate and I:E ratio, as its calculated. This may be of disadvantage in some clinical scenario.
3. This mode is not able recognize dead space ventilation or shunts to make adjustments to ventilation.
4. As there is no backup mode during weaning on this mode, there is a risk of hypoventilation and hypercapnia if patient is kept on the lower percent of minute ventilation support.

Remark

The automation in ASV has a high potential to select adequate ventilatory patterns based on the condition suffered by the patient, i.e. normal lungs, restrictive or constrictive diseases. It takes into account of spontaneous breathing, and it is useful to prevent tachypnea, the development of auto-PEEP, and excessive dead-space ventilation. ASV has been studied in controlled mode, intermittent mandatory and support mode. Several clinical studies showed as compared to clinician setting, ASV chose lesser tidal volume and higher respiratory rate in controlled mode. Further studies have shown that ASV adapts to change in patient position, double or single lung anaesthesia, causes less air trapping in COPD, and longer studies have shown that ASV ventilates an anaesthetised person as well as patient in acute respiratory failure well.[25–28] Study which compared NIV support of PSV with ASV demonstrated that both are viable options without significant differences in mortality.[29]

SUMMARY

Two important challenges with positive pressure mechanical ventilation is to provide adequate gas change with avoiding VILI and comfort of patient while on ventilator. Introduction of closed loop feedback in ventilators have given rise to these NOVEL modes that tend to address much of the issues of conventional modes. However, quest for an ideal mode still continues. None of the mode are complete in itself and have shown better clinical outcomes. Also, these modes are patented by particular company, hence their wide spread use is restricted. Clinicians needs to understand basics of these modes and their indication, so as to use them appropriately when encountered. The tables under respective mode will help to decode the modes in terms of control, trigger, limit and cycling. Further introduction of artificial intelligence (AI) may make the understanding more complex in future but so do the next generation understanding, they say!.

References

1. Slutsky AS. History of Mechanical Ventilation. From Vesalius to Ventilator-induced Lung Injury. Am J Respir Crit Care Med. 2015 May 15;191(10):1106–15.
2. Platen, P.v., Pomprapa, A., Lachmann, B. et al. The dawn of physiological closed-loop ventilation—a review. Crit Care 24, 121 (2020). https://doi.org/10.1186/s13054-020-2810-1.
3. Singh PM, Borle A, Trikha A. Newer nonconventional modes of mechanical ventilation. J Emerg Trauma Shock. 2014;7(3):222-227. doi:10.4103/0974-2700.136869.
4. Al-Hegelan M, MacIntyre NR. Novel modes of mechanical ventilation. Semin Respir Crit Care Med. 2013;34(4):499-507. doi:10.1055/s-0033-1351123.
5. Silvia Valente Barbas, Carmen, and Sergio Nogueira Nemer. 'Advanced Modes of Mechanical Ventilation'. Mechanical Ventilation, IntechOpen, 12 Jan. 2022. Crossref, doi:10.5772/intechopen.100283.
6. MacIntyre NR, Sessler CN. Are there benefits or harm from pressure targeting during lung-protective ventilation? Respir Care 2010;55(2):175–180, discussion 180–183.
7. Kallet RH, Campbell AR, Dicker RA, Katz JA, Mackersie RC.Work of breathing during lung-protective ventilation in patients with acute lung injury and acute respiratory distress syndrome: a comparison between volume and pressure- regulated breathing modes. Respir Care 2005;50(12):1623–1631.
8. Amato MB, Barbas CS, Bonassa J, Saldiva PH, Zin WA, de Carvalho CR. Volume-assured pressure support ventilation (VAPSV). A new approach for reducing muscle workload during acute respiratory failure. Chest. 1992;102(4):1225-1234. doi:10.1378/chest.102.4.1225.
9. Taniguchi C, Victor ES, Pieri T, Henn R, et al. Smart CareTM versus respiratory physiotherapy-driven manual weaning for critically ill adult patients: a randomized controlled trial. Crit Care. 2015 Jun 11;19(1):246. doi: 10.1186/s13054-015-0978-6.
10. Ou-Yang LJ, Chen PH, Jhou HJ, Su VYF, Lee CH. Proportional assist ventilation versus pressure support ventilation for weaning from mechanical ventilation in adults: a meta-analysis and trial sequential analysis. Crit Care 2020:24:556 .
11. Pantazopoulos I, Mavrovounis G, Mermiri M, Kampolis C. Proportional assist ventilation versus pressure support ventilation for weaning from mechanical ventilation in adults: weaning success and mortality. Crit Care 2021:25:200 .
12. Kataoka J, Kuriyama A, Norisue Y, Fujitani S. Proportional modes versus pressure support ventilation: a systematic review. Ann Intensive Care 2018:8:123.
13. Jonkman AH, Rauseo M, Carteaux G, Telias I, Sklar MC, Heunks M et al. Proportional modes of ventilation: technology to assist physiology. Intensive Care Med 2020. https://doi.org/10.1007/s00134-020-06206-z.
14. Kumar B, Vijayaraghavan T, Hamed S, Jain A, Chimunda T, T, Elias I et al. Evidence supporting clinical use of proportional assist ventilation: a systematic review and meta-analysis of clinical trials. J Intensive care Med 2018:1-9.

15. Kacmarek RM, Villar J, Parrilas D, Alba F, Solano R, Liu S et al. Neurally adjusted ventilatory assist in respiratory failure: a randomized controlled trial. Intensive Care Med 2020: https:// doi. org/10.1007/s00134-020-06181-5 .
16. Sinderby C, Beck J. Neurally adjusted ventilatory assist (NAVA):an update and summary of experiences. Neth Crit Care 2007;11:243-252.
17. Swindin J, Sampson C, Howatson A. Airway pressure release ventilation. BJA Educ. 2020;20(3):80-88. doi:10.1016/j.bjae.2019.12.001.
18. Zhou, Y., Jin, X., Lv, Y. et al. Early application of airway pressure release ventilation may reduce the duration of mechanical ventilation in acute respiratory distress syndrome. Intensive Care Med 2017; 43: 1648–59.
19. Chang HK. Mechanisms of gas transport during ventilation by high-frequency oscillation. J Appl Physiol 1984;56(3):553–563.
20. Young D, Lamb SE, Shah S, et al. High-frequency oscillation for acute respiratory distress syndrome. N Engl J Med. 2013;368(9):806-813. doi:10.1056/NEJMoa1215716.
21. Ferguson ND, Cook DJ, Guyatt GH, et al. High-frequency oscillation in early acute respiratory distress syndrome. N Engl J Med. 2013;368:795–805.
22. Sklar MC, Fan E, Goligher EC. High-Frequency oscillatory ventilation in adults with ARDS: Past, present, and future. Chest 2017;152(6): 1306–17. doi: 10.1016/j.chest.2017.06.025.
23. Clark RH, Null DM, Gerstmann DR. Prospective randomized comparison of high-frequency oscillatory and conventional ventilation in respiratory distress syndrome. Pediatrics 1992;89(1): 5–1.
24. OTIS AB, FENN WO, RAHN H. Mechanics of breathing in man. J Appl Physiol. 1950 May;2(11):592-607 : Mead J, Takishima T, Leith D. Stress distribution in lungs: a model of pulmonary elasticity. J Appl Physiol. 1970 May;28(5):596-608. doi: 10.1152/ jappl.1970.28.5.596. PMID: 5442255.
25. Laubscher TP, Frutiger A, Fanconi S, Brunner JX. The automatic selection of ventilation parameters during the initial phase of mechanical ventilation. Intensive Care Med 1996;22(3):199–207.
26. Belliato M, Palo A, Pasero D, Iotti GA,Mojoli F, Braschi A. Evaluation of the adaptive support ventilation (ASV) mode in paralyzed patients. Int J Artif Organs. 2004;27(8):709–716.
27. Tassaux D, Dalmas E, Gratadour P, Jolliet P. Patient-ventilator interactions during partial ventilatory support: a preliminary study comparing the effects of adaptive support ventilation with synchronized intermittent mandatory ventilation plus inspiratory pressure support. Crit Care Med 2002;30(4):801–807.
28. Linton DM, Potgieter PD, Davis S, Fourie AT, Brunner JX, Laubscher TP. Automatic weaning from mechanical ventilation using an adaptive lung ventilation controller. Chest 1994;106(6): 1843–1850.
29. Sehgal IS, Kalpakam H, Dhooria S, Aggarwal AN, Prasad KT, Agarwal R. A Randomized Controlled Trial of Non-invasive Ventilation with Pressure Support Ventilation and Adaptive Support Ventilation in Acute Exacerbation of COPD: A Feasibility Study. COPD. 2019 Apr;16(2):168-173

CHAPTER 23

Hazards of Mechanical Ventilation

❒ Viswesvaran Balasubramanian ❒ Sumita Agrawal

INTRODUCTION

Mechanical ventilation is one of the most commonly used life saving modalities for patients with critically illness and respiratory failure. Though lifesaving, it is associated with hazards related to intubation and ventilation which can lead to longer duration of mechanical ventilation, lengthier stays in the intensive care unit (ICU) and hospital, increase in healthcare costs, and increased risk of morbidity and mortality. The complications related to intubatuion and mechanical ventilation can be broadly classified into:

Ventilator induced lung injury:

- Ventilator-associated tracheobronchitis
- Ventilator-associated pneumonia
- Tracheal stenosis

History

John Fothergill had postulated way back in the 18th century that mouth-to-mouth resuscitation may be preferable to mechanical ventilation because "the lungs of one man may bear, without injury, as great a force as those of another man can exert; which by the bellows cannot always be determined".[1] It is almost two centuries since then that we have proved that ventilator-induced lung injury is indeed one of the major contributing factors to increasing morbidity and mortality in patients with ARDS. It was the 1952 polio epidemic, where the structural damages to the lungs in patients treated with mechanical ventilation were documented.[2] A new terminology called "respirator lung" came to be in use in 1967 when patients on mechanical ventilation started showing changes in the lungs in terms of alveolar infiltrates and hyaline membrane formation.[3]

Definition

The damage caused to the airways, lung parenchyma and the alveolar-capillary membrane due to mechanical ventilation's positive pressure effects is broadly termed as Ventilator-induced lung injury (VILI). When the cause of damage to the lungs cannot be proven definitely due to mechanical ventilation, i.e. a causal relationship between the lung damage and ventilation cannot be achieved, it is called ventilator-associated lung injury (VALI).

Pathogenesis[4–6]

Four main mechanisms that cause VILI are:

1. High tidal volumes and pressures lead to overdistention causing increased stress and strain at the alveolar epithelium and airways
2. Shear stress-related injury due to cyclic inflation and deflation of alveoli.
3. Stress-related injury at the capillary level and heart-lung interactions causing endothelial damage
4. The release of cytokines due to stress and strain in the alveolar units and in the systemic circulation.

Types of VILI are recognized are:

Volutrauma: The injury caused to the lungs as a result of overdistention due to high tidal volumes is defined as volutrauma. This overdistention leads to an increase in transpulmonary pressure **(Fig. 23.1)** (the difference between the alveolar pressure and the intrapleural pressure in the pleural cavity) which causes pulmonary capillary stress failure contributing to VILI **(Fig. 23.2)**. This is especially true for lungs with heterogeneous consolidation like ARDS, lung fibrosis, or atelectasis. In these lungs, each breath delivers a disproportionate amount of tidal volume to different alveoli. This leads to regional over distention thus causing VILI.[7] This can be further understood by the concept of 'baby lung'—a nominee which was introduced for ARDS lungs where the normally aerated tissue is reduced to the size of a lung of a 5–6-year-old child. The size of the baby lung depends on the severity of ARDS.[8] Again, it is important to note that this is not an anatomical concept but more of a functional concept which also explains the improvement in oxygenation seen in patients when put in prone positioning **(Fig. 23.3)**. Prone positioning causes a redistribution of the aerated alveoli thus improving

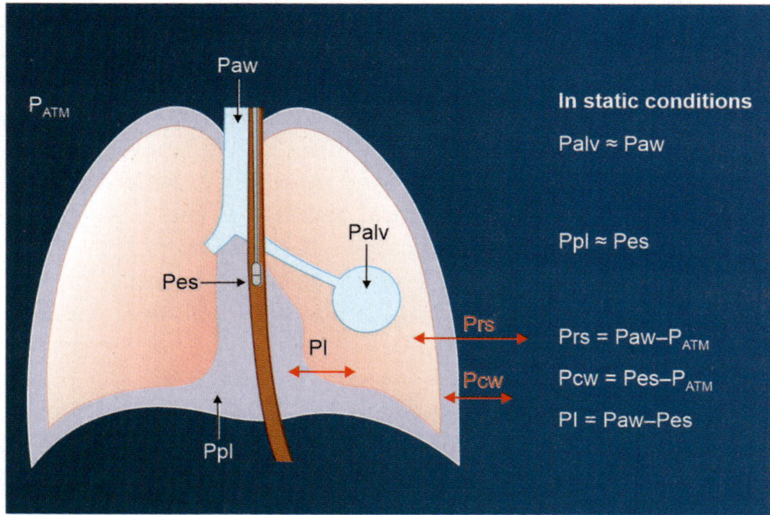

Fig. 23.1: P_{ATM}, atmospheric pressure; Paw, airway pressure; pes, esophageal pressure; Palv, alveolar pressure; Ppl, pleural pressure; Prs, transrespiratory pressure; Pcw, trans-chest wall pressure; Pl, transpulmonary pressure[25]

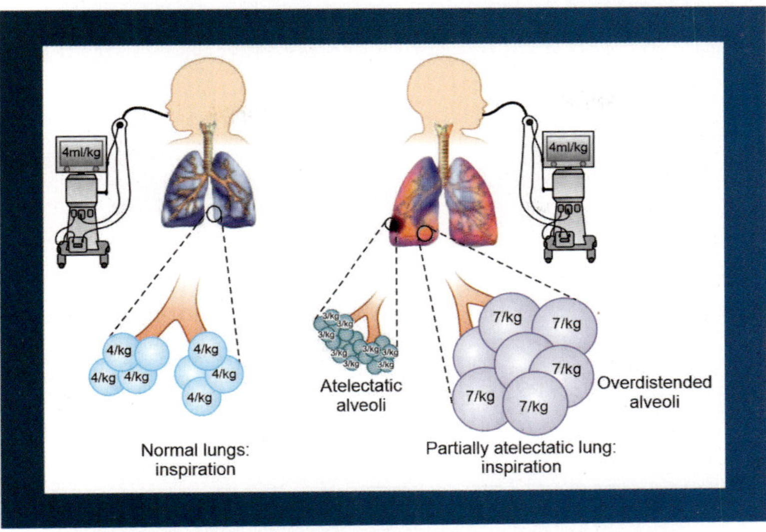

Fig. 23.2: Lung inspiration (pulmonary stress failure)[26]

lung compliance.[9] Although the earlier studies done in animal models did prove that high volume strategy led to severe lung injury, the ARDS network trial of the year 2000 definitively prove that low tidal volume (6 vs. 12 mL/kg predicted body weight [PBW]) and low plateau airway pressures (≤30 vs. ≤50 cmH_2O) improved survival in patients with ARDS.[10] Studies have shown that each ml increase in tidal volume above 6 ml per kg of ideal body weight has increased risk of VILI (OR 1.3, 95% CI 1.12–1.51).[11]

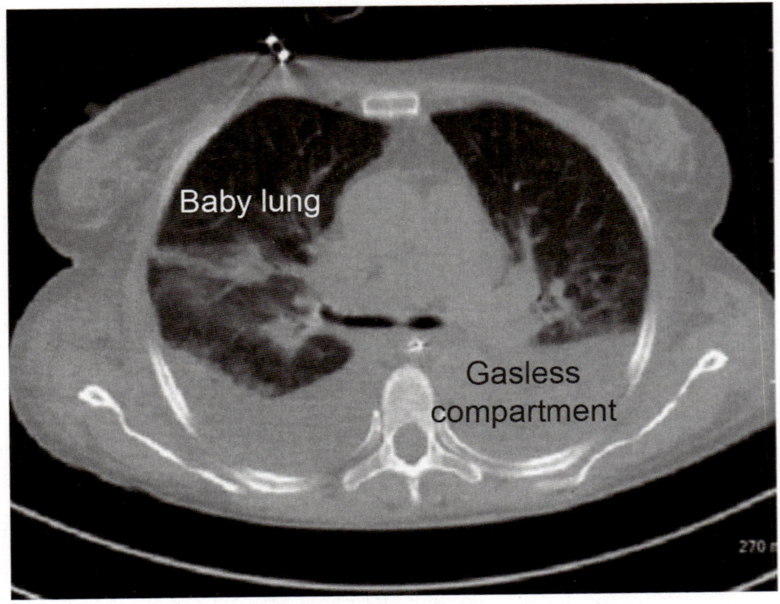

Fig. 23.3: ARD (CT Scan)[26]

Barotrauma: Barotrauma refers to alveolar rupture resulting as a result of increased trans alveolar pressure (the difference between alveolar pressure and the pressure in the adjacent interstitial space) in patients on mechanical ventilation. The alveolar rupture leads to air leaking in adjacent spaces including interstitium leading to pneumothorax, pulmonary interstitial emphysema, pneumomediastinum, and subcutaneous emphysema.[12] Other rare manifestations include pneumoperitoneum, air embolization, and tension lung cysts.

Risk factors for barotrauma include:

1. Underlying lung induced: COPD, ILD, ARDS, and necrotizing infections
2. Mechanical ventilation-induced: High transpulmonary pressure (airway pressure minus the pleural pressure), high tidal volumes, and high intrinsic PEEP leading to dynamic hyperinflation.

Again, the ArdsNET trial demonstrated that keeping the plateau pressures at <30 cm H_2O decreased mortality risk.[10] The concept of driving pressure is also used to prevent barotrauma. Driving pressure is defined as the difference between plateau pressure and PEEP. It can also be obtained by dividing tidal volume by static compliance of the respiratory system (C_{rs}) **(Fig. 23.4)**.[13] A meta-analysis done by Amato, *et al.* where more than 3500 patients were included showed that driving pressure was the ventilator variable that has been associated best with decreased mortality.[14] Ventilator strategies directed at driving pressure in ARDS patients are commonly used in order to prevent lung injury.

Atelectrauma: It has been seen that repeated opening and closing of collapsed alveoli leads to damage to adjoining non-collapsed alveoli and airways due to the force of shear stress. This is called atelectrauma.[6] An effective way to prevent this is by applying

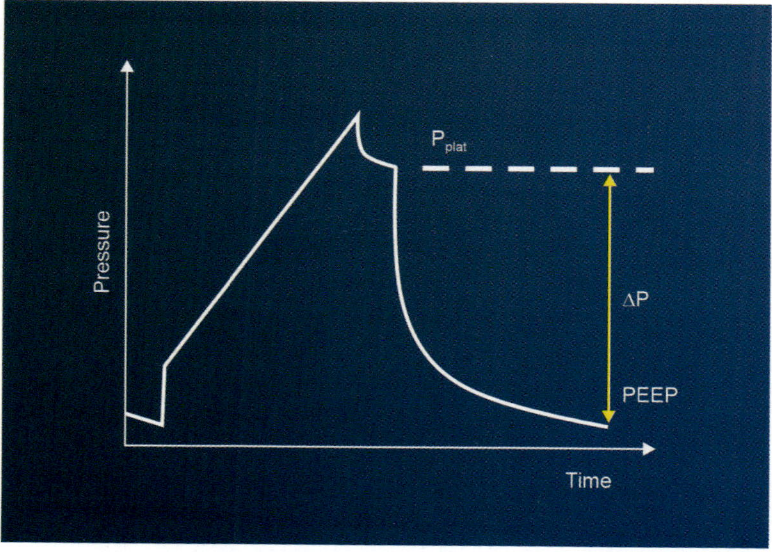

Fig. 23.4: Driving pressure (ΔP) = plateau pressure (P_{plat})–positive end-expiratory pressure (PEEP)[13]

optimal PEEP. Applying less PEEP will cause the repeated collapse of alveoli and higher PEEP will cause over distention resulting in barotrauma.[6,15]

Biotrauma: Ventilation leads to mechanical stress resulting in release of inflammatory mediators from lung tissue. The normal balance between proinflammatory cytokines and anti-inflammatory mediators is thus disturbed. This enhanced inflammatory system causes cell damage, surfactant dysfunction or deficiency or both. It also leads to activation of the coagulation cascade causing coagulopathy and the spill of these cytokines in the systemic circulation leads to other organ dysfunction as well. In addition to causing direct injury to lung tissue there is injury to other organs. This response is called biotrauma.[6]

Cardiovascular complications: Mechanical ventilation also leads to various heart-lung interactions which can be detrimental to the cardiovascular stability of the patient. During mechanical ventilation, the blood flow to the pulmonary vessels decreases during inspiration as a result of positive pressure, which causes increased pulmonary artery pressures and consequently decreased cardiac output. The blood flow on the other hand increases during expiration. This cyclical variation in blood flow causes damage to the pulmonary capillary endothelium and ultimately leads to capillary stress failure. This injury results in increase capillary permeability causing influx of protein and water which causes pulmonary edema.[6, 16]

Large volumes delivered during mechanical ventilation compresses the heart, collapse of pulmonary capillaries adjacent to the alveoli and increase in pressure difference between airway and pleura raised pulmonary artery pressure thus decreasing the cardiac output.[16]

Diagnosis

A patient on mechanical ventilator can have worsening of oxygen saturation due to multiple reasons like pulmonary edema, ventilator induced lung infections, pulmonary embolism. Hence, there needs to be a high index of suspicion to detect ventilator induced lung injury. Many a times, two or more of these conditions may even overlap in the same patient.

Examination

A thorough bedside examination is needed needs to rule out new-onset bronchospasm, localized decrease in air entry or presence of crackles or bronchial breathing. Lower limb swelling to rule out deep venous thrombosis, development of ascites and raised intra-abdominal pressure also needs to be seen. History of drug allergy or blood product transfusion needs to be elicited. Ventilatory settings need to be checked to look for any contributing factors for acute lung injury.

Investigations

Radiology

Chest Xray very commonly will show diffuse opacities present bilaterally. Other causes of worsening oxygen saturation like pneumothorax, pulmonary edema, VAP, tube position can also be ruled out via chest X-ray.

A CT scan thorax may show heterogeneous consolidation and atelectasis with focal areas of hyperlucencies suggestive of alveolar overdistension.

ECG and ECHO needs to be done to rule out cardiac causes of pulmonary edema.

Others

Total cell count, endotracheal aspirates for bacterial cultures and associated fever will help in diagnosis of VAP.

D-dimers, lower limb venous Doppler and if indicated a CT pulmonary angiogram may help in diagnosis of pulmonary thromboembolism.

Bronchoscopy may be needed in certain cases where collapse lung is suspected due to mucus or blood clot plugging.

Management

Prevention is the key to manage VILI. We learnt from the ARDSNET trial that low tidal volume strategy of 6 ml/kg of predicted body weight(PBW) prevents overdistension of the alveoli. This trial had proven that there are improved mortality rates when lower tidal volumes are used as compared to higher tidal volumes (i.e., 12 ml/kg of predicted body weight).[10] In non-ARDS patients as well, meta-analysis of 15 small randomized control trials and 5 large observational studies have shown similar findings.[18] Hence, low tidal volume ventilation targeting low plateau pressures and driving pressures should be the goal of the ventilator strategy plan. When non-invasive ventilation is given to patients with mild to moderate ARDS, they can generate excessive efforts leading to high tidal volumes, which can cause harm to the lung. In these cases, early intubation is recommended.[4]

PEEP plays an important role in the ARDS ventilatory management. It prevents atelectrauma and improves oxygenation. But higher PEEP may cause overdistention and be detrimental in causing barotrauma and deranged heart-lung interactions. Hence, it needs to be carefully titrated such that optimal alveolar opening is present at the end of expiration. The most widely used and recommended way to select optimal PEEP is as adopted at the landmark ARDS Nett trial which gives PEEP for a given FiO_2.[10] Other methods of titration are those using the pressure-volume curve analysis, transpulmonary pressure measurements using esophageal manometer to calculate the pleural pressures or use of CT, and ultrasound pictures. These methods have been studied in various clinical trials but a definite benefit of these is still lacking. Another method to prevent PEEP decruitment during suctioning is to use closed suction catheters in mechanically ventilated ARDS patients.[4]

The use of a neuromuscular agent in ARDS patients plays multiple roles in decreasing VILI. It helps in synchronizing the ventilation, decreases auto-triggers, and excessive patient-related efforts thus avoiding lung trauma, and in turn, decreases the cytokine levels thus preventing barotrauma. The ACURASYS trial published in 2010 enrolled 340 patients and showed a mortality benefit of approximately 10% at 28 days and 90 days in patients of ARDS who were given neuromuscular agents for 48 hours.[19]

Prone position ventilation helps by decreasing the heterogeneity between the lung units thereby protecting the lung from injury and improving the oxygenation **(Fig. 23.5)**.[20] A meta-analysis done of seven trials including a total of 1724 patients had

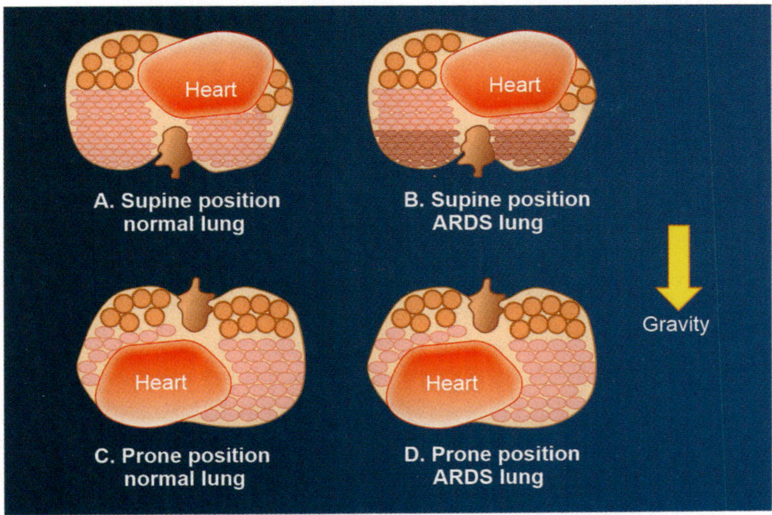

Fig. 23.5: Cross-section of the lungs. (A) Normal lung in supine position; (B) Acute respiratory distress syndrome lung in supine position; (C) Normal lung in prone position; (D) ARDS lung in prone position. Circles represent alveoli. Shaded circles indicate alveoli with infiltrates[9]

shown an absolute reduction in mortality by 10 % in patients of severe hypoxemia with ARDS having a PaO_2: FiO_2 ratio < 100.[21] The landmark PROSEVA trial is the landmark trial on prone positioning in ARDS patients done on 466 patients with severe ARDS with a PaO_2: FiO_2 ratio < 150. This trial also showed a significant mortality difference of 16.8 % at day 28 as compared to patients who were supine.[22] The largest of the meta-analyses published in March 2014 by Tonelli, *et al.* where they included 159 RCTs and 29 meta-analyses to see the effect of various modalities in cases of ARDS, also suggested that prone-position ventilation has survival benefit in cases of severe ARDS.[23]

Partial or total extracorporeal support (ECMO/ECCO has been a newer strategy that is being considered to prevent ventilator-induced lung injury. However, data regarding their clinical benefits is still less at this stage and more studies are needed before getting this into active practice.[24]

VENTILATOR-ASSOCIATED PNEUMONIA

Introduction

Ventilator-associated pneumonia (VAP) is one of the most important cause of ICU-acquired infection with incidences varying from 5 to 40% depending on the setting and diagnostic criteria.

VAP is defined by infection of the pulmonary parenchyma in patients exposed to invasive mechanical ventilation for at least 48 h and is a part of ICU-acquired pneumonia. Increased incidence of VAP is seen amongst trauma, COPD and ARDS patients. Amongst ARDS patients, incidence is higher amongst patients requiring extracorporeal membrane oxygenation (ECMO) (35%) vs those requiring only mechanical ventilation (29%). Though mortality in patients with VAP is primarily driven by patients' underlying conditions and illness severity, VAP is associated with prolonged duration of mechanical ventilation and prolonged ICU stay.

Etiology

Microorganisms causing VAP may vary depending on the duration of mechanical ventilation, length of hospital and ICU, timing and cumulative exposure to antimicrobials, the local ecology, and the occurrence of any potential epidemic phenomena in a given ICU. Major gram-negative microorganisms attributed to VAP include *Pseudomonas aeruginosa, Escherichia coli, Klebsiella pneumoniae,* and *Acinetobacter* species\while *Staphylococcus aureus* is the major Gram-positive microorganism associated with VAP. Though it was previously hypothesized that early-onset VAP (within the first 4 days of hospitalization) in previously healthy patients not receiving antibiotics usually involves normal oropharyngeal flora, current evidence suggest MDR pathogens may also be isolated in early-onset VAP, especially amongst those with antimicrobial exposure within the preceding 90 days. However, MDR pathogens are the likely causative organisms in late-onset VAP (occurring after at least 5 days of hospitalization) and amongst those patients with high risk factors . High risk factors include prior colonization or infection with MDR pathogens, ARDS and acute renal replacement therapy preceding VAP and patients with septic shock at time of diagnosis of VAP. Though uncommon, certain viruses and fungi are attributed VAP. Evolving evidence suggest that Aspergillus infection as causative organism for late VAP in patients with recent history of influenza.

The potential role of other viruses such as herpes simplex virus, cytomegalovirus and respiratory syncytial virus are still debated.

Diagnosis

The diagnosis of VAP is traditionally defined by the concomitant presence of the three following criteria: Clinical suspicion, new or progressive and persistent radiographic infiltrates, and positive microbiological cultures from lower respiratory tract specimens. Though Clinical Pulmonary Infection Score (CPIS) which is based on 6 variables (temperature, blood leukocytes, tracheal secretions aspect, oxygenation, radiographic infiltrates, and semiquantitative cultures of tracheal aspirates with Gram stain) was initially used to improve diagnostic accuracy, recent guidelines do not recommend CPIS to diagnose VAP and emphasizes need to suspect VAP in patients with clinical signs of infection when at least two of the following criteria are met. The criteria include new onset of fever, purulent endotracheal secretions, leukocytosis or leucopenia, increase in minute ventilation, decline in oxygenation, and/or increased need for vasopressors to maintain blood pressure. None of the biomarkers such as C-reactive protein, procalcitonin or soluble triggering receptor expressed on myeloid cells (sTREM-1) are recommended for VAP diagnosis as they lack sufficient accuracy.

For diagnosis of VAP, meta analysis of 5 randomized trials comparing invasive microbiological sampling techniques with quantitative cultures versus non-invasive sampling methods with either quantitative or semiquantitative cultures did not find any differences in patients' outcomes. The recent American Thoracic Society Guidelines suggest non-invasive sampling with semiquantitative cultures to diagnose VAP, rather than invasive sampling with quantitative cultures and rather than non-invasive sampling with quantitative cultures. ATS also suggest that high quality Gram stain from a respiratory specimen with numerous and predominant organisms provides support for the diagnosis of VAP. However, the absence of microorganisms on Gram stain, does not reliably exclude VAP, and review of culture results are emphazised. For patients who received antibiotics prior to microbiological sampling, procalcitonin can be used as a guide to rationalise use of antibiotics. Recommendations suggest to stop antibiotics at 48–72 h if the procalcitonin level is <0.5 ng/mL or has decrease of more than 80% as compared to the peak value.

Recent studies have evaluated the role of multiplex PCR as compared to conventional microbiological methods for diagnosis of VAP and found a concordance rate between the two techniques of 50–60% for pathogen identification, and of 70–75% for identifying resistance.[85–88] However, disadvantages associated with routine use of PCR include the risk of detection of DNA of non-viable organisms, non-pathogenic organisms and detection of pathogens at non-pathogenic thresholds.

Prevention

Contrary to earlier recommendations, current evidence suggest that selective oral and digestive decontamination may not be effective in ICUs with high baseline rates of antibiotic resistance, and subglottic secretion drainage may not shorten duration of mechanical ventilation or ICU length-of-stay . Though existing scientific evidence is limited, elevating the head of the bed to prevent reflux of gastric secretions into the lungs is the most commonly practiced intervention and may lower VAP rates. Evidence is also emerging to support putting patients in the lateral Trendelenburg as a better way to prevent VAP by recruiting gravity to carry oral secretions away from the lungs.

Adherence to VAP prevention bundle interventions like avoiding intubation and minimizing exposure to invasive ventilation by using high flow oxygen or non-invasive ventilation as alternatives to intubation, lightening sedation, using spontaneous breathing trials to prompt early extubation, and early mobilization is associated with earlier extubation and lower mortality rates.

Treatment

Intravenous (IV) antimicrobial therapy remain the cornerstone of VAP treatment. Factors determining the choice and timing of antibiotics include severity of the current illness, type and number of underlying diseases and their severity, risk factors for MDR pathogens, and the local pattern of antimicrobial susceptibility. The risk factors for MDR pathogens include high (>25%) local prevalence of pathogen resistance, antibiotic therapy in the previous 90 days, hospital stay >5 days, septic shock at VAP onset, ARDS prior to VAP onset, acute renal replacement therapy prior to VAP onset and previous colonization with MDR pathogens. While the initial empiric treatment is influenced by disease severity (i.e., mortality risk) and risk factors of MDR pathogens, the definitive treatment is focussed on targeting the isolated pathogen to limit the side effects of broad-spectrum antibiotics.

For non-immunocompromised patients with early-onset VAP and no risk factors for MDR pathogens monotherapy with narrow-spectrum antibiotic (non-pseudomonal third generation cephalosporin) can be tried. For all others, empiric treatment should include a broad-spectrum β-lactam targeting *Pseudomonas aeruginosa* and/or ESBL producing

Enterobacteriaceae (ceftazidime, cefepime, piperacillin–tazobactam or a carbapenem) plus a non-β-lactam antipseudomonal agent, such as aminoglycosides (amikacin or tobramycin) or fluoroquinolones (ciprofloxacin or levofloxacin).

References

1. Fothergill J. Observations of a case published in the last volume of the medical essays of recovering a man dead in appearance, by distending the lungs with air. Philosophical Transactions 1744;43: 275–81.
2. Lassen HC. A preliminary report on the 1952 epidemic of poliomyelitis in Copenhagen with special reference to the treatment of acute respiratory insufficiency. Lancet 1953;1:37–41
3. Respirator lung syndrome. Minn Med 1967;50:1693–705.
4. AK AK, Anjum F. Ventilator-Induced Lung Injury (VILI) [Updated 2022 Sep 19]. In: StatPearls [Internet]. Treasure Island (FL): StatPearls Publishing; 2022 Jan-. Available from: https://www.ncbi.nlm.nih.gov/books/NBK563244/.
5. Carrasco Loza R, Villamizar Rodríguez G, Medel Fernández N. Ventilator-Induced Lung Injury (VILI) in Acute Respiratory Distress Syndrome (ARDS): Volutrauma and Molecular Effects. Open Respir Med J. 2015 Jun 26;9:112–9.
6. Slutsky, AS, & Ranieri, VM (2013). Ventilator-Induced Lung Injury. New England Journal of Medicine, 369(22), 2126–36.
7. Beitler JR, Malhotra A, Thompson BT. Ventilator-induced Lung Injury. Clin Chest Med. 2016 Dec;37(4):633-646.
8. Gattinoni L, Pesenti A. The concept of "baby lung". Intensive Care Med. 2005 Jun;31(6):776–84.
9. Agrawal SP, Goel AD. Prone position ventilation in Acute Respiratory Distress Syndrome: An overview of the evidences. Indian J Anaesth. 2015 Apr;59(4):246–8.
10. The Acute Respiratory Distress Syndrome Network. Ventilation with lower tidal volumes as compared with traditional tidal volumes for acute lung injury and the acute respiratory distress syndrome. N Engl J Med 2000;342:1301–8.
11. Gajic O, Dara SI, Mendez JL, Adesanya AO, Festic E, Caples SM, Rana R, St Sauver JL, Lymp JF, Afessa B, Hubmayr RD. Ventilator-associated lung injury in patients without acute lung injury at the onset of mechanical ventilation. Crit Care Med. 2004 Sep;32(9):1817–24.
12. Diaz R, Heller D. Barotrauma and Mechanical Ventilation. [Updated 2022 Aug 1]. In: StatPearls [Internet]. Treasure Island (FL): StatPearls Publishing; 2022 Jan. Available from: https://www.ncbi.nlm.nih.gov/books/NBK545226/
13. Williams EC, Motta-Ribeiro GC, Vidal Melo MF. Driving Pressure and Transpulmonary Pressure: How Do We Guide Safe Mechanical Ventilation? Anesthesiology. 2019 Jul;131(1):155–63.
14. Amato MB, Meade MO, Slutsky AS, Brochard L, Costa EL, Schoenfeld DA, Stewart TE, Briel M, Talmor D, Mercat A, Richard JC, Carvalho CR, Brower RG. Driving pressure and survival in the acute respiratory distress syndrome. N Engl J Med 2015; 372:747–55
15. Cipulli F, Vasques F, Duscio E, Romitti F, Quintel M, Gattinoni L. Atelectrauma or volutrauma: the dilemma. J Thorac Dis. 2018 Mar;10(3):1258-1264. doi: 10.21037/jtd.2018.02.71. PMID: 29707275; PMCID: PMC5906244.
16. Pinsky MR. Cardiopulmonary Interactions: Physiologic Basis and Clinical Applications. Ann Am Thorac Soc. 2018 Feb;15(Suppl 1):S45-S48. doi: 10.1513/AnnalsATS.201704-339FR. PMID: 28820609; PMCID: PMC5822394.
17. Fan E, Del Sorbo L, Goligher EC, *et al.* An Official American Thoracic Society/European Society of Intensive Care Medicine/Society of Critical Care Medicine Clinical Practice Guideline:

Mechanical Ventilation in Adult Patients with Acute Respiratory Distress Syndrome. Am J Respir Crit Care Med 2017;195:1253–63.

18. Serpa Neto A, Cardoso SO, Manetta JA, Pereira VG, Espósito DC, Pasqualucci Mde O, Damasceno MC, Schultz MJ. Association between use of lung-protective ventilation with lower tidal volumes and clinical outcomes among patients without acute respiratory distress syndrome: a meta-analysis. JAMA. 2012 Oct 24;308(16):1651–9.
19. Papazian L, Forel JM, Gacouin A, Penot-Ragon C, Perrin G, Loundou A, Jaber S, Arnal JM, Perez D, Seghboyan JM, Constantin JM, Courant P, Lefrant JY, Guérin C, Prat G, Morange S, Roch A., ACURASYS Study Investigators. Neuromuscular blockers in early acute respiratory distress syndrome. N Engl J Med. 2010 Sep 16;363(12):1107–16.
20. Agrawal SP, Goel AD. Prone position ventilation in Acute Respiratory Distress Syndrome: An overview of the evidences. Indian J Anaesth. 2015 Apr;59(4):246-8. doi: 10.4103/0019-5049.155004. PMID: 25937653; PMCID: PMC4408655.
21. Beitler JR, Shaefi S, Montesi SB, Devlin A, Loring SH, Talmor D, *et al.* Prone positioning reduces mortality from acute respiratory distress syndrome in the low tidal volume era: A meta-analysis. Intensive Care Med. 2014;40:332–41
22. Guérin C, Reignier J, Richard JC, Beuret P, Gacouin A, Boulain T, Mercier E, Badet M, Mercat A, Baudin O, Clavel M, Chatellier D, Jaber S, Rosselli S, Mancebo J, Sirodot M, Hilbert G, Bengler C, Richecoeur J, Gainnier M, Bayle F, Bourdin G, Leray V, Girard R, Baboi L, Ayzac L; PROSEVA Study Group. Prone positioning in severe acute respiratory distress syndrome. N Engl J Med. 2013 Jun 6;368(23):2159–68.
23. Tonelli AR, Zein J, Adams J, Ioannidis JP. Effects of interventions on survival in acute respiratory distress syndrome: An umbrella review of 159 published randomized trials and 29 meta-analyses. Intensive Care Med. 2014;40:769–87
24. Leligdowicz A, Fan E. Extracorporeal life support for severe acute respiratory distress syndrome. Curr Opin Crit Care 2015;21:13–9.
25. Umbrello M, Chiumello D. Interpretation of the transpulmonary pressure in the critically ill patient. Ann Transl Med 2018;6(19):383. doi: 10.21037/atm.2018.05.31
26. Kalikkot Thekkeveedu, R.; El-Saie, A.; Prakash, V.; Katakam, L.; Shivanna, B. Ventilation-Induced Lung Injury (VILI) in Neonates: Evidence-Based Concepts and Lung-Protective Strategies. J. Clin. Med. 2022, 11, 557. https://doi.org/ 10.3390/jcm11030557
27. Intensive Care Med (2016) 42:663–673 DOI 10.1007/s00134-015-4200-8.

CHAPTER 24

Non-Invasive Ventilation

R Vijai Kumar

INTRODUCTION

History

Almost 80 years ago (1940) a clinician and a few investigators in Bellevue Hospital near Manhattan, New York City, USA, started using a strange looking contraption along with an anesthetic mask to treat cases of respiratory failure. Motley is credited with using this non-invasive ventilation (NIV) on people with pneumonia, pulmonary edema, Guillain-Barré syndrome, and acute asthma with varied success.[1] In course of time, as Invasive Mechanical Ventilation started gaining popularity, NIV was relegated to backbenches for a short time. Forty years later, Professor Sullivan Colin Edward, Honorary Physician at Royal Prince Alfred Hospital, Sydney, Australia, discovered that nasal Continuous Positive Airway Pressure (CPAP) is beneficial to patients with Obstructive Sleep Apnea (OSA).[2,3] Eventually, as clinical research and technological advances progressed shoulder to shoulder, CPAP devices became better and better and paved way to Bilevel Positive Airway Pressure (BiPAP) machines. With rapid advances on the field of biomedical engineering, NIV machines currently match technically almost in all areas of Invasive Mechanical Ventilators, and at the same time offer all the advantages.

Definition

It is defined as providing ventilation without the use of an invasive airway (endotracheal tube).

Advantages of Non-invasive Ventilation

It is rather paradoxical and an irony that all the disadvantages of invasive mechanical ventilation are in fact advantages of NIV. This was a major reason that pulmonologists and critical care physicians world over were quick to realise the drastic reduction in morbidity and mortality in their patients. They started expanding the indications for NIV as they continued to accumulate experience in the use of this method of ventilation. Non-invasive ventilation can truly be considered as an important milestone in the management of respiratory failure **(Box 24.1)**.[4]

Mechanism of Efficacy of NIV

Non-invasive ventilation by virtue of augmenting the respiratory effort, can unload the respiratory respiratory muscles, especially the diaphragm. NIV by increasing the alveolar ventilation, can improve the gas exchange. This can be seen improved oxygenation and decreasing partial pressure carbon dioxide in the blood ($PaCO_2$).

Cardiopulmonary Interactions

As a result of changes in the intrathoracic pressures and changes in lung volumes, certain reciprocal changes occur in the heart. During a spontaneous breathing, and during inspiration, a negative intrathoracic pressure develops inside the thorax, and the blood gets sucked into the right atrium (RA) through superior vena cava and inferior vena cava. However, the reverse is the case for a patient on NIV. The positive pressure is transmitted across the intrathoracic compartment, resulting in decreased venous return into the right heart, and thus reduced right ventricular output into the pulmonary arteries. However, this effect is more pronounced in hypovolemic patients.

Box 24.1

Invasive Mechanical Ventilation	Non-invasive Ventilation
Intubation with endotracheal tube	Intubation not required
Natural defense system bypassed	Defense system intact
Extreme discomfort to patient	Minimal discomfort
Patient needs significant sedation	Minimal/no sedation
High nosocomial infections	Negligible infections
Volutrauma/Barotrauma	No such complication
Longer ICU/hospital stay	Shorter ICU/hospital stay
More morbidity	Lesser morbidity
Higher mortality	Lesser mortality
Higher healthcare cost	Lesser healthcare cost

Ventilators: Non-invasive ventilators basically generate pressure with a turbine or a pump. If the pressure generated is continuous throughout the respiratory cycle, then it is a Continuous Positive Airway Pressure (CPAP) machine. The pressure generated can be higher during inspiration and lower during expiratory phase, thus providing a bilevel pressure and hence called Bilevel Positive Airway Pressure (BiPAP) machines. Pressure from the non-invasive ventilators is carried through ventilator circuits, and delivered into the mask (interface). Patient can inhale the high-pressure air through nose/mouth into his lungs. Usually these are single tube circuits. The expired air from the patient escapes through expiratory port (intentional leak) placed near the mask. A continuous flow of air during expiration prevents rebreathing. A pressure of 4 cm H_2O is desirable to prevent rebreathing. Newer machines have the expiratory port on the interface rather than in the circuit. Provisions are available to add oxygen into the circuits. Even regular intensive care unit (ICU) ventilators can be used to provide Non-invasive ventilation. However, the ICU ventilators have two separate circuit limbs for inspiration and expiration separately.

Non-invasive ventilators come equipped with trigger sensitive to pressure and flow. Several modes like spontaneous mode (S), timed mode (T) and ST mode are available. These machines are capable of compensating for leaks to a great extent. NIV machines switch from inspiration to expiration as the flow drops (flow cycled). Some machines do the cycling automatically. The current NIV machines are as good as the ICU ventilators[6] as they are capable of providing all the sophisticated monitoring and chip-based algorithms **(Box 24.2)**.

Box 24.2: NIV machines

- Continuous positive airway pressure (CPAP) machine
- Bilevel positive airway pressure (BIPAP) machine
- Home NIV machines
- ICU ventilators (to be used for NIV)
- Have all modes (S/T/ST/PS/PC)
- Have leak compensation
- Have chip-based algorithms
- Can display fraction of inspired oxygen (FiO_2)
- Have monitoring capabilities
- Have alarms
- Operate on A/C and D/C power
- Can run on batteries (4 hr/8 hr/16 hr)

Indications

In experienced hands, NIV can virtually be used in almost all major situations, where a regular invasive ventilation can be thought of. However, it is important to appreciate the fact that the interface is a mask sitting on the nose/mouth/face and not an endotracheal tube. It is also important to realise that the patient needs to be at least partially conscious and not in a coma. Most of the experience on NIV was gained by pulmonologists who treated acute exacerbations of chronic obstructive pulmonary disease (COPD). After remarkable success shown by the randomised clinical trials (RCT) in these group of patients, certain basic do's and don'ts were understood, and eventually were extrapolated to other causes of respiratory failure, including cardiogenic pulmonary edema **(Box 24.3)**.

Box 24.3: Indications for non-invasive ventilation

- Acute exacerbation of COPD
- Cardiogenic pulmonary edema
- Respiratory failure in HIV
- Respiratory failure in immunologically compromised patients
- Post operative (general anesthesia) respiratory compromise
- Neuromuscular disorders of chest wall
- Guillain-Barré syndrome
- Respiratory failure due to kyphoscoliosis
- Postextubation respiratory failure
- Weaning failure
- Acute severe asthma in the emergency room

Contraindications

As discussed earlier, there are two very important factors which can limit the use of non-invasive ventilation. First, non-invasive ventilation is delivered through an interface attached to the face of patient, and the second, the patient should be reasonably conscious and oriented (Glasgow Coma Scale >8) **(Box 24.4)**.

Box 24.4: Glasgow Coma Scale

Eye Response	
Eyes open spontaneously	4
Eyes open to verbal command	3
Eyes open to pain	2
No eye opening	1
Motor Response	
Obeys command	6
Localises pain	5
Withdraws from pain	4
Flexion response to pain	3
Extension response to pain	2
No motor response	1
Verbal Response	
Oriented	5
Confused	4
Inappropriate words	3
Incomprehensible words	2
No verbal response	1

Many of the contraindications actually, are relative and only a few are absolute contraindications **(Box 24.5)**.

Box 24.5: Contraindications for non-invasive ventilation

- **Absolute**
- Cardiac arrest
- Coma
- Arrhythmia with compromised hemodynamics
- Shock with major organ failure
- Surgery on face/neck/oesophagus
- Trauma face/neck/head
- Severe deformity of Face
- Upper airway obstruction
- **Relative**
- Confused/agitated/uncooperative patient
- Uncontrolled/severe vomiting
- Copious AW secretions/inability to cough and expectorate
- Impaired consciousness (GCS <8)
- Severe acidosis (pH <6)

Modes

It is easier to understand, the different modes delivered by the NIV ventilators, if we can look at what makes the machine to initiate an inspiratory breath into patient's lungs (trigger), how is the volume of air delivered to the lungs (control), and what makes the machine to stop pushing the air (cycling).

Trigger

The ventilator needs a signal/trigger from the patient, to initiate inspiratory flow. The trigger can be a drop in the pressure in the (proximal) airways. This trigger is seen in the older ventilators. Recent ventilators have a flow trigger, that is a slight drop in the flow of air towards the end of expiratory phase, is detected by the machine, which can trigger the inspiration. Sometimes there can be a false triggering due to air leaks. However, newer machines can counter these air leaks (compensate) and thus prevent this anomaly.

Control

The body of inspired air travels from machine and into the lungs. This is mostly pressure limited, that is controlled by a set pressure as determined by the operator. Earlier ventilators were volume controlled, however the newer maches have a hybrid facility where both pressure and volume can be contolled by the operator.

Cycling

Cycling is a signal which makes the machine to end inspiration and allow expiration. Cycling from inspiration to expiration can happen when the inspiratory flow drops (flow cycled), or when the operator sets a time limit for inspiration (time cycled), the familiar I:E ratio.

1. Volume targeted ventilation mode: The ventilator delivers a preset volume of air during inspiration (tidal volume). However, flow, time, pressure will be determined as per the volume delivered. This mode is not a popular mode.
2. Pressure targeted ventilation: This is a popular mode in non-invasive ventilation. A preset pressure for the inspiration is selected. Higher pressure is delivered in the beginning of inspiration, gradually decelerating towards the expiration.

Continuous Positive Airway Pressure (CPAP)

The NIV machine maintains a constant preset pressure throughout the respiratory cycle (inspiration and expiration). There is no trigger and no cycling. Patient can inhale as much air as he wants, flow and time are as per patient's effort. This constant pressure in the circuit and airways creates an effect of air splint and thus collapsed upper airways are kept open. Also, the CPAP opens the collapsed and under ventilated alveoli, increases functional residual capacity (FRC), to improve oxygenation, and mitigate right to left intrapulmonary shunt.

For these reasons CPAP is useful in treating Obstructive Sleep Apnea (OSA) and Congestive Heart Failure (CHF). CPAP in patients with CHF can decrease the left ventricular afterload, and can improve cardiac output. In both situations the usual pressure needed is around 10 cm H_2O (**Fig. 24.1**).

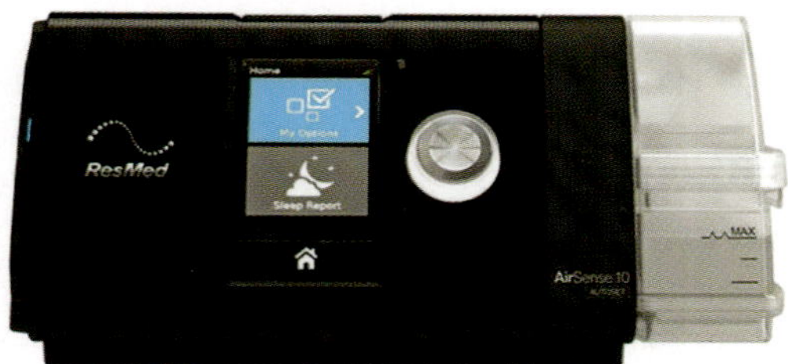

Fig. 24.1: Continuous positive airway pressure machine

Bilevel Positive Airway Pressure (BiPAP)

This mode is used widely in critical care units. As the term denotes, there are two different pressures delivered by the machine, a higher-pressure during inspiration during expiration. It is triggered by pressure and flow, and cycled by flow, and limited by pressure which is preset.

Thus, machine needs to be preset with Inspiratory Positive Airway Pressure (IPAP) and Expiratory Positive Airway Pressure (EPAP). The difference between the two pressures is the pressure support (PS) in the language of the conventional Invasive Mechanical Ventilators. Tidal Volume (TV) varies as per patient's effort, compliance, airway resistance.

It is important to keep the EPAP low (usually ⅓ of IPAP) to generate a good pressure support. An often-used scenario is 12/4 (of IPAP/EPAP). EPAP is synonymous with Positive End Expiratory Pressure (PEEP) in the language of conventional Mechanical Ventilators.[7]

BiPAP is most useful in Acute Exacerbation of COPD (AECOPD), and in all those situations where a good tidal volume is required to wash out the excessive CO_2 from the circulation.

Sometimes due to poor effort from the patient, the desired tidal volume and hence minute volume may not be achieved. To overcome this difficulty the machine calculates TV of a few breaths and increases the inspiratory pressure thereby to augment the TV and thus achieve a preset minute volume (MV). For this reason, this added feature is called Average Volume Assured Pressure Support[8] (AVAPS). This feature goes by different names in machines of different companies.

Machines are available with features of BIPAP spontaneous/timed/controlled mode, etc. (**Fig. 24.2**).

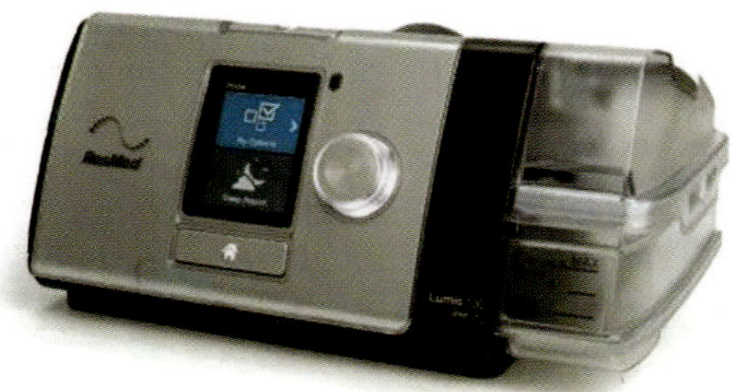

Fig. 24.2: Bilevel positive airway pressure machine

Interfaces

The machines described above will use room air and generate compressed high pressure flow. This is transmitted through the a very soft yet non-collapsible tubing. These tubes (22 mm) are made from a durable polyolefin elastomer material (that is latex, BPA and phthalate-free). The universal connectors are made with flexible thermoplastic elastomer. These tubes are connected to a mask through which the patient receives the high-pressure air. The masks (interfaces) come in several sizes (Small, Medium and Large) to fit different size/shape of patient's face/head. These masks are held by soft straps and fixed with a Velcro tape. Although several masks of several descriptions are available for use (nasal, oro-nasal, full face, helmet, etc.), in the hospital scenario, it is best to use an oro-nasal mask **(Figs 24.3 and 24.4)**. Oro-nasal mask is the best choice for first time users and sick patients who need efficacy more than comfort in a short duration of time. In the earlier times these masks were made with plastic, however all current generation masks are made with silicone. The part which touches the skin is made of even softer (cushion) silicone.

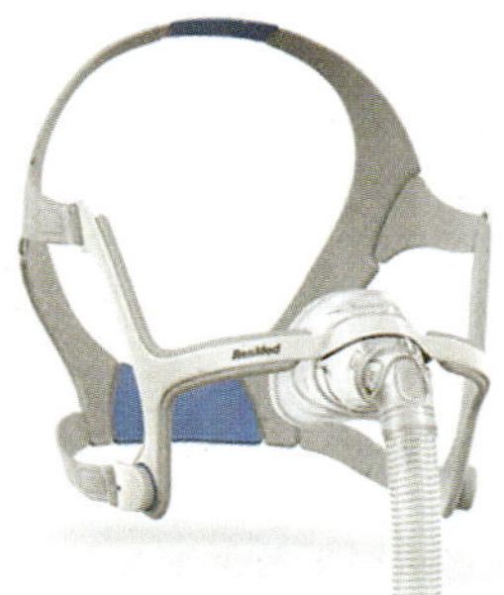

Fig. 24.3: Oro-nasal mask

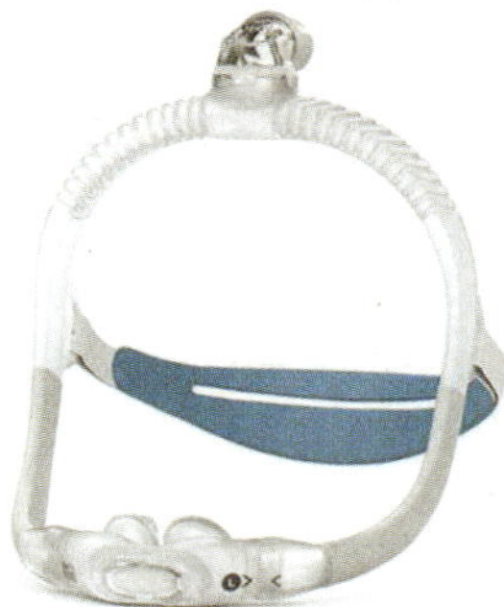

Fig. 24.4: Nasal pillows

Technique of Applying the Mask: The method of applying the mask on the face of the patient is by far the most important part of non-invasive ventilation which decides a successful outcome **(Box 24.6)**.

Box 24.6: Important steps for applying the mask on the patient

1. Make sure the appropriate (CPAP/BIPAP) machine is available
2. Connect the machine to power source, and switch it on
3. Select the appropriate setting (pressure)
4. Obtain necessary consent from patient/family
5. Explain to patient the procedure to patient/family
6. Reassure the patient
7. Select the right fit mask
8. Make sure the connections from the machine to to the mask via the tubing is secure and free from leaks
9. Hold the mask in your hand and gently place it on the face of patient (do not fasten the straps)
10. Hold the mask for a few minutes on the face of of the patient (15 to 30 minutes), and keep talking to the patient sitting next to him gently and softly. The blast of air will make some patients uncomfortable, and some patients become claustrophobic on applying the mask
11. When the patient becomes comfortable and accepts the mask, gently strap the mask (head gear), using the 2 finger rule.
12. Make sure that there are no wrinkles in the soft part of silicone mask. Wrinkles and folds appear if the mask is tightened too much

Complications of Interfaces

Applying the mask too tight can cause discomfort, air leaks due to folds in the silicone lining. Sometimes because of the pressure, sores/ulcers can occur on the bridge of the nose (**Fig. 24.5**). One can use the 2 finger rule (inserting 2 fingers near the temple and gently applying the straps (**Fig. 24.6**). Applying an adhesive tape over the bridge of the nose also minimizes the risk of pressure sores (**Fig. 24.7**).

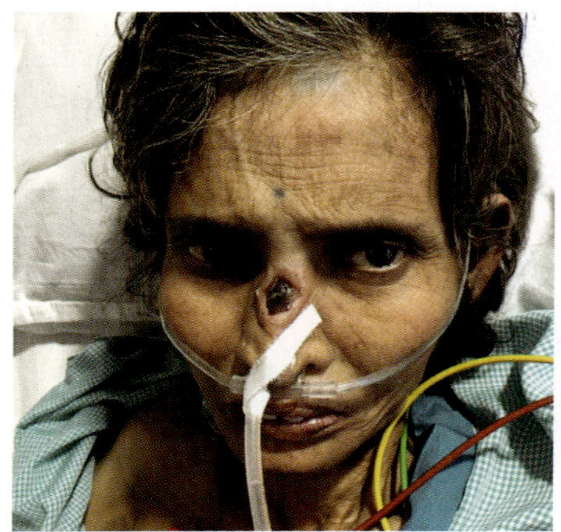

Fig.24.5: Skin necrosis caused by mask over nasal bone

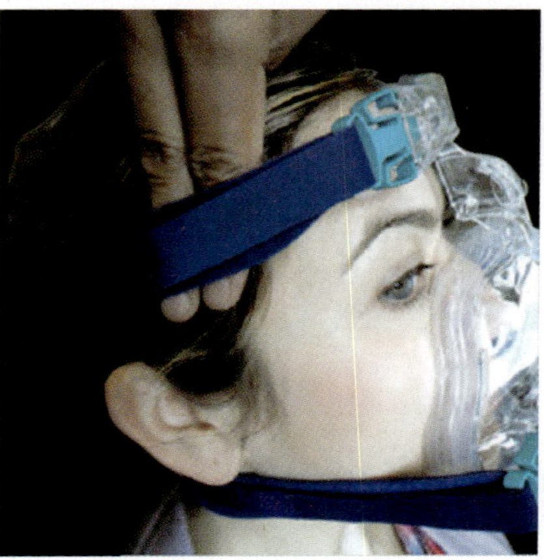

Fig. 24.6: Two finger rule (insert 2 fingers and gently fix the straps)

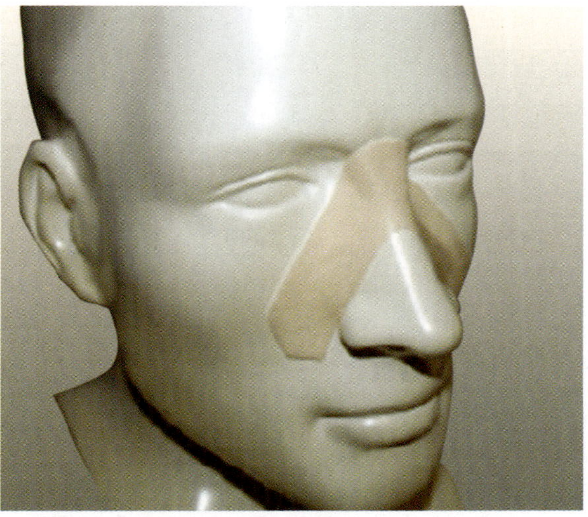

Fig. 24.7: Foam tape placed over bridge of nose

Adjuvant therapies although the main purpose of non-invasive positive pressure ventilation (NIPPV) is to provide ventilatory support, a variety of adjuvant therapies and procedures also can be performed to augment the outcomes (**Box 24.7**).

Box 24.7: Adjuvant therapies/interventions

- Oxygen
- Aerosol (nebulisers)
- Metered dose inhalers
- Bronchoscopy

Oxygen

Most patients of respiratory failure need supplemental oxygen. Oxygen can be delivered through many entry points in the system (directly into the NIV machines, tubing or a port provided in the mask). Current technology allows the clinician to monitor oxygen delivery (SpO_2) through the monitoring panel fixed on the machine. As per the basic principles of management of respiratory failure, it is important to maintain the SpO_2 around 90%, thus the arterial blood oxygen can remain around 60 mm Hg.

Nebulisation

Many important drugs can be delivered through nebulization [Nebulus Cloud (Greek)]. Short acting β_2 agonists (SABA), Long acting β_2 agonists (LABA), Short acting muscarinic agents (SAMA), Inhaled corticosteroids (ICS), Antibiotics (e.g. Tobramycin) as and when needed, and as frequently as needed, without removing the NIV mask and without disturbing the tubing arrangement. Special nebulization ports are provided in some masks available in the market (**Figs 24.8 and 24.9**).[9]

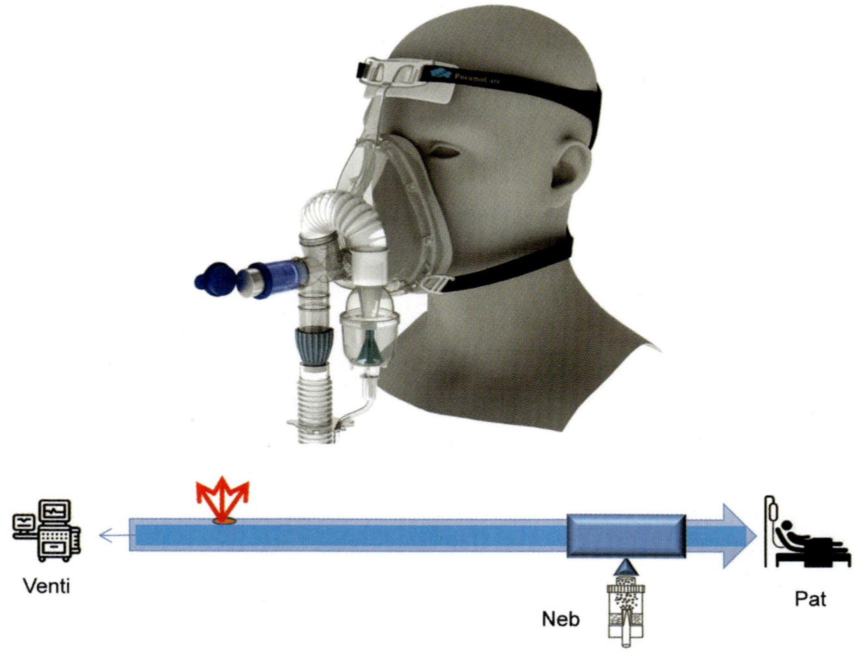

Figs 24.8 and 24.9: In line aerosol delivery
Courtesy: Pneumo Care (Deepak Chander)

Metered Dose Inhalers (pMDI)

Almost all drugs delivered through nebulization are also available in the pMDI form. As some studies have shown 10 pMDIs can be as effective as the nebulization. And in fact, they are simpler to deliver. Many tubing inlets provide a port for facilitating the inhaler. There are special spacer devices available to be attached/inserted into the tubing of NIV system.

Fiberoptic Bronchoscopy

There are many situations in the ICU where a patient admitted for an infectious cause or a noninfectious cause, may need a bronchoscopy. It may be to sample the tracheobronchial secretions, or to clear thick mucus impacting the airways making NIV ineffective. It can even be a therapeutic bronchoscopy for the same indications as an office day care. Foreign body extractions, restoring lumen for a stenotic trachea or bronchus also can be undertaken, however these procedures are desirable to perform after an endotracheal intubation. Special NIV masks are available **(Fig. 24.10)** for inserting the bronchoscope either orally or through the nasal route.

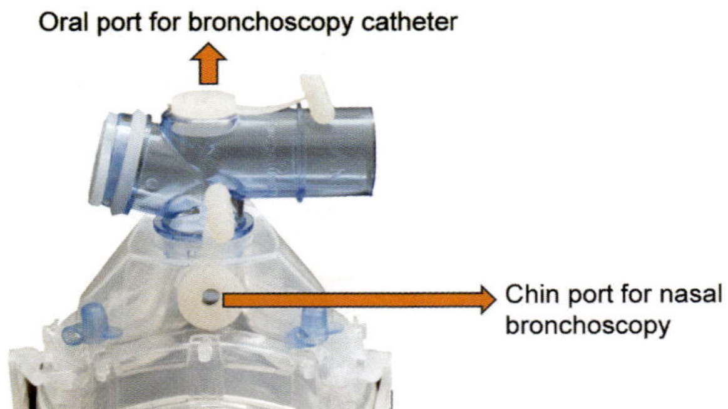

Fig 24.10: NIV mask. *Courtesy*: Pneumocare (Deepak Chander)

NIV in Type 1 Resp Failure

Most common pathophysiological reason for type1 respiratory failure is a ventilation perfusion mismatch (V/Q mismatch). Typically where the ventilation is good but perfusion is inadequate or the other way, that is perfusion is good but ventilation is faulty. Most such cases of V/Q mismatch is resolved with administration of 100% oxygen. An example of decreased ventilation is an airway disease like asthma or COPD. And an example of decreased perfusion is interstitial lung disease or typically pulmonary embolism. Sometimes shunts where the deoxygenated blood comes back into arterial circulation (called shunt) can cause severe hypoxemia. The shunt can be inside the heart (Atrial septal defect, Ventricular septal defect, etc.), or in the lung (Arteriovenous malformations). Appropriately the shunts are called intracardiac or intrapulmonary. Administration of oxygen (even 100%) will not rectify the hypoxemia unless the shunts are rectified **(Box 24.8)**.

Box 24.8: Type 1 respiratory failure (causes)

- **Airway**
- COPD
- Asthma
- Bronchiectasis (rare)

Interstitial
- Pneumonia
- Pulmonary edema
- Interstitial lung diseases
- Pneumoconiosis
- ARDS

Pleura
- Pneumothorax (tension)
- Pleural effusion (massive)

Vascular
- Pulmonary thromboembolism
- FAT/Air Embolism
- Pulmonary Hypertension

Rationale for use of NIV in Hypoxemic Respiratory Failure

NIV improves alveolar ventilation (opens the collapsed alveoli, and keeps them open), improves oxygenation, exerts pressure on the alveolar walls to expel the excess fluid. This advantage is achieved by Inspiratory Positive Airway Pressure (IPAP) which in mechanical ventilation language is called Peak End Expiratory Pressure (PEEP). That is the reason Continuous Positive Airway Pressure (CPAP) works well in these situations.[11] A classic example of hypoximec respiratory failure is Cardiogenic Pulmonary Edema. Several studies have shown the beneficial effect of NIV in cardiogenic pulmonary edema. In a randomised study, symptoms and metabolic disturbances resolved rapidly.[12] A meta-analysis of 24 studies involving cases of acute cardiogenic pulmonary edema, showed that NIV decreased hospital mortality and need for endotracheal intubation.[13]

NIV in Type 2 Respriatory Failure

Use of NIV in type 2 respiratory failure is a historical milestone. Several trials and randomised clinical trials have shown that NIV can dramatically improve and relieve the symptoms of respiratory failure, correct the blood gas abnormalities, and also correct the acidemia **(Box 24.9)**. The trials have also shown to reduce hospital stay, reduce ICU stay and reduce cost of treatment. Need for intubation and connecting to mechanical ventilator has been significantly reduced.

The pathophysiology can be due to the following 3 reasons:

1. Reduced respiratory drive: Due to drug overdose, anaesthesia, diseases of medulla, or any injury/infection to brain.
2. Diseases of respiratory muscles (chiefly diaphragm), nerves, anterior horn cells: Examples are trauma to chest (flail chest), kyphoscoliosis, poliomyelitis, myopathies and Guillain-Barré syndrome.

3. Excessive inspiratory muscle load: Classic example is acute exacerbation of COPD, where the respiratory muscles are overworked and fatigued, leading to decreased respiratory drive, in the background of generalized airway narrowing

Box 24.9: Benefits of NIV in acute/chronic type 2 respiratory failure

- NIV can relieve the symptoms of respiratory failure (dyspnea)
- Pressure support (PS) plays an important role
- PS is the difference between IPAP and EPAP
- PS drives the tidal volume (TV) and minute volume (MV)
- EPAP also stabilizes the upper airway (maintains patency)
- Corrects intrinsic PEEP
- Washes out CO_2
- Rests the respiratory muscles (diaphragm)
- Recruits collapsed alveoli
- Improves V/Q mismatch
- Corrects hypoxemia
- Corrects the acidemia
- Reduces hospital stay
- Reduce ICU stay
- Reduces cost of treatment
- Reduces need for intubation/ventilation

NIV in Acute Exacerbation of COPD

Use of NIV in this indication has dramatically changed the outcome. There is a severe muscle fatigue (especially the diaphragm), bronchospasm, and air trapping which in turn causes dynamic hyperinflation in these patients. This results not just hypoxia, but retention of carbon dioxide, and the blood $PaCO_2$ starts increasing. NIV reverses all these pathophysiological abnormalities.

Evidence

Plant and his associates in 2000 have shown very convincingly that bilevel NIV is very effective. In the landmark trial from United Kingdom the authors have randomised 236 patients with acute exacerbation of COPD into two groups of 118 each. Inclusion criteria was a respiratory rate of >23 per minute, pH of between 7.25 and 7.35, $PaCO_2$ >6 kPa All patients had similar demographic and clinical parameters. One group received the standard care, while the other group were treated with Bilevel NIV. Patients were followed up until death or discharge. Thirty patients (27.1%) got intubated while in the NIV group 18 (15.3%) needed intubation. There was a significant difference in in-hospital mortality, 24 (20.3%) patients died in the standard care, while 12 (10.2%) died in the NIV group. Arterial Blood Gas (ABG) analysis was done at baseline, 1 hour and 4 hours after initiating NIV. Success was predictable with improvement in pH and respiratory rate (RR) at 4 hours NIV treatment.

Several other studies validated these outcomes. Keenan, *et al.* 15 in their review of literature concluded that NIV reduces need for intubation, complications, overall mortality, and length of hospital stay. Various authors have initiated NIV on very severe

COPD exacerbations (pH <7.25), and surprisingly, the outcomes were very good **(Box 24.11)**. Intubation rates came down by 34%, inhospital mortality by 12%, and absolute reduction in length of stay by 5.59 days. Most studies have concluded that improvement in pH and $PaCO_2$ after 2 hours of NIV is predictive success.[16–18]

Box 24.10: Advantages of NIV in AECOPD

- Decreased need for intubation
- Reduced in-hospital mortality
- Reduced hospital stays
- Reduced overall cost
- Reduced hospital acquired infections
- Improvement in pH and $PaCO_2$ after 2 hours is predictive success

Box 24.11: NIV in extended indications

- ARDS
- Postoperative respiratory distress
- Pneumonia in immunocompromised patients
- Patients who refuse mech ventilation
- Extubation failures
- Obstructive sleep apnea
- Neuromuscular diseases
- Chest wall deformities
- Flail chest
- Palliative care
- Respiratory support during transport
- During procedures in ICU
- During interventional pulmonary procedures

Monitoring

The first 2 to 4 hours are crucial while the patient is on NIV, and very close monitoring is vital to decide either success or failure of NIV. Monitoring the patient for clinical parameters and also by Arterial Blood Gas (ABG) analysis is important. The clinician at the end of the magic 2 hours must decide, if continuation of NIV is beneficial to the patient. Delay causes increased mortality.[19] Bedside clinical monitoring is of utmost importance and can never be replaced with lab investigations.

It is desirable to keep an exclusive unit for patients who are on NIV, and the unit can be manned by respiratory therapists and nurses who are familiar with the standard operating procedures (SOP) and all the protocols. Exclusive special charts can be made available where all pertinent information is documented. Experience has shown that such dedicated units have a better success rates **(Box 24.12)**.

Weaning

General principles of weaning are very similar to those practiced for invasive mechanical ventilation. The most important underlying tenet is that "Has the reason for which the NIV was initiated, been resolved?"

Box 24.12: What to monitor while on NIV

Bedside

- General demeanor of the patient
- Consciousness level
- GCS score
- Is the patient comfortable
- Any vomiting
- Any copious expectoration
- Visible respiratory distress
- Respiratory rate (<23 p mt)
- Hemodynamically stable
- Check urine output (1 ml/kg/hr)
- Hydration
- Nutrition

Mask

- Is it fitting well (any leaks)
- Are there any undue pressure points

Blood Gases (ABG)

- Is the pH improving (compared to base line)
- Is the $PaCO_2$ improving (compared to base line)
- Oxygenation (SpO_2 88–90%)
- Transcutaneous CO_2 (desirable/not essential)

Machine

- Make sure the pressures are right (IPAP/EPAP)

All the clinical and laboratory parameters which were disturbed or deranged should have been normalized. The criteria for weaning are a commonsense points **(Box 24.13)**.

Box 24.13: Criteria for weaning

pH	>7.35
SpO_2	±+90%
Resp rate	<23 p mt
Herat rate	<100 p mt
Diastolic blood pressure	±100 mmHg

References

1. Motley HL, Werko L, Cournand A, Richards DW. Observations on the clinical use of intermittent positive pressure. J Aviation Med 1947;18(5):417–35.
2. Pierson DJ. Non-invasive positive pressure ventilation: history and terminology. Respir Care 1997;42(3):370–79.
3. Sullivan CE, Berthon-Jones M, Issa FG, Eves L. Reversal of obstructive sleep apnea by continuous positive airway pressure applied through the nose. Lancet 1981;1(8225):862-865.
4. Nava S, Hill N. Non-invasive Ventilation in acute respiratory failure. Lancet.2009;374 (9685):250–9.
5. Schettino GP, Chatmongkolchart S, Hess DR, Kacmarek RM, Position of exhalation port and mask design affect CO_2 rebreathing during positive pressure non-invasive ventilation Critical Care Medicine 2003:31(8);2178–21.

6. Miyoshi E, Fujino Y, Uchiyama A, Mashimo T, Nishimura M, Effects of gas leak on triggering function, humidification, and inspiratory oxygen fraction during non-invasive positive pressure ventilation Chest 2005:128 (5);3691–98.
7. Rabec C, Rodenstein D, Leger P, Rouault S, Perrin C, Gonzalez-Bermejo J, *et al.* Ventilator modes and settings during non-invasive ventilation: effects on respiratory events and implications for their identification. Thorax.2011;66(2)170–8.
8. Briones Claudett KH, Briones Claudet M, Chung Sang WongM, Nuques Martnez A, Soto Espinoza, R, Montalvo M, *et al.* Non-invasive mechanical ventilation with average volume assured pressure support (AVAPS) in patients with chronic obstructive pulmonary disease and hypercapnic encephalopathy BMC Pulm Med 2013; 13:12.
9. Ari A. Aerosol Therapy in Pulmonary Critical care. Resp Care. 2015;60 (6): 858–79.
10. Nava S, Karakurt S, Rampulla C, *et al.* Salbutamol delivery during Non-invasive mechanical ventilation in patients with chronic obstructive pulmonary disease: A randomised controlled study. Intensive care Medicine 2001;27: 1627–35.
11. MacIntyre NR. Physiologic effects of Mechanical ventilation. Respiratory Care.2019; 64 (6):617–28.
12. Gray A, Goodcare S,Newby DE, Masson M, Sampson F, Nicholl J, *et al.* Non-invasive ventilation in acute cardiogenic pulmonary edema. N Eng J Med. 2008; 359:142–51.
13. Berbenetz N, Wang Y, Brown J, Godfrey C, Ahmad M, Vital FMR, *et al.* Non invasive Ventilation in acute cardiogenic pulmonary edema. Cochrane database Syst Rev 2019: (4): CD 005351.
14. P K Plant, J L Owen, M W Elliott: Thorax 2001;56:708–12.
15. Keenan SP, Sinuff T, Cook DJ, Hill NS. Which patients with acute exacerbation of chronic obstructive pulmonary disease benefit from non-invasive positive pressure ventilation? A systematic review of literature Ann Int Medicine 2003;138 (11):861–70.
16. Diaz GG, Alcaraz AC, Talavera JC, Perez PJ, Rodriguez AE, Cordoba FG, *et al.* Non-invasive positive pressure ventilation to treat hypercapnic coma secondary to respiratory failure. Chest 2005;127 (3):952–60.
17. Confalonieri M, Garuti G, *et al.* A chart of failure risk for non-invasive ventilation in patients with COPD exacerbation Eur Resp J.2005;25(2)348–55.
18. Scala R, Naldi M, Archinucci I, Coniglio G, Nava S, Non-invasive positive pressure ventilation in patients with acute exacerbation of COPD and varying levels of consciousness. Chest 2005;128(3)348–55.
19. Antonelli M, Conti G, Moro M, Esquinas A, Gonzalez-Diaz G, Confalonieri M, *et al.* Predictors of failure of non-invasive positive pressure ventilation in patients with acute hypoxemic respiratory failure: a multi-center study. Intensive Care Medicine 2001; 27 (11):1718–28.

CHAPTER 25

Nutritional Assessment

❑ Subba Reddy K ❑ Raj Kumar Jupally

Nutrition is an important aspect in management of critically ill patients who are on mechanical ventilator support. Critical illness is often associated with a catabolic stress state and inadequate nutrition can lead to complications such as increased infectious morbidity, loss of lean body mass and increase in hospital length of stay. Adequate nutritional intervention has shown to attenuate metabolic response to stress and favorably modulate immune responses. Examining critically ill patients will help in deciding the strategy of nutritional support to fulfill the macro- and micro-nutrient requirements. Route of feed administration (enteral or parenteral) needs to be decided based on the assessment of hemodynamic status and gastrointestinal functioning. Prospective observational study, conducted in Indian multidisciplinary ICU, involving adult critically ill patients requiring mechanical ventilation for greater than 48 hr showed that 36.1% of patients were at nutritional risk and only 29.6% of patients achieved nutritional adequacy. Underfeeding in mechanically ventilated patients results in respiratory muscle weakness, decreases respiratory epithelium regeneration thereby increasing the days on mechanical ventilation on the otherhand overfeeding increases carbon dioxide production and is also known to increase the days on mechanical ventilation. Thus proper nutrition protocols can reduce morbidity in ICU.

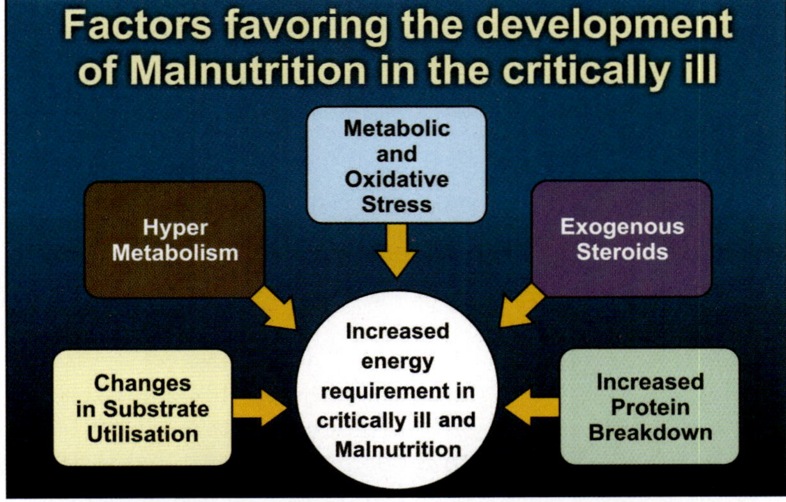

Fig. 25.1: The factors favoring the development of malnutrition in the critically ill

NUTRITIONAL ASSESSMENT

Nutritional assessment is detailed evaluation of nutritional status of the patient. Nutritional assessment should be done by Intensivist and Dietician during inter disciplinary team rounds. Nutritional history like decreased intake, decrease in physical performance and weight loss for 3–6 months before admission can be taken from the family members for the patients on mechanical ventilator support. All hospitalized patients are required to undergo an initial nutrition screen within 48 hours of admission. However, patients at higher nutrition risk in an ICU setting require a full nutrition assessment. Many screening and assessment tools are used to evaluate nutrition status, such as Mini Nutritional Assessment, Malnutrition Universal Screening Tool, Nutritional risk screening 2002 (NRS), Short Nutritional Assessment Questionnaire, Malnutrition Screening Tool, Subjective Global Assessment (SGA). Patients at risk are defined by an NRS 2002 >3 and those at highrisk with a score ≥5 or a NUTRIC score ≥5 (if interleukin-6 is not included, otherwise >6). Among the assessment tools available, subjective global assessment (SGA) is inexpensive, quick and can be conducted at the bedside. Indicators such as anthropometrics or total body fat evaluation are not accurate to assess the nutrition status in ICU. The measurement of plasma concentrations of Albumin, Prealbumin, Transferrin, Retinol binding protein lacks specificity. Wherever feasible, computed tomography or ultrasonography can be used to assess the lean muscle mass. ASPEN 2016 guidelines recommend to use NRS 2002, NUTRIC score but the recent ESPEN 2021 guidelines disagree with the use of these tools and recommend to use general clinical assessment until a well validated tool is available.

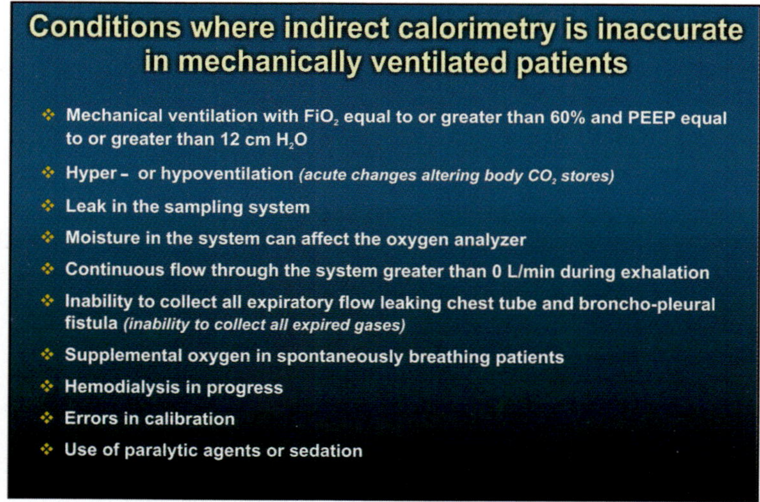

Fig. 25.2: The conditions where indirect calorimetry is inaccurate in mechanically ventilated patients[6]

ROUTE

Enteral route is more physiologic, providing nutritional benefits without adversely affecting structural–functional integrity of gut and intestinal microbial diversity. Enteral tube feeding can be done with different techniques that include nasogastric (NG) feeding using fine tubes, nasojejunal (NJ) feeding, and percutaneous endoscopic

Box 25.1: Contraindications to enteral feeding

- Severe acidosis
- Shock
- Uncontrolled upper gastrointestinal bleeding
- Bowel ischemia
- Intestinal obstruction
- High output enteric fistula without distal feeding access
- Abdominal compartment syndrome
- Gastric aspirate >500 ml/6 hr

gastrostomy(PEG) feeding. Early enteral nutrition, within 48 hr, is preferred over parenteral nutrition in a mechanically ventilated patients. Contraindications to enteral feeding are severe acidosis, shock, uncontrolled upper gastrointestinal bleeding, bowel ischemia, intestinal obstruction, high output enteric fistula without distal feeding access, abdominal compartment syndrome, gastric aspirate >500 ml/6 hr **(Box 25.1)**. In patients with gastric intolerance pro-kinetic agents (Erythromycin, Metoclopramide) are to be considered before proceeding to post-pyloric feeding. ESPEN 2021 recommends continuous feeds over bolus feeds. Early and progressive parenteral nutrition can be provided instead of no nutrition in patients with contraindications for EN in severely malnourished patients, whereas in other patients who are not severely malnourished it can be started within three to seven days. ASPEN 2016 recommends that in patients at either low or highnutrition risk, use of supplemental parenteral nutrition be consideredafter 7–10 days if unable to meet >60% of energy andprotein requirements by the enteral route alone.

Estimating Energy and Protein Requirements

Indirect calorimetry is considered as gold standard for the measurement of energy requirements **(Fig. 25.3)**. However, cost and convenience remain the issue with indirect calorimeter. If calorimetry is not available, using VO_2 (oxygen consumption) from pulmonary arterial catheter or VCO_2 (carbon dioxide production) derived from the ventilator will give a better evaluationon energy expenditure than predictive equations (EE =VCO_2*8.19). Predictive equations like Penn State, Ireton-Jones, Swinamer, Harris-Benedict, MifflinSt Jeorare less accurate in obese and underweight patients. Most commonly energy requirement in Indian ICUs are estimated based on simple weight based estimates. Energy requirementis approximately 20 25 kcal/kg/day in acute phase of critical illness followed by 25 30 kcal/kg/day in recovery phase. ASPEN 2021 update suggest to consider enteral nutrition with 12–25 kcal/kg/day in the first 7–10 days of ICU stay.Hypocaloric enteral feeding (60% 70% of target energy requirements, or 11 14 kcal/kg actual body weight or 22 25 kcal/kg ideal body weight) in obese surgical patients was associated with shorter length of ICU stay, improved nitrogen balance, and reduced use of antibiotics. Protein requirement in adult critically ill patients is 1.2–2 gm/kg/day. Intravenous lipids should not exceed 1.5 gm/kg/day including all non-nutritional lipid sources. ASPEN 2021 Update suggests there's no difference between mixed oil lipid injectable emulsions (medium chain triglycerides, fish oil, olive oil, mixture of oils) and 100% soybean oil for patients requiring parenteral nutrition **(Fig. 25.3)**.

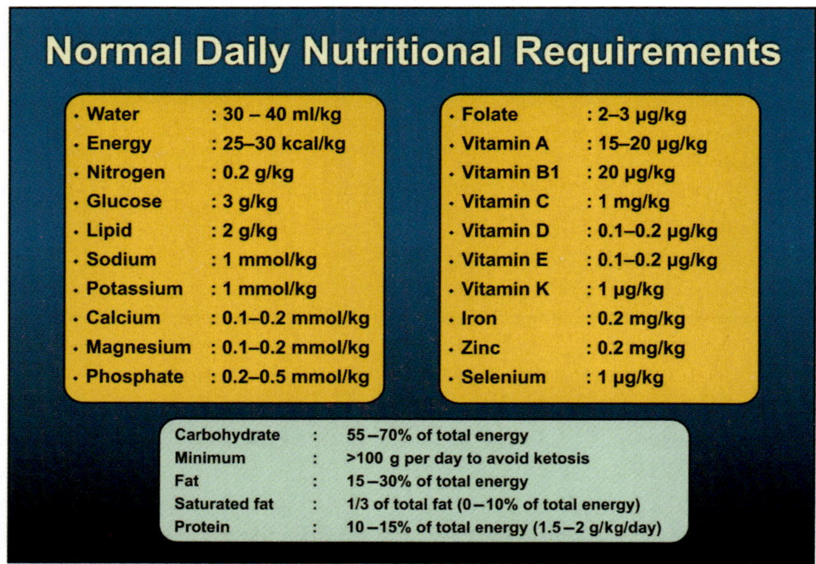

Fig. 25.3: The normal RDA[2]

Selection of Appropriate Enteral Formula

The composition of EN products varies greatly. Considering the basic macro- and micro-nutrient requirements of the patients, polymeric formula feeds are designed. Blenderized tube feeding formula (BTF) is typically prepared at kitchen by blending food or meals into a liquid feed. BTF may be completely prepared from homemade food or a combination of food and standard formula. Limitations of blenderized feeds include high microbial contamination, inconsistency in amount and supply of nutrients (16–50%), higher osmolality and viscosity and possibility of blockage of the feeding tube. Indian society of critical care medicine in its position statement has recommended standard polymeric formula feed over blenderized tube feeding as it avoids inconsistency in nutrient levels.

Enteral Feeding and Diarrhea

Passage of three or more loose/liquid stools per day is defined as diarrhea. Patients with persistent diarrhea may benefit with the use of mixed fiber-containing or soluble fiber-supplemented or small peptide-based semi-elemental formula feeds. Apart from changing the enteral feeding formula, simultaneous workup for infective causes of diarrhea is to be done.

Micronutrients

Pre-existing micronutrients' deficiency should beevaluated. Patients on formula feeds may not require additional micronutrients, vitamins and trace elements, if they areon complete and balanced formula feeds. Micronutrients can be supplemented in patients on blenderized feeds and those on PN.

Immune-enhancing enteral nutrition

Inflammatory/oxidative stress responses and impaired immune function may be favorably modulated by immune modulating nutrients such as omega 3 fatty acids, selenium, and antioxidants (**Fig. 25.4**). Patients suffering from trauma, traumatic brain injury (TBI)and ARDS may be prescribed immune modulating nutrients. Glutamine supplementation has been shown to reduce nosocomial infections and length of hospital stay in critically ill surgical patients, without showing reduction in mortality (**Fig. 25.4**).

Summary of selected immune modulating nutrients, including their probable mechanisms and beneficial effects in critically ill patients

Nutrient	Effects	Mechanisms
Omega-3 fatty acids	Reduce inflammation Lead to production of less inflammatory prostaglandins and leukotrienes	Enhance immunity–Effect signal transduction and gene translation through incorporation into cells
Glutamine	Enhances wound healing	Fuel for enterocytes and lymphocytes
Arginine	Enhances wound healing	Precursor to collagen and nitric oxide
Antioxidants	Reduce oxidative stress	Neutralize reactive oxygen species and reactive nitrogen species

Fig. 25.4: The summary of immunomodulating nutrients[9]

Pulmonary Failure

Previously low carbohydrate/high fat formulations was designed to reduce carbon dioxide production and alter respiratory quotient in acute respiratory failure patient but recent studies have shown that its not beneficial and even ASPEN 2016 Guidelines recommend that these formulas should not be used in such patients. Energy dense, fluid restricted enteral nutrition to be considered in patients with acute respiratory failure who shows signs of volume overload. Serum phosphate levels should be monitored closely and replaced appropriately if needed.

Conclusion

Nutrition is a very important aspect of patient care in critical illness. Use of appropriate nutritional support is cost effective as it reduces length of stay, infectious morbidity. Optimal nutritional management to prevent and treat nutritional deficiencies should become part of routine management. Nutrition is a part of multitude of treatments and therapies that are optimally applied by a multidisciplinary team of professionals. Once thought of only as nutritional support, these supplements have now been regarded as important therapy in ICU care. Do not miss feeding as it becomes harder to catch up on later.

References

1. Mehta Y, Sunavala JD, Zirpe K, Tyagi N, Garg S, Sinha S, *et al.* Practice guidelines for nutrition in critically ill patients: A relook for Indian scenario. Indian J Crit Care Med 2018;22:263–73.
2. Guidelines for the Provision and Assessment of Nutrition Support Therapy in the Adult Critically Ill Patient: Society of Critical Care Medicine (SCCM) and American Society for Parenteral and Enteral Nutrition (ASPEN) 2016
3. Guidelines for the provision of nutritional support therapy in the adult critically ill patients: ASPEN 2021 update.
4. ESPEN guideline on clinical nutrition in the intensive care unit 2019.
5. Maday KR. The importance of nutrition in critically ill patients. JAAPA 2017;30:32–7.
6. Hensurd DD. Nutrition screening and assessment. Med Clin North Am 1999;83:1525–46
7. Prado CM, Heymsfield SB. Lean tissue imaging: A new era for nutritional assessment and intervention. JPEN J Parenter Enteral Nutr 2014;38:940–53.
8. Guttormsen AB, Pichard C. Determining energy requirements in the ICU. Curr Opin Clin Nutr Metab Care 2014;17:171–6.
9. Bajwa SJ. The underestimated nutritional aspects of micronutrients supplementation in intensive care. J Med Nutr Nutraceut 2013;2:114–6.
10. Anker SD, John M, Pedersen PU, Raguso C, Cicoira M, Dardai E, *et al.* ESPEN guidelines on enteral nutrition: Cardiology and pulmonology. Clin Nutr 2006;25:311–8.

CHAPTER 26

Heart–Lung Interactions during Mechanical Ventilation

❒ Balasubrahmanyam CH ❒ Palepu B Gopal

INTRODUCTION

The idea of this review is to understand the complex interplay between the heart and lungs while functioning as a single unit to meet the body's demands. In 1733, Hales *et al* first demonstrated heart-lung interactions in mares by using glass tube manometers to measure circulatory variations during respiratory cycles.[1] During the latter half of the 19th century, intense debate arose regarding Cardiorespiratory interactions such as pulsus paradoxus as the relevance of pleural pressure was recognised.[2] Cardiorespiratory interplay can be critically deranged by neurally mediated phenomena, such as respiratory sinus arrhythmia, or because of effects of altered gas exchange (e.g. hypoxic and hypercapnic pulmonary vasoconstriction) in the context of lung disease or high-altitude exposure, besides the direct mechanical interdependence between lung, heart, and circulation.[3,4]

APPLIED CARDIORESPIRATORY PHYSIOLOGY BASICS

Understanding the heart–lung interactions has led to the physiologic foundations of modern cardiovascular resuscitation of the critically ill.

From a simplistic viewpoint, it is interesting to note that the human circulatory system can be simplified into two main components—the circuit and the pump.

The circuit is represented by a systemic vascular tree consisting of arterial resistance and venous capacitance vessels **(Fig. 26.1)**.

Whereas the right and left ventricles act as serial pumps linked by the pulmonary and systemic vasculature. They work together in parallel within the pericardial reserve through their electrical and mechanical synchronisation.

The heart and lung interplay occurs because of their structural housing within the same thoracic cavity and as such, the heart can be described as a "pressure chamber within a pressure chamber" **(Fig. 26.2)**.[5]

The compliance of the lung (C_L), Chest wall (C_{CW}), along with the compliance and filling of intrathoracic blood vessels and heart chambers modify the effects of lung volume, alveolar (P_{ALV}), pleural (P_{PL}) and pericardial pressure (P_{PER}) on cardio-circulatory function and vice versa.

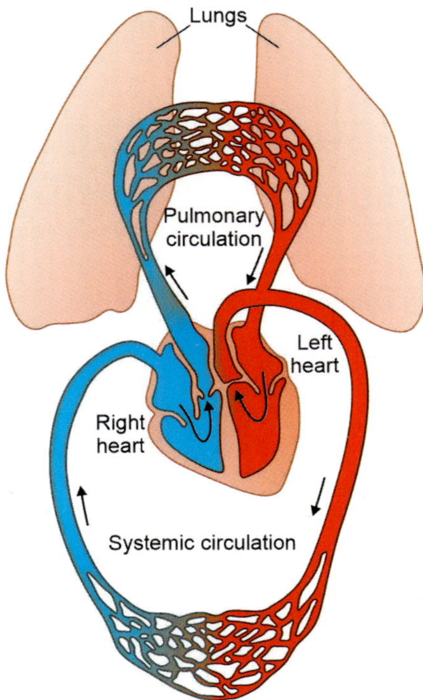

Fig. 26.1: Systemic vascular tree

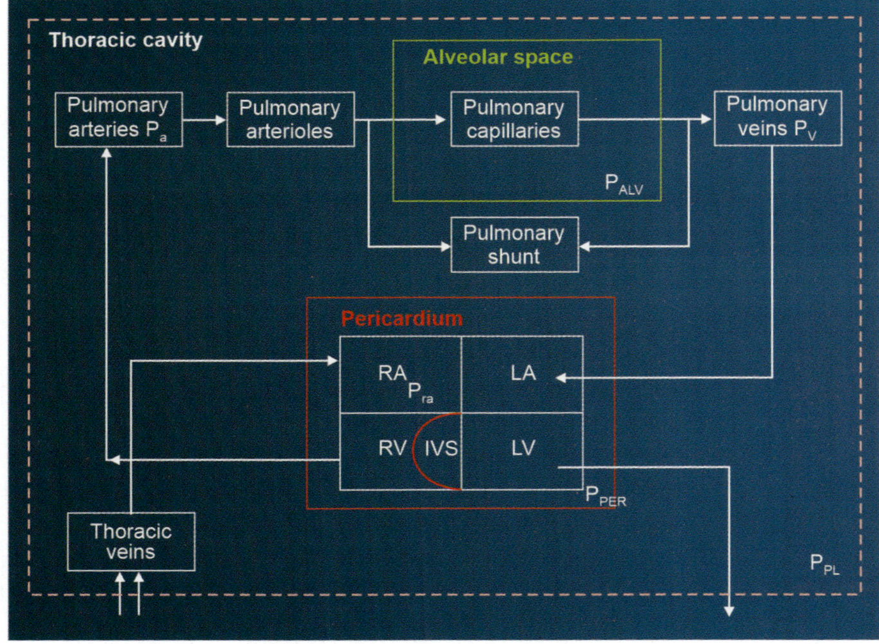

Fig. 26.2: Pressure chamber within a pressure chamber

Intracavitary and Transmural Pressures

Pressure measurements in clinical settings with fluid-filled catheters are not absolute and depend on the chosen zero level. It is crucial to note that when measuring pressure in clinical settings using fluid-filled catheters, the chosen zero level is conventionally set as the right atrium with atmospheric pressure as the reference point. **However, this practice can lead to significant errors when assessing intrathoracic pressures because the surrounding pressure within the thorax is the pleural pressure (P_{PL}) not atmospheric.** As PPL changes relative to atmospheric pressure over the respiratory cycle, it can significantly impact the gradient for venous return and preload, as well as afterload. Therefore, when evaluating heart-lung interactions, it is of utmost importance to consider PPL to avoid erroneous measurement readings.[7,8]

The intracavitary pressure, for example, of the right atrium, is the pressure measured against the atmosphere (right atrial pressure, P_{ra}), that is, against the zero reference. The term transmural pressure (P_{TM}) refers to the pressure difference between the inside of a cavity, relative to the atmosphere and the surrounding pericardium (P_{PER}) outside, which is also relative to the atmosphere. For the right atrium (Fig. 26.3), the transmural pressure (P_{raTM}) would therefore be:

$$P_{raTM} = P_{ra} - P_{PER}$$

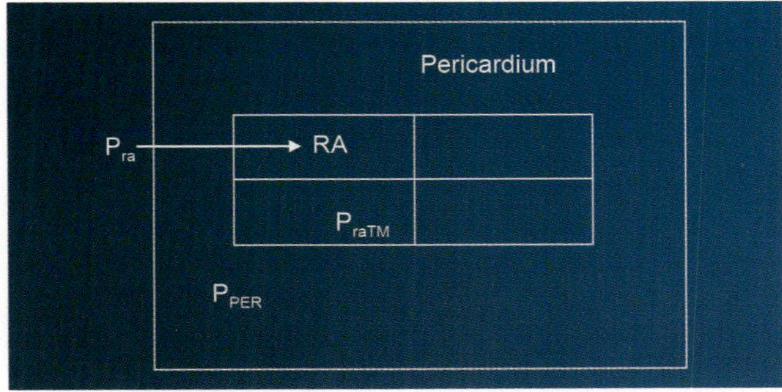

Fig. 26.3: Transmural pressure in the right atrium

The lungs, surrounded by a bilayered pleura enclosed within the chest wall and the diaphragm ensures mechanical coupling of the lung to the chest wall. Pleural pressure {P_{PL}} acts as the surrounding pressure of the lung and cardiac structures and is negative during spontaneous breathing. Hence transpulmonary pressure is the difference between alveolar {P_{ALV}} and Pleural pressure {P_{PL}} (Fig. 26.4).

$$(P_{TP} = P_{ALV} - P_{PL})$$

The transpulmonary pressure plays a critical role in defining the lung volume, and it depends on the compliance of the lung within the chest wall.

The total compliance of the respiratory system is defined by Lung (C_L) and chest wall compliance (C_{CW}).

$$(1/C_{RS} = 1/C_L + 1/C_{CW})$$

During spontaneous inspiration, assuming the vocal cords are open, PPL becomes more negative through the contraction of the diaphragm and accessory respiratory muscles and end-inspiratory lung volume is defined by P_{PL} and C_{RS}, since P_{ALV} equals atmospheric pressure.

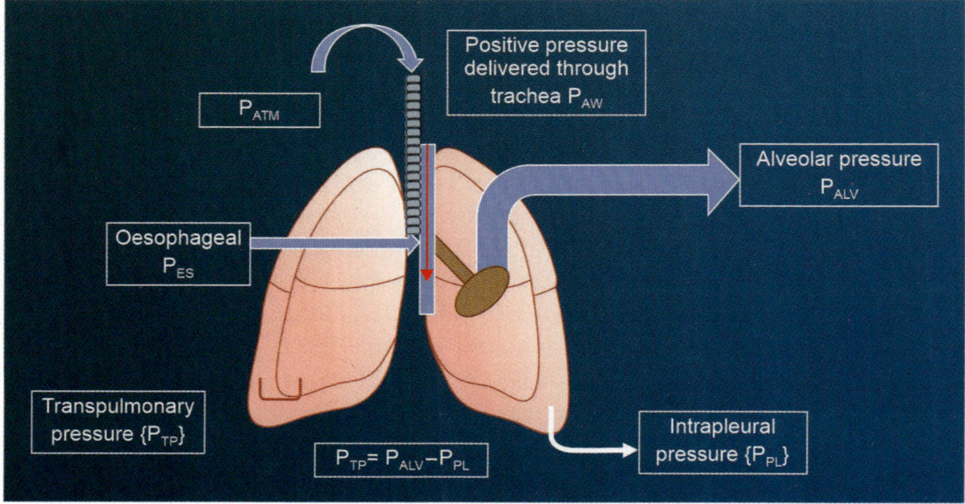

Fig. 26.4: Transpulmonary pressure

Blood flow through the lungs depends on the driving pressure which is mean pulmonary artery pressure [mPAP] – mean left atrial pressure [LAPm] and pulmonary vascular resistance (PVR).[9]

Pulmonary vessels are more compressible as they are more compliant than systemic vessels and act as starling resistors, which change their diameter and the related resistance to flow according to their surrounding pressure.[10]

Therefore, blood flow through the pulmonary vasculature depends on extravascular pressure (increased P_{ALV} or P_{PL}), and diminished transmural pulmonary vascular pressure, resulting in an increased PVR.[11]

The lowest PVR during the respiratory cycle is found at end-expiration, where the lung is at its functional residual capacity (FRC) because the resistance of alveolar vessels equals the resistance of extra-alveolar vessels at this point (**Fig. 26.5**).

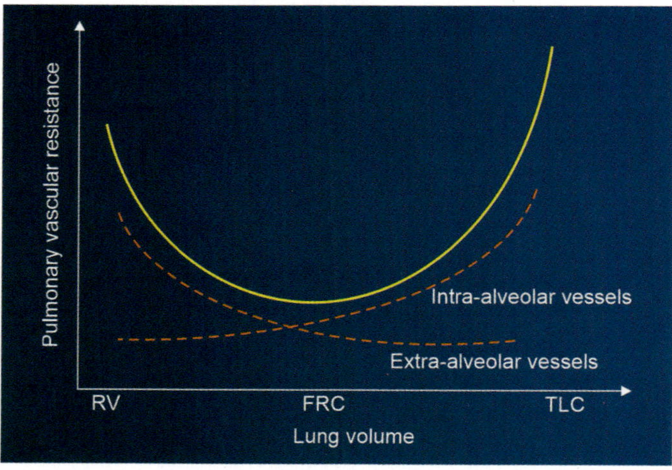

Fig. 26.5: Lowest PVR is at the end of expiration

A conceptual description of pulmonary blood flow based on driving pressure and P_{AL}, which divided the lungs into different zones, as introduced by J.B. West.[12]

In the upright healthy person, zone 2 ($P_a > P_{AL} > P_v$) and zone 3 ($P_a > P_v > P_{AL}$) conditions can be found (**Fig. 26.6**).

Zone 3 conditions are characterised by continuous blood flow since PTM along the vascular bed is always positive. Whereas, in regions with zone 2 conditions, PTM becomes negative at the capillary level and vessel collapse occurs. Blood flow is regulated by the intermittent collapse of the vessel, which depends on respiratory fluctuations of PAL.

Zone 1 conditions ($P_{AL} > P_a > P_v$) with no vascular blood flow can be observed in the lung apex of healthy upright subjects.

West's seminal animal studies utilised a continuous-flow pump setup as in Zone 3. It remains uncertain whether the pulmonary pressure-flow relationship with pulsatile blood flow is correctly depicted by West's concept.

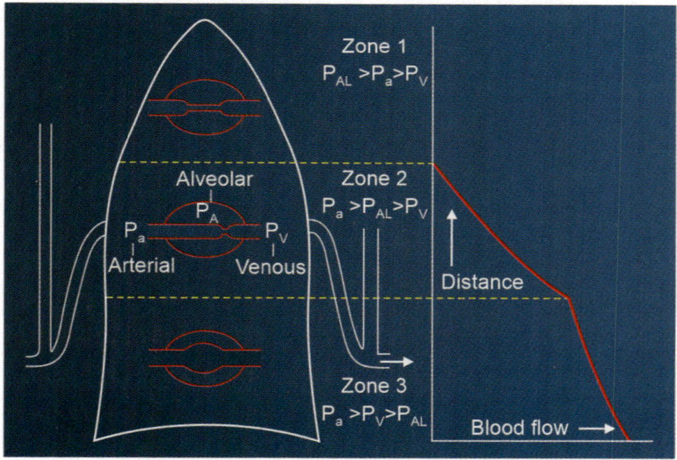

Fig. 26.6

Effect of Mechanical Ventilation on ITP

During controlled mechanical ventilation, PPL is positive throughout the respiratory cycle, because of the application of positive end-expiratory pressure (PEEP) and the absence of spontaneous breathing efforts, whereas in unforced spontaneous breathing, PPL always remains negative.

The physiological consequences of these changes in PPL and PTP are manifold:

i. Elevated P_{AL} combined with the recumbent position alters pulmonary blood flow by creating lung areas with zone 1 conditions (compression of alveolar vessels) and increasing the proportion of areas with zone 2 conditions, leading to increased Pulmonary Vascular Resistance and dead space ventilation with loss of Functional Residual Capacity.

ii. Increased intrathoracic pressure (ITP) reduces the transpulmonary pressure (P_{TM}) of large intrathoracic blood vessels such as venae cavae and thoracic aorta, thereby diminishing intrathoracic blood volume.

iii. The intrathoracic pressure (ITP) also plays a crucial role in the interplay between the heart and lungs. It gets transmitted to the pericardium in the cardiac fossa where the heart is trapped and exposed to elevated ITP.

Effect of Intrathoracic Pressure on Cardiac Function

To approach and understand cardiovascular physiology and heart-lung interactions it is essential to become familiar with determinants of venous return and the right ventricular functioning status.

Preload is right ventricular end-diastolic wall stress. Intrathoracic pressure (ITP) is the pressure surrounding the heart.

So right atrial pressure (Pra) relative to right ventricular (RV) filling is best quantified as Pra minus ITP referred to as transmural pressure and left ventricular (LV) ejection pressure is estimated as arterial pressure minus ITP.

Preload

Venous return (VR) as described by Arthur Guyton was VR = $(P_{msf}-P_{ra})/RVR$ (resistance to venous return). Roughly 70% of the blood volume resides within the veins (also called capacitance vessels) as a reserve pool. Most of this blood volume resides in the vessels at near zero PTM, referred to as **unstressed Volume**. The blood volume that creates positive PTM in the systemic circuit is named **stressed volume** and is represented by the mean systemic filling pressure (P_{msf})[13] which is the elastic recoil pressure generated around the stressed volume by the systemic vascular tree (**Fig. 26.7**).

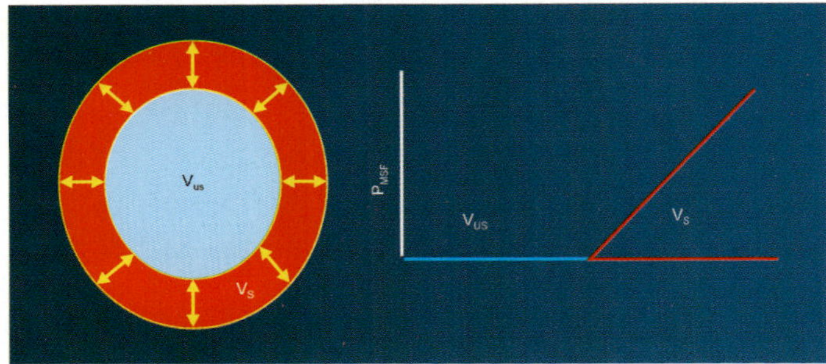

Fig. 26.7

Mean systemic filling pressures (P_{msf}) can be measured at a circulatory standstill and is therefore independent of myocardial properties. It is influenced by the expansion or reduction of stressed volume by a change of total intravascular volume and recruitment or derecruitment of unstressed volume through increased or decreased vessel tone. P_{msf} is constant throughout the cardiac cycle due to the large compliance of the vascular system and is assumed to be unaltered during the respiratory cycle. *Changes in ITP will vary both transmural Pra and transmural LV pressure, while neither venous driving pressure (P_{msf}), nor arterial pressure are affected by isolated changes in ITP.*

Therefore, the changes in ITP can markedly alter these pressure gradients by altering transmural Pra and transmural LV pressures both cyclically during breathing and the steady state but not the pulmonary arterial to left atrial pressure gradient because that entire circuit is within the thorax. *Thus, changes in ITP have profound effects on the systemic circulation whereas the pulmonary circulation is immune unless lung volumes also change.*

Contractility and the Starling Curve

Contractility is described as the intrinsic ability of the myocardium to generate force and contract which is regulated by the Ca^{2+} concentration in myocytes as well as the transfer of Ca^{2+} ions from the sarcoplasmic reticulum to the cytoplasm and vice versa. The availability of Ca^{2+} ions is tightly regulated by the sympathetic nervous system via β1-adrenoceptors.

An increase in heart rate per se can also increase contractility (Bowditch effect).[14] Contractility is load dependent, so sudden afterload elevation increases contractility (Anrep effect) and by Starling's law of the heart, increasing preload recruits' contractile reserves.[15]

It is unclear for now whether there is a direct effect of mechanical ventilation on myocardial contractility, but from an intensivist's clinical perspective, the direct effects of mechanical ventilation on contractility appear far less important compared to its effect on pre- and afterload.

Starling's law of the heart states that myocardial work varies with the initial length of the cardiomyocytes.[16] Pre-stretching of sarcomeres will result in a more vigorous contraction up to a maximum effect, but upon further stretching contractility will no longer increase, but possibly reduce.

Interpreting starling curves suggests that P_{ra} acts as right ventricular preload. The original experimental study of Patterson's and Starling's makes it apparent that it was not P_{ra} that was primarily altered, but venous return. P_{ra} increased because of more volume in the right atrium due to increased venous return, and P_{ra} rose more rapidly when ventricular contractile reserve was reached.[17] Therefore, we can point out that in the Starling curve, Pra or central venous pressure does not reflect a pure preload signal, but the node of interaction between cardiac function and VR function (**Fig. 26.8**), black dot).

Cardiac function curves are graphical analyses of the venous return function and cardiac output with superimposition of the venous return function curve (blue) and the Frank-Starling (cardiac output) curve (red). In an equilibrated system, the intersection between these two curves is right atrial pressure. Venous return reaches its maximum when the right atrial pressure (P_{ra}) is near zero. The venous return function curve intersects the x-axis at zero blood flow, where it represents the mean systemic filling pressures (P_{msf}).

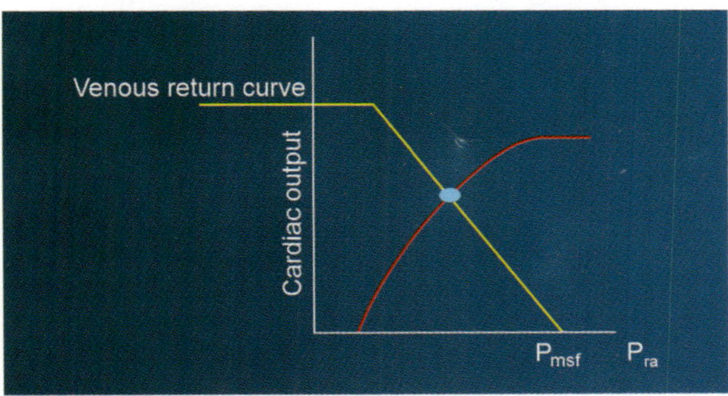

Fig. 26.8

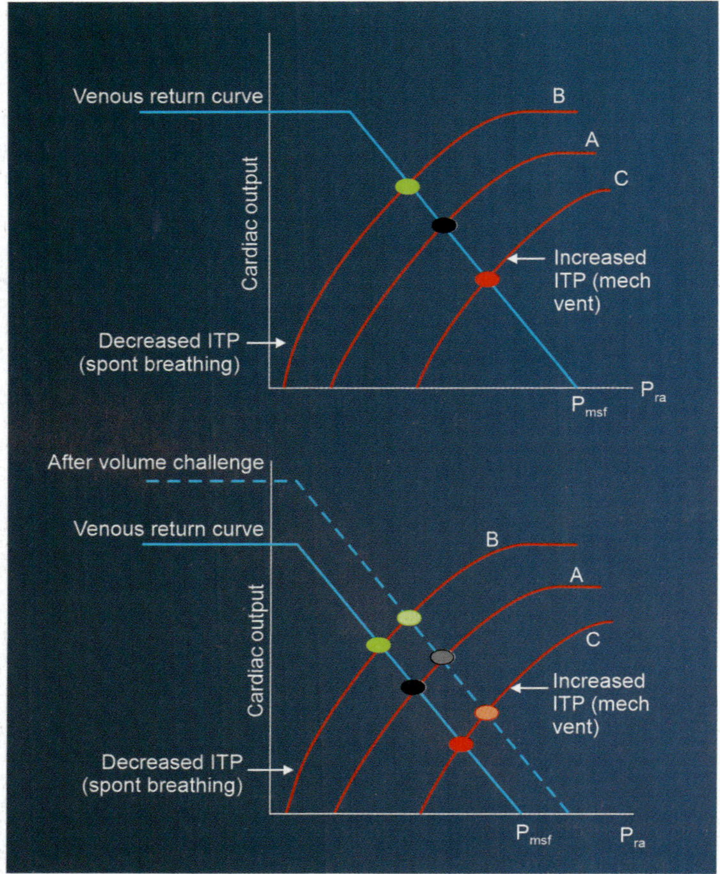

Fig. 26.9

During spontaneous breathing, PPL becomes more negative in inspiration. Right atrial pressure (P_{ra}) drops during inspiration, and creates a higher-pressure gradient for venous return, resulting in higher venous return. Accordingly, in the new state, the Starling curve is shifted to the left (curve B).

The opposite will happen with mechanical ventilation. Pleural Pressure (P_{PL}) increases with mechanical inflation of a tidal volume and is partially transmitted to the right atrium whose intracavitary pressure rises. The Starling curve is shifted to the right (curve C).

In the case of volume responsiveness, the Venous Return function curve is shifted upwards and to the right and reaches a new equilibrium (dotted blue line with resulting grey P_{ra}).

With spontaneous inspiration, pleural pressure and P_{ra} drop, while transmural P_{ra} will rise. The Starling curve is shifted to the left (B) . A new equilibrium point is reached (light green P_{ra}), and cardiac output will rise despite lower P_{ra}.

With mechanical inspiration and positive intrathoracic pressure, the opposite happens (C). Lower cardiac output despite a higher P_{ra} (light red) is observed.[13]

It should be kept in mind that a healthy heart normally works on the steep part of the Starling curve. Volume responsiveness is therefore a normal phenomenon. In the intensive care unit (ICU), only around 50 to 60% of patients are volume responsive. Volume responsiveness may not always mean that the patient needs volume. This must be cross-checked with other parameters and clinical situations.

Ventricular Afterload

Afterload is defined as the force opposing the ventricular ejection of blood. Afterload can be evaluated by assessing ventricular wall tension or vascular resistance and impedance.[18]

LV Afterload

The work of the ventricle is impacted by the aortic elastance ($\Delta P/\Delta V$), which refers to the ability of the aorta to temporarily expand and release some of the stroke volume. Additionally, the overall resistance of the arterial vascular tree also plays a role in determining the workload of the ventricle. The stiffer the aorta, as, for example, in older hypertensive subjects, and the higher the arterial resistance, the bigger the work the left ventricle must deliver to maintain a certain cardiac output.

Intrathoracic pressure (ITP) swings during spontaneous breathing cause only minor cyclic changes in left ventricular afterload, but a Müller manoeuvre can considerably affect cardiac output.[19]

Spontaneous breathing	Inspiration→Decrease ITP→Increases left ventricular afterload
Mechanical ventilation	Tidal breathing→change In P_{PL}→increased LV transmural pressure of the left ventricle and, to a lesser extent, fall of the intrathoracic part of the aorta, while transmural pressure (P_{TM}) in the abdominal aorta remains higher→net LV afterload reduction

In spontaneous breathing, inspiration-associated increase in LV afterload is one of the major mechanisms thought to be operative in the weaning-induced LV ischemia because of increased LV afterload and myocardial O_2 consumption and supports the application of continuous positive airway pressure (CPAP) or pressure support (PS) ventilation with PEEP in mechanically ventilated patients to decrease LV afterload, in the treatment of acutely decompensated left ventricular failure.[20]

Right ventricular afterload: The right heart is described more as a flow generator than a pressure generator owing to its low-pressure ejection into a compliant pulmonary vasculature. So, the right ventricular afterload is more accurately measured using measuring pulmonary vascular elastance or impedance. Intrathoracic pressure (ITP) changes can strongly affect transmural pulmonary vascular pressure and PVR, and thereby right ventricular afterload.

$$\text{PVR} = (\text{mPAP} - \text{PAOP})/\text{CO}$$

Spontaneous breathing	Inspiration→negative P_{PL}→distends pulmonary vasculature→reduces right ventricular afterload
Mechanical ventilation	Tidal breathing→increases P_{PL}→reduces transmural pulmonary vascular pressure →elevates right ventricular afterload

Pulmonary vascular resistance during mechanical ventilation increases mostly in those areas of the lung where zone 1 and zone 2 conditions, with negative PTM and intermittent or continuous pulmonary vascular collapse, are created.

Right ventricular afterload is highly sensitive to cyclical tidal inflation with positive pressure ventilation, this explains why mechanical ventilation may sometimes result in right ventricular failure, especially in individuals with pre-existing right ventricular dysfunction or severe hypoxic pulmonary vasoconstriction as in ARDS.[21,22]
Acute elevations of afterload are poorly tolerated by the right ventricle as compared with the left ventricle, which possesses much higher contractile reserves.[23]

During the respiratory cycle, at end-expiration, i.e. at FRC will find the lowest PVR. Below and above FRC, the PVR rises.[24]

Effect of Lung Volume

In mechanical ventilation, inspiration-associated over-inflation of lung volume will increase pulmonary vascular resistance and thus increase RV afterload. Thus, using large tidal volume ventilation can impede RV ejection.[25] This effect gets annulled by using lung-protective tidal volume routinely in ventilated patients.

Changes in PPL affect lung west zone 1, where alveolar pressure (P_{ALV}) exceeds pulmonary artery pressure (P_{PA}) and zone 2 where P_a exceed P_{ALV} but P_{ALV} exceeds pulmonary venous pressure (P_v).[26] During mechanical inspiration delivery of positive Ppl can create more zone 1 and 2 areas, altering pulmonary blood flow to zone 3 areas, increasing resistance and RV afterload and causing both an increased dead space ventilation and potential increased shunt blood flow.[27] This effect is due primarily to the increases in lung volume caused by positive pressure breathing, rather than the increases in P_{ALV} perse. For example, if tidal volume is kept constant but chest wall compliance is markedly reduced, no change in pulmonary blood flow occurs. Similarly, in subjects with decreased lung compliance (e.g. ARDS) the effects of increased P_{ALV} are often blunted.[28] However, it is interesting to note that ARDS is typically associated with an increase in pulmonary arterial pressure, which is independent of mechanical ventilatory strategies. This means that RV afterload may still be increased due to hypoxic vasoconstriction from pulmonary oedema and lung injury, rather than a high P_{ALV} exceeding P_{PA}.

Ventricular Interdependence

The anatomical differences between the right and left ventricles are significant, with the left ventricle being spherical and having a spiral arrangement of muscle fibres that allow for the efficient generation of high pressures.[29] In contrast, the right ventricle is partially wrapped around the left ventricle and has a thin free wall, which is not well-suited for high-pressure work but is adapted to the low-resistance pulmonary vasculature. Interestingly, the contraction of the interventricular septum, which consists of muscle fibres attributed to the left ventricle, plays a crucial role in supporting right ventricular ejection.[30,31] This structural dependency of the two ventricles has important clinical implications.

It is interesting to note that the shared septum and the pericardial constraint, play a significant role in the interplay between the diastolic pressure of one ventricle directly affecting the diastolic filling of the other,[32] biventricular lusitropy (i.e. active relaxation and diastolic filing). Constrained with space to expand, increased filling of one ventricle leads to decreased diastolic compliance of the other.[33] When there is an increase in right ventricular volume, left ventricular filling declines. This phenomenon can occur in various scenarios, such as elevated right ventricular afterload (e.g. pulmonary embolism, pulmonary hypertension) or disease-aggravated respiratory physiological changes (e.g. pericardial effusion) or mechanical ventilation.

The respiratory cycle has a significant impact on the end-diastolic ventricular volume (EDV) and pressure (EDP) of the left and right ventricles. During normal conditions, EDV and EDP change in opposite directions in both ventricles. The changing stroke volumes of the left and right ventricles with each heartbeat also vary with the respiratory cycle, with the sum of stroke volumes of the right ventricle being equal to the left ventricular output on average. This dynamic interplay is possible due to the compliant pulmonary vasculature and venous capacitance vessels.[33] Clinical examples of interventricular dependence include pericardial tamponade or status asthmaticus, which can cause a sudden increase in right ventricular EDV during inspiration, impairing left ventricular filling and stroke volume and leading to an exaggerated inspiratory drop in peripheral arterial pressure (pulsus paradoxus).

Heart–lung Interactions: Clinical Application and Pitfalls

Functional Haemodynamic Monitoring

Functional hemodynamic monitoring refers to a type of monitoring that is conducted to evaluate the effectiveness of treatment. It involves using a repetitive and known physiological perturbation to drive a readout physiological signal that defines cardiovascular reserve. This type of monitoring is considered functional because it implies a therapeutic application and can provide valuable insights into the patient's cardiovascular function and response to treatment. By measuring cardiovascular reserve, clinicians can make informed decisions about the most appropriate treatment options for their patients.

Assessment of Preload Reserve and Volume Responsiveness

Assessment of preload reserve and volume responsiveness based on Heart-lung interactions in three different approaches:

i. Pulse Pressure Variation (PPV) and its variants,
ii. Echocardiographic assessment of the caval veins, and
iii. Estimation of Mean Systolic Filling Pressure (MSFP) with ventilator manoeuvres.

Pulse Pressure variation and its variants

During mechanical ventilation, the cyclical change in PPL causes right atrial pressure (RAP) to rise in inspiration and fall with exhalation leading to a drop in venous return and right ventricular stroke volume in inspiration and vice versa in expiration resulting in varying right ventricular stroke volume with a time delay, referred to as pulmonary transit time.

We know from interventricular interdependence that LV stroke volume depends on RV stroke volume, so this resultant RV stroke volume variation with pulmonary transit time is what we see in the pulse pressure variation {difference between systolic and

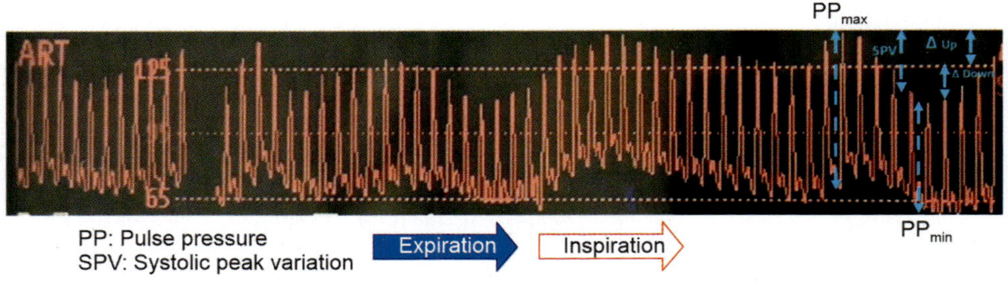

Fig. 26.10

diastolic arterial pressure}in the arterial pressure curve. These variations indicate to us that the heart is working on the steep part of its Starling curve and volume expansion should increase cardiac output **(Fig. 26.10)**.

Systolic pressure variation {SPV} was first described by Perel as a surrogate of Hypovolemia in animal models. Bedside assessment was refined to stroke volume variation {SVV} and Pulse pressure variation {PPV}.

$$PPV = (PPV_{max}–PPV_{min})*100/(PPV_{max} + PPV_{min})*0.5$$

In septic patients, Michard and colleagues in their study[34] concluded a good prediction of fluid responsiveness with a PPV ≥12%.

Pitfalls of PPV

The concept of PPV of the arterial pressure only takes into account preload and stroke volume changes in the right ventricle and neglects the passage of blood through the lungs. PPV is affected by any factor that interferes with the pulmonary vasculature or function.

Factors that influence PPV include any spontaneous respiratory effort[35], tidal volume (needs to be larger than 8 ml/kg),[36] respiratory rate and pulmonary transit time,[37] the CRS[38] and absence of sinus rhythm and frequent ectopic beats. Monnet, *et al.*[39] showed that the predictive value of PPV was related to the compliance of the respiratory system and if the compliance was <30 ml/cmH_2O, PPV was less accurate in predicting fluid responsiveness.

A novel test was proposed by Myatra, *et al.*[40] The 'tidal volume challenge' to improve the reliability of PPV during low tidal volume ventilation. The test involves transiently increasing tidal volume from 6 ml/kg PBW to 8 ml/kg PBW for one minute and observing the change in PPV (ΔPPV_{6-8}) from baseline (PPV_6) to that at 8 ml/kg PBW (PPV_8). The ΔPPV_{6-8} after performing the tidal volume challenge is recorded. A ΔPPV_{6-8} greater than 3.5% predicts fluid responsiveness with high accuracy. The change in PPV after giving a fluid bolus (ΔPPVfb) also accurately confirmed fluid responsiveness with an AUROC of 0.98 (sensitivity 94% and specificity 100%) with a cut-off value of 1.5%.

The failing right ventricle is a major limitation of using PPV to assess fluid responsiveness. In this scenario, increased afterload during mechanical inspiration can cause smaller stroke volumes and lead to arterial pressure fluctuations despite adequate fluid volume. This is because the right ventricle is responsible for pumping blood to the lungs and any dysfunction in this process can impact the left ventricle's stroke volume. Therefore, it is important to consider other factors in addition to PPV when assessing fluid responsiveness in patients with right ventricular dysfunction.[41] To avoid deleterious volume loading, PPV should not be seen as a marker of volume responsiveness per se,[42] but rather as an indicator of left ventricular function depending on right ventricular stroke volume. Immediate evaluation of right ventricular function is mandated whenever volume expansion fails to increase cardiac output.

A negative PPV does not necessarily mean that a patient does not need volume if a patient's blood volume is centralised owing to endogenous or exogenous vasoconstriction with concomitant insufficient tissue perfusion. Vasoconstriction shifts volume from the unstressed volume pool (V_{us}) to the stressed volume pool (V_s) to maintain venous return. In such a scenario, volume expansion may lead to a decrease in vasopressor dose requirement and restoration of tissue perfusion by normalising unstressed volume and reducing vasoconstriction.

Finally, regarding the impact on clinical decision-making, it needs to be emphasized that a potential increase in cardiac output in response to fluids does not mean that the patient needs an increase in fluids.

Echocardiographic Assessment of Volume State

Respiratory variations of the diameters of the superior (ΔSVC)[43] and inferior caval veins(ΔIVC) or variations in the aortic flow velocity (ΔV_{max} Ao)[44] have been reported to predict fluid responsiveness in ventilated patients. Vignon P, *et al*[45] published a large cohort study which showed ΔVmaxAo had the best sensitivity (79%) and ΔSVC (84%) the best specificity in predicting fluid responsiveness. ΔSVC had greater diagnostic accuracy than ΔIVC and ΔPP, but its limitation was a requirement of transoesophageal echocardiography for its measurement (**Fig. 26.11**).

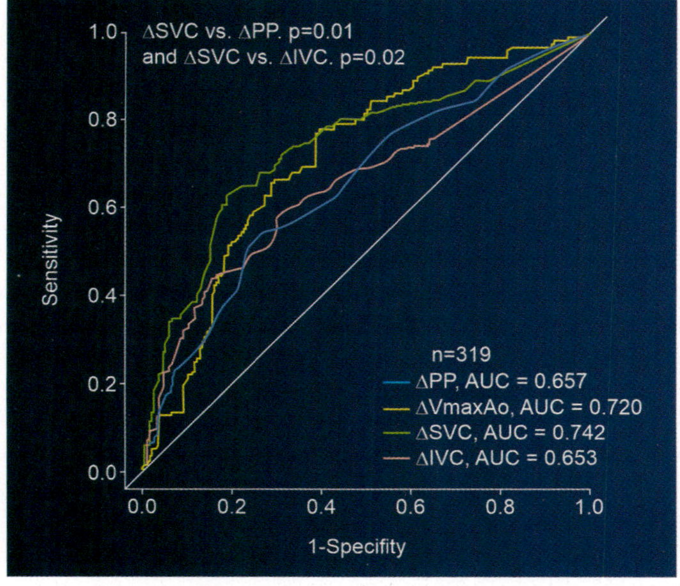

Fig. 26.11

The rationale for the high specificity of ΔSVC is its anatomical positioning before the right heart rendering it to be primarily independent of right heart function. Still, ΔSVC diameter changes depend on the airway pressure change and, therefore, tidal volume. Overall, these dynamic echocardiographic predictors are as accurate and modest as PPV and need the same prerequisites as PPV regarding the need for fluid administration except that they can be used in patients with cardiac arrhythmias.

Estimation of mean systemic filling pressure (P_{msf}) with respiratory manoeuvres.

Physiological concepts of the construction of venous return curves by stepwise increases in RAP and decreasing cardiac output with increasing airway pressure were developed in animal models by Versprille and Pinsky.[46]

Estimates of P_{msf} with increasing pressures in inspiratory hold manoeuvres have lately been used at the bedside[47] in cardiac and septic ventilated ICU patients.

Though these methods show a good correlation with mathematical estimates of P_{msf}, whether inspiration influences P_{msf} is an ongoing, unresolved debate,[48] which warrants caution in the application of these methods. The concept holds great clinical promise since direct measurement of right atrial pressure and MSFP may help to guide fluid resuscitation and warrants further research.

In summary, it is important to understand the interplay between the heart and lungs, especially in patients who require mechanical ventilation. Failure to recognize and address this interplay can lead to severe clinical deterioration. However, by understanding the individualized determinants of these interactions, one can deconvolute the more complex presentations and treat patients more efficiently, particularly in cases involving advanced ventilatory modes and varying levels of cardiac and pulmonary insufficiency leading to dramatic clinical deterioration if not recognised.

References

1. Smith IB. The Impact of Stephen Hales on Medicine. J R Soc Med. 1993 Jun 7;86(6):349–52.
2. Barr J. The effects of respiration on the circulation; and the pulsus paradoxus VEL pulsus inspiratione intermittens. BMJ. 1907 Apr 20;1(2416):913–8.
3. Yasuma F, Hayano J ichiro. Respiratory Sinus Arrhythmia. Chest. 2004 Feb;125(2):683–90.
4. Dorrington KL, Talbot NP. Human pulmonary vascular responses to hypoxia and hypercapnia. Pflugers Archiv - European Journal of Physiology. 2004 Oct 19;449(1):1–15.
5. Mahmood SS, Pinsky MR. Heart-lung interactions during mechanical ventilation: the basics. Ann Transl Med. 2018 Sep;6(18):349–49.
6. Magder S. Right Atrial Pressure in the Critically Ill. Chest. 2017 Apr;151(4):908–16.
7. Magder S, Verscheure S. Proper Reading of Pulmonary Artery Vascular Pressure Tracings. Am J Respir Crit Care Med. 2014 Nov 15;190(10):1196–8.
8. Marini JJ, Culver BH, Butler J. Mechanical effect of lung distention with positive pressure on cardiac function. Am Rev Respir Dis. 1981 Oct;124(4):382–6.
9. Naeije R. Pulmonary vascular resistance. Intensive Care Med. 2003 Apr 28;29(4):526–9.
10. Permutt S, Riley RL. Hemodynamics of collapsible vessels with tone: the vascular waterfall. J Appl Physiol. 1963 Sep 1;18(5):924–32.
11. West JB, Dollery CT, Naimark A. Distribution of blood flow in isolated lung; relation to vascular and alveolar pressures. J Appl Physiol. 1964 Jul 1;19(4):713–24.
12. West JB. Blood Flow to the Lung and Gas Exchange. Anesthesiology. 1974 Aug 1;41(2):124–38.

13. Magder S. Volume and its relationship to cardiac output and venous return. Crit Care. 2016 Dec 10;20(1):271.
14. Lakatta EG. Beyond Bowditch: the convergence of cardiac chronotropy and inotropy. Cell Calcium. 2004 Jun;35(6):629–42.
15. Cingolani HE, Pérez NG, Cingolani OH, Ennis IL. The Anrep effect: 100 years later. American Journal of Physiology-Heart and Circulatory Physiology. 2013 Jan 15;304(2):H175–82.
16. Berlin DA, Bakker J. Starling curves and central venous pressure. Crit Care. 2015 Dec 1;19(1):55.
17. Patterson SW, Starling EH. On the mechanical factors which determine the output of the ventricles. J Physiol. 1914 Sep 8;48(5):357–79.
18. Borlaug BA, Kass DA. Invasive Hemodynamic Assessment in Heart Failure. Heart Fail Clin. 2009 Apr;5(2):217–28.
19. Buda AJ, Pinsky MR, Ingels NB, Daughters GT, Stinson EB, Alderman EL. Effect of Intrathoracic Pressure on Left Ventricular Performance. New England Journal of Medicine. 1979 Aug 30;301(9):453–9.
20. Pinsky MR. Cardiovascular Issues in Respiratory Care. Chest. 2005 Nov;128(5):592S-597S.
21. Mekontso Dessap A, Boissier F, Charron C, Bégot E, Repessé X, Legras A, *et al*. Acute cor pulmonale during protective ventilation for acute respiratory distress syndrome: prevalence, predictors, and clinical impact. Intensive Care Med. 2016 May 9;42(5):862–70.
22. Pinsky MR. Determinants of pulmonary arterial flow variation during respiration. J Appl Physiol. 1984 May 1;56(5):1237–45.
23. Matthews J, McLaughlin V. Acute Right Ventricular Failure in the Setting of Acute Pulmonary Embolism or Chronic Pulmonary Hypertension: A Detailed Review of the Pathophysiology, Diagnosis, and Management. Curr Cardiol Rev. 2008 Feb 1;4(1):49–59.
24. Whittenberger JL, McGregor M, Berglund E, Borst HG. Influence of state of inflation of the lung on pulmonary vascular resistance. J Appl Physiol. 1960 Sep 1;15(5):878–82.
25. Vieillard-Baron A, Loubieres Y, Schmitt JM, Page B, Dubourg O, Jardin F. Cyclic changes in right ventricular output impedance during mechanical ventilation. J Appl Physiol. 1999 Nov 1;87(5):1644–50.
26. West JB. Understanding pulmonary gas exchange: ventilation-perfusion relationships. J Appl Physiol. 2004 Nov;97(5):1603–4.
27. Grbler MR, Wigger O, Berger D, Blchlinger S. Basic concepts of heart-lung interactions during mechanical ventilation. Swiss Med Wkly. 2017 Sep 12;
28. Jardin F, Genevray B, Brun-Ney D, Bourdarias JP. Influence of Lung and Chest Wall Compliances on Transmission of Airway Pressure to the Pleural Space in Critically Ill Patients. Chest. 1985 Nov;88(5):653–8.
29. Voorhees AP, Han H. Biomechanics of Cardiac Function. In: Comprehensive Physiology. Wiley; 2015. p. 1623–44.
30. Haddad F, Hunt SA, Rosenthal DN, Murphy DJ. Right Ventricular Function in Cardiovascular Disease, Part I. Circulation. 2008 Mar 18;117(11):1436–48.
31. Haddad F, Doyle R, Murphy DJ, Hunt SA. Right Ventricular Function in Cardiovascular Disease, Part II. Circulation. 2008 Apr;117(13):1717–31.
32. Taylor R, Covell J, Sonnenblick E, Ross J. Dependence of ventricular distensibility on filling of the opposite ventricle. American Journal of Physiology-Legacy Content. 1967 Sep 1;213(3):711–8.
33. Magder S, Guerard B. Heart–lung interactions and pulmonary buffering: Lessons from a computational modelling study. Respir Physiol Neurobiol. 2012 Jul;182(2–3):60–70.

34. Michard F, Boussat S, Chemla D, Anguel N, Mercat A, Lecarpentier Y, *et al*. Relation between Respiratory Changes in Arterial Pulse Pressure and Fluid Responsiveness in Septic Patients with Acute Circulatory Failure. Am J Respir Crit Care Med. 2000 Jul 1;162(1):134–8.
35. Magder S. Clinical Usefulness of Respiratory Variations in Arterial Pressure. Am J Respir Crit Care Med. 2004 Jan 15;169(2):151–5.
36. de Backer D, Heenen S, Piagnerelli M, Koch M, Vincent JL. Pulse pressure variations to predict fluid responsiveness: influence of tidal volume. Intensive Care Med. 2005 Apr 8;31(4):517–23.
37. de Backer D, Taccone FS, Holsten R, Ibrahimi F, Vincent JL. Influence of Respiratory Rate on Stroke Volume Variation in Mechanically Ventilated Patients. Anesthesiology. 2009 May 1;110(5):1092–7.
38. Mesquida J, Kim HK, Pinsky MR. Effect of tidal volume, intrathoracic pressure, and cardiac contractility on variations in pulse pressure, stroke volume, and intrathoracic blood volume. Intensive Care Med. 2011 Oct 8;37(10):1672.
39. Monnet X, Bleibtreu A, Ferré A, Dres M, Gharbi R, Richard C, *et al*. Passive leg-raising and end-expiratory occlusion tests perform better than pulse pressure variation in patients with low respiratory system compliance*. Crit Care Med. 2012 Jan;40(1):152–7.
40. Myatra SN, Monnet X, Teboul JL. Use of 'tidal volume challenge' to improve the reliability of pulse pressure variation. Crit Care. 2017 Dec 21;21(1):60.
41. Wyler von Ballmoos M, Takala J, Roeck M, Porta F, Tueller D, Ganter CC, *et al*. Pulse-pressure variation and hemodynamic response in patients with elevated pulmonary artery pressure: a clinical study. Crit Care. 2010;14(3):R111.
42. Vieillard-Baron A, Chergui K, Augarde R, Prin S, Page B, Beauchet A, *et al*. Cyclic Changes in Arterial Pulse during Respiratory Support Revisited by Doppler Echocardiography. Am J Respir Crit Care Med. 2003 Sep 15;168(6):671–6.
43. Vieillard-Baron A, Chergui K, Rabiller A, Peyrouset O, Page B, Beauchet A, *et al*. Superior vena caval collapsibility as a gauge of volume status in ventilated septic patients. Intensive Care Med. 2004 Sep 26;30(9).
44. Feissel M, Mangin I, Ruyer O, Faller JP, Michard F, Teboul JL. Respiratory Changes in Aortic Blood Velocity as an Indicator of Fluid Responsiveness in Ventilated Patients With Septic Shock. Chest. 2001 Mar;119(3):867–73.
45. Vignon P, Repessé X, Bégot E, Léger J, Jacob C, Bouferrache K, *et al*. Comparison of Echocardiographic Indices Used to Predict Fluid Responsiveness in Ventilated Patients. Am J Respir Crit Care Med. 2017 Apr 15;195(8):1022–32.
46. Jansen JR, Maas JJ, Pinsky MR. Bedside assessment of mean systemic filling pressure. Curr Opin Crit Care. 2010 Jun;16(3):231–6.
47. Maas JJ, Geerts BF, van den Berg PCM, Pinsky MR, Jansen JRC. Assessment of venous return curve and mean systemic filling pressure in postoperative cardiac surgery patients*. Crit Care Med. 2009 Mar;37(3):912–8.
48. Chihara E, Hashimoto S, Kinoshita T, Hirose M, Tanaka Y, Morimoto T. Elevated mean systemic filling pressure due to intermittent positive-pressure ventilation. American Journal of Physiology-Heart and Circulatory Physiology. 1992 Apr 1;262(4):H1116–21.

CHAPTER 27

Extracorporeal Membrane Oxygenation (ECMO)

❒ Sambit Sahu ❒ Rakesh Venuturumilli

Extracorporeal Membrane Oxygenation (ECMO) is a treatment modality for respiratory and/or cardiac support.

ECMO as a treatment modality evolved from cardiopulmonary bypass which has long been used as a short term cardiorespiratory support during surgery. The evolution of technology from short-term operative theatre support to long-term support in the critical care setting was arduous. Robert Bartlett known as the Father of modern ECMO did extensive work and was the first to use it in a neonate, a baby girl of an illegal immigrant in the USA. The girl was named 'Esperenza' meaning 'hope'. Her survival was the spark which started the ECMO revolution. ECMO was initially used in neonates with meconium aspiration syndrome and later in the treatment of other causes of respiratory failure with good success.

ECMO in adult Acute respiratory distress syndrome (ARDS) was initially associated with poor clinical outcomes limiting its use in few centres in the world. The first trial to show mortality benefit with the use of ECMO in respiratory failure was the CESAR trial conducted in the UK in 2009. The release of the trial results coincided with the global H1N1 swine flu pandemic. The strong evidence base led to the widespread use of ECMO as a rescue strategy for severe ARDS. The ongoing novel coronavirus (COVID-19) pandemic has increased the usage of ECMO and has shown good overall result in patient outcome.

Today ECMO is an established mode of treatment for severe ARDS with good outcomes in the right patients when done in centres which have expertise in managing this modality.

Case Scenario

A-33-year-old male presents with respiratory distress to Emergency Room. Initial workup is suggestive of influenza pneumonia with the following CT scan **(Fig. 27.1)**. Pulse oximetry shows saturation of 85% ON 15 L/min on high flow face mask. The patient is subsequently intubated for type 1 respiratory failure and ventilated as per ARDS guidelines. He is difficult to ventilate with lung protection strategies and proned in view of P:F ratio <100. There is minimal response to proning with no major improvement in oxygenation and increasing CO_2 retention.

This is a patient in whom mechanical ventilation cannot achieve oxygenation and CO_2 targets and may actually cause ventilator induced lung injury (VILI).

He needs to be referred for ECMO.

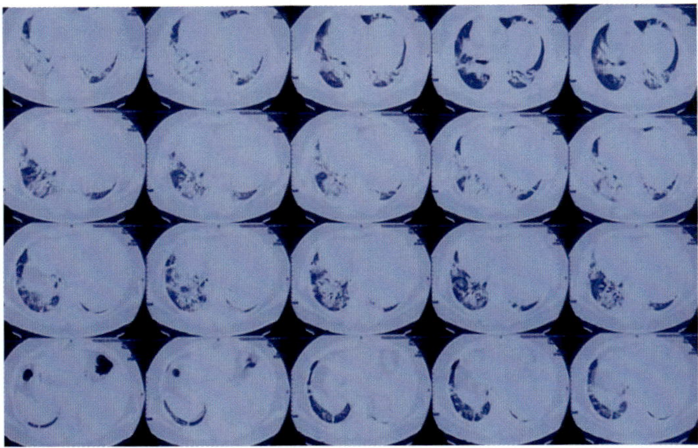

Fig. 27.1

What is ECMO: ECMO is an extracorporeal therapy where blood passes through a centrifugal pump, over a membrane to oxygenate and decarboxylate the blood and is returned into the body.

Types of ECMO:

1. Veno-venous ECMO (V-V ECMO): For pulmonary support
2. Veno-arterial ECMO (V-A ECMO): For cardiac support
3. Veno-arterio-venous ECMO (V-A-V ECMO): For pulmonary and cardiac support

ECMO Circuit

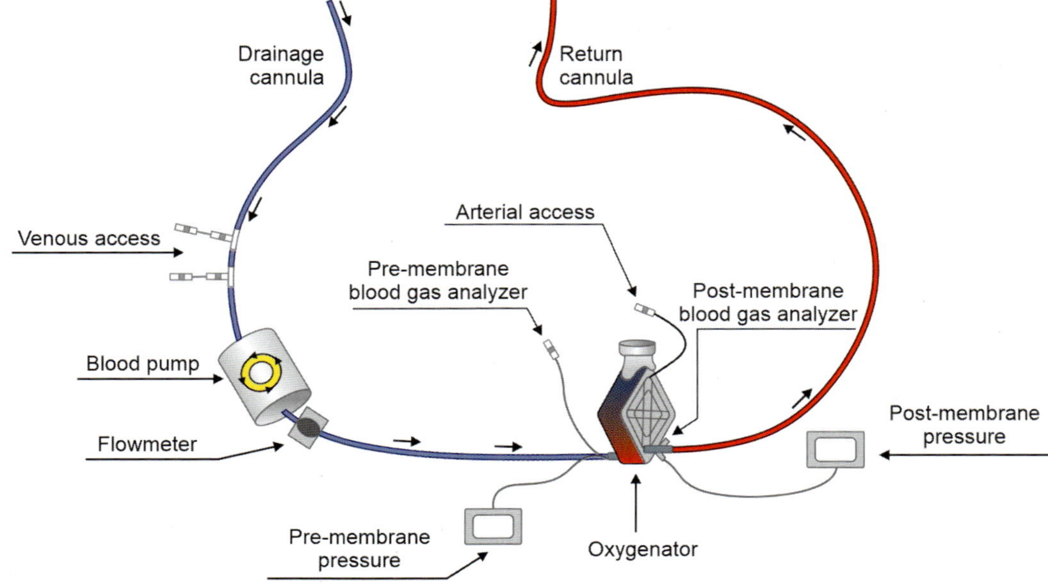

Fig. 27.2

Indications

V-V ECMO

1. Potentially reversible cause of respiratory failure
2. Severe hypoxia : P: F ratio <100
3. Severe hypercapnia with pH <7.2 despite adequate ventilation adjustment
4. Murray score > 3.0

Contraindications

1. Refractory multiorgan failure (relative contraindication)

V-A ECMO

1. Postcardiotomy stunning/difficult to wean off bypass
2. Cardiogenic shock refractory to medical management (high ionotropic score)
3. Post CPR myocardial stunning
4. Pulmonary embolism causing cardiovascular collapse
5. Fulminant myocarditis

It is important to note that ECMO is a method of organ support rather than treatment. It can be used as:

a. Bridge to recovery
b. Bridge to transplant
c. Bridge to ventricular assist device (VAD)
d. Bridge to decision making

A potential patient for ECMO needs to be referred early to the service to give him the best chance at recovery while reducing ongoing ventilator induced lung injury. Various scoring systems are available to determine if the patient needs ECMO.

1. P:F ratio: The most commonly used ARDS stratification tool but it lacks specificity
2. Murray score: Used in ARDS patients, it consists of 4 criteria
   a. Quadrants of lung involved
   b. P:F ratio
   c. PEEP
   d. Lung compliance

This is the most commonly used score for centralised ECMO referral and triaging in centres with high ECMO load.

Prognostication scores: Other scores such as the Respiratory ECMO Survival Prediction(RESP) score is used for prediction of in hospital survival of patients requiring V-V ECMO, survival after V-A ECMO (SAVE) score for patients on V-A ECMO.

ECMO Physiology

V-V ECMO

In V-V ECMO, venous blood is drained, oxygenated and returned back to the venous system which then passes through the pulmonary circulation and ends up in the systemic circulation. Therefore, part of the venous return to the heart is oxygenated. The oxygenator is a membrane consisting of ploymethyl pentene (PMP) with a high surface area which has blood on one side and gas flow on the other side. It acts as the alveolar membrane to enable gas exchange.

Oxygenation is determined by the fraction of delivered oxygen (FiO_2) and blood flow, while carbon dioxide (CO_2) removal is determined by the sweep gas flow.

V-A ECMO

In V-A ECMO the return cannula is placed in one of the major arteries, most commonly the femoral artery and, therefore, provides arterial perfusion to the organs in cases where the heart is not able to maintain perfusion (cardiogenic shock).

The native cardiac output is measured by a right radial arterial catheter preferably, as it is the first branch of the aorta, it is more likely to receive output from the native heart.

Due to the differences in oxygenation from the patients lung and the ECMO circuit, a differential oxygenation (upper half of the patient being cyanosed and lower half normal) may be seen. This is called Harlequin syndrome.

In the case of peripheral V-A ECMO because the return flow is in the opposite direction of the cardiac output, it increases the afterload of the heart. Precautions must be taken to prevent stagnation of blood in the left ventricle which can clot. This is treated either by increasing ionotropic drugs, a Ventricular Assist Device (VAD), Intra-aortic balloon pump (IABP) or direct left ventriculostomy.

Management of ECMO

Insertion

Insertion is usually done by Seldinger method using ultrasound and/or fluoroscopy to guide positioning of cannula. The drainage cannula is a multistage cannula up to 31Fr depending on the diameter of the vessel. The drainage cannula is inserted into the femoral vein with the tip lying near the hepatic vein drainage in the inferior vena cava. The return cannula is inserted either in the IVC or the right internal jugular vein with the tip lying at the IVC RA junction or the SVC RA junction. In case of VA ECMO the percutaneous return cannula is inserted into the femoral artery. During insertion after the guidewires are in place the patient needs to be anticoagulated with heparin and an ACT of >200 seconds must be maintained.

Complications during insertion:

a. Bleeding
b. Arterial puncture
c. Vessel dissection
d. Retroperitoneal haematoma
e. Pneumothorax

Initiation

Once the cannula is in place and good flow is confirmed, the primed ECMO circuit is connected. The flow is slowly increased along with gas flow in a ratio of 1:0.5 to 1:2

Complications during initiation

a. Hypotension
b. Flow problems
c. Air embolization
d. Cardiac tamponade

Once good flow is confirmed, the blood flow and sweep gas flow is adjusted to targets of oxygenation and decarboxylation.

After adequate gas exchange is achieved, mechanical ventilation is changed to lung rest settings, usually SIMV mode (pressure control) with PC: 10, PEEP: 10, frequency: 10 and FiO_2: least possible.This prevents further VILI. In case of V-A ECMO, inotropic support is decreased to minimum possible level.

Maintenance

Monitoring and managing a patient on ECMO is a labour intensive process requiring highly trained manpower. Given the complexity of pathology and equipment, the use of checklists and protocols reduce the chances of missing vital part of management.

Daily Examination

Patient

1. Pupillary examination
2. Return cannula site check for position, bleeding
3. Chest examination for air entry, pneumothorax
4. Femoral site check for cannula position
5. Peripheral pulses of the leg (especially in case of V-A ECMO)

Circuit

1. Pump RPM and flow
2. Colour change in drainage and return cannula
3. Circuit and membrane check for thrombi using flashlight test
4. Pre- post- and transmembrane pressure (DELTA pressure)

Labs

1. ABG from patient
2. Pre- and postmembrane ABG as and when required
3. Patient ACT (target 160–180 seconds)
4. CXR as and when required
5. Routine labs (like any other critically ill patient in ICU)

Problems encountered with V-V ECMO and troubleshooting

1. **Chattering of circuit:** This happens when the flow is obstructed due to the collapse of the vessel around the drainage cannula. This can be rectified by improving the volume status of the patient or by reducing the negative pressure created by the circuit, i.e. reducing RPM.

2. **Recirculation:** Seen when returned blood drains out through the drainage cannula without entering the systemic circulation either because the drainage and return cannulae are in proximity or the negative pressure generated by the drainage cannula is very high. The patient is hypoxic despite adequate flows. It is diagnosed by the absence of colour change in the tubing (both drainage and return cannulas are of same colour usually bright red). This is managed by reducing the flow, to reduce negative pressure and by adjusting cannula position. Acceptable recirculation is around 30%. Imaging after initial cannulation to confirm distance of 15 cm between the cannula tips decreases chances of recirculation.
3. **Hypoxia:** This may be due to inadequate flow or recirculation as described above or increased demand in the body (increased VO_2) causing an increase in shunt. If the patient has increased requirement this can be addressed by decreasing the basal metabolic rate of the patient. This is achieved by treating fever, sedation and paralysis or by using beta blockers to decrease cardiac output.

Management of anti-coagulation: Exposure of blood to the extracorporeal circuit activates the clotting pathways and requires anticoagulation to prevent circuit clotting and incidence of embolic events the most common anticoagulant used is unfractionated heparin. It has the advantage of being short acting, easy titrability and non-organ dependent metabolism. Disadvantage includes possibility of heparin induced thrombocytopenia (HIT).

Its activity is measured using either activated clotting time (ACT) or anti Xa levels.

Disadvantages include bleeding and heparin induced thrombocytopenia.

In patients with suspected heparin induced thrombocytopenia, bivalirudin or argatroban are the choice of anticoagulation.

Patients in VA ECMO need a higher level of anticoagulation as compared to V-V ECMO and also have a higher risk of ischaemic and bleeding complications.

ECMO related changes in pharmacokinetics

ECMO increases the volume of distribution of drugs (Vd), there is also increased drug sequestration in the circuit. The intense inflammation which the patients have due to the underlying disease and due to ECMO, changes the protein binding and distribution of drugs. This may lead to increase in drug requirement, leading to decreased efficacy. In case of antibiotics, increased incidence of resistance.

ECMO Weaning

V-V ECMO weaning: Once the patient's lungs start recovering, the support provided by the ECMO can be reduced by reducing the FiO_2 and sweep gas flow. Oxygenation usually returns earlier than CO_2 exchange. Weaning needs close monitoring in the form of blood gases, clinical examination of the patient and radiological monitoring in the form of CXR and CT scan. Once the sweep gas flow is reduced to 0 L/min the patient is completely dependent on his lungs and blood continues to flow through the circuit without any gas exchange. This is called trial off. If the patient tolerates being trialled off for 24 hr, then he can be decannulated. Hemostasis after venous decannulation can be achieved by local pressure and simple sutures.

V-A ECMO weaning: weaning of ECMO for cardiac support involves daily echo to look for cardiac function recovery. Once this is documented, ECMO flow can be reduced. This increases preload to the heart and decreases afterload. Evaluation of cardiac function involves looking for increase in cardiac output, lactate clearance, etc. If the patient tolerates weaning to minimum flows of 2 L/min (IDLE flow) then he can be taken temporarily off ECMO using a bridge in circuit. Once patient has shown to tolerate being off ECMO, he can be decannulated. Arterial decannulation requires surgical closure.

The turnaround time for VA ECMO is days to weeks whereas for VV ECMO it is generally weeks.

Emerging Indications for ECMO

ECMO has evolved from a research intervention to a niche intervention to rescue therapy to the present day standard of care for respiratory and cardiac support. Newer indications for ECMO are being studied and as physicians become comfortable with this therapy, its indications grow.

Evolving indications including

1. Low flow ECMO, Extracorporeal CO_2 removal ($ECCO_2R$) for hypercapneic respiratory failure and to deliver ultra-protective ventilation to lungs.
2. Management of pulmonary hypertensive crisis
3. Use in extracorporeal CPR in patients in cardiac arrest
4. Use of ECMO to prevent physical deconditioning associated with mechanical ventilation.
5. Use of ECMO in brain dead patients for better organ retrieval

The future of ECMO is one where one single machine could replace the entire function of the lung with minimal complications which can be mobile and has very little effect on the quality of life of the individual.

ECMO is a complex life support system which when used in the correct patient can have a good clinical outcome. As with many high risk interventions it has specific indications and complications. It needs a good understanding of physiology and expertise and a dedicated team to manage and achieve desired outcomes. It has dramatically changed the management of respiratory failure and its use has been increasing since the onset of the global coronavirus pandemic. The present state of ECMO is the result of years of lab research and clinical use which continues to happen to this day with newer indications and modifications to this therapy.

Further Reading

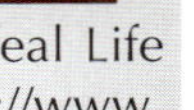

1. Brogan, TV, Lequier, L, Lorusso, R, MacLaren, G, & Peek, G (2017). Extracorporeal Life Support: The ELSO Red Book. (1 ed.) Extracorporeal Life Support Organization. https://www.elso.org/Publications/RedBook5thEdition.aspx.
2. Hadaya J, Benharash P. Extracorporeal Membrane Oxygenation. JAMA. 2020;323(24):2536. doi:10.1001/jama.2020.9148.
3. Venturumilli R, Vala PK. ECMO for Circulatory Support. Indian Journal of Clinical Cardiology. 2022;3(2):103–110. doi:10.1177/26324636221103703.

CHAPTER 28

Transporting a Patient on a Ventilator

❐ Uthara Vijai Kumar ❐ Jayaprakash Narayana Reddy

Transport of patients on a mechanical ventilator increases the risk of serious harm to the patient. A structured process conducted by a well trained and a well prepared team with adequate communication between team members plays an important role in ensuring safety of the patient being transported. Intra- and inter-hospital patient transfer is an important aspect of patient care that is often necessary to ensure prompt diagnosis and treatment. This includes transferring a patient within the hospital premises for a diagnostic procedure or to a different facility for better or advanced care. The primary objective is to avoid any disruption of medical care. Since transfer of a sick patient may induce various physiological changes in the patient that can affect the outcomes, it should be initiated in a systematic manner following all protocols from evidence based guidelines.

Transporting a patient on the ventilator from one location to another is one of the frequently undertaken tasks by healthcare professionals in acute medicine. This can be challenging as patients are moved to a different setting that may carry a risk of adverse events such as deterioration of physiological parameters, malfunctioning of equipment and displacement of lines and tubes. Incorrect operation of tools and failure of equipment can be contributing risk factors. Patients on mechanical ventilation while being transported, are at high risk of physiological worsening leading to organ failure.

Caring for a patient who is on a ventilator requires additional staff such as respiratory therapists and nurses trained in critical care. It is the same set of people who carry out the herculean task of transporting the patient safely between two locations.

Key Components of a Transport of Ventilator Patients

- Decision to transport
- Pre-transport preparation
- Transport vehicle and equipment
- Personnel who accompany the patient
- Transfer
- Handover

Decision to Transport

A decision on transfer can be taken only if healthcare professionals at both places have a mutual agreement. The decision on how to transport depends on the urgency of transfer, availability of experienced personnel to handle the patient and equipment.

Local SOP (standard operating procedure) should be prepared that will reflect referral patterns and expertise available at various centers.

Pre-transport Preparation

Reasonable stabilization of the patient prior to transfer is important to avoid complications during transit. In addition to full access to patient clinical details including history and examination, pre-transport monitoring should include electrocardiography, arterial oxygen saturation, blood pressure by intra-arterial monitoring and hourly urine output. If there is history of trauma, the need for an intra-abdominal drain or a chest drain should be assessed before commencing transport. If the patient is likely to develop respiratory failure, it is important to secure the airway before departure.

Appropriate drugs for analgesia and sedation should be administered as well as kept ready to take along. A patient who has persistent hypotension despite resuscitation should not be moved until any on-going blood loss has been identified and controlled. Long bone fractures should be stabilized to prevent limb ischemia. A nasogastric tube should be in place, all lines and tubes should be secured. These are important steps that should not be overlooked in an attempt to speed up the transfer because it can be very difficult to deal with problems that may arise once the journey has commenced.

Transport Vehicle

Vehicles used for transport should have good trolley access, adequate lighting and temperature control. It should be able to accommodate paramedical staff along with the patient. The time taken to mobilize, geographical factors, weather, traffic conditions and cost are important factors for a successful and uneventful transfer. Transport by road is the most preferred because it is cost effective, allows easy patient monitoring, rapid mobilization and is not affected by bad weather. For longer journeys, a flight transfer should be considered. Helicopters for journeys of 80–200 km or where access is difficult although they provide a less comfortable environment when compared to a road ambulance or an aircraft, more expensive and holds a poor safety record. Contact numbers of local ambulance services should be available in all ICU and emergency departments of all hospitals.

Equipment

Devices must be battery powered, robust and lightweight. Ambulance services have advanced greatly. A portable monitor with a big and clear display should be available to monitor heart rate, oxygen saturation, blood pressure end tidal carbon dioxide and temperature by non-invasive and invasive methods. A portable mechanical ventilator with disconnect alarms that provides variable oxygen concentrations, respiratory rates, tidal volumes, positive end expiratory pressure levels and inspiratory-expiratory ratios should be available. The transport vehicle should carry sufficient oxygen to last the duration of the transfer and a reserve. Alarms should be audible as well as visible due to ambient noise during transport. Suction apparatus and a defibrillator should be available. Syringe pumps with long battery life, a warming blanket and a mobile phone are a few other things that should be made available within the transport vehicle. All those assisting with the transfer should be familiar with the equipment, their use and where they are being kept within the vehicle.

Personnel who Accompany the Patient

An able physician, usually an anesthetist experienced in resuscitation, airway care and other organ support should accompany the patient. Assistance should be sought from another physician, paramedic, a trained nurse familiar with intensive care procedures and equipment.

Transfer

Admittedly, the same level of care should be maintained in the intensive care unit as it is almost impossible to interfere with transport. Monitoring of arterial oxygen saturation, expired carbon dioxide tensions, heart rate, temperature, and arterial pressure should be continuous. Non-invasive measurement of blood pressure affected by movement Therefore, intra-arterial monitoring is recommended. The transfer should be smooth and not at high speed. A record should be maintained at the time of transfer. Even with careful preparation, unexpected clinical emergencies can occur; the vehicle should be stopped at the first safe opportunity to facilitate patient handling.

Handover

On arrival, there should be direct communication between the transfer team and the receiving team. A detailed record of the patient's history, treatment and events during transfer should be handed over. A record of all investigations with their interpretation should be presented. The transfer team should maintain a record of all events for future audit. The receiving hospital should provide refreshments and arrange for them to return to base.

Further Reading

1. AARC Clinical Practice Guideline: In-Hospital Transport of the Mechanically Ventilated Patient-2002.
2. Monitoring during transport, Respiratory Care, June 2020.
3. Transport of the Ventilator-supported patient-Principles and Practice of Mechanical Ventilation-Chapter 27.

CHAPTER 29

Role of Bronchoscopy while on Ventilator

❐ Nagarjuna Maturu ❐ Rinoosha BR

INTRODUCTION

Flexible bronchoscopy is an important tool in respiratory medicine. Its use in critical care is also increasing owing to its diagnostic and therapeutic capabilities. Indications for FB in ICU includes removal of mucous plugs, blood clots, management of massive hemoptysis and for obtaining samples for microbiological samplings.

The knowledge of the unique features of intensive care unit patients, as well as indications and contraindications for the procedure, is paramount in achieving optimal results, while minimizing potential risks and complications. Performing bronchoscopy in an unstable patient, often on mechanical ventilation, requires awareness of the specific pathophysiological impact of the procedure. This in turn determines respiratory and cardiovascular derangements frequently observed during the procedure.

The critical patient often has one or more organ failures, which makes him or her a high-risk patient for the procedure. Moreover, as respiratory system involvement is a common feature, regardless of the precipitating factor of critical illness, the risk of respiratory failure is not negligible.

How Bronchoscopy is Different in ICU

The ICU environment is different from a well-equipped bronchoscopy suit.The area around the patient bed is often more crowded and limited due to other ICU equipment. There may be on spot non-availability of all the bronchoscopy accessories and certain ancillary devices, e.g. fluoroscopy, as a result the procedure may be interrupted several times.

The patients in ICU are sicker with one or more unstable organ systems as compared to those undergoing routine bronchoscopy, hence, they are at higher risk of iatrogenic hypoxemia and respiratory failure.

Although, it is true that the critically ill patients are more susceptible to developing complications during bronchoscopy, yet as compared to the spontaneously breathing patients, the mechanically ventilated patients are paradoxically less at risk because their airway is secured.

INDICATIONS

In the ICU, mostly basic bronchoscopy is performed with examination of tracheobronchial tree, bronchoalveolar lavage (BAL), brushing, and forceps biopsy as the primary techniques.

It is recommended that ICU must be equipped to perform urgent FOB for a range of diagnostic and therapeutic indications **(Table 29.1)**.

The most common indication of bronchoscopy in ICU is removal of retained secretion in 45% cases followed by microbiological sampling in 35% cases.[1] However, many a times bronchoscopy is performed for the diagnostic as well as therapeutic purposes simultaneously at the same time.[2]

Table 29.1

Diagnostic Indications	Therapeutic Indications
✦ Pneumonia – Immunocompromised host, – Hospital acquired or ventilator acquired – Non-resolving pneumonia	✦ Atelectasis and collapse
✦ Diffuse parenchymal lung disease	✦ Excess airway secretions
✦ Airway trauma – Intubation injury – Blunt thoracic injury – Postoperative	✦ Foreign body removal
✦ Acute inhalational injury or burns	✦ Difficult intubation
✦ Stridor	✦ Double lumen endotracheal tube placement
✦ Localized wheeze	✦ Massive hemoptysis – Application of glue – Tamponade – Double lumen endotracheal intubation
✦ Trachea esophageal fistula	✦ Bronchopleural fistula closure – Application of glue, sealants or spigots
✦ Aspiration	✦ Tracheoesophageal fistula closure – Stent
✦ Atelectasis and collapse	✦ Obstructing endobronchial neoplasms (malignant and benign) – Laser photoresection – Electrocautery debulking – Cryotherapy – Endobronchial brachytherapy
✦ Hemoptysis	✦ Strictures and stenoses – Dilatation – Stents
✦ Suspected foreign body	
✦ Airway stricture and stenosis	
✦ Benign and malignant neoplasms	

CONSENT, ANESTHESIA AND SEDATION DURING BRONCHOSCOPY IN ICU

Patient's selection is of paramount importance. Educating the patient or the next of kin regarding the risks and benefits of the procedure is the first essential step.

During the administration of anesthesia for bronchoscopy in the ICU, multiple factors for each individual patient must be reviewed. The level of sedation (minimal, moderate, deep, or general anesthesia) used during bronchoscopy can vary based on the procedural settings, complexity and duration of the procedure (advanced diagnostic or therapeutic bronchoscopy).

To achieve the required level of sedation, the chosen pharmacological sedative should be administered by titration of small incremental doses to the desired clinical and physiological effect. This is particularly important in patients where the arm–brain circulation time is prolonged (e.g. heart failure).

In the elderly, dose adjustments are particularly important due to the reduced hepatic metabolism and renal function, reduced tissue and blood esterases and increased sensitivity to a given concentration of drug.

Patients in shock have decreased hepatic metabolism and decreased renal clearance which affects the clearance of the drug.

Dose adjustments are required in patients who are on drugs which have interactions with the pharmacological sedative agents that may lead to enhancement or inhibition of the effects.

CONSENT

Verbal and written information explaining indications, procedure, and potential complications should be provided.

If the patient does not have capacity to make decisions, next of kin should be approached to obtain informed consent.

In the elective bronchoscopy, solid/fatty food should be avoided for 8 hours and light/non-fatty food and non-human milk should be avoided for 6 hours. Clear liquids like water, fruit juice without pulp are allowed up to 2 hours prior to the procedure.[3,4]

For patients on mechanical support or patients requiring emergency bronchoscopy, aspiration of stomach content with naso-/orogastric tube just prior to the procedure may be sufficient to prevent aspiration.[5]

VENTILATION AND ANESTHESIA

The patient could be conscious non-hypoxemic, conscious with hypoxemia and/or hypercapnia, conscious and requiring NIV, and conscious on spontaneous invasive ventilation, with altered sensorium that may require active measures to help maintain airway patency or sedated and/or paralyzed on controlled invasive ventilation.

It is important to preoxygenate patient before administering anesthesia.

Patients already requiring oxygen supplementation may be escalated to NIV to prevent worsening hypoxemia and preventing invasive ventilation.[6]

In patients with NIV, there is very minimal evidence to support the role of sedation; however, some authors propose the use of propofol during bronchoscopy in these patients.[7]

Patients on spontaneous mode of ventilation on invasive ventilation may be switched over to controlled mode prior to bronchoscopy.

Fraction of inspired oxygen should be increased to 100% prior to procedure. A sedation level which allows ventilation without patient fighting it is necessary to be achieved to prevent hypoxemia.[6]

PREMEDICATION FOR BRONCHOSCOPY

- Routine administration of anticholinergics as premedication for bronchoscopy is not recommended. Anticholinergics lack any clinical benefit and increase risk of hemodynamic changes.[8]
- Nebulized bronchodilators should be considered in patients with asthma prior to bronchoscopy.[6]

PHARMACOLOGICAL AGENTS FOR SEDATION DURING BRONCHOSCOPY

Benzodiazepines

- Benzodiazepines have a lengthy record of safety and efficacy in bronchoscopy and are widely used for sedation.[9] These drugs enhance the effect of the γ-aminobutyric acid (GABA) and have sedative, hypnotic, anxiolytic, anticonvulsant, and muscle relaxing properties.
- They are metabolized in the liver via the cytochrome P450 3A4 and 3A5 system and excreted mainly in the urine and have relatively minimal cardiovascular depressant effects.
- Midazolam is the most frequently used drug in this group because of its advantages of rapid onset of action, rapid time to peak effect, and short duration of action. It can be safely and effectively used in combination with opiates.[8]
- It may cause a slight decrease in arterial blood pressure and increase in heart rate with reduction in vagal tone and thus result in heart rate variability.
- The ventilatory drive is depressed and apnea may occur with higher doses of midazolam, especially in those with co-morbidities and when used in combination with other respiratory depressants.
- Lorazepam and diazepam are the other drugs in this group which have been used for bronchoscopy.
- The doses used for sedation of midazolam, lorazepam, and diazepam are 0.01–0.1 mg/kg, 0.03–0.05 mg/kg and 0.04–0.2 mg/kg, respectively.
- Flumazenil, is a competitive antagonist of benzodiazepines at the GABA receptor and is used for reversal of benzodiazepine effects.[8] The dosage for reversal of sedation is 0.2 mg, repeated every 60 seconds up to 1 mg as bolus and 0.1–0.4 mg/h for continuous infusion till reversal of effects of benzodiazepine.

Opioids

- Opioids are frequently used along with benzodiazepines during bronchoscopy for their analgesic, antitussive, and sedative properties.
- The complementing properties of opioids with benzodiazepines help in improving conditions for the bronchoscopists by improving patient tolerance of the procedure and reduction in the amount of other pharmacological sedatives.[9]
- Opioids bind to mu (μ), kappa (κ), delta (δ), and sigma (σ) receptors that are found in the brain, spinal cord, peripheral sensory neurons, and gastrointestinal tract. They are mainly metabolized by the liver and excreted by the kidneys.
- Due to renal elimination, opioids may accumulate in patients with renal failure leading to prolonged sedation and ventilatory depression.[9]

- In high doses, they lead to bradycardia and associated hypotension but do not lower cardiac contractility.
- The effects on the respiratory system are more significant, particularly reduction of the respiratory rate resulting in ventilatory depression. Due to the effects opioids on the respiratory centers in the brainstem the apneic threshold is increased and the hypoxic drive is reduced.
- Fentanyl is the most widely used opioid because of its rapid onset of action and elimination half-life that makes it suitable for use in bronchoscopy.
- The recommended dose of fentanyl in moderate sedation is 50–200 µg followed by supplemental doses of 50 µg when used alone, however, when co-administered with other agents, an initial dose of 25–50 µg is recommended with supplemental doses of 25 µg as required until the desired effect is achieved or a total dose of 200 µg has been reached.[9]
- Naloxone is used for the reversal of respiratory depression due to opioids. The intravenous dose for reversal of opioid respiratory depression and over sedation is usually 100–200 µg (1.5–3 µg/kg) with supplemental doses of 100 µg every 2 minutes until reversal occurs to the desired level of respiration and consciousness.

Propofol

- Propofol is a short-acting anesthetic agent with rapid onset of action, short initial distribution half-life (2–8 minutes) and gets rapidly metabolized by the liver.
- It acts by binding to the β-subunit of the γ-aminobutyric acid A (GABA-A) receptor resulting in hyperpolarization of the postsynaptic membrane.[10]
- It is an effective agent for sedation in bronchoscopy and can achieve similar sedation, amnesia and patient tolerance compared with the combined administration of benzodiazepines and opioids.
- It is important to remember the dose dependent hemodynamic effect of propofol which could cause hypotension and decreased cardiac output as well as the development of propofol infusion syndrome though rare.
- Propofol can cause respiratory depression and apnea even at induction doses and it can inhibit the hypoxic ventilator drive even at dose used for conscious sedation. For induction of sedation, a dose of 0.5–1 mg/kg over 1–5 minutes is usually required followed by maintenance concentrations of 1.5–4.5 mg/kg/h.
- It is reported that sedation with propofol in comparison to midazolam has similar efficacy and safety but faster onset of action and more rapid recovery with propofol along with improved patient tolerance to the procedure.[11] It is important to know that there is no antagonist available for reversal of action of propofol and there is narrow therapeutic window between moderate sedation and anesthesia with propofol.

Other Pharmacological Sedative Agents

- Dexmedetomidine which is a selective α_2-agonist has been shown to be safe and effective for conscious sedation during intubation using flexible bronchoscopy.[12]
- A study reported dexmedetomidine in comparison with midazolam provides better oxygen saturation and is equally tolerated for conscious sedation in postoperative patients undergoing bronchoscopy.

- Remifentanil and fospropofol are the other emerging pharmacological sedative agents for inducing moderate sedation for bronchoscopy.[13]

TOPICAL ANESTHESIA

- Topical airway anesthesia is an important component of flexible bronchoscopy as it provides the patient with additional comfort and tolerability along with sedation.
- Local anesthesia of the nares, oropharynx, and hypopharynx allows comfortable passage of the bronchoscope to the upper airway.
- Topical anesthesia of the airways beyond the glottis depresses the cough reflex and allows the bronchoscopist to comfortably visualize the airways and perform the procedures.[14]
- Lidocaine (or lignocaine) is the most commonly used topical anesthetic during flexible bronchoscopy because of its efficacy in suppressing cough, short half-life, wide safety margin, and minimal tissue toxicity.
- It is metabolized by the liver and may have side effects at serum levels greater than 5 µg/mL.
- British Thoracic Society recommends no greater than 8.2 mg/kg cumulative dose of lidocaine.[15]
- Cardiac and neurologic toxicities, namely circumoral paraesthesia, seizures, and cardiac arrhythmias, are dose-related and can occur if serum lidocaine level exceeds 5 mg/L.
- Particularly at risk are patients with advanced age, impaired liver function or congestive heart failure although, no dose adjustment is required for renal failure.
- Spray-as-you-go technique is effective in delivering lidocaine to the vocal cords and trachea depending upon the procedure and mode of ventilatory support.
- Nebulization can be used as a technique for delivering lidocaine to the airway.
- 1–2% lidocaine solution should be used for spray-as-you-go administration.[16]

PATHOPHYSIOLOGICAL CHANGES DURING BRONCHOSCOPY IN ICU

The vast majority of the ICU patients receive some form of mechanical ventilation either by noninvasive bilevel positive airway pressure (NIV) or via an endotracheal tube (ETT) or tracheostomy tube (T tube). Bronchoscopy is an invasive procedure that may cause or trigger a series of pathophysiologic consequences on the respiratory mechanics, gas exchange, and hemodynamics.

SIZE OF BRONCHOSCOPE AND AIRWAY

- In a non-intubated patient, a 5.7 mm outer diameter bronchoscope occupies only 10% of the total cross-sectional area of the trachea,[17] as a result generates endotracheal pressures similar to those in patients without bronchoscopy which are –5 cm H_2O during inspiration and +3.5 cm H_2O during expiration.[18]
- On the other hand, bronchoscope passed through an ETT or tracheostomy tube generates pressures of –10 to +9 cm H_2O during inspiration and expiration, respectively.

- Therefore, the bronchoscope diameter and its relation with the airway diameter play an important role in causing airflow obstruction in intubated patients. The increase in airway pressures during bronchoscopy is related to the internal diameter of the trachea and outer diameter (OD) of bronchoscope.[18]
- A bronchoscope with OD of 5.7 mm occupies 40% of cross-sectional area of 9 mm ETT whereas 51% and 66% of cross-sectional area of 8 mm and 7 mm ETT respectively, signifying that smaller the diameter of ETT, more is obstruction to airflow during bronchoscopy.
- This not only compromises the ability to ventilate the patient, but it makes the procedure considerably more difficult for the bronchoscopist, because the narrow artificial airway decreases the maneuverability of the bronchoscope.
- In practice, one needs a substantially larger ETT in order to be able to advance the bronchoscope without difficulty while maintaining adequate ventilation.
- It is recommended to use an ETT of an internal diameter at least 2 mm larger than the OD of the bronchoscope. The choice of using a narrow bronchoscope has a potential disadvantage of lesser aspiration capacity as compared with those of a larger size.

Respiratory Mechanics

- A flexible bronchoscope with an outer diameter of 5.7 mm occupies approximately 10% of the cross-sectional area of the trachea and 15% of the cross-sectional area at the cricoid ring in an adult patient. The immediate consequence is some degree of airway obstruction.
- In a conscious, spontaneously breathing patient, this obstruction is mild to moderate, perfectly tolerated, and does not induce significant intra-tracheal pressure variations.
- However, in the ventilated patient, the obstructive effect of the flexible bronchoscope is added to that of the ETT. This obstruction leads to a significant increase in airway resistance, which in turn generates significant intra-tracheal pressure variations during the respiratory cycle.
- When the patient is ventilated in a volume control (VC) mode, the increase in Raw during bronchoscopy will result in increases in the Peak inspiratory pressures (PIP) and positive end expiratory pressures (PEEP).
- These pressure changes increase the risk for barotrauma, auto-PEEP and significant hemodynamic instability. On the other hand, pressure control (PC) ventilation has little effect on pressures, but it may severely limit the delivered tidal volume
- Lindholm, *et al.*[19] described the cardiorespiratory effects of fiberoptic bronchoscopy (FOB) in 38 patients. During the procedure, peak tracheal pressures varied between 18 cm H_2O and 60 cm H_2O, while PIP varied between 28 cm H_2O and 80 cm H_2O. Even though PEEP was discontinued during the procedure, auto-PEEP averaging 10.4 cm H_2O was present in all but five patients immediately on insertion of the bronchoscope. The auto-PEEP occurs during bronchoscopy due to impedance to expiratory flow and insufficient time for complete expiration.[19]
- Usually PEEP remains below 20 cm H_2O in an 8 mm ETT. A PEEP of up to 35 cm H_2O has been recorded with a 7 mm ETT.
- The reduction in delivered tidal volume is a direct result of obstruction of the airway by the bronchoscope and, if the high-pressure limit setting is reached, the ventilator

prematurely cycles from the inspiratory to the expiratory phase, resulting in a further decrease in delivered Vt.[20]

- Suction applied through the bronchoscope also decreases the delivered tidal volume. As much as 200–300 mL of the Vt can be removed during each suction period.
- Although Vt falls dramatically in all cases during bronchoscopy, but returns to pre-bronchoscopic values immediately on its removal, especially in VC mode.
- In the PC mode, the presence of the bronchoscope in the airway results in a reduction in delivered Vt similar to that observed in the VC mode when the high-pressure limit is not readjusted.
- A common practice among bronchoscopists is to transiently withdraw the bronchoscope for brief periods to allow the patient unobstructed ventilation. This would expose the lung to risk of very high Vts, and thus the potential for barotrauma.
- It is, therefore, important that the inspiratory pressure level be reduced to pre-bronchoscopic values before the bronchoscope is removed from the ETT.

Gas Exchange

- Transient deterioration of gas exchange due to partial obstruction of the airway is one of the most common problems encountered during bronchoscopy. This is largely due to reductions in lung volumes and FRC, which may produce alveolar closure during bronchoscopy.
- Another mechanism is reflex bronchospasm induced by stimulation of sub-epithelial vagal receptors in the upper airway.
- Utilization of short-suction periods of no more than 3 seconds and adequate topical anesthesia should minimize the hypoxic response to these two stimuli.
- Post-procedure, these gas exchange abnormalities return to baseline values, from about 15 minutes to several hours depending upon the severity of parenchymal disease.[19]

Cardiovascular Effects

- Although bronchoscope does not directly affect the cardiovascular system, it may cause significant cardiac as well as hemodynamic changes. Lindholm, *et al.*[19] reported an increase in cardiac output reaching 50% during the procedure, and returning to baseline in 15 minutes after its completion. Schiffman, *et al*. demonstrated sinus tachycardia is the most common hemodynamic consequence during bronchoscopy observed in 55–58% patients followed by sinus bradycardia in 5–8%, premature ventricular contraction in 8%, and atrial premature contraction in 3–5% patients.[21]
- These hemodynamics effects during bronchoscopy are attributed to multiple factors. There is reflex sympathetic discharge caused by mechanical irritation of the airways
- Hypoxemia and/or elevation of $PaCO_2$ lead to increase in vascular tone. Increase in PIP, development of auto-PEEP and rise in intrathoracic pressure may affect the venous return
- All these effects are usually well tolerated by most patients but they can be very deleterious in patients with compromised cardiac function, increased systemic blood pressure, or increased intracranial pressure.

Bronchoscopy Assisted by Noninvasive Ventilation

Noninvasive ventilation (NIV) is the provision of assisted ventilation without an artificial airway, it not only improves gas exchange but also reduces the work of breathing, prevent ETI and need for intensive care unit (ICU) admission in selected cases of acute respiratory failure.

The commonly used modes during NIV include continuous positive airway pressure (CPAP), which is the application of uniform airway pressure throughout the respiratory cycle or bi-level positive airway pressure (BiPAP) where the pressure can be applied at two levels namely the inspiratory positive airway pressure (IPAP) and expiratory positive airway pressure (EPAP). The IPAP augments the inspiratory flow and pressure, thereby increases the tidal volume and unloads the inspiratory muscles.[23] The EPAP decreases dead space ventilation and improves alveolar ventilation, re-expands flooded alveoli and counteracts intrinsic positive-end expiratory pressure.[24] The EPAP also prevents micro-atelectasis with resultant increase in FRC, thereby placing the respiratory pressure–volume characteristics in a more favorable position.

The use of NIV during FOB has been associated with significant improvement in SpO_2 in majority of the studies in contrast to the fall of SpO_2 while performing FOB without ventilatory support.[25]

In the first study on NIV-assisted bronchoscopy, Antonelli, *et al.* performed bronchoalveolar lavage (BAL) in immunocompromised patients with pneumonia and severe hypoxemia (PaO_2/FiO_2 <100 mm Hg). There are significant improvements in PaO_2/FiO_2 ratios during bronchoscopy and BAL was diagnostic in all eight cases; six patients survived to hospital discharge.[26]

Maitre, *et al.* randomized 30 patients with hypoxemia (PaO_2 <125 mm Hg) to receive either high flow oxygen by mask or CPAP during bronchoscopy. The CPAP group had significantly high SpO_2 values compared to oxygen group. In the other group, patients experienced hypoxemia during the bronchoscopy, and five patients (compared to none in the CPAP group) required ventilatory assistance.[27]

In a randomized trial comprising of patients with nosocomial pneumonia, the NIV was found to improve oxygenation and hemodynamic tolerance when compared to oxygen supplementation during bronchoscopy. NIV improved PaO_2/FiO_2 by 82%, whereas in oxygen group PaO_2/FiO_2 declined by 10% during bronchoscopy and further 10% in the hour after the procedure.[28]

Recently, Agarwal, *et al.* published a case series of NIV-assisted bronchoscopic lung biopsy in six patients with diffuse pulmonary infiltrates and hypoxemia (median PaO_2/FiO_2 164.5 mm Hg). FOB was well tolerated and all subjects maintained SpO_2 greater than 92% during the procedure.[29] One subject required ETI due to hemoptysis, which stopped in 24 hours. A definite diagnosis was obtained in five of the six subjects; there was no pneumothorax.

Indications for Noninvasive Ventilation-Assisted Bronchoscopy

Noninvasive ventilation-assisted bronchoscopy is indicated in any patient who requires FOB and BAL (and/or bronchial biopsy and/or transbronchial lung biopsy) for diagnostic purposes and is hypoxemic (PaO_2/FiO_2 ≤300 mm Hg).[30,31] In general, this would include:

1. Patients with acute hypoxemic respiratory failure, diffuse (or focal) parenchymal infiltrates,
2. Patients at high-risk of post-bronchoscopy respiratory failure including patients with severe COPD, expiratory dynamic airway collapse, obstructive sleep apnea and obesity hypoventilation syndrome.
3. Pediatric subjects who are at risk for hypoxemia and hypercapnia due to the smaller diameter of airways and greater tendency for airway collapse.
4. Bronchoscopy may also be indicated for diagnostic purposes or bronchial toileting in patients who are already receiving NIV.

Contraindications for Noninvasive Ventilation-assisted Bronchoscopy

- Shock (SBP <90 mm Hg) or need for vasopressors
- Uncontrolled hypertension (SBP >180 mm Hg)
- Severe respiratory failure (pH <7.25, $PaCO_2$ >80 mm Hg, PaO_2/FiO_2 <150 mm Hg)
- Recent (<4 weeks) acute coronary syndrome or unstable cardiac arrhythmias
- Coagulation abnormalities (thrombocytopenia < 30,000/µL, INR >2)
- Contraindications for NIV: Reduced level of consciousness, significant
- Psychomotor agitation, recent facial or esophageal surgery, inability to tolerate face mask
- SpO_2 <90% despite NIV.

Setting

- Noninvasive ventilation-assisted FOB can be performed either in the ICU (or high dependency unit) or bronchoscopy suite.
- Continuous monitoring of heart rate, electrocardiogram and pulse oximetry during the procedure is mandatory.
- Arterial blood gas analysis is recommended before, during and 15 minutes after the procedure to document the adequacy of gas exchange.

Noninvasive Ventilation Interfaces

- The interfaces used to provide NIV during FOB are nasal masks, oronasal masks and helmet mask.
- The choice depends on the expertise of the unit and the availability of the interface.
- A universal swivel adapter with soft cap prevents air leak from the face mask and facilitates the introduction of the bronchoscope. Specially customized masks for introducing the bronchoscope with nasal or oral ports are also available.[32]

Noninvasive Ventilation Protocol

- Noninvasive ventilation can be delivered either by using a critical care ventilator or portable NIV equipment and always it is preferable to have an NIV delivery device with in-built oxygen blender which delivers precise and high concentrations of oxygen.
- The bronchoscope is inserted through a universal swivel adapter attached to the mask to prevent air leak during the procedure.

- To allow easy entry of the bronchoscope, the mask is initially held by the assistant over the patient's face and adjusted to facilitate the passage of the scope from the nose to the vocal cords, and is secured to the patient's face with elastic straps.
- Once the bronchoscope enters the trachea. The NIV support should be initiated with ventilatory parameters set at EPAP of 5 cm H_2O, IPAP of 10–15 cm H_2O and FiO_2 of 1 commencing 15 minutes before the bronchoscopy.
- The ventilatory parameters are adjusted to maintain a SpO_2 greater than 92% throughout the procedure. The patient ventilator synchrony, air leaks, tidal volume and respiratory rate must be closely monitored during the procedure.

Patient Position

- The procedure is performed in the standard fashion with the patient lying supine and the operator standing behind the patient. In patients who are unable to lie supine,the procedure can be performed with the patient at 45° with the operator standing in front of the patient.

Bronchoscopy Preparation and Procedure

- Patients should be well prepared for the bronchoscopy procedure. They are initially nebulized with 2.5 ml of 4% lignocaine for 15 minutes prior to the procedure.
- Lignocaine spray (10%) is sprayed twice over the oropharynx. Approximately 5 ml of 2% lignocaine gel is administered in the nasal cavity prior to the introduction of the bronchoscope.
- Thereafter, patients receive 2 mL aliquots of 1% lignocaine solution delivered through the bronchoscope one of each at the vocal cord, tracheal carina, and in the right and left main bronchus, using the "spray-as-you-go" technique.
- Routine use of sedatives before or during the procedure is not recommended so as to avoid the risk of cardiorespiratory depression.[26] Thus, patient tolerance to both NIV and awake bronchoscopy is paramount.
- While obtaining bronchoscopic lung biopsy, the EPAP should be reduced to zero and PS to 10 cm H_2O to prevent pneumothorax.[29]
- The duration of the procedure should be limited to the shortest possible time required to obtain the necessary samples. In previous studies, the median duration of NIV-assisted bronchoscopy with BAL and NIV-assisted bronchoscopic lung biopsy was about 8 and 11.5 minutes, respectively.[29]
- Noninvasive ventilation is usually continued for 30 minutes after the procedure.
- Subsequently, the patient can be oxygenated by high flow air-entrainment mask under close monitoring for the next 1–2 hours.

Complications

- The use of NIV with high pressures can cause gastric distension by air which predisposes the risk of aspiration.
- Agitation and lack of cooperation from the patient worsens the patient-ventilator synchrony and result in respiratory distress.
- There can be refractory hypoxemia and hypercapnia during the procedure, which may necessitate intubation and mechanical ventilation. Thus, the necessary resuscitative

equipment and expert personnel should be readily available for tackling this emergency.
- Cardiac arrhythmias and myocardial ischemia can be precipitated during the procedure, which can be avoided by meticulous patient selection and avoidance of hypoxemia.
- A recent prospective multicenter observational study reported the performance of 169 FOB procedures in ICU patients with a $PaO_2/FiO_2 \leq 300$ mm Hg[33] in which it was found that following FOB there was increase in ventilatory assistance in 59 (35%) patients, of which 25 (15%) required ETI
- Bronchoscopic lung biopsy may be complicated by hemoptysis, pneumothorax and pneumomediastinum. Routine point-of-care ultrasonography and chest radiograph must be performed to exclude these complications.

Bronchoscopy during Mechanical Ventilation

Bronchoscopy in ventilated patients is now an essential tool in modern ICUs, with a comprehensive approach balancing safety and ensuring outcomes. Bronchoscopy in mechanically-ventilated patients can have diagnostic or therapeutic applications.

Preprocedure Preparation

- A review of the indication for bronchoscopy, appropriate imaging and written informed consent
- A careful assessment of the propensity for cardiorespiratory worsening and planning for the same, including availability of a skilled and experienced operator for troubleshooting
- Stop enteral feeding at least 4 hours before a semi urgent procedure. In case of emergency procedures, empty the stomach contents prior to the procedure by nasogastric tube aspiration.
- Medications including topical anesthetic agents (lignocaine 1–2%), sedatives and hypnotics (midazolam, morphine/fentanyl, propofol, etc.), short acting neuromuscular blocking agents (atracurium and vecuronium) and hemostatic agents (iced saline and epinephrine)
- Due to the alterations in the cardiorespiratory parameters during bronchoscopy in mechanically ventilated patients, monitoring during and after bronchoscopy is very important. Monitoring includes blood pressure (invasive as needed), pulse oximetry, electrocardiogram for heart rate and rhythm, ventilatory parameters like tidal volume, minute ventilation and peak inspiratory pressures.[34]
- It is important to ensure that all equipment essential for bronchoscopy in mechanically ventilated patients is readily available at the bedside of the patient
- A typical bronchoscopy preparation table contains local anesthesia agents, sterile saline, hemostatic agents, and tools such as forceps, brush, needle, catheter mount and mucus trap for specimen collection.

Procedure

- It is important to ensure adequate sedation and use of neuromuscular blocking agents, as needed.

- Patients with bronchial asthma and chronic obstructive pulmonary disease (COPD) who are prone to bronchospasm, use of nebulized bronchodilators like salbutamol can reduce the risk of bronchospasm, rise in peak airway pressures and barotrauma
- The FiO_2 should be increased to 100% prior to the procedure and maintained for at least an hour after the procedure to ensure adequate oxygenation and oxygen saturation greater than 90% at all times
- In patients where it is not possible to maintain oxygen saturation greater than 90%, with FiO_2 greater than or equal to 90% before the procedure, bronchoscopy should be performed only after careful review of the indications and risks involved. Often, common pathological conditions such as atelectasis, lobar/lung collapse, excessive secretions and hemoptysis can severely impair gas exchange.
- Bronchoscopy can help clear secretions and blood clots rapidly, and in alleviating hypoxemia can be a lifesaving procedure. In such difficult situations, bronchoscopy should be done by the most experienced operator
- Ventilator parameters need to be adjusted prior to the procedure to ensure delivery of adequate tidal volume and respiratory rate (minute ventilation) to prevent hypercapnia, and maintain oxygenation. In patients with pressure control mode of ventilation, the pressure control is adjusted to compensate for the elevated airway resistance due to presence of the scope in the ETT, and maintain the tidal volume. In patients on volume control mode of ventilation, the alarm settings for peak airway pressure need to be adjusted. Positive end-expiratory pressure (PEEP) should be zero during the procedure, or if not safe, should be reduced by at least half. The peak airway pressures pre- and post-bronchoscopy should be noted.
- The ETT should be at least 2 mm greater than the outer diameter of the bronchoscope, and can be replaced with a larger diameter tube as needed. If the ETT cannot be replaced, a smaller sized scope should be used.
- The catheter mount, comprising of a rubber diaphragm with central orifice attached to the swivel adapter is used as a conduit for the procedure to ensure a tight seal and minimize the loss of tidal volume.
- The bronchoscopist should ideally stand at the head end of patient, for easy navigation and understanding of the anatomy of the tracheobronchial tree.
- Use of an oral airway/bite block is essential to prevent damage to the bronchoscope due to biting, especially if sedation is used without paralysis
- The bronchoscope should be adequately lubricated prior to insertion using a thin layer of jelly. Bronchoscope is then gently introduced in the endotracheal tube through the swivel adapter.
- For ensuring airway anesthesia, topical lignocaine (2%) should be instilled in the trachea, at the carina and both main bronchi. This is in line with an important axiom in bronchoscopy, namely "stay behind your anesthesia".
- In case of desaturation, hypotension or arrhythmias, the procedure should be temporarily stopped and if vitals return to normal, the procedure can be started only after careful re-appraisal of the risk-benefit ratio. In borderline patients, a strategy of short runs rather than a single prolonged procedure can be followed.
- Use intermittent brief suction for 3 seconds or lesser, to avoid hypoxemia.

- The amount of bronchoalveolar lavage (BAL) fluid or washings to be instilled should be carefully decided based on the condition of the underlying lung parenchyma, the extent of pre-existing hypoxemia and propensity for worsening.
- Use of smaller amounts is particularly useful in patients with pre-existing severe hypoxemia. In patients with pre-existing hypoxemia, a quick procedure with the mucus trap already attached to the bronchoscope with smaller aliquots of saline can reduce postprocedure worsening of hypoxemia.[2]
- For patients with high FiO_2/PEEP requirement, the procedure should be done by an experienced operator with adequate sedation and paralysis. The procedure should be done in the shortest possible time, with limited suctioning and volume of instilled saline washings recommended over BAL. Recruitment maneuvers may be required postprocedure to ensure adequate oxygenation in case of life-threatening desaturation.

Postprocedure Care

- Monitoring of vital parameters with special attention for possible desaturation, hypercapnia and worsening respiratory distress.
- Frequent clinical reviews with monitoring for bronchospasm are required.
- Monitoring of peak and plateau airway pressures, which should revert to baseline over time.
- Postprocedure blood gas analysis to look for hypercapnia is not mandated, unless clinically indicated.
- Precise documentation and reporting of details must be done, including premedications, procedure details, complications, postprocedure advice and the relevant endobronchial pictures.
- Prompt dispatch of samples collected after proper labeling with details of tests required and brief clinical history.
- Cleaning and disinfection of the scope along with the leak test to check for any possible damage to the scope.

Technical Aspects

In patients under mechanical ventilation, there are a number of practical recommendations that must be met according to the pathophysiological considerations outlined above. They relate mainly to the adaptation of the ventilatory circuit and the adjustment of ventilator parameters:

1. Anesthetize the tracheobronchial tree properly
2. Sedate the patient (add muscle relaxation in selected cases);
3. The ETT should have an inner diameter of at least 8.0 mm; the difference between the inner diameter of the ETT and the outer diameter of the flexible bronchoscope should be ≥2 mm. If the patient is intubated with an ETT <8.0 mm, and tube change is not a viable option, then a pediatric or an ultrathin bronchoscope can be used;
4. Use a swivel adapter to minimize VT loss through the circuit;
5. Ventilate on volume control mode. Triggered modes are not generally recommended because ventilation will not be guaranteed unless the peak pressure limit is increased to ensure that the desired VT is delivered.

6. Pressure-control ventilation will also result in a reduced VT, unless the inspiratory pressure level is increased to compensate for high airway resistance during the procedure.
7. Exhaled VT must be continuously monitored (ensure that it is similar to pre-bronchoscopic levels during the procedure). In addition to the increase in VT, increase the ventilator rate, if necessary, to maintain adequate ventilation;
8. Set PEEP to 0 cmH_2O (if this is not feasible, reduce the PEEP level by 50%). Despite concern over derecruitment, this measure is proposed by most investigators to avoid dangerous hyperinflation and barotrauma, as generation of auto-PEEP during the examination is well documented;
9. Increase FiO_2 to 1.0, starting 5 to 15 minutes before the procedure, for adequate preoxygenation. Maintain FiO_2 at 1.0 during and up to 1 hour after FB, with the purpose of keeping SaO_2 as close to 100% as possible;
10. Set the peak inspiratory flow level to ≤60 L/min;
11. Visually monitor the magnitude of thoracic excursions during the procedure;
12. Apply suction only for short periods (3 s or less).

Monitoring during Bronchoscopy in ICU

- Basic monitoring during bronchoscopy includes SpO_2, BP, and HR monitoring; of these SpO_2 is the most vulnerable.
- Critically ill patients are at risk of developing hypoxemia even with trivial manipulations of the airway. It is, therefore, recommended to increase FiO_2 to 1.0 well before the start of the procedure.[8]
- FOB may cause arrhythmia in the critically ill, thus monitoring of HR, preferably with a continuous electrocardiography (ECG) monitoring is essential.
- BP monitoring is also essential as both hypertension and more commonly hypotension may occur during the procedure. Hypertension may indicate an inadequately sedated patient, inadequate topical analgesia or a rising CO_2.
- Hypotension may be a consequence of sedation, increased inspiratory pressure, high auto-PEEP or even hypoxia, and arrhythmias.
- In ventilated patients, monitoring of a ventilator parameters will usually be in progress. Of these, $EtCO_2$, ventilator inspiratory pressure, FiO_2, and PEEP are the most important parameters that should be monitored specifically during the conduct of bronchoscopy.
- $EtCO_2$ monitoring is useful in order to maximize the safety of the procedure.
- Modest increase in $EtCO_2$ are of little significance in most patients even in the critically ill; however, it may have a significant impact in patients with raised intracranial pressure (e.g. traumatic head injury).
- In these situations, increase in tidal and minute volume during bronchoscopy will minimize surges in end-tidal and arterial CO_2. Additionally, frequent withdrawals of bronchoscope (i.e. "rest periods" during bronchoscopy) usually help to maintain adequate alveolar ventilation and limit rise in $PaCO_2$. Adequate sedation will also help to improve minute ventilation and, therefore, reduce CO_2 increase during the procedure.

References

1. Olopade CO, Prakash UBS. Bronchoscopy in the critical-care unit. Mayo Clinic Proceed. 1989;64:1255–63.
2. Bronchoscopy in ICU. A Practical Guide / Manoj K Goel, Ajay Kumar, Gargi Maitra.
3. Practice Guidelines for Preoperative Fasting and the Use of Pharmacologic Agents to Reduce the Risk of Pulmonary Aspiration: Application to Healthy Patients Undergoing Elective Procedures: An Updated Report by the American Society of Anesthesiologists Task Force on Preoperative Fasting and the Use of Pharmacologic Agents to Reduce the Risk of Pulmonary Aspiration. Anesthesiology 2017;126:376–93.
4. Dobson G, Chow L, Filteau L, *et al*. Guidelines to the Practice of Anesthesia - Revised Edition 2020. Can J Anaesth 2020;67:64–99.
5. Lee JC, Williams GW, Kozar RA, *et al*. Multitargeted Feeding Strategies Improve Nutrition Outcome and Are Associated With Reduced Pneumonia in a Level 1 Trauma Intensive Care Unit. JPEN J Parenter Enteral Nutr 2018;42:529–37.
6. Du Rand IA, Blaikley J, Booton R, *et al*. British Thoracic Society guideline for diagnostic flexible bronchoscopy in adults: accredited by NICE. Thorax. 2013;68(Suppl 1): i1–44.
7. Esquinas A, Zuil M, Scala R, Chiner E. Bronchoscopy during non-invasive mechanical ventilation: a review of techniques and procedures. Archivos de Bronconeumología (English edition). 2013;49(3):105–12.
8. Wahidi MM, Jain P, Jantz M, *et al*. American College of Chest Physicians consensus statement on the use of topical anesthesia, analgesia, and sedation during flexible bronchoscopy in adult patients. Chest. 2011;140(5): 1342–50.
9. José RJ, Shaefi S, Navani N. Sedation for flexible bronchoscopy: current and emerging evidence. Eur Respir Rev. 2013;22(128):106–16.
10. Morgan GE, Mikhail MS, Murray MJ, *et al*. Clinical pharmacology: inhalational anesthetics. In: Morgan GE, Mikhail MS, Murray MJ (Eds). Clinical Anesthesiology: New York, NY: McGraw Hill; 2002. pp. 155–78.
11. Clark G, Licker M, Younossian AB, *et al*. Titrated sedation with propofol or midazolam for flexible bronchoscopy: a randomised trial. Eur Respir J. 2009;34(6):1277–83.
12. Bergese SD, Khabiri B, Roberts WD, *et al*. Dexmedetomidine for conscious sedation in difficult awake fiberoptic intubation cases. J Clin Anesth. 2007;19(2):141–4.
13. Ryu JH, Lee SW, Lee JH, *et al*. Randomized double-blind study of remifentanil and dexmedetomidine for flexible bronchoscopy. Br J. Anaesth. 2012;108(3):503–11.
14. Morris MJ, Kwon HP, Zanders TB. Monitoring, sedation, and anesthesia for flexible fiberoptic bronchoscopy. In: Haranath SP (Ed). Global Perspectives on Bronchoscop. Rijeka: InTech Open Access Publisher; 2012.
15. British Thoracic Society Bronchoscopy Guidelines Committee. British Thoracic Society guidelines on diagnostic flexible bronchoscopy. Thorax. 2001;56(Suppl. 1):i1–21.
16. Kaur H, Dhooria S, Aggarwal AN, *et al*. A randomized trial of 1% vs. 2% lignocaine by the spray-as-you-go technique for topical anesthesia during flexible bronchoscopy. Chest. 2015;148(3):739–45.
17. Jolliet P, Chevrolet JC. Bronchoscopy in the intensive care unit. Intensive Care Med. 1992;18:160–9.
18. Shennib H, Baslaim G. Bronchoscopy in the intensive care unit. Chest Clin North Am. 1996;6:349–61.
19. Lindholm C, Ollmann B, Snyder J, Millen E, Grenvik A. Cardiorespiratory effects of flexible fiberoptic bronchoscopy in critically ill patients. Chest. 1978;74:362–7.

20. Lawson RW, Peters JI, Shelledy DC. Effects of fiberoptic bronchoscopy during mechanical ventilation in a lung model. Chest. 2000;118:824–31
21. Schiffman PL, Westlake RE, Fourre JA, Leonard ET. Arterial oxygen saturation and cardiac rhythm during transoral fiberoptic bronchoscopy. J Med Soc N J. 1982;79: 723–6
22. Brochard L, Mancebo J, Elliott MW. Noninvasive ventilation for acute respiratory failure. Eur Respir J. 2002;19:712–21.
23. Hess DR. The evidence for noninvasive positive-pressure ventilation in the care of patients in acute respiratory failure: a systematic review of the literature. Respir Care. 2004;49:810–29.
24. Katz JA, Marks JD. Inspiratory work with and without continuous positive airway pressure in patients with acute respiratory failure. Anesthesiology. 1985;63:598–07
25. Agarwal R, Khan A, Aggarwal AN, Gupta D. Bronchoscopic lung biopsy using noninvasive ventilatory support: case series and review of literature of NIV-assisted bronchoscopy. Respir Care. 2012;57:1927–36.
26. Antonelli M, Conti G, Riccioni L, Meduri GU. Noninvasive positive-pressure ventilation via face mask during bronchoscopy with BAL in high-risk hypoxemic patients. Chest. 1996;110:724–28.
27. Maitre B, Jaber S, Maggiore SM, Bergot E, Richard JC, Bakthiari H, *et al*. Continuous positive airway pressure during fiberoptic bronchoscopy in hypoxemic patients. A randomized double-blind study using a new device. Am J Respir Crit Care Med. 2000;162:1063–67.
28. Antonelli M, Conti G, Rocco M, Arcangeli A, Cavaliere F, Proietti R, *et al*. Noninvasive positive-pressure ventilation vs. conventional oxygen supplementation in hypoxemic patients undergoing diagnostic bronchoscopy. Chest. 2002;121:1149–54
29. Agarwal R, Khan A, Aggarwal AN, Gupta D. Bronchoscopic lung biopsy using noninvasive ventilatory support: case series and review of literature of NIV-assisted bronchoscopy. Respir Care. 2012;57:1927–36.
30. Murgu SD, Pecson J, Colt HG. Bronchoscopy during noninvasive ventilation: indications and technique. Respir Care. 2010;55:595–600.
31. Esquinas A, Zuil M, Scala R, Chiner E. Bronchoscopy during non-invasive mechanical ventilation: a review of techniques and procedures. Arch Bronconeumol. 2013;49:105–12.
32. Heunks LM, de Bruin CJ, van der Hoeven JG, van der Heijden HF. Non-invasive mechanical ventilation for diagnostic bronchoscopy using a new face mask: an observational feasibility study. Intensive Care Med. 2010;36:143–47.
33. Cracco C, Fartoukh M, Prodanovic H, Azoulay E, Chenivesse C, Lorut C, *et al*. Safety of performing fiberoptic bronchoscopy in critically ill hypoxemic patients with acute respiratory failure. Intensive Care Med. 2013;39:45–52.
34. Du Rand IA, Blaikley J, Booton R, Chaudhuri N, Gupta V, Khalid S, *et al*. BTS Guideline for diagnostic flexible bronchoscopy in adults. Thorax. 2013;68:i1–44

CHAPTER 30

Tracheostomy

❐ Vajrapu Rajendra ❐ Maneendra Singarapu

INTRODUCTION

Tracheostomy is performed in approximately 10–15% of patients who are admitted to intensive care units (ICU). A tracheostomy is defined as creating an artificial airway passage in the anterior neck directly into the trachea, and kept open via a tracheostomy tube.

Indications

Emergency

a. Acute upper airway obstruction in whom endotracheal intubation is not possible(angioedema, anaphylaxis, hematoma, infection, submandibular space infections, retropharyngeal abscess, foreign body, etc.),
b. Laryngeal trauma
c. Difficult airway
d. Facial trauma (LeFort III fracture)
e. Post-cricothyroidotomy

Elective

a. Patients who require prolonged ventilation
b. Patients having weaning difficulty from ventilator support
c. Patients with respiratory and bulbar muscle weakness with a risk of recurrent aspiration
d. Decreased or incompetent clearance of trachea-bronchial secretions
e. Patients with refractory severe obstructive sleep apnea
f. Patients with congenital anomalies of larynx like severe subglottic stenosis
g. Head and neck surgeries or treatments involving airway compromise and postoperative edema
h. Ca larynx

Contraindications

Absolute Contraindications

- Cervical instability
- Uncontrolled coagulopathy

- Infection at planned insertion site
- Operator inexperience.
- End of life issues
- Past history of resection of cervical trachea

Relative Contraindications

- Difficult anatomy due to any tumor, hematoma or any previous neck surgeries (relative contraindications for percutaneous tracheostomy)
- Severe ARDS requiring high PEEP
- Hemodynamic instability
- Coagulopathy
- Close proximity of burns or surgical wounds.

ANATOMIC LANDMARKS

- **Thyroid notch:** It is the superior aspect of the larynx in the midline.
- **Cricothyroid membrane:** A palpable depression between cricoid and thyroid cartilages for an emergent cricothyrotomy.
- **Cricoid cartilage:** It is the junction of the larynx and trachea. The skin incision is typically placed 1–2 cm inferior to the cricoid.
- **Sternal notch:** A palpable landmark to identify the thoracic inlet. It is important to palpate here to the possibility of a high-riding innominate artery that may be encountered during tracheostomy **(Fig. 30.1A and B)**.

Preparation

- Verify patient identity and consent
- Check labs and coagulation parameters
- Open tracheostomy usually done in operation theatre under general anesthesia or concious sedation.
- local anesthetic is infiltration with lidocaine or lidocaine with epinephrine (lidocaine 1% with 1:150,000 parts epinephrine) can be used.
- The selected tracheostomy should be checked for any air leaks, ideally under sterile saline or water
- In situations where aerosolization of respiratory secretions is a concern (open tuberculosis/Covid-19), appropriate specialized personal protective equipment is necessary for the team, and the procedure should be performed in a negative-pressure room.
- Extra length tracheostomy tubes for obese patients are required.

Personnel

- For open tracheostomy
  - Surgeon and assistant
  - Anesthesiologist
  - Nurse
  - Scrub assistant

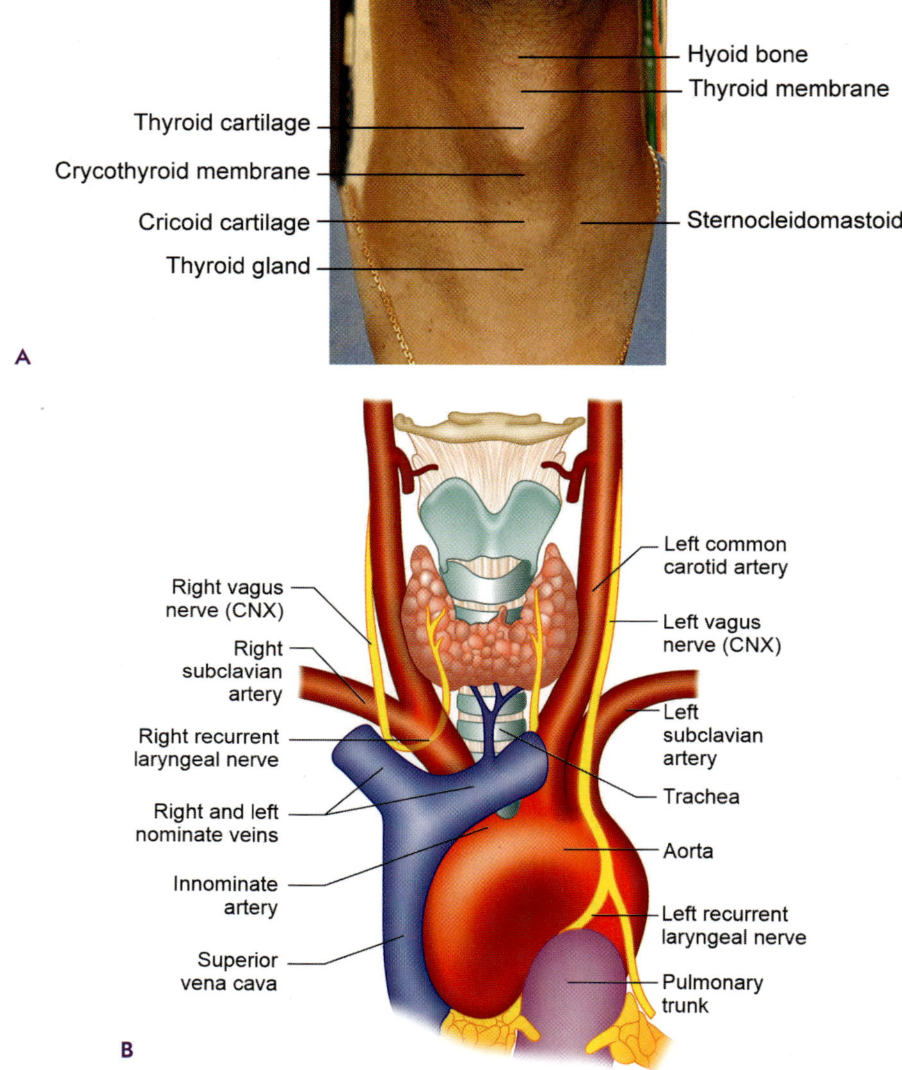

Fig. 30.1A and B: Anatomy of neck

- For percutaneous tracheostomy at bedside
  - Intensivist
  - Airway assistant
  - Bronchoscopist

Equipment

Resuscitation equipment, suction and suction catheters, mechanical ventilator

- **For open tracheostomy**
  - OT equipment (OT table, anesthesia machine, etc.)

- Tracheostomy set with different sizes of tracheostomy tubes
- Cautery

- **For percutaneous tracheostomy at bedside**
  - Tracheostomy set with different sizes of tracheostomy tubes
  - Fibreoptic bronchoscope
  - Ultrasound machine
- **Drugs**
  - Anesthesia drugs like sedatives, paralysing agents, inhalation anesthetics, resuscitation drugs like atropine, adrenaline, etc.
  - Local anesthetics
- **Monitoring**
  - ECG
  - $ETCO_2$
  - SpO_2
  - NIBP
  - Respiratory rate
  - FiO_2
  - Airway pressure
  - Expired tidal volume and minute ventilation
- **Position**
  - After anesthesia or conscious sedation and If no neck instability neck extension with a pillow below the shoulder and head supported by ring to open up the anterior neck surface anatomy clearly (**Fig. 30.2**).

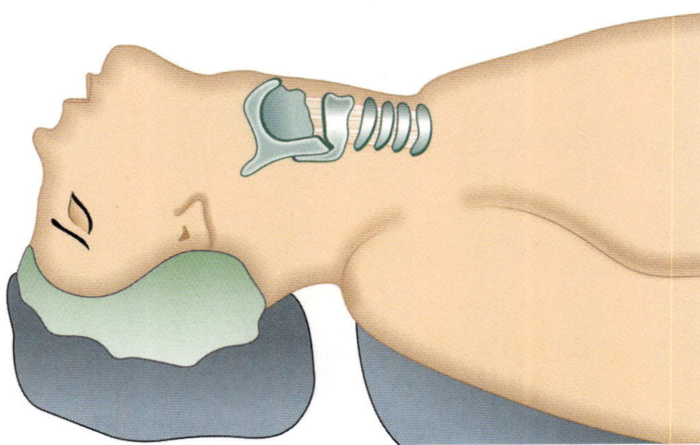

Fig. 30.2: Positioning for tracheostomy

Procedure

- After local sterile preparation and draping
- Palpate the neck to identify thyroid cartilage, cricoid cartilage, and the sternal notch. The ideal location for placement of the tracheostomy tube is between the second and third tracheal rings. Palpate the neck to identify the pulse of a high-riding innominate artery, open tracheostomy is preferred in patients with a high-riding innominate artery.

- **Open tracheostomy**

  A skin incision is then marked in the midline anterior neck 1 to 2 cm inferior to the carotid cartilage. A horizontal or vertical incision may be utilized.

  The incision is extended through the platysma muscle to expose the strap muscles (sternohyoid and sternothyroid), identify the median raphe. The strap muscles are then retracted laterally, exposing the cricoid cartilage and thyroid gland. The thyroid isthmus is identified and ligated, if necessary. Hemostats can be utilized to cross-clamp the isthmus, and oversewing each stump with a silk suture to ensure hemostasis. A cricoid hook is then placed under the cricoid cartilage to elevate the larynx and trachea into the operative field.
- The second and third tracheal rings are identified.
- Stay ligatures may be placed laterally to facilitate traction on the trachea for tube placement, as well as tube security in the postoperative period. An incision is made between the second and third rings, and tracheostomy tube placed.

The first ring is avoided to decrease the risk of subsequent stenosis. With the tube in place, it is connected to the anesthesia circuit, and end-tidal CO_2 confirmed. Only then is the cricoid hook released. The tracheostomy tube is secured with a soft trans-cervical tie as well as sutured to the anterior neck skin.

PERCUTANEOUS DILATATIONAL TRACHEOSTOMY(PDT)

Special Considerations

Bronchoscopic guidance can make PDT more safer procedure as it can visualize needle entry point and prevent posterior wall rupture. Low incidence of pneumothorax, pneumomediastinum or paratracheal placement.

Ultrasound guidance: By using linear array high frequency probe the neck can be examined prior to reveal any aberrant blood vessels in the path of the needle. In obese real time guidance can be used (**Fig. 30.3**).

The basic principle is trachea is punctured using a hollow needle, guidewire is advanced into the airway and then over the guidewire dilatation and eventually tracheostomy tube placement is performed.

Two common techniques used for PDT are:

1. **Ciaglia blue rhino single dilator technique:** When initially introduced by ciaglia in 1985, multiple separate dilators were used which was consolidated into a single dilator technique which simplified insertion process and time.

   Once the entry site is identified by palpation, a small incision is made and after minimal dissection, needle is inserted into the trachea and dilatation made using a punch tapered dilator followed by tube insertion and securing.
2. **Griggs technique:** It uses a forceps called griggs forceps which has grooves to slide over the wire. Using griggs forceps trachea is identified and guidewire insertion done and trachea is dilated and a tracheostomy tube placed.

Steps

1. Prior preparation and positioning and plan discussion with team members.
2. Keeping the patient on 100% FiO_2 and appropriate ventilator settings.

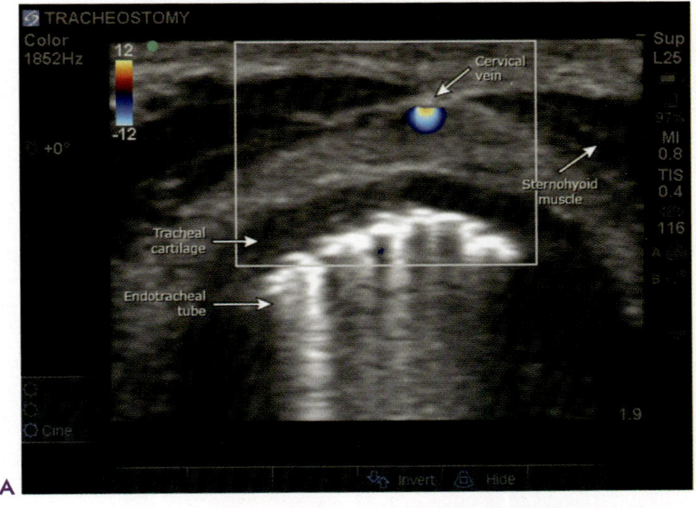

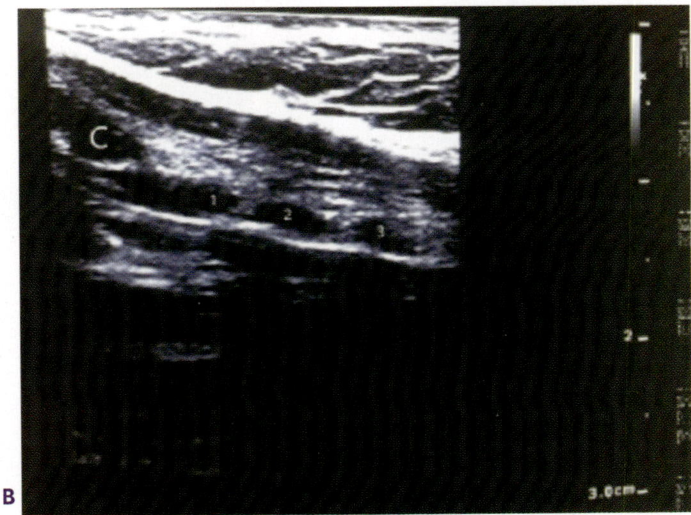

Fig. 30.3A and B: Ultrasound images transverse and longitudinal views

3. Ensure adequate sedation, analgesia and muscle paralysis and positioning
4. Deflate the ET cuff and withdraw the ET tube under laryngoscopic vision until cuff is visualized at just below the vocal cords and then reinflate the cuff.
5. Clean and drape the patient as per sterile protocols.
6. Identify the site of insertion.
7. Inflitrate the skin using local anaesthesia containing vasoconstrictor.
8. Making a 2–2.5 cm tranverse incision at proper and planned site.
9. Blunt dissection of subcutaneous fat and pretracheal tissue with mosquito forceps.
10. Advance a 14 gauge sheathed introducer needle into the trachea with non-dominant hand stabilizing the trachea.
11. Tracheal placement confirmed by aspiration-air bubbles into the saline filled syringe and if available visualization through the bronchoscope.

12. Withdraw the needle and insert the seldinger guidewire through the plastic sheath.
13. Dilate the insertion site using a dilator or griggs forceps.
14. After adequate dilation, dilator removed and tracheostomy tube inserted over the guide wire.
15. Placement of tracheostomy tube Is confirmed by $EtCO_2$ graph, 5-point auscultation and if available bronchoscope.
16. ET tube deflated and removed after thorough suctioning.
17. Tracheostomy tube is then sutured and fixed in place with the help of tie provided with kit.
18. Chest X-ray is done to rule out any pneumothorax or pneumomediastinum.

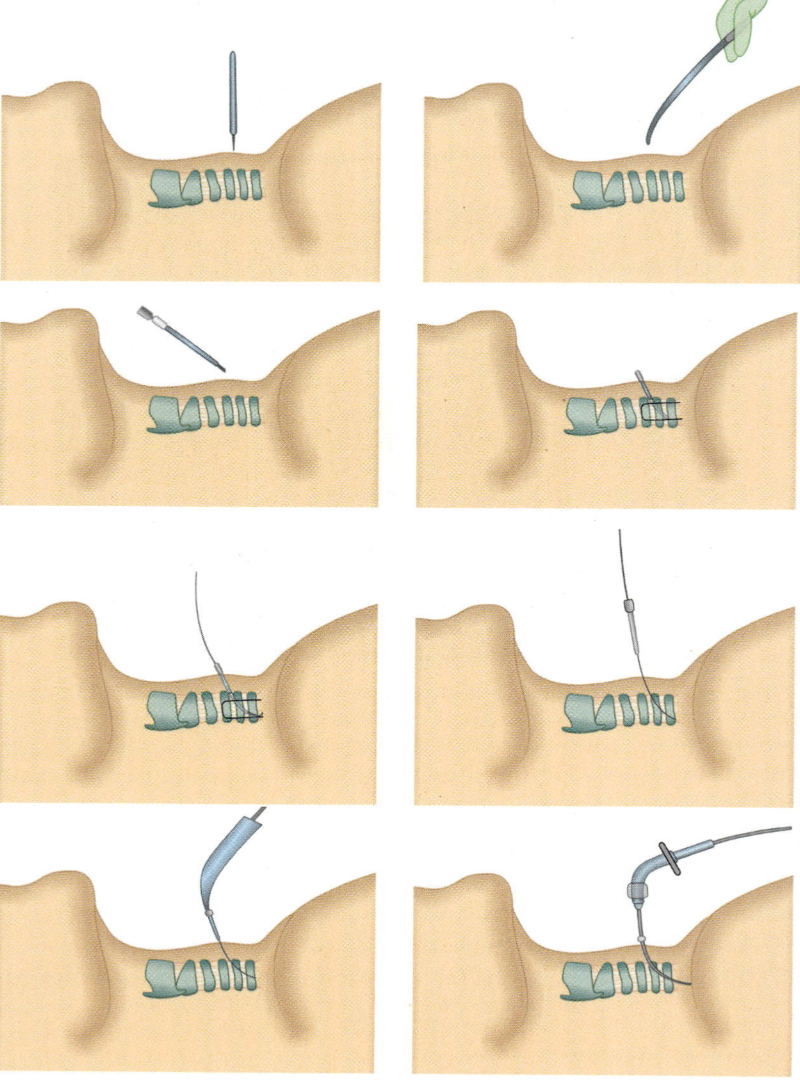

Fig. 30.4: Steps of tracheostomy

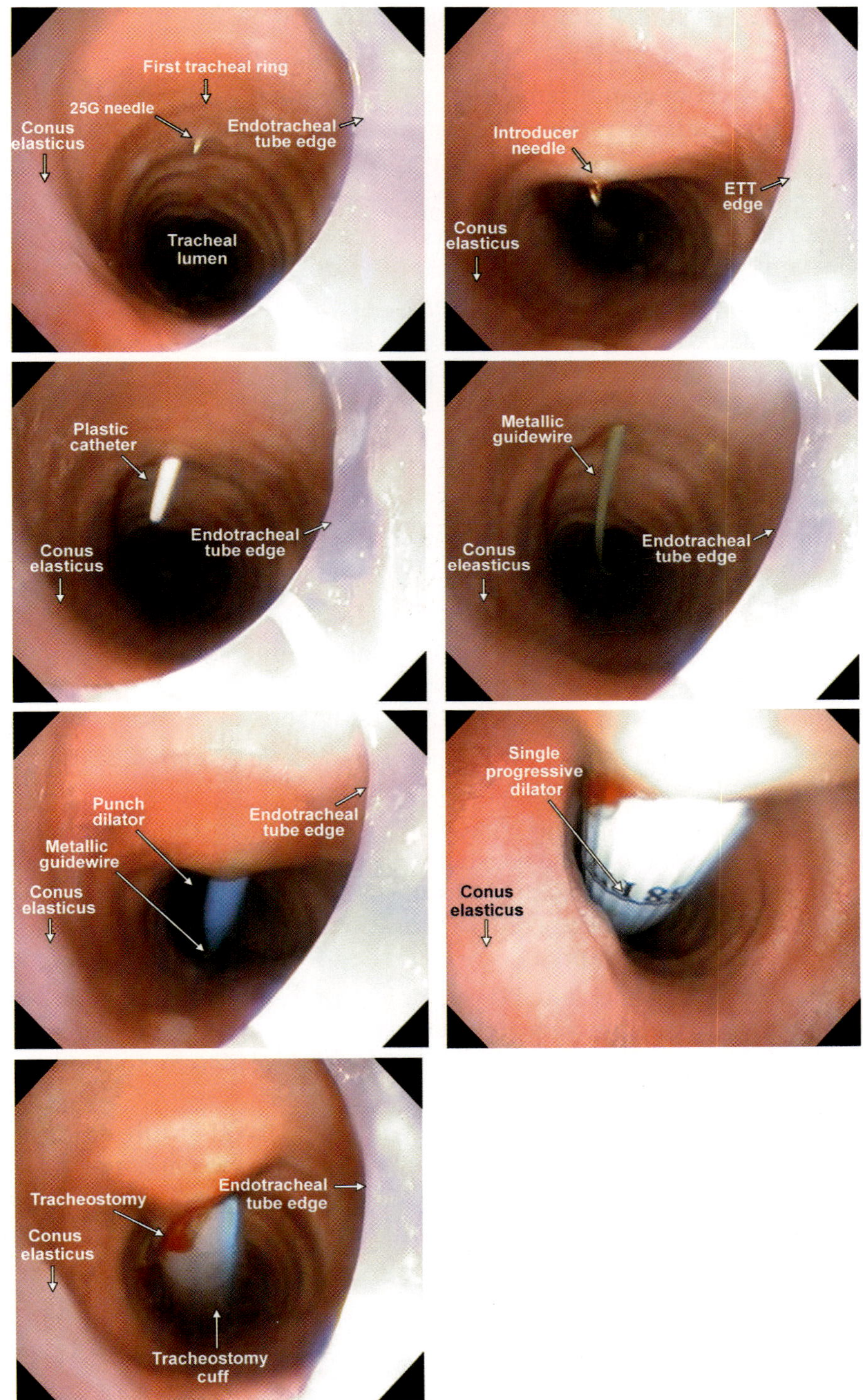

Fig. 30.5: Bronchoscopic views

SURGICAL VERSUS PERCUTANEOUS TRACHEOSTOMY

Both surgical tracheostomy(ST) and PDTs can be performed safely in critically ill patients with a low incidence of complications. A meta-analysis of 22 studies (1,608 patients) demonstrated no significant difference in rates of mortality, intraoperative hemorrhage, and postoperative bleeding between the two procedures.

Another meta-analysis that included 1,795 procedures found no significant difference in the risk of a potentially life-threatening event. There was also no significant difference in complications of false passage or subglottic stenosis in another large meta-analysis.

In addition to comparable safety, PDT offers several benefits compared to ST. PDT has been shown to have a lower rate of wound infection and stoma infection, shorter procedural time and decreased costs. One prospective observational study identified significantly lower rates of tracheal tube obstruction(1.0% vs. 3.6%, P=0.007) and displacement (1.3% vs. 4.8%, P=0.002)with PDT compared to ST. There is also a lower rate of unfavorable scarring with PDT.

COMPLICATIONS

Intraoperative

- Bleeding is the most common complication due to injury to anterior juglar veins or thyroid ima artery or thyroid isthmus, usually self-limited or can be controlled with the use of measures such as the application of pressure or the use of hemostatic agents, if not controlled needs surgical exploration and ligation of the bleeding vessels.
- The purse-string suture usually done just prior to tracheostomy tube insertion may help to control bleeding from the skin.
- In open tracheostomy airway fire may occur due to the presence of high concentrations of oxygen in the anesthetic tubing and an ignition source provided by the electrocautery unit, If a fire occurs, the entire circuit should be removed from the patient, and the patient bagged with a mask until the tracheostomy is placed. The aerodigestive tract should then be evaluated for any potential thermal injury
- Difficulties commonly encountered during the procedure may be due to the skin incision being too small, inadequate neck extension, suboptimal dilation, incorrect selected tracheostomy tube size, or lack of enough lubrication for tracheostomy tube placement.
- It is important that ventilation is not performed through the ETT with the tracheostomy cuff inflated to minimize the risk of developing pneumomediastinum.
- Avoid kinking of guidewire, guidewire movements should always be smooth and easy.

Early Postoperative Period

- Acute obstruction of the tracheostomy tube may be caused by blood or mucus.
- Postoperative protocols involving scheduled flexible tracheal suctioning, use of humidified oxygen, and scheduled replacement or cleaning of the inner cannula (daily) can minimize the risk of complete obstruction.

Inadvertent Decannulation and Obstruction of the Tracheostomy

- Rare, but can be managed by securing the airway through oral endotracheal intubation.
- Insertion of a new tracheostomy tube through a tract that has not fully matured should not be attempted. Reintubation can be required to re-establish a definitive airway and is best performed via flexible laryngoscopy through the tracheostomy tube to visually confirm an intralumenal placement.
- Obstruction may be distal tip of the tracheostomy tube exits the tracheal lumen and rests in the soft tissue or a false-passage.

Pneumothorax/Pneumomediastinum

- An X-ray chest should be obtained and a chest tube placed if indicated
- Remove the tracheostomy tube if confirmed to be in a false track and secure the airway with endotracheal intubation

Tracheoinnominate Fistula

- Tracheoinnominate fistula is a very rare but potentially devastating complication, occurring in less than 1% of tracheostomies but with an estimated mortality of 80%. The event may be preceded by a sentinel bleed, a pulsatile bleed from the stoma, which stops spontaneously. The bleed may then recur several days later with subsequent exsanguinating hemorrhage. Several risk factors have been identified, which include placement of the tracheostomy below the third tracheal ring, the presence of a more cephalad (high-riding) innominate artery, and placement of an improperly sized tube (either too large in diameter or of an improper length) which places excessive pressure on the anterior tracheal wall behind the sternum. The treatment is surgical or endovascular stenting as well as embolization.

Late Complications

- Pressure necrosis due to over-inflation of the cuff of the tracheostomy tube. These are rarer than in the past due to advancements in low-pressure cuffs and the awareness of cuff pressure as a risk factor. Tracheostomy cuff pressure should be measured regularly to prevent this occurrence, ideally at a maximum of 20 cm H_2O. High pressure in the trachea can lead to necrosis of the wall due to ischemia. Subsequent healing results in scarring and stenosis. Stenosis can be treated in several ways, both endoscopic and open.
- Tracheoesophageal fistula
- Tracheal stenosis
- Persistent tracheocutaneous fistula
- Laryngotracheal malacia

TRACHEOSTOMY CARE

- *Heat moisture exchanger (HME):* For example, thermal humidifying filters, Swedish nose, artificial nose, filter, thermovent T.
- Suction and wound care protocols

- Monitoring oxygenation and ventilation adequacies
- Nutrition and psychological assistance

EARLY VS LATE TRACHEOSTOMY

Early tracheotomy is defined as intervention no more than 7 days after initiation of mechanical ventilation. In a meta-analysis (3145 individuals), early tracheotomy improved VAP, ventilator, and ICU days, but not short-term all-cause mortality.

Another meta-analysis suggests that early tracheostomy in traumatic brain injury **(TBI)** patients could help in reducing duration of mechanical ventilation, ICU and hospital length of stay, contribute to a lower exposure to secondary injuries and nosocomial adverse events, increasing the opportunity of patients' early rehabilitation and discharge.

DECANNULATION

Decannulation to be considered in patients once respiratory mechanics are adequate, mechanical ventilation is no longer needed, oxygen requirement reduced, upper airway obstruction is resolved, airway secretions are controlled, and swallowing has been evaluated. Presence of an intact sensorium coordinated swallowing and protective coughing are often the minimum requirements for a successful decannulation.

Decannulation failure is the need to reinsert an artificial airway within 48 to 96 hours of planned tracheostomy removal and acceptable a 2 to 5% failure rate.

Endoscopic assessment is essential particularly in tracheostomized patients who have failed to achieve decannulation through conventional protocols.

Johns Hopkins Criteria for Decannulation

1. Patient should not be dependent on a ventilator.
2. Patient's mental status should be to the level of alert and responsive and should be able to manage their oral secretions without a risk of aspiration.

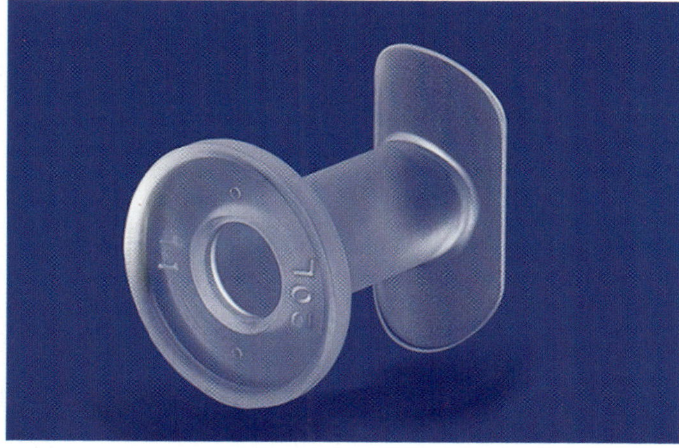

Fig. 30.6: Tracheostomy retainer

3. Should not require frequent suctioning for tracheal secretions.
4. Patient should be able to cough and clean his/her tracheal secretions.
5. The patient should have their tracheostomy tube downsized to a size 4 Shiley or similar tracheostomy tube and they should not have breathing difficulty in the presence of this tube.
6. The size 4 Shiley or similar tube should be occluded (with a trach plug/cork) for twelve hours during the day with close monitoring by the nursing staff with no evidence of respiratory difficulty or requiring of suctioning of the trach tube.
7. Once the patient is seen to tolerate the steps in item # 6 above, their trach is plugged for 24 hours and they are monitored for respiratory difficulty or suction requirement.

References

1. Szmuk P, Ezri T, Evon S, Roth.u, Katz J. A brief history of tracheostomy and tracheal intubation. Intensive care med 008:34:222–8
2. Ciaglia P, Firschring R, Syniec C. Elective percutaneous dilatational tracheostomy—a new and simple bedside procedure. Chest 1985;87:715–9.
3. Raimondi N, Vidal MR, Calleja J, Quintero A, Cortes A, Celis E, *et al*-Evidence based guidelines for use of tracheostomy in critically ill.
4. Huang CS, Chen PT, Cheng SH, Chen CK, Hsu PK, *et al*. relative contraindications for percutaneous tracheostomy.
5. Delaney A, Bagshaw Sm, Nalos M. PCDT vs ST in critically ill patients a systematic review and metaanalysis. Critcare 2006;10:R55.
6. Al Ansari M, Hijazi MH. Clinical review:Percutaneous dilatational tracheostomy. Crit care 2006;10:202.
7. Griggs WM, worthley LI, Gilligan JE, Thomas PD. A simple percutaneous technique. Surg Gynecol obstet. 1990;170:543–5.
8. Fantoni A, Ripamonti D. A non derivative non surgical tracheostomy:The translaryngeal method. Intensive care med. 1997;23:386–92
9. JAMA Otolaryngol Head Neck Surg. 2021;147(5):450–59.
10. J. Clin. Med. 2021, 10(15), 3319.
11. Stelfox, H.T., Crimi, C., Berra, L. *et al*. Determinants of tracheostomy decannulation: an international survey. Crit Care 12, R26 (2008).
12. Swain SK, *et al*. Int J Otorhinolaryngol Head Neck Surg. 2021 Jun;7(6):1083–88.
13. Whitmore KA, *et al*. BMJ Open Resp Res 2020;7:e000651.
14. J Thorac Dis, 2021;13(8):5251–60.
15. J Thorac Dis, 2017;9(Suppl 10):S1128–S1138
16. J Thorac Dis, 2021;13(8):5261–76.
17. Trouillet, *et al*. Ann. Intensive Care (2018) 8:37.
18. Tanaka, *et al*. Journal of Intensive Care (2022) 10:19.

CHAPTER 31

Setting up an ICU

❐ Pavan Gorukanti ❐ Sricharan G

Intensive care unit (ICU) is the critical heart of the hospital, catering to the sickest and most vulnerable patients. This confined area provides special expertise and the facilities for various organ supports, noninvasive, invasive monitoring and uses the skills of specially qualified and trained medical, nursing and other personnel for the management of these sick patients.[1]

Since humble beginnings in 1950s, intensive care units have evolved over time significantly, embracing the latest technology, multidisciplinary care, diagnostic and management strategies to cater to ever more complex and sicker patient cohorts. And over the years, intensive care management has become more standardized with established protocols and guidelines to help with everything from setting up ICUs, staffing, daily functioning, treatment and management strategies and holistic care of the patient, through national and international societies and consensus guidelines.[2–4]

In emerging countries like India and the developing world where healthcare delivery is through diverse players like Government, Private, Public-Private or a combination, in varied setups ranging from smaller lower-acuity setups in remote places to the most complex tertiary hospitals in major cities and financial burden being borne by Government, Corporates, Private insurance, Out-of-pocket or a combination, ICU care delivery necessarily needs to be customized and tailored taking all the above into account while trying to ensure the minimum acceptable care and trying to match the best evidence based practices as far as possible.

Infrastructure of an ICU

ISCCM consensus on ICU planning and design classifies ICU into Level I, II, IIIA and IIIB based on increasing level of support system. It recommends Level I for 50–100 bedded hospitals, Level II for 100–150 bedded hospitals and Level IIIA, Level IIIB to >150 bedded hospitals.[2,5]

Intensive care unit area can be divided into four zones namely:

- **Patient care zone:** This includes the area around patients bed
- **Observation area:** This includes the central nursing station and other equipment required for nursing support like drug trolleys, crash cart, etc.
- **Support area:** This includes doctors' offices, duty rooms, toilets, stores, etc.
- **Family support area:** This includes waiting area, counselling rooms, etc.

Patient Care Zone

The spectrum of ICUs in India varies from Dormitory like ICU with beds separated with clean colored curtains, to that of ICUs with separate cubicles for each bed. Even though ICUs with individual isolation cubicles for each bed may be ideal, it may not be cost effective enough to warrant its execution in all ICUs.

- The recommended patient care zone area should be 150 – 200 square feet with ISCCM recommending an area of 150 square feet for Indian ICUs.
- It is recommended that at least one or two of the ICU beds be isolation cubicles with transparent wall to facilitate the monitoring of the patient.
- These isolation rooms are for immunocompromised or infected patients.
- In case of isolation rooms with positive or negative pressure isolation, the recommended area is 200–250 square feet.[6]
- International societies like ESICM and ANZICS recommend an ante chamber of at least 30 square feet for each isolation room with a wash basin and racks for gowns before entering the isolation area.[3,4]
- Positive pressure isolation: These are for patients who are immunocompromised like neutropenic or post-transplant patients with positive pressures ranging between 2.5 Kpa and 8 Kpa.
- Negative pressure isolation: These are for patients harboring infections which are transmissible by droplets (<5 microns) with pressure differential of 2.5 Kpa between corridor and cabin.[2]
- For solid organ and hematopoietic stem cell transplanted patients, HEPA filtration is required
- All the ICU beds should be equipped with oxygen, air and suction ports preferably via a central system. According to ISCCM guidelines, each tertiary (Level III) ICU bed should have at least 3 oxygen, 2 air and 2 suction outlets
- Each ICU bed should be equipped with at least 6 fifteen ampere sockets and 20 five ampere sockets as per AIA guidelines.[7] It is preferable that all the electrical sockets have uninterrupted power supply (UPS), if not at least half of them should have UPS
- The power sockets ideally should be distributed on either side of the bed to facilitate minimal interference in nursing care. The head end should be free from the wall to facilitate procedures such as endotracheal intubation and central venous catheterization. This can be facilitated by a stalactite structure coming down from the roof which has all the electrical outlets and central gas outlets. But this is expensive.[3]
- Ideally each patient isolation cubicle should have a communication system like an audible alarm, buzzer, etc. needed for patient's communication (**Figs 31.1 to 31.3**).[2]

Environmental Requirements

Heating Ventilation and Air Conditioning (HVAC)[2,7]

All ICUs should be fully air conditioned and ventilated with temperature regulation. Air should always flow from clean to dirty areas. The number of air exchanges recommended is as follows:

- 6 air exchanges per hour per room with 2 exchanges comprising of outside air
- Cubicles should have 15 air exchanges per hour

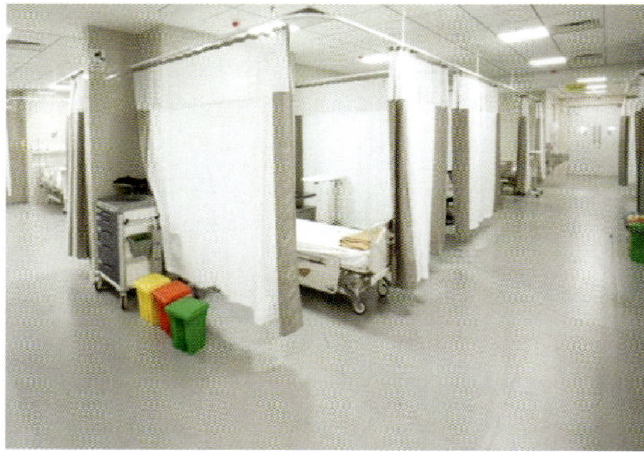

Fig. 31.1: Dormitory style ICU

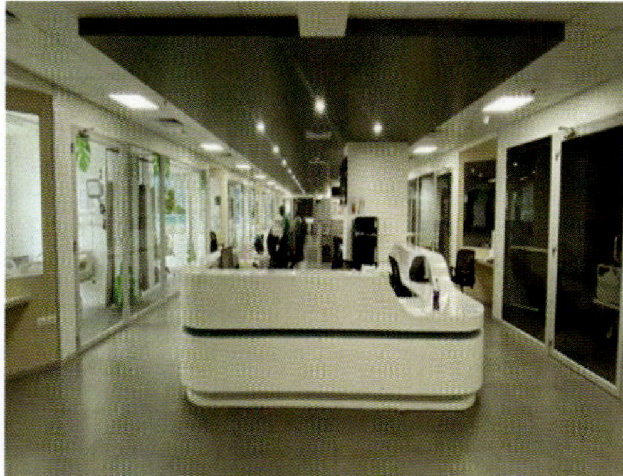

Fig. 31.2: Central nursing station

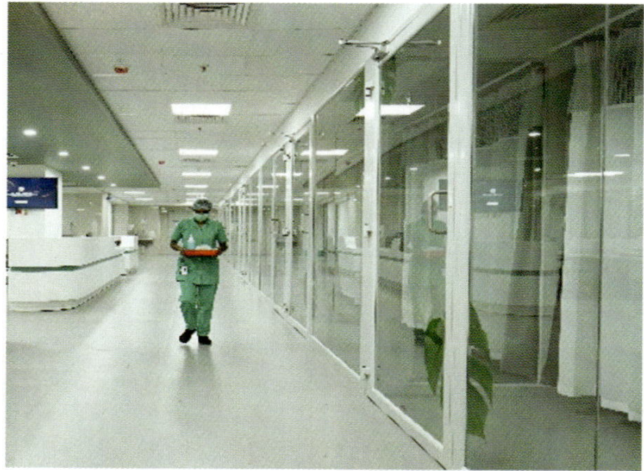

Fig. 31.3: Cubicle isolation style ICU

- Dirty utility, laboratory should have 5 air exchanges per hour
- Other staff areas need 2 air exchanges per hour

Lighting[2,8]

It is recommended to have access to outside natural light as much as possible.[2,3] Artificial lighting is also used as needed.

- For procedures like inserting central venous catheters, spotlighting with 150 foot-candles of brightness is recommended
- For general patient care, overhead lighting with at least 20 foot-candles of brightness is recommended

Noise control[2,9]

- The recommendation by International noise Council is to restrict noises to 45 dBA in day time, 40 dBA in evening and 20 dBA at night

Similarly ISCCM suggests guidelines on, Observation areas, Support areas, Laboratory and Family support areas.[2]

Manpower

Medical, nursing and allied manpower would vary quite a bit based on acuity of care, and in smaller vs tertiary set ups with various national and international guidelines for recommendations.[2–4]

The various healthcare and allied healthcare personnel involved in the smooth running of a tertiary level ICU include:[2,3]

Medical Staff

Table 31.1	
Director/HOD	✦ Responsible for clinical decision making and administrating the various human resources ✦ Also a part of Infection prevention and Control Committee, CPR Committee, Quality control and oversees the correct execution of various standard operating procedures with the help of other members of the said committees
Consultant intensivists	✦ 1 intensivist per ICU of 12–15 beds ✦ Responsible for formulating and implementing plan of care in association with the primary or attending physicians where applicable ✦ As per hospital policy, consultant intensivist may be available round the clock for ICU services
Medical trainees	✦ Trainees from various specialties who want to undergo intensive care training shall be working full time in the ICU under the guidance of consultant intensivist

Nursing Staff

Table 31.2	
ICU head nurse	✦ Makes sure that the hospital protocols were followed stringently and also review the periodic quality control and infection related audits ✦ Makes plans with the intensivist on nursing education and improving nursing care protocol compliance ✦ Should not be involved in individual patient nursing care
Staff nurse	✦ Intensive care nurses undergo formal training from hospital, state/national critical care nursing body and has to go through rigorous training and assessments for competence in intensive care nursing ✦ The ideal nurse to patient ratio for a critically ill/mechanically ventilated/ MODS patient should be 1:1.For less sick patients the nurse to patient ratio can be more liberal ✦ ISCCM recommends nurse to patient ratio not less than 2:3 in a level III critical care unit[2]
Nurse trainees	✦ Nurses under training shall perform any bedside care only under supervision of qualified nurses

Allied Health Care Personnel[2,3]

Table 31.3

Type	Role	Number
Respiratory therapist	✦ Assist management of patients on respiratory support, etc.	1/ICU
Physiotherapist	✦ Chest and limb physiotherapy ✦ Mobilization, ambulation, rehabilitation, etc.	1–2/ICU
Other technicians	✦ Phlebotomist ✦ Dialysis technician ✦ Perfusionists for ECMO	On call to ICU, available 24×7 in hospital
Pharmacist	✦ Oversee prescription orders ✦ Document and report ADR ✦ Discuss with intensivist on possible interactions	1/ICU in normal working hours
Biomedical engineer	✦ Troubleshoot biomedical equipment ✦ Discuss and demonstrate new equipment	1/ICU on call
Nutritionist	✦ Optimize feeding and nutrition of critically ill patients ✦ Formulate diet plan along with intensivist	1/ICU in working hours
Housekeeping staff	✦ Observes and adheres to protocols for infection control and disinfection of surfaces and equipment ✦ Cater to sanitary needs of critically ill patients	As many as needed
Security guards	✦ Control and protect from emotionally charged patient related crowd ✦ Maintains visitor discipline	As many as needed
Medical social worker	✦ Helps patient kith and kin by counselling	On call

Operating Procedures

A typical intensivist's day workflow is as below:

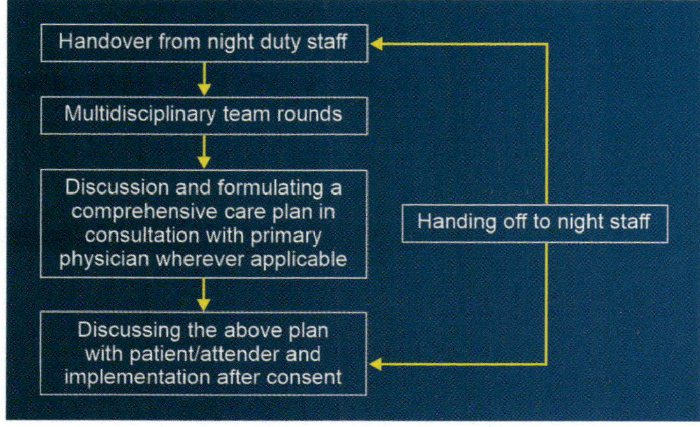

Fig. 31.4

There are protocols and bundles based on national/international/hospital guidelines in place to ensure the safe and comprehensive treatment of the patient like:

- ICU admission and discharge criteria
- Infection prevention and control:
  - Notification of hospital acquired infections
  - Formulating infection control practices and ensuring adherence
  - VAP/CAUTI/CLABSI bundles
  - Infection control audits
  - Formulating hospital antibiogram
  - Antimicrobial stewardship, etc.
- Quality control and assessment
  - Monitor hospital/critical care societies recommended standard quality parameters with internal and external audits
- Patient care bundles for sepsis, glucose management, CHF, acute stroke, pre, post-transplant care bundles, etc. depending on hospital policy to assist compliance. The reason for treatment plans at variance with established protocols, if any, should also be documented in those bundles
- Patient and family feedback questionnaires

Importance of Patient Communication in ICU

Adequate patient and/or family communication is the cornerstone of good intensive care facility to increase patient/family satisfaction and decrease chances of physical/verbal confrontations and medico-legal litigation.[10]

Daily and as required transparent communication of the condition, progress, prognosis and other patient queries in patients own/understandable language (using translator services where applicable) and confirming with the patient's/family that they clearly understand the condition and plan of care and they are not confused/intimidated by medical terminologies.[10] It is always best practice to explain and take informed consents in patient's native language.

Financial Aspects in Intensive Care

With increasing complexity and latest medical advances including but not limited to prolonged mechanical ventilation, ECMO, CRRT and latest life-saving medication, etc. could be a major financial burden in most countries but particularly so in a country like India where a significant proportion of population has to pay, out-of-pocket for their healthcare expenses in a private hospital setup with the chance of financial bankruptcy.

Hence it is extremely important to keep the patient/family updated about the financial implications of all treatment decisions regularly and obtain their consent while explaining the alternative options at every stage.

End of Life and Palliative Care

Many patients in the ICU may have, multiple comorbidities, advanced age, compromised quality of life with poor functional status and continued aggressive intensive care may be, against the wishes of patient, strain on resources of the ICU and financial burden for the patient/family and hence the importance of discussion about goals of care including options for a more palliative care approach if so desired, for such patients but always with full informed consent with patient/family. Palliative care specialists, social workers, spiritual and religious services, NGOs, government agencies, hospital ethics committees may also greatly assist with this complex end of life care decision making and management.[11]

CLOSED VS OPEN ICUs[12]

- **Closed ICU:** In which the intensivist is responsible for all aspects in patient care including admission, discharge and in ICU management
- **Open ICU:** In which the "primary clinician" is responsible for patient care in co-ordination with intensivist

There are a number of studies comparing the outcomes of closed and open ICUs

Li, *et al*. analysed the outcomes of patients before and after intensivists are assigned for complete patient care which showed significantly lower mortality after intensivist assignment.[13] Multiple retrospective analyses showed similar results.[14–16]

However, some other studies like that by Chowdhury, *et al*. concluded that hybrid ICU models with well written and executed protocols, adequate nurse to patient ratio and round the clock availability of intensivist shall reduce mortality in cost effective manner.[17]

eICU

Electronic Intensive Care Unit or eICU is a form of telemedicine where state-of-the-art monitoring technologies are employed and the patients are taken care of by remotely located intensivists. This form of telemedicine has proved fruitful by various studies:

Rosenfeld, *et al*. conducted a prospective observational study before and after introducing telemedicine critical care services which showed decrease in mortality.[18]

A meta-analysis conducted by Young, *et al*. concluded that telemedicine coverage by intensivist resulted in decrease in ICU mortality but not in hospital mortality and also decrease in ICU LOS but not hospital LOS.[19]

In a single center study by Lilly, *et al*. use of eICU was associated with decreased adjusted odds of mortality, hospital LOS, and lower rates of preventable complications.[20]

Suggestions for Smooth Running of a Modern ICU

- Constant monitoring of adequacy of physical infrastructure, technology as per the latest guidelines and updating/redesigning wherever required
- Manpower staffing planning for routine functioning and during surges, nights, weekends, holidays, etc.
- Multidisciplinary role clarity, communication and coordination
- Internal and external audit of quality parameters to maintain highest standards
- Transparent communication on all aspects of patient care, including financial implications, alternatives, patient support and robust patient redressal services
- Discharge planning, end of life, palliative care wherever applicable early in the course of admission

References

1. https://www.ics.ac.uk/ICU/Guidance/PDFs/Archive-Core_Standards_for_ICU#:~:text=An Intensive Care Unit (ICU,of patients with lifethreatening conditions.
2. Rao B, Mittal K, Khilnani G, *et al*. Indian Society of Critical Care Medicine Experts Committee Consensus Statement on ICU Planning and Designing, 2020. Indian J Crit Care Med. 2020;24(S1):S43-S60. doi:10.5005/jp-journals-10071-G23185.
3. Valentin A, Ferdinande P. Recommendations on basic requirements for intensive care units: structural and organizational aspects. Intensive Care Med. 2011;37(10):1575. doi:10.1007/s00134-011-2300-7.
4. ANZICS guidelines. https://cicm.org.au/CICM_Media/CICMSite/CICM-Website/Resources/Professional Documents/IC-1-Minimum-Standards-for-Intensive-Care-Units_1.pdf
5. ICS guidelines. https://www.cc3n.org.uk/uploads/9/8/4/2/98425184/2021-03__levels_of_care_second_edition.pdf.
6. Chaudhury H, Mahmood A, Valente M. Advantages and Disadvantages of Single-Versus Multiple-Occupancy Rooms in Acute Care Environments. Environ Behav. 2005;37(6):760-786. doi:10.1177/0013916504272658.
7. AIA guidelines. https://fgiguidelines.org/wp-content/uploads/2015/08/2001guidelines.pdf
8. Kaufman JE, Haynes H, others. IES Lighting Handbook; Reference Volume and Application Volume.; 1981.
9. Balogh D, Kittinger E, Benzer A, Hackl JM. Noise in the ICU. Intensive Care Med. 1993;19(6):343-346. doi:10.1007/BF01694709.
10. Hall DE, Prochazka A V, Fink AS. Informed consent for clinical treatment. CMAJ. 2012;184(5):533-540. doi:10.1503/cmaj.112120.
11. Patel F, Sharma S, Khosla D. Palliative care in India: Current progress and future needs. Indian J Palliat Care. 2012;18(3):149. doi:10.4103/0973-1075.105683.
12. Gutsche JT, Kohl BA. Who should care for intensive care unit patients? Crit Care Med. 2007;35(Suppl):S18-S23. doi:10.1097/01.CCM.0000252907.47050.FE.
13. Li TC, Phillips MC, Shaw L, Cook EF, Natanson C, Goldman L. On-site physician staffing in a community hospital intensive care unit. Impact on test and procedure use and on patient outcome. JAMA. 1984;252(15):2023-2027. http://www.ncbi.nlm.nih.gov/pubmed/6481908
14. Reynolds HN, Haupt MT, Thill-Baharozian MC, Carlson RW. Impact of critical care physician staffing on patients with septic shock in a university hospital medical intensive care unit. JAMA. 1988;260(23):3446-3450. http://www.ncbi.nlm.nih.gov/pubmed/3210284.
15. Brown JJ, Sullivan G. Effect on ICU Mortality of a Full-time Critical Care Specialist. Chest. 1989;96(1):127-129. doi:10.1378/chest.96.1.127.
16. Pronovost PJ, Angus DC, Dorman T, Robinson KA, Dremsizov TT, Young TL. Physician Staffing Patterns and Clinical Outcomes in Critically Ill Patients. JAMA. 2002;288(17):2151. doi:10.1001/jama.288.17.2151.
17. Chowdhury D, Duggal AK. Intensive care unit models: Do you want them to be open or closed? A critical review. Neurol India. 65(1):39–45. doi:10.4103/0028-3886.198205.
18. Rosenfeld BA, Dorman T, Breslow MJ, *et al*. Intensive care unit telemedicine: Alternate paradigm for providing continuous intensivist care. Crit Care Med. 2000;28(12):3925-3931. doi:10.1097/00003246-200012000-00034.
19. Young LB, Chan PS, Lu X, Nallamothu BK, Sasson C, Cram PM. Impact of Telemedicine Intensive Care Unit Coverage on Patient Outcomes. Arch Intern Med. 2011;171(6). doi:10.1001/archinternmed.2011.61.
20. Lilly CM. Hospital Mortality, Length of Stay, and Preventable Complications Among Critically Ill Patients Before and After Tele-ICU Reengineering of Critical Care Processes. JAMA. 2011;305(21):2175. doi:10.1001/jama.2011.697

CHAPTER 32

Maintenance of Ventilators

Anil Kumar Chillimuntha

All living things breathe in and out. Living means breathing. As human beings, we breathe constantly and involuntarily without even realizing it. We often do not realize the importance of breathing until there is a threat to breathing due to any pathological condition. Accordingly, ventilation is done for patients in the ICU. When a newborn baby or an old comatose patient is administered medical gases, every breath is monitored carefully. In all such cases, the health of these patients is dependent on reliably functioning ventilators and a constant supply of medical gases. Medical gases are indispensable in a hospital system. Using high-pressure cylinders at the patient bedside was a costly and risky proposition, therefore, most hospitals moved to a centralized system where pressure could be monitored and controlled efficiently as per the need. Medical gas pipeline system (MGPS) is supposed to be safe, convenient, cheap, and cost-effective. Therefore, a hospital requires a well-maintained medical gas management system which is well-planned, installed and undergoes stringent regular preventive maintenance.

The Respiratory Care Practitioner working in the ICU should take complete responsibility for every breath a patient takes. It is ensured that the prescribed medical gas is supplied to patients uninterrupted, with the highest levels of quality, and at the right pressure, available 24 × 7, all 365 days a year.

Medical gases such as oxygen, compressed air, nitrous oxide and carbon dioxide are majorly used in a hospital. Of these gases, compressed air and oxygen are produced in the hospital, distributed, and monitored. Around 200 m^3 of medical gases are required daily in a 300 bedded hospital. Nearly 10 km long copper pipelines are installed in the hospital to distribute these gases and supply them to around 600 gas terminal units. From the stage of production to consumption by a patient, all the components need to work cohesively with the highest standards maintaining uninterrupted supply with multiple redundancies.

The altercation of critical components is visible after a specified time of its functioning. Therefore, regular preventive maintenance is mandated. The equipment maintenance is done by an experienced biomedical engineer who is employed by the healthcare organization. There is often a lack of cooperation between the technical and medical personnel which leads to a term coined as "technical desert." A respiratory therapist, being a part of the medical staff, needs to collaborate with them in the interest of patients and their working environment in the ICU. The biomedical engineer does essential service independently based on his capabilities and relies on collaboration with outside after-sales service engineers. Therefore, an annual maintenance contract or a comprehensive maintenance contract needs to be done with the manufacturing company or a third party. Some of the core responsibilities of a respiratory therapist are to ensure the ventilators function optimally for which he must do good surveillance, detection and corrective actions and implement necessary training with feedback analysis. Preventive maintenance is significantly affordable and cheaper than reactive maintenance.

MEDICAL GAS SYSTEM

The medical gas system is an engineering area. Oxygen therapy started in the year since 1867. Gases used for human consumption in a hospital are strictly controlled by legislation and the prescribed quality standards such as ISO 7396-1/2 Origin European Nations (e.g. Italy, Spain, France, etc.); (National Fire Protection Association) NFPA99-Origin, USA; (Health Technical Memorandum) HTM2022/0201. Origin, UK. These medical gases are listed as drugs in Indian, European, Japanese, and USA pharmacopoeia or National Formulary of these countries. These are considered drugs and are regulated by FDA through statutory specifications.

Maintenance of the Medical Gas System

Medical gas systems are major life-saving systems in any healthcare organization. It is not enough to purchase a quality product. Proper preventive maintenance is important because even the best equipment fails if not properly maintained. This warrants a need for a good monitoring and maintenance plan to ensure the smooth functioning of mechanical ventilation systems in the ICUs. Gradually and subtly, the use of medical gases under high pressure usually makes them vulnerable to unexpected breakdowns. Therefore, a preventive maintenance plan and a regular monitoring checklist are the need of the hour. The MGPS should be designed in such a way that it ensures and increases safety for the ICU patient. It is very crucial and imperative to ensure the smooth running of a hospital's medical gas system. A well-maintained medical gas system with quality assurance will create the needed confidence and trust in using mechanical ventilation by the Intensivist, Respiratory Therapist, Nurse, and other healthcare personnel who provide care for patients in the ICU.

The medical gas system in a hospital involves a large array of things such as the medical oxygen system, the medical air systems, and the medical vacuum system, the medical pipeline system with pendants, bed head panels and medical gas outlets.

The most vital lifesaving central medical oxygen system encompasses a wide range of things. Firstly, the sources of medical oxygen for a hospital are the traditional Oxygen Cylinders of varied sizes connected through the Manifold, Dura Cylinders with Vaporizers, and Liquid Medical Oxygen with Vaporizers and Oxygen Generation Plants (OGP). They all are linked to an automatic changeover and control panel with an alarm system. The medical air system with all its components has compressors, reservoirs, dryers, filters, and a control panel with alarms. The medical vacuum system contains vacuum pumps, a reservoir, filters, and a control panel. The piped medical gas system is color coded as per international standards and has area valve service units, isolation valves, area alarm panel and master alarm panels. At the patient's bedside, there are pendants or bed head panels with medical gas outlets.

Medical Air System

The medical air is a blending agent for oxygen delivery to patients in ICU at different concentrations. It is considered as a drug manufactured on-site. The compressed air consists of oxygen, carbon monoxide, nitrous oxide, nitric oxide, Sulphur dioxide and humidity. It is supplied at 370–400 kPa with a flow rate of 40 and 80 liters per minute at each terminal unit in the ICU. The components of the medical air system contain compressors, reservoirs, dryers, filters, and control panels with alarms.

Compressors

Every compressor has a meter that shows the number of hours it has been used. Every compressor or pump should have redundancy or backup, which means every primary supply should have a secondary supply or a companion that is either duplexed or multiplexed based on the capacity and need in the ICU. They are kept on standby in the event of a failure or demand shortage. Based on the number of hours the compressor is run, there must be a change of oil and filters.

Usually, there is a minimum of three filters needed for the delivery of medical air to the patient's bedside. First, is the pre-filter with a filtration size of 5 or 1 micron. The second filter is a fine or bacterial filter which filters up to 0.01 micron. The third filter is usually a coal filter. With the help of these filters, we can get IS/ISO7396-1 medical air quality. The intake air filtration system is the first line of defense for the protection of the compressor. A clean filter ensures smooth functioning with good cooling and low energy consumption. A clogged dirty filter reduces efficiency and leads to a reduction in the life of the lubricant. So, make sure that filters are changed at a regular frequency to ensure the needed filtration and output is generated as per applicable standards. The change of filter is dependent on the ambient environment around the compressor. A weekly check on the air filter is mandatory.

Oil filter maintenance is also needed to prevent damage to the compressor. It removes from the lubricant the dirt and particulate matter along with abrasives. When this oil filter is changed regularly it increases the life of the lubricant and reduces the wear and tear of the moving parts. It also protects the air and oil separator which is usually there in a rotary screw compressor. Usually, this oil filter is changed every 2000 hr. Some compressors use a long-life filter so checking the manufacturer's specifications and keeping it on the checklist will ensure proper preventive maintenance.

Some compressors use oil, and some are oil-free. If it is an oil compressor check for the condition of the oil and whether the requisite levels are being maintained and monitored regularly. The use of oil indicates worn-out parts in the compressor.

The rotary screw compressors have an oil/air separator that removes the oil particulate matter from the air stream. The particulate matter buildup and further accumulation of contaminants will increase the pressure drop across the oil/air separator. As a thumb rule, for every 2 PSIG increase in the pressure drop raises brake horse power use by 1%. Servicing the separator regularly will keep low the oil carryover and will increase the lubricant life too by reducing its consumption of it.

Synthetic lubricants have a life, and they hold up to any kind of harsh environment and thereby protect the compressor. Synthetic lubricants can become corrosive and form varnishes due to the breakdown of the lubricant. Therefore, regular oil checks and analyses need to be conducted and incorporated into the preventive maintenance checklist.

The belts and mechanical connections are checked to detect wear and tear and to identify if there is a labored pump operation. The drains are checked for the patency of accumulated water inside them. Air is compressed inside the compressor, and this wrings humidity from the air and forms water. There must be a clear path for this water to get drained otherwise the water can back up into the compressor and damage it.

The voltage and amperage are checked to verify the adherence to operating specifications as per manufacturer. The motor taking more than the required electricity will wear out the parts and cause labored operation. The audio-visual indicators are checked to see if they will light up when a faulty condition arises. Likewise, all the audio alarms are checked to ensure they are working as per set points. The operating temperature of the compressor needs to be monitored to prevent burnout. The valves and rings are checked for in the compressor regularly, especially in the reciprocating compressors.

After cooler or air cooler maintenance check for dirt accumulation on the compressed air system needs to be done regularly. When they are clogged with particulate matter and become dirty, the cooler loses its ability to dissipate heat and cool the medical-grade air produced. This heat buildup causes increased temperature leading to damage to the compressor, and a decrease in the life of the lubricant. The actual due point is measured and checked to ensure the patient takes in the right concentration of air with humidity. The dew point is the amount of water in the output. The dew point alarms are set and checked for functioning. A certain amount of water in the air helps in the easy breathing of the patient but excessive water will cause uneasy, labored breathing and clogging of the pipes and equipment. The room that houses the compressors needs to be well-ventilated to prevent build-up of heat inside the room. Explosions and fires occur very often in these places if proper preventive maintenance is not done. Therefore, the necessary fire-mitigating systems need to be installed and monitored for emergencies.

Mostly like all high-powered equipment in the industry, compressors require safety measures in place to keep the operators and staff protected.

MEDICAL GAS PIPELINE SYSTEM (MGPS)

The medical gas pipeline system supplies gases from the source of onsite manufacturing and storage to the patient's bedside through a mechanism of the pipeline distribution system. Each medical gas must be supplied through a different designated pipeline system that is placed and traversing next to each other closely. Therefore, during installation, it is ensured to see that no cross-connections are done which can be life-threatening. Tests are also conducted after installation to ensure this cross-connection has not occurred.

The different pipeline system has various color coding to enable identification during maintenance. Piped oxygen is supplied at 4 bar (400 kPa) which range from 3.8–4.2 at the terminal end where a patient is located. A pressure drop of 5% is factored in during the design. During the design and installation, a principle of design from "inside to outside" is adhered to. The average rate of consumption is assumed to be 10 liters per minute in a ward and 100 liters per minute in an ICU or operation theatre.

Pipeline Nomenclature and Material

There is a "main hospital pipeline" that supplies from the source, i.e. manifold to the hospital building. It is also sometimes called the "main trunk line." Connected to this is the "feeder pipeline" which comprises "Risers" that are vertically and horizontally connected to the branch pipeline. Usually, a "branch pipeline" or distribution pipeline connects one single floor and does not go vertical. It connects to a drop pipe where there's distribution through terminal units.

These pipelines are usually made of medical-grade copper. When the copper is phosphorous deoxidized, processed and made non-arsenical, it conforms to BSEN 1412:1996 grade CW024A (Cu-DHP). The copper pipes are round, seamless, and size conforming to BS EN 13348. It is used because there is no sagging or distortion of the pipeline distribution system when laid vertically or horizontally. The material temper for the tailpiece is R220 and R250 half-hard for pipes of outer diameter 12–54 mm. The copper pipes with an outer diameter of 76 mm are R290 hard. The following copper pipe specifications are mandated as per EN 13348.

PIPELINE TESTING

All the tubing, valves and other fittings should be inspected for oil, grease, or any combustible material. While brazing the copper pipe connections, the interior parts need to be purged with nitrogen continuously. A flux-less silver copper-phosphorous brazing alloy (CP 104) which conforms to BS EN 1044:1999 standards is used. The MGPS pipeline should be properly secured at sufficient intervals. When copper pipes pass through walls, partitions, and floors we need to keep the sleeves secured **(Table 32.1)**. This table is an indicative measurement of the same. Before installing the terminal outlets, blow the free particles from the pipeline.

Table 32.1 : The medical gas pipeline testing procedures

Tests	Procedures
Blow down	Lines are blown clear oil-free dry nitrogen
Initial press test	System is subjected to 1.5 times working pressure to check leaks
Standing press test	System is subjected to 20% higher pressure for 24 hr
Piping purge	Purging of each outlet until there is no discoloration of the white cloth held over it
Cross-connection test	One gas system at a time using O_2 analyzer
Final tie-in test	Active vacuum pipeline joints are tested using an ultrasonic leak detector

Validation of MGPS

The validation of the medical gas pipeline system is done by pressure testing and leak locating. Cross-connection testing is also done to ensure each pipeline is supplying the intended gas and not a mixture of gases. The tests are performed before validating a medical gas system safe for patient use. The main aim of these tests is to always maintain and safeguard the well-being of patients.

Color Coding of MGPS

The pipelines are colored and standardized internationally. Throughout the world, medical gas pipeline color coding is used as a gas identifier. This provides identification of gas running in a pipeline during any kind of maintenance. We cannot identify gases with our naked eye. Using a different gas for a different function can be life-threatening for a patient. Therefore, color coding and labeling are done. There is a ground color and color band.

Ground colors are applied throughout the length for a minimum of two meters. The color bands are placed at intersection points and places where direction changes. It is also done midway through each pipeline and near the valves. When there is a long stretch of pipeline, color bands are placed at every fifty-meter interval. Color bands are also placed at the beginning and end of every pipeline.

The color coding is different for USA and India. In India, we follow the ISO system. **Figure 32.1** depicts the different color coding of USA and ISO.

Gas	U.S. Color code	ISO Color code
Carbon dioxide	Grey	Grey
He-O_2	Brown and green	Brown and white
Instrument air	Red (USA only)	
Medical air	Yellow	Black and white
Nitrogen	Black	Black
Nitrous oxide	Blue	Blue
O_2-He	Green and brown	White and brown
Oxygen	Green	Green
Vacuum (suction)	White	Yellow
WAGD (Evac)	Purple	Purple

Fig. 32.1: The medical gas pipeline color coding for USA and India

Area Valve Service Units (AVSU) and Medical Terminal Units

The gas pipeline distribution system encompasses the different areas of the hospital. Therefore, a problematic area is cut off from the other distribution system for service and maintenance. The area cut-off valve enables smooth functioning of the pipeline distribution system. The medical terminal units are located at the end-user where the final delivery of medical gas is provided. Terminal units are provided to ensure single-hand insertion and removal of the probe. Usually, the probes are pushed to insert. The terminal unit has a leak-proof press-to-release mechanism. There is a self-sealing valve that is disengaged. There is a non-return valve that is useful for servicing and repairing. The front plate is color coded for easy identification.

Non-interchangeable screw thread connectors (NIST) are used. A Diameter-Indexed Safety System (DISS) is used. It uses non-interchangeable threaded fittings to connect at the terminal unit. A gas-specific connector is used at the terminal unit. Dimensions of the male part of the connector are gas specific. It is employed to safeguard against the installation of wrong connectors to the terminal unit.

Bed head panels are used to dispense gases at the patient's bedside. The terminal units are housed in them. They also house two oxygen, two air, and two vacuum suction terminal units as per requirement. Most of the bed head panels incorporate plug points, nurse call systems, suction apparatus, flow meters and sometimes even reading light.

Manifold Room

The manifold should be in a spacious, well-ventilated room, located at the outer wall of the hospital to enable the loading and unloading of cylinders and for service convenience. Provision of a raised level loading bay reduces any kind of cylinder handling hazards. Access to this room should not be from patient rooms or corridors. It should preferably have an open-air enclosed system.

The room for the manifold is different from the room that holds compressors and medical air storage tanks. It is preferable to have two doors, with one of them providing accessibility and ease of transportation of cylinders. They must be free of any kind of obstruction and no oily substances should come in contact with the cylinders. The internal walls and doors should be preferably non-combustible and fire-resistant as per BS476-4:1970 and BS476 Parts 20–23 (1987). The manifold area cylinders are secured through a safety chain with sufficient space to house full and empty cylinders. No oily substances or inflammable chemicals are stored or kept near these cylinders.

Medical Oxygen

Medical oxygen is a life-saving gas that needs to be distributed from the source to the patient's bedside. Oxygen is an essential medicine. Only high-quality oxygen which is of medical grade is needed for patient administration. The oxygen ecosystem involves the devices and equipment needed to produce, monitor, and distribute oxygen to the patient's bedside.

The sources of oxygen are traditional oxygen cylinders, liquid medical oxygen and through oxygen generation plants. The uninterrupted supply of oxygen is ensured by using a primary, secondary, and reserve supply. Usually, liquid oxygen is preferred as a primary source and cylinders in the manifold are kept as secondary. The manifold room houses the oxygen cylinders.

Oxygen Cylinders

Oxygen can be compressed and stored in varied sizes of cylinders. The cylinders are filled at an oxygen manufacturing facility and transported to the hospital. The cylinders are connected to the manifold system and oxygen is delivered to patients through a network of the piping system. Cylinders also can be used directly at the patient's bedside too provided they are properly secured to the wall through chains or a trolley.

Trouble shooting for some common problems that occur with cylinders is shown in Table 32.2.

Table 32.2: Trouble shooting for oxygen cylinders and its accessories

Problem or fault	Possible cause	Solution
No oxygen is flowing	✦ Empty cylinder ✦ Flowmeter Knob or cylinder flow valve is closed ✦ Faulty regulator	✦ Replace cylinder ✦ Open the valves, and then check the meter registers flow ✦ Close all the valves and replace the regulator
Leakage from cylinder or flowmeter	✦ Cylinder is not connected to pressure regulator property ✦ Faulty or missing washeer between regulator and cylinder ✦ Flowmeter seal damaged or loose ✦ Cylinder faulty	✦ Tighten all fittings ✦ Replace the washer. ✦ Replace sealing of the washer and realign the flowmeter ✦ Label faulty cylinder and take appropriate action
Leakage cannot be iocated	✦ Leakage too small to be heard	✦ Apply detergent solution (NOT oily soap) to the joints. There will be bubbles at the leakae point. Clean/replace the washer and tighten the joint.
Flowmeter ball not moving, yet oxygen is flowing	✦ Faulty flowmeter	✦ Close all the valves, disconnect flowmeter, and clean the flowmeter. Reconnect and test. If problems perissts, replace the flowmeter
Pressure gauge does not show pressure, yet oxygen is flowing	✦ Faulty pressure gauge	✦ Replace pressure gauge

Liquid Medical Oxygen (LMO)

Liquid oxygen is a cryogenic liquid which is pale blue and is a compressed form of oxygen. Liquid medical oxygen is installed in a hospital where there is a large requirement of oxygen for patients. It is the most economical way of storing and supplying oxygen which is 95 % pure while the rest of it is argon gas. It is a low-pressure, high-flow supply system, vacuum-insulated vaporizer (VIE). There is a need for special equipment to manage and store oxygen. The tank is made up of stainless-steel inner vessel and an outer vessel, with insulation in between them. There is pressure control equipment to control the pressure and flow. LMO is stored at a temperature of –150° to –170°C and a pressure of 10.5 bars. The cold oxygen is warmed when it comes out and enters a vaporizer which is a coil of copper tubes. As the oxygen gets warmer the pressure increases. At a temperature of 15° and atmospheric pressure, we can see that the liquid oxygen supplies 842 times its volume as a gas. **Figure 32.2** depicts the components of the LMO tank.

All the LMO tanks are powder and vacuum insulated in the annular space. They are equipped with various circuits to monitor pressure buildup and relief, product withdrawal, and vacuum levels.

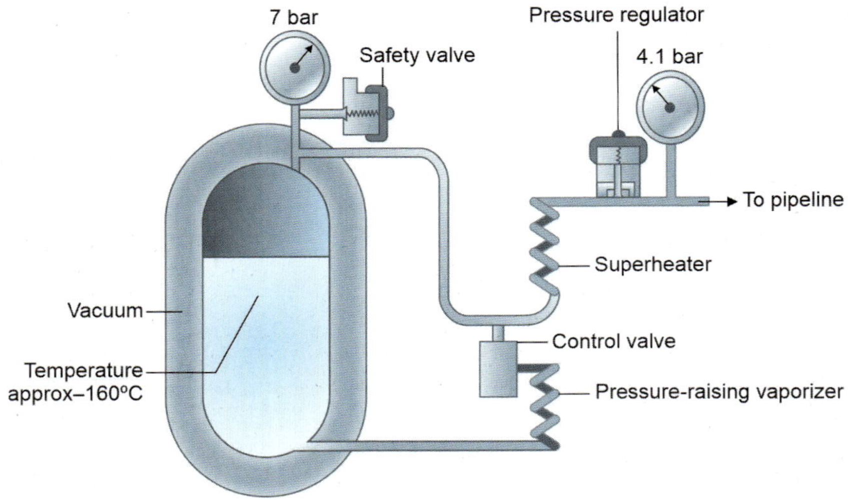

Fig. 32.2: Components of liquid medical oxygen tank

They are designed as per national and international standards such as:

- HTM02-01 Medical gas pipeline system—Part A, Design, installation, validation, and verification.
- AIGA049/17-Guideline to medical oxygen supply system for healthcare facilities.
- NFPA55–2016-Chapter 9, Bulk oxygen systems.

The LMO tank is insulated well, but the tank always absorbs the surrounding heat which causes the liquefied gas to evaporate. This increases the pressure inside the tank and activates the safety pressure relief valve which will vent oxygen into the atmosphere. Therefore, if liquid oxygen is left unused for a long time, a lot of oxygen is lost. That is why a proper size LMO tank will be cheaper only when there is a constant demand and usage of oxygen and not much oxygen will be vented out. Usually, the liquid oxygen is stored for not more than a week or two.

The liquid medical oxygen is supplied by an external party which comes at regular intervals to refill the tank. Liquefied oxygen is a compressed gas stored in liquefied form in a specially designed container. In India, the license is procured from the Petroleum and Explosive Safety Organization (PESO).

The manifold functions on a high-pressure low flow system. Usually, ten cylinders are fixed to one manifold, where cylinders are kept always vertical and secured by chains to provide safety. Typically, an oxygen gas manifold system, from the terminal unit to the manifold room, consists of the terminal unit which has bed head panels and then area alarm panels.

Cryogenic Liquid Cylinders (Dura)

It is a vacuum-jacketed, insulated pressure cylinder. To protect from the pressure buildup, it has a pressure relief valve and rupture disks. They operate in pressures of 100–350 PSIG (24 Atms). It has capacities between 80 and 450 liters of liquid oxygen. In India, we usually get Dura cylinders with a capacity of 180–250 liters. They come with a warranty of 2–3 years. The liquid oxygen can get converted into gaseous form when passed through a vaporizer.

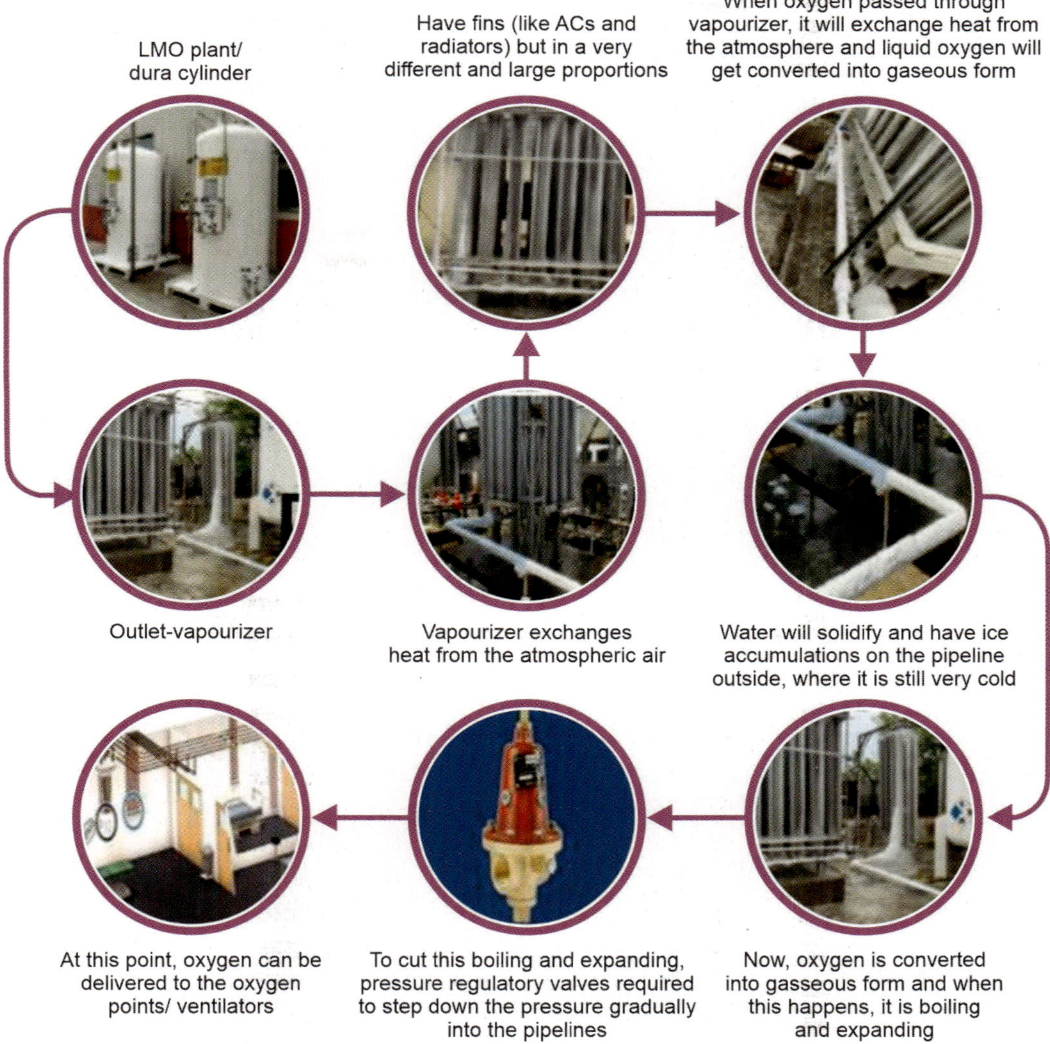

Fig. 32.3: The working plan of an LMO tank and Dura cylinder

The prerequisite for LMO tank installation is large, open uncovered land availability where civil work is in progress. Typically, a space of W x L of (9 m x 15 m) is needed without any utility overhead cables crisscrossing. The applicable licenses from PESO are availed for filling, storage, and operation. There must be sufficient space needed to have a crane to unload and install the huge LMO tank and vaporizer. There must be good fencing with a gate around the installation along with fire safety equipment, water connection, lightning safety device, earthing pit, and safety signages. Some of the drawbacks of LMO are the need for adequate infrastructure, logistical constraints of the supply chain with supply constraints, and the need for cylinder backup supply. It has a high installation cost and has a heavy dependency on the maintenance of piping with a risk of leakage. Maintenance checks must be carried out to ensure that abrasive and solvent-cleaning materials are not being used. To clean the external surfaces using a damp cloth soaked in a mild soap solution is recommended. Detergent and surfactant solutions are not recommended. Phenol or halogenated disinfectant solutions that release chlorine are not to be used.

The service personnel diagnose many faults. Some of the faults require a simple solution. Most of the faults for trouble shooting can be avoided by performing regular preventive maintenance.

Table 32.3: Troubleshooting of LMO tank

	Possible cause	Remarks/rectification action
Failure to reach or maintain operating pressure	✦ Excessive withdrawal ✦ Liquid level too low ✦ Leaks on outer piping ✦ Safety valves do not close ✦ Strainer at inlet of pressure building regulator clogged ✦ Improper adjustment of regulator, or regulator defective	✦ Increase capacity of pressure building ✦ refill tank ✦ Seal ✦ Replace ✦ Clean ✦ Correct adjustment or replace regulator—see Maintenance section
Erroneous or irregular contents gauge readings	✦ Bypass valve not closed or leaking ✦ Wron adjustment ✦ Leaking in differential pressure pipes or connections ✦ Gauge damaged or leaking	✦ Close or replace ✦ Readjust ✦ Seal ✦ Replace, or return to manufacturer for repair
Main safety valve leaking	✦ Dirt or ice under disk cone	✦ Repair/replace
Inner vessel bursting disk has burst	✦ Bursting disk with too low pressure ✦ Corrosion or material fatigue	✦ Replace ✦ Replace
Shut-off valves leaking	✦ Valve seat loose ✦ Damaged seat or cone	✦ Tighten ✦ Replace seat
Loss of vacumm	✦ Leak on vacuum bursting disk ✦ Leaking measuring socket	✦ Replace ✦ Seal
Wron or incorrect vacuum gauge reading	✦ Gauge not properly calibreated ✦ Batteries have no charge ✦ Defective vacuum gauge tube	✦ Calibrate ✦ Replace ✦ Replace

Oxygen Generation Plant (OGP)

Pressure swing adsorption (PSA) is a method followed by OGP which produces medical-grade oxygen. PSA is a process where ambient air passes through a molecular sieve made of zeolite granules and membranes. They have a large surface area available to separate oxygen and nitrogen. It contested the remaining oxygen for purity up to 93%.

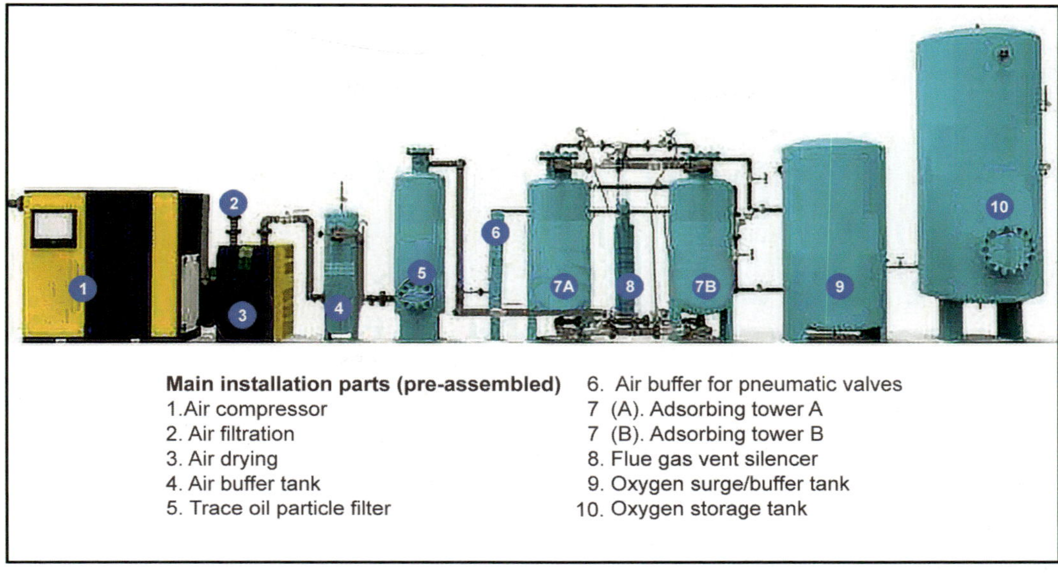

Fig. 32.4: Layout of pressure swing adsorbent plant

The atmospheric air is compressed when it is passed through the compressor. This compressed air moves to the first filter that removes impurities and water particles. Then the air moves through an air dryer where it is refrigerated at 2°–7°C, effectively removing the water vapor. Then the air moved to the sieve containers or adsorbent towers where it passes through different filters and membranes which remove foreign and carbon particles. The adsorbent towers with zeolite sieves selectively adsorb nitrogen to provide concentrated oxygen. The oxygen is then passed through bacterial filters and other filters. The oxygen generated is stored under pressure in a storage container and is ready for delivery to patients through the medical gas pipeline system.

Table 32.4: Common Issues occurring in OGP and their troubleshooting

Issue	Troubleshooting
Displays not showing up	Check the power supply connection and tension
Tower status LED not changing	Change the controller
LEDS status change but tower not switching	Check the coil connection at DIN* and terminal connector in the controller check the solenoid valve
No purging	✦ Check the solenoid valve ✦ Check the exhaust valve ✦ Clean the silencer (muffler) continuous purging at tower 1A—shuttle not closing ✦ Check pilot air for exhaust valve ✦ Check exhaust valve piston if it is stuck
High purge loss	✦ Check oulet shuttle clossing ✦ Check for silencer choke

Contd.

Table 32.4: Common Issues occurring in OGP and their troubleshooting (Contd.)

Issue	Troubleshooting
High pressure drop across generator	✦ Pre-filter may be clogged. Check and replace filter elements ✦ Check whether the generaor is being overflowed.
Oxygen analyser (Purity) issue	✦ Follow the flow diagram given by the manufacturer
Low operating pressure	Lower than normal operating pressure may indicate any of the following, ✦ A restriction in the suction air intake filter, which limits the amount of air pass through it to the generator. Clean the air filters free from foreign materials ✦ An improperly operating circuit board or solenoid valve. Confirm that the circuit board and solenoid valves function properly. ✦ A leak in the unit, which allows system pessure to escape. Perform leak test in the unit. ✦ A compressor with reduced output. Ensure that the oxygen concentration level at the desired liter flow is within Trident's specifications. If it is below specifications, replace or repair the compressor
High operating pressure	Higher than normal operating pressure may indicate any of the following: ✦ A restrictive muffler, which does not allow the waste (purge) gas to exit the system freeely. Operate the unitl with the muffler disconnected to see if the operating pressure returns to nomral. ✦ An improperly operating circuit board or solenoid valve. Confirm that the circuit board and solenoid valves function properly. ✦ A restrictive diffuser, which does not allow the inlet feed air as well as exhaust air from the generator. Check the diffuser and correct it. ✦ Contaminated sieve beds. Change the sieve beds.
Leak test operation	✦ Shut off the oxygen application/consumption ✦ Let the plant run in manual mode, untill the oxygen tank pressure reaches a minimum of 5 bar ✦ Turn the mode slector switch to stand-by/off, and the PSA generator will stop after a little while, when the actual operation cycle is completed. ✦ Shut off the feed air supply ✦ If coal tower is installed, close of oil indication tube. If fitted with purity monitoring probe close of the pressure reduction valve on probe inlet. ✦ Read and note the pressure P1 in product tank, column 1, column 2, column 3 if present and feed air tank ✦ Let the plant stand still (rest) and isolatedin pressurized condition for an hour

Contd.

Table 32.4: Common Issues occurring in OGP and their troubleshooting

Issue	Troubleshooting
	✦ After an hour read and note the pressure P2 in product tank, column 1, column 2, column 3 if present and feed air tank ✦ Then determine an eventually pressure drop as the difference between P1 and P2 for each component. ✦ The Leak test is right, if the pressure drop after one hour pressurized isolation is less than 0.1 bar. In case of leaks they must not cause more than 0.1 bar pressure drop per hour. ✦ If closed open for coal tower oil indication tube and rest the pressure reduction valve on probe inlet 1.0 bar
DIN (Deutsches institue füur Nomung)—A DIN connector is an electrical connector that was originally standardized in the early 1970s by the Deutsches institut für normung (DIN), the German national standards organization.	

Before maintenance and checking for troubleshooting issues, make sure the MGPS are connected to a minimum of three independent sources of oxygen. The generator should be having a minimum of 95% uptime with preventive service assurance from the vendor. The PSA plant should be operated by trained personnel. A minimum of 2–3 personnel is to be trained on how to operate the plant. Ensure that the vendor who installed the PSA plant should be contracted with and must have sufficient spares. There should be sufficient ventilation since the compressor generates hot air exhaust which eventually raises the temperature inside the PSA plant room thereby causing the malfunction of the plant. If ventilation is not possible keep sufficient exhaust fans to throw out hot air and bring in fresh air. Ideally, there must be two compressors for a PSA plant.

The minimum pressure at the oxygen outlet should be a minimum of 4.2 psi pressure to service ventilators in the ICU. To ensure the uninterrupted seamless working of the PSA plant, monthly inspection checks for drying and regeneration cycles are functioning appropriately. The silencers must be checked every month to ensure that they are not clogged. Replace filter elements every six months. Each year check for the condition of valve seals. During the entire preventive maintenance, the compressor and the generator should be shut down. Before changing the desiccant, make sure all the personnel wear a mask to avoid ingestion of fine dust. Bypass the oxygen supply to the secondary line and disconnect the power supply to the generator. Make sure the inlet to the air supply is closed and then depressurize both towers. Loosen the dummy present in the desiccant port located near the bottom of the tower. Remove the old desiccant and keep the new one. Before the filter element is changed, ensure that there is a requirement for replacement. Repair all leaks by tightening all connections. Make sure the unit is cycling appropriately. Some of the common troubleshooting issues are mentioned below.

Automatic Control Panel

The changeover from the primary source to the secondary and reserve or vice versa is done automatically by this control panel. It is based on pneumatic pressure measured by the pressure valves placed at the control panel. There is a pneumatic relief valve in the

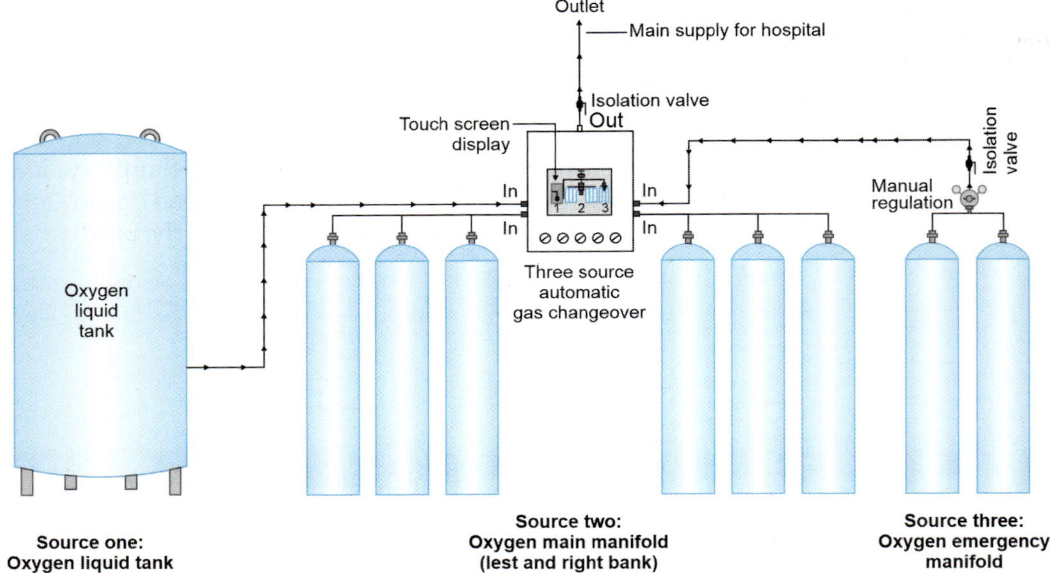

Fig. 32.5: A Schematic diagram of automatic control panel

main distribution line. There are also visual audio alarms for alerting the workers. The master alarm panel is kept in a strategic place to alert the on-duty manifold technician. The alarm is usually set for a 10–15% pressure drop.

NABH Standards for Medical Gas System

The National Accreditation Board for Hospitals and Healthcare providers is set up by the Quality Council of India, a Government of India initiative to establish and operate accreditation for hospitals. The country presently follows the fifth edition which was recently released. They specify a commitment, core and achievements to be met for fulfilling the standards. The standards and objective elements related to the medical gas system are found in the 5th Edition book "NABH Accreditation Standards for Hospitals 2020", Chapter 8, "Facility Management System (FMS). As per these standards, it is required for a hospital to provide medical gases along with safe water and ventilation. As per FMS Standard 6, **Table 32.5** depicts the list of objective elements that are related to the medical gas system.

Table 32.5: NABH standards for medical gas system

Commitment	a	Written guidance governs the implementation of procurement, handling, storage, distribution, usage, and replenishment of medical gases
Core	b	Medical gases are handled, stored, distributed and used in a safe manner
Commitment	c	The procedures for medical gases address the safety issues at all levels
Core	d	Alternate sources for medical gases, vacuum and compressed air are provided for, in case of failure
Commitment	e	The organisation regularly tests the functioning of these alternate sources
Commitment	f	There is an operational, inspection, testing and maintenance plan for piped medical gases, compressed air and vacuum installation

There is also an exclusive ISO standard ISO 7361-1:2007 which discusses the installation, operation, and maintenance of the medical gas system.

Conclusion

A beautiful article is titled "With every breath you take thank the ocean." More than half of the oxygen we breathe comes from marine photo synthesizers. Similarly, in a hospital setting, we can boldly say, "With every breath, you take thank the Respiratory Care Practitioner." If work is done with this spirit, the hospital can ensure the production and safe delivery of medical gases to ICU patients.

CHAPTER 33

Talking to Family and Counselling

❒ Sai Praveen Haranath

INTRODUCTION

The orderly chaos of an intensive care unit is only matched by the constant alarms that percolate the area. Patients and their families are often thrown suddenly in the middle of this confusing and emotionally charged environment. Among several decisions that constitute critical care, the mechanical ventilator takes a central role. Ever since mechanical ventilation gained importance in the polio crisis in Denmark.[1] It has managed to save lives while creating extreme stress among families and providers.

The cardinal questions have been whether to intubate and ventilate and subsequently prophesizing the ideal time to liberate the patient from the glorified air pump. In this chapter an approach to discuss the role of the ventilator with families and patients will be outlined with practical examples of case scenarios. Language that can be used with appropriate translation to the local language of the patient will be suggested. The ethics of mechanical ventilation will be discussed and the impact of the often prohibitive cost reviewed. There will also be principles discussed which can be applied in any healthcare setting especially when a patient is critically ill. Cultural variations and syntax as well as grammar will be different for various languages and the evidence and essence must not be lost in translation.

At the heart of a patient counseling session or family meeting to update the next of kin is the need for communication. This is generally verbal but like all forms of efffective communication there is a need for clarity, brevity and honesty. Trust must be built since patient care depends on decisions made at this meeting. Delayed decisions or deferred decisions can have serious health consequences for critically ill patients.

Practical Considerations

Mechanical ventilators, their noisy features, the cacophony of the ICU can be daunting and disorienting to families and patients. Explaining why we use ventilators in simple language is helpful. Likewise speaking in an even tone, while seated and making eye contact are ideal best practices. Adequate time to explain the process, encouraging questions and making sure there is a realistic understanding of risks and benefits.

The family will need at least daily updates but often in a critically ill patient this may need to be done several times a day. Crucial decisions when mechanically ventilating a patient may need consent and these possibilities should be discussed before hand rather than urgently.

As shown in the algorithm some simple principles can be followed when talking with families and this will improve communication.

Clear Complete Compassionate Collaborative Confident	Family and patient counseling: The five 'C' approach

NIV

Chronic obstructive pulmonary disease (COPD) is the fourth leading cause of death in the world.[2] In one randomized controlled study evaluating the effectiveness of a short-term cognitive behavioral therapy intervention on NIV acceptance and adherence in patients with COPD, the intervention significantly improved NIV adherence and Quality of Life, with mild short-term anxiety improvement.[3]

It appears that this may be an area of research to improve use of mechanical ventilators in this group of patients.

Cultural Factors

While trust and acceptance of medical therapy may be variable in different societies, it is also important to learn about the varied cultural factors that impact understanding the use of mechanical ventilation. Language used when speaking to families must be simple to comprehend. Low health literacy is very common and one article noted that over 90 million Americans may fit this criteria.[4]

Adults

The patient or family counseling for most adults can be done in a standard manner. This will include introduction of the critical care team and the consultant under whom the patient has been admitted of it is an open ICU. In addition consulting providers like pulmonology and other subspcialties should ideally be present to clarify any questions. Practically this would be a very difficult coordination exercise since there is limited time to have everyone in one location. However, in certain situations it is imperative for the whole team to be present especially if there has been a major change in status, a change in plan of care, conflict between providers of conflict with patient families.

Children

Family counseling when children are sick may involve some differences from an adult approach. As shown in a study on parent perspectives, individualized approach with incorporation of varied perspectives of the particular family was important. End of life descriptions by clinicians were vividly intimidating. Clearly, a lot more needs to be done collaboratively in this sad situation where foregoing or withdrawing mechanical ventilation may be discussed.[5]

Who does the Counseling?

Ideally the provider closest to the patient must build rapport with the family and provide daily and periodic updates. In an era of shifts and rapid turnover this may not be possible. In this situation detailed and accurate handovers are important. When a care team changes it will help to have the outgoing team introduce the incoming team and explain that the plan of care has been shared. This may seem like a lot of work but will play a big role in avoiding loss of trust as well as patient safety.

The resident doctor or fellow, the attending consultant, the critical care consultant, nurse, social worker and patient family must meet everyday to discuss the plan of care. Adequate time to explain and answer questions is essential.

Having the family appoint a spokesperson who may or may not be the legal next of kin can help alleviate difficulties from varying language competency and literacy levels. Simple language and appropriate emotion will be important in ensuring that nothing is lost in translation. Likewise, any information not available or questions where an immediate answer is not available will need to be proactively followed up with the family by the healthcare team.

When should the Counseling be Done?

Patients often have a period of time in the hospital outside the ICU where the respiratory status begins to decline. The bedside team should initiate discussion on potential ICU transfer as well as the need for noninvasive or invasive mechanical ventilation. The ICU team members can try to assist the ward team in this process when evaluating patients for transfer. This also helps possibly prevent some patient transfers if critical care expertise is used to assist the patient in the ward.

Clinical example 1: A 56-year-old patient with COPD exacerbation from influenza is on the medical ward. He has worsening hypercapnia from enthusiastic oxygen use. The ICU or pulmonary evaluating team can try to mitigate a transfer by adjusting down the oxygen delivery to a minimum level. In this situation the counseling can be done by the ICU team or the pulmonary team.

Elderly

The physiologic reserve of elderly patients may be decreased and many patients with impending respiratory failure will need mechanical ventilation. Family members to decide on next steps will often be unclear on what needs to be done. Many patients may be unresponsive or unable to offer any meaningful insight into their wishes at this stage. It is hence extremely important to have these discussions early on in the admission and even as an outpatient. Mechanical ventilation can be dangerous and while prolonging life may increase the pain and suffering that patients endure.

A picture is said to be worth a thousand words and in this era a video is perhaps a close simulation of an experience. In decision making for end of life care, one randomized study of patients with dementia showed that a video depiction of advanced dementia led more patients to choose comfort care rather than opt for measures like critical care or mechanical ventilation.[6]

Likewise, explanatory videos on mechanical ventilation can go a long way in clarifying the process for families and patients.

Values

Paternalism versus autonomy has always been an issue central to the practice of ethical medicine. As technology progresses and definitions of disease as well as social behavior changes, new challenges arise. Critical care is at the forefront of such challenges due to the extreme circumstances-whether it is the physiologic precipice that patients face or economic mountains they must surmount for complete care. Family and patient counseling will have to deal with some of these concepts and introduce them with examples. They may include ideas of futile care, life prolongation, palliative care and balancing patient wishes and clinical circumstances.[7]

Can trust be measured? Apparently so, as a recent study showed. Shared decision making in a US hospital context improved trust.[8] These are structured behaviors that can be systematically employed in a family counseling session or as is commonly called, a family meeting.

Costs

Some of the key questions families ask is about the cost of intensive care. Most countries have a serious problem with access and supply of good quality critical care beds and trained providers. The cost of critical care is very high.[9]

In general it is helpful to outline the components of critical care that add to the daily cost. These include more expensive antibiotics, more extensive investigations, in depth monitoring by nurses and doctors, cost of mechanical ventilation, added expenses of complications and additional staff resource utilization. The duration of critical care also comes into factor and an approximate expected timeline for various diseases can be suggested. As an example a patient on a ventilator may take a week to recover with pneumonia but someone with ARDS may take two weeks and also require a tracheostomy. Simple procedure based intensive care stays such as a postoperative patient with a perforated appendix who has prompt surgery may be expected to only have a short duration of intensive care while on the ventilator. It is also important to set expectations that none of the time lines are hard and fast and may vary depending on each patient and their progress. Trust with the family is critical to build to avoid any notion that care in the ICU is being unnecessarily prolonged. Also, many patients need to be in the ICU even after coming off the ventilator and this can be mentioned early on. They may need non-invasive ventilation that can only be safely done in the ICU in many hospitals but there are situations where these patients can be moved to a step down unit or high dependency unit and even have remote monitoring using newer monitoring devices.

When speaking with families, an even tone can be used with complete and accurate information conveyed. Even in times of uncertainty families and patients look for reassurance and confidence in the clinician. Explaining the pros and cons of an approach honestly will allow families to understand the process of critical care. The discussion is collaborative—the options to be used if ventilation does not help the patient or the time that the meeting should occur as well as decisions on who may be allowed to visit the patient are taken by the family and clinician together.

Overall compassion, empathy and genuine concern for the patient must be visible and felt by the patient and their family and demonstrated by the entire healthcare team. Health literacy is variable and barriers of language, understanding, hearing, accents and general chaos and noise can impair family meetings and efforts to address these are essential. Despite all efforts the message may not be clear and one study showed great variance between family understanding of prognosis and what was conveyed by the clinician.[10]

Listen

Data suggests that in outpatient settings a diagnosis can be reached in X percent of patients if the physician listens to the patient for Y seconds. Likewise listening to the concerns of the family or the patient may alleviate some of the stress of critical illness which often occurs in a setting of sleep deprivation, urgency and unfamiliar surroundings. Time was the biggest constraint in patient and family engagement in both clinical and research situations.[11]

Eye Contact

One of the key tenets of communication is to maintain eye contact and sit at the level of the patient. This may be difficult in many situations but having a dedicated counseling room would be ideal. Many hospitals now require audiovisual recording of these interactions with the permission of the family for medico-legal protection.

Aggressive Families

Defusing tense situations with a calm voice and a dedicated social worker and if needed security staff will protect medical staff and premises. Violence against health care providers and institutions is illegal as per the law. Mock training in counseling that is polite, compassionate, accurate and complete is one way to enhance these skills.

Specific Situations

Financial Constraints

In situations where families decide to transfer a patient to lower cost settings or for insurance coverage purposes it is critical that this is done with patient safety as the primary driver. A patient with ARDS is often on high PEEP settings and possibly vasopressors. Such a patient may be unstable to transfer and these details must be shared with families and documented. Lowering the cost of care by stopping unnecessary and often overlooked tests or medicines should be done on a continuous basis. Social workers and admission/hospital administrators should counsel families on methods to control cost and avoid fiscal losses. In developing countries like India where a large part of healthcare is paid for by patients it is a responsible healthcare practice to have a clear outline on daily costs and some laws mandate these are prominently displayed. Only 41% have some form of health insurance as per the National Family Health Survey 5.[12]

Newer methods of insurance coverage, crowdsourcing of funding assistance, deferred payment, bank loans are some options. Unfortunately healthcare expense is responsible for 2.2% of families falling below the poverty threshold.[13] Charitable institutions, government and public sector hospitals often have excellent care facilities and may be great options for many patients at a lower cost. However, they need to be strengthened with partnership and the COVID pandemic showed may positive areas that collaboration can help improve. A statement I like to often use is that most people cannot afford more than two weeks of critical care even with health insurance. This is based on the approximate cost per ICU stay of $2818 US dollars overshooting most insurance coverage limits.[14]

Terminally ill Patients

End of life care is stressful for families and providers as seen even in the recent COVID crisis.[15] Many terminally ill patients may need to have minimal medical interventions while the focus of care switches to comfort and relief of symptoms. Mechanical ventilator use can be stopped and the patient extubated. While there may be some ambiguity in the understanding and application of relevant laws there are good resources in India now available to discuss this in more depth. The Indian Society of Critical Care Medicine has an excellent guideline with suggestions on language to be used when speaking to families.[16] Families should be counseled on what to expect as the ventilator is disconnected and terminal extubation is performed. Air hunger, respiratory distress, management of wheezing, secretions and beeping alarms need to addressed. Families can be told that relief of pain and dyspnea will be done continuously.

Prolonged Respiratory Support

Some patients require long durations of mechanical ventilation. This may or may not involve tracheostomy as was seen during the COVID pandemic. Daily counseling on progress, setting a plan in place for milestones that will indicate liberation from mechanical ventilation as well as sharing information on the other aspects of critical care that are essential to recovery will be helpful. In a recent article an important item for a checklist was providing an update on weaning progress.[17]

Complications during Mechanical Ventilation

Various complications may occur during the process of intubation and mechanical ventilation. These include misplaced tubes in the esophagus or right mainstem, pneumothorax, hypotension, bradycardia, cardiac arrest and ventilator associated pneumonia. Longer term issues such as difficulty weaning and subglottic stenosis may occur. Some of these may need to be discussed before intubation or when the event occurs. Prevention is ideal by adopting safe practices. However when an event has occurred it is optimal to stabilize the patient first and then inform the family as well as the hospital administration as per local policy. A very simple patient information booklet is available from the American Thoracic Society.[18]

Participation in Research

There is a need for better approaches to patient and family counseling. As patient centered care is now becoming the standard there are studies incorporating patient and family opinions.

Investigational Therapy

Families may ask about investigational or non-approved therapies. During the COVID pandemic there has been an onslaught of new medications and approaches. Families have cited media reports and word of mouth information to request various forms of treatment. In the mechanical ventilation area innovators have built various devices to conserve limited ventilator availability. Different forms of oxygen delivery were also explored. These topics may need to be discussed when counseling and adherence to hospital and regional governmental as well as medical board policies on using these investigational options is needed.

Non Evidence Based Therapies

As with investigational treatment options, non standard approaches will need to be discussed on a case by case basis weighing risk of harm with patient satisfaction as well as impact on care for the patient.

Prayer

Patients on mechanical ventilators desire to communicate their needs through gestures, writing or head movements. They can be counseled on the progress of their illness and their liberation from mechanical ventilation. One study showed that they even may want to communicate non medical requests like a need for prayer.[19]

Conclusion

Family engagement in the care of the patient can improve outcomes.It may involve simple things like medication management.[20] Strategies to involve families in understanding the role of the healthcare team in preventing ventilator associated pneumonia may be one example of further engaging families beyond just counseling.[21,22] Groups have been exploring the role of patient engagement for better outcomes.[23] Ultimately engagement may help with the patient experience and along with technology will likely be better for patients and their families.[24]

Ultimately communication with patients and families is a very human act, filled with compassion to enable some clarity and solace at what is a very stressful and emotionally charged time for most. There are many ways to do this but the simpler the better and just as with children there will be many teachable moments as well as frustration. However, there will always be an opportunity to learn more about the person who till then may have been just a patient without identity on a ventilator.

Clinical Example 2: Let us consider the following situation and analyze the principles that will apply. The counseling of patients and their relatives will need to always be done in a calm and compassionate manner. It should be recorded, documented and structured. There should be time for answering questions and facts shared as far as possible. A dedicated counseling location is mandatory.

A 70-year-old male presents with a history of COPD and infected with influenza. His children are abroad and he has been admitted with a severe exacerbation due to the infection. He has on non invasive ventilation with IPAP 14, EPAP 8 and FiO_2 60%. He is tachypneic, febrile and confused. His next of kin is his wife who has a good understanding of his wishes and shared that he would never want to be placed on a ventilator. His children are already making arrangements to arrive at the hospital but will take about 36 hours to reach.

In this situation what would be the ideal next steps?

While there are no right answers the principles to be followed are those that intersect between the legal requirements and patient treatment. If there is clear documentation that the patient does not want advanced life support that must be honored. However, the counseling must explain the possible disease trajectory, the need for medication to decrease the work of breathing, the possibility of intubation with supportive care till the children arrive, the possibility of worsening despite all measures as well as the risks and possible benefits of mechanical ventilation. Each location may have different regulations but there are good guidelines available (ACCP, ISCCM, Palliative Care Society).

Algorithm for Family and Patient Counseling on Mechanical Ventilation

1. Identify clinical team and patient, family, legal decision maker.
2. Explain reason for counseling and identify spokesperson from family to communicate.
3. Give overall history, pause for understanding and have family explain any other history. Use the opportunity to listen about functional status of the patient and level of health literacy. Explain all medical terms and offer to answer questions
4. Specifically for mechanical ventilation the process of intubation. Alternatives such as HFNC or NIV and benefits and risks are to be explained. The need for sedation, paralysis, restraints, enteral tubes, urinary catheters, central lines as well as benefits and complications of these are to be explained. In addition the possibility of tracheostomy in future if needed may be also brought in. In general this is a lot of information to process and must be documented. Despite best efforts the details will need to be repeated multiple times due to lack of understanding fatigue and information overload for patients and families
5. Daily progress on sedation vacation, spontaneous breathing trials and overall requirement of ventilatory support can be conveyed in general terms. For literate or medically trained family members more details may be needed but in general they must be allowed to maintain their role as family and not be unnecessarily burdened with details.
6. The risk of ventilator related complications including pneumothorax, infection, tube dislodgment and blocks must be watched for and family reassured that these are being monitored
7. Weaning and liberation from mechanical ventilation will need to be discussed on a daily basis and progress or lack of progress conveyed to the next of kin

References

1. West JB. The physiological challenges of the 1952 Copenhagen poliomyelitis epidemic and a renaissance in clinical respiratory physiology. J Appl Physiol (1985). 2005 Aug;99(2):424–32. doi: 10.1152/japplphysiol.00184.2005. PMID: 16020437; PMCID: PMC1351016.
2. [WHO. The World Health Report 2000: Health Systems: Improving Performance. Geneva, Switzerland: World Health Organization; 2000.
3. Volpato E, Banfi P, Pagnini F. Promoting Acceptance and Adherence to Noninvasive Ventilation in Chronic Obstructive Pulmonary Disease: A Randomized Controlled Trial. Psychosom Med. 2022 May 1;84(4):488-504. doi: 10.1097/PSY.0000000000001053. Epub 2022 Feb 10. PMID: 35149638; PMCID: PMC9071031.
4. Riley, JB, Cloonan, P, Norton, C (2006). Low Health Literacy. Critical Care Nursing Quarterly, 29 (2), 174–78.
5. Bogetz JF, Munjapara V, Henderson CM, Raisanen JC, Jabre NA, Shipman KJ, Wilfond BS, Boss RD. Home mechanical ventilation for children with severe neurological impairment: Parents' perspectives on clinician counselling. Dev Med Child Neurol. 2022 Jul;64(7):840-846. doi: 10.1111/dmcn.15151. Epub 2022 Jan 26. PMID: 35080259.
6. Volandes AE, Paasche-Orlow MK, Barry MJ, Gillick MR, Minaker KL, Chang Y, Cook EF, Abbo ED, El-Jawahri A, Mitchell SL. Video decision support tool for advance care planning in dementia: randomised controlled trial. BMJ. 2009 May 28;338:b2159. doi: 10.1136/bmj.b2159. PMID: 19477893; PMCID: PMC2688013.

7. Lee J, Ward NS. Emerging Ethical Challenges in Critical Care for the 21st Century: A Case-Based Discussion. Semin Respir Crit Care Med. 2019 Oct;40(5):655-661. doi: 10.1055/s-0039-1698408. Epub 2019 Dec 11. PMID: 31826266.
8. Lincoln TE, Buddadhumaruk P, Arnold RM, Scheunemann LP, Ernecoff NC, Chang CH, Carson SS, Hough CL, Curtis JR, Anderson W, Steingrub J, Peterson MW, Lo B, Matthay MA, White DB. Association between shared decision-making during family meetings and surrogates' trust in their ICU physician. Chest. 2022 Nov 3:S0012-3692(22)04043-0. doi: 10.1016/j.chest.2022.10.028. Epub ahead of print. PMID: 36336000.
9. Turner HC, Hao NV, Yacoub S, *et al*. Achieving affordable critical care in low-income and middle-income countries.BMJ Global Health 2019;4:e001675.
10. Chiarchiaro J, Buddadhumaruk P, Arnold RM, White DB. Quality of communication in the ICU and surrogate's understanding of prognosis. Crit Care Med. 2015 Mar;43(3):542-8. doi: 10.1097/CCM.0000000000000719. PMID: 25687030; PMCID: PMC4336600.
11. Burns KEA, McDonald E, Debigaré S, Zamir N, Vasquez M, Piche-Ayotte M, Oczkowski S; Canadian Critical Care Trials Group. Patient and family engagement in patient care and research in Canadian intensive care units: a national survey. Can J Anaesth. 2022 Dec;69(12):1527–36. doi: 10.1007/s12630-022-02342-w. Epub 2022 Nov 7. PMID: 36344874; PMCID: PMC9640777.
12. [https://main.mohfw.gov.in/sites/default/files/NFHS-5_Phase-II_0.pdf].
13. Peters, David H.; Yazbeck, Abdo S.; Sharma, Rashmi R.; Ramana, G. N. V.; Pritchett, Lant H.; Wagstaff, Adam.
Better health systems for India's poor: findings, analysis, and options (English). Health, nutrition, and population series Washington, DC: World Bank Group. http://documents.worldbank.org/curated/en/997121468034140238/Better-health-systems-for-Indias-poor-findings-analysis-and-options.
14 Peter JV, Thomas K, Jeyaseelan L, Yadav B, Sudarsan TI, Christina J, Revathi A, John KR, Sudarsanam TD. Cost of Intensive Care In India. Int J Technol Assess Health Care. 2016 Jan;32(4):241-245. doi: 10.1017/S0266462316000398. Epub 2016 Sep 9. PMID: 27608529.
15. Chen C, Wittenberg E, Sullivan SS, Lorenz RA, Chang YP. The Experiences of Family Members of Ventilated COVID-19 Patients in the Intensive Care Unit: A Qualitative Study. Am J Hosp Palliat Care. 2021 Jul;38(7):869-876. doi: 10.1177/10499091211006914. Epub 2021 Apr 1. PMID: 33789492; PMCID: PMC8020036.
16. Mani RK, Amin P, Chawla R, Divatia JV, Kapadia F, Khilnani P, Myatra SN, Prayag S, Rajagopalan R, Todi SK, Uttam R. Guidelines for end-of-life and palliative care in Indian intensive care units' ISCCM consensus Ethical Position Statement. Indian J Crit Care Med. 2012 Jul;16(3):166-81. doi: 10.4103/0972-5229.102112. PMID: 23188961; PMCID: PMC3506078.
17. Rose L, Istanboulian L, Amaral ACK, Burry L, Cox CE, Cuthbertson BH, Iwashyna TJ, Dale CM, Fraser I. Co-designed and consensus based development of a quality improvement checklist of patient and family-centered actionable processes of care for adults with persistent critical illness. J Crit Care. 2022 Dec;72:154153. doi: 10.1016/j.jcrc.2022.154153. Epub 2022 Sep 26. PMID: 36174432.
18. https://www.thoracic.org/patients/patient-resources/resources/mechanical-ventilation.pdf accessed December 18,2022.
19. Duffy EI, Garry J, Talbot L, Pasternak D, Flinn A, Minardi C, Dookram M, Grant K, Fitzgerald D, Rubano J, Vosswinkel J, Jawa RS. A pilot study assessing the spiritual, emotional, physical/environmental, and physiological needs of mechanically ventilated surgical intensive care unit patients via eye tracking devices, head nodding, and communication boards. Trauma Surg Acute Care Open. 2018 Sep 19;3(1):e000180. doi: 10.1136/tsaco-2018-000180. PMID: 30246152; PMCID: PMC6144907.

20. Tobiano G, Mackie BR. Routine activities in the intensive care unit provide opportunities for family engagement. Aust Crit Care 2021; 34: 113–5. https://doi.org/10.1016/j.aucc.2020.05.002
21. https://rtmagazine.com/disorders-diseases/critical-care/ards/a-successful-vap-prevention-program/
22. Berger Z, Flickinger TE, Pfoh E, Martinez KA, Dy Sm. Promoting engagement by patients and families to reduce adverse events in acute care settings: a systematic review. BMJ Qual Saf 2014; 23: 548–55. https://doi.org/10.1136/bmjqs-2012-001769
23. Patient-Centered Outcomes Research Institute. The value of engagement. Available from URL: https://www.pcori.org/ engagement/value-engagement (accessed June 2022).
24. Prey JE, Woollen J, Wilcox L, *et al*. Patient engagement in the inpatient setting: a systematic review. J Am Med Inform Assoc 2014; 21: 742–50. https://doi.org/10.1136/amiajnl-2013-002141.

CHAPTER 34

Thoracic Ultrasound in Ventilated Patients

❒ Manjush Karthika ❒ Chris Sara Mathew

ABSTRACT

Since the last two decades, point-of-care ultrasound is integrated in the critical care settings across the world, due to its clinical significance. Regarding ventilated patients, respiratory assessment using ultrasound facilitates the diagnostic accuracy in various areas such as airway management, lung aeration, abnormal presentations related to lung and pleura, optimizing ventilator settings, heart lung interactions and weaning from mechanical ventilation.

INTRODUCTION

Diagnostic ultrasound is a point-of-care imaging tool that is regularly used in acute care settings. Although radiology physicians are the first-hand practitioners of ultrasound, still with the scope of its relevance in intensive care units (ICUs), the critical care physicians have also started mastering this practice. The multidisciplinary team comprising of nurses and respiratory therapists alongside the physicians, are actively involved in the care of ICU patients.[1] Their scope of practice differs; however, the role of these professionals is pivotal in the management of ventilated patients, from intubation to extubation. Since mechanical ventilation is vital for many critically ill patients[2], the initiation, monitoring and discontinuation are of utmost importance, to balance the patient outcome. While switching from spontaneous breathing to positive-pressure ventilation and vice versa, a series of physiological changes including changes in intrathoracic pressure may alter the heart, lung, and diaphragm interactions. During the liberation phase from ventilator, any such altered dysfunction may even lead to weaning failure.[3] Ultrasound, because of its superior diagnostic accuracy, has been used to identify some of the risk factors or complications such as weaning failure and extubation failure, associated with mechanical ventilation. For example, echocardiographic evidence of poor left ventricular diastolic function is an indicator of potential weaning failure, and lung aeration loss defined by lung ultrasound is an accurate predictor of respiratory distress in post-extubation phase. Literature suggests that the utility of echocardiography and LUS are useful in predicting the accuracy of weaning outcomes.[4] On the other hand, in some patients with normal cardiorespiratory mechanics, diaphragmatic evaluation can predict weaning outcome, as some of these patients are presented with diaphragmatic dysfunctions.[5] This chapter details the importance of airway, lung, cardiac and diaphragmatic ultrasound in the management of the mechanically ventilated critically ill patients.

PHYSICS AND TECHNICAL DETAILS

The frequencies of ultrasound waves are higher than the upper limit of the human audible range, i.e., 2–20 kHz. Diagnostic ultrasound in medical science typically uses frequencies that range between 2 and 20MHz. Ultrasound waves are generated by piezoelectric crystals present under the the head of the ultrasound probe.[6] The probe which used by the operator to examine a specific body part for visualization is the transducer. The piezoelectric crystals are arranged in a row just beneath the scanning interface of the probe. When electrical energy is conducted through these crystals of the transducer, it deforms the crystals resulting in the production of ultrasound waves. These waves are then transmitted, attenuated, absorbed, reflected, refracted, and diffracted by the adjacent tissues or medium.[7] Crystals spend only 1% of the time for generating the sound waves from the tissues and the remaining 99% for processing the returning echo thus effectively translating them for image.[8] Although most of the energy is reflected back, the difference in the acoustic impedance of various tissues changes the ultrasound signal strength. This provides information regarding the location and characteristics of tissues, and these data are processed into grayscale images, on which the technology of ultrasound is based.[9] Another aspect is echogenicity, i.e., the presentation of various tissues/media upon the transmission of ultrasound waves.[10] Hence the images produced will be of different contrast when the ultrasound waves pass through tissues of different echogenicity. Based on which the images are classified as hyperechoic (white), hypoechoic (gray), anechoic (black), and isoechoic (echogenicity similar as the neighbouring structure). As the energy sources are different, the production and interpretation of ultrasound images differ from those of radiographic images. Most of the modern ICU ultrasound machines are usually portable, lightweight, and have built-in memory to store images and videos. Various types of probes are available based on the design, size, and frequency and the most utilized in the acute care settings are linear, curvilinear, and phased array probes (**Fig. 34.1**).[1]

- Linear array probes: This is a high frequency probe with frequency ranging between 5 and 18 MHz, designed specifically for examination of superficial structures such as trachea, pleura, and blood vessels.
- Curvilinear array probes: This is a low frequency probe with frequency range between 1 and 5 MHz, designed for examination of structures lying deeper such as diaphragm, abdomen, and pelvis. This is also useful in the assessment of effusions, consolidated lung, and the diaphragm because of good penetration and large sector width.
- Phased array probes: This also is a low frequency probe with frequency range 1 and 5 MHz, specifically designed for echocardiography. These probes have a small footprint for fitting between the ribs to demonstrate all the signs of LUS, but the image clarity of the images is not as good compared to linear or curvilinear probes

Even though most of the ultrasound machines are similar in their operational features, there are difference in their designs based on different manufacturers. Hence it is important for the clinicians to become familiar with the modes and control interface of the specific machine before the scan.

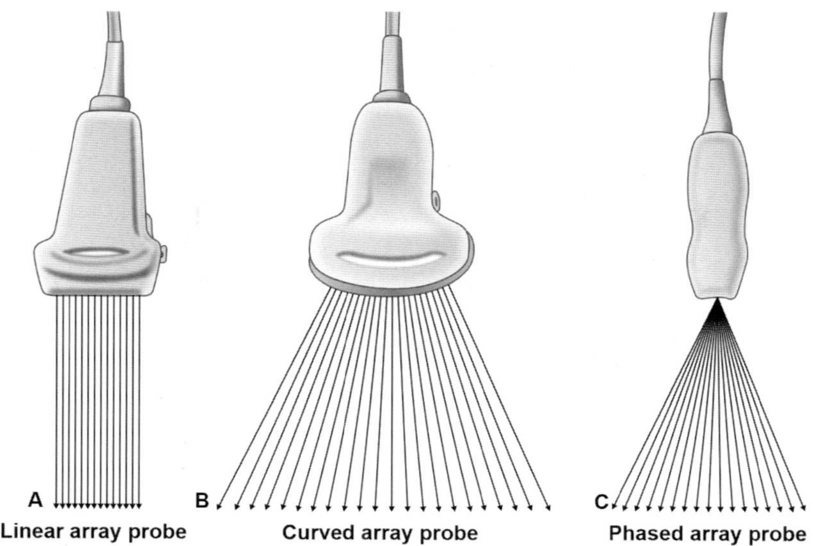

Fig. 34.1: Different types of ultrasound probes[1]

AIRWAY ULTRASOUND

Traditionally tracheal intubation is confirmed by methods such as direct visualization, chest rise, 5-point auscultation, colorimetry, esophageal detector devices, and by the end-tidal CO_2 detection which is the gold standard for the same.[11] Ultrasound has gained popularity in airway management, specifically in the confirmation of endotracheal intubation with the real time scan using a linear ultrasound probe longitudinally and transversely on the anterior aspect of the neck at the level of the cricothyroid membrane, cricoid cartilage, and tracheal cartilages. In the longitudinal scan, the cricoid cartilage will appear as a hypoechoic hump, and the tracheal cartilages appear as a "string of beads", with the thyroid cartilage and cricothyroid membrane on upward sliding of the probe **(Fig. 34.2)**. In the transverse plane tracheal rings forms the air-mucosal interfaces and comet tail artifacts are seen **(Fig. 34.3)**. The cricoid cartilage appears as an inverted 'U' in the transverse plane **(Fig. 34.4)**. The reverberation artifacts produced by the air-mucosal interface will be seen at the tracheal level images.[12]

When the endotracheal tube, passes through the trachea, it will appear as a bright hyperechoic fluttering structure, producing comet-tail artifacts due to acoustic shadowing. The esophagus is identifiable deep on the left side of the trachea if the patient is asked to perform swallow movement before the induction.[13] If the tube enters the esophagus, the collapsed appearing esophagus will appear dilated with a bright hyperechoic curved line with distal dark shadow, on the left-posterior side of the trachea. This will appear as two tracts, hence the name 'double tract sign' **(Fig. 34.5)**.[14].

Another important use of airway ultrasound is the determination of endotracheal tube insertion depth by measuring distance between the proximal edge of the endotracheal tube cuff and vocal cords. Although the role of ultrasound in ETT insertion depth was put forward in 1987,[15] there remains a paucity of literature support on this, except

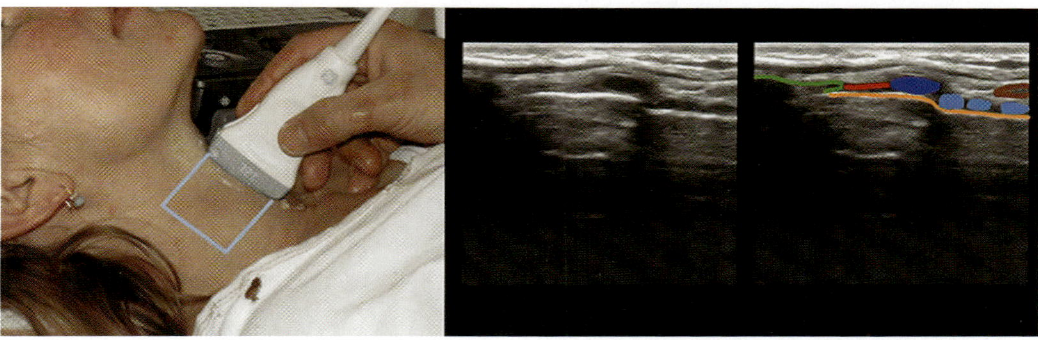

Fig. 34.2: The longitudinal airway approach: (1) thyroid cartilage (green); (2) cricothyroid membrane (red); (3) cricoid cartilage as a 'hypoechoic hump' (dark blue) and (4) the tracheal cartilages appear as a 'string of beads' light blue)[54]

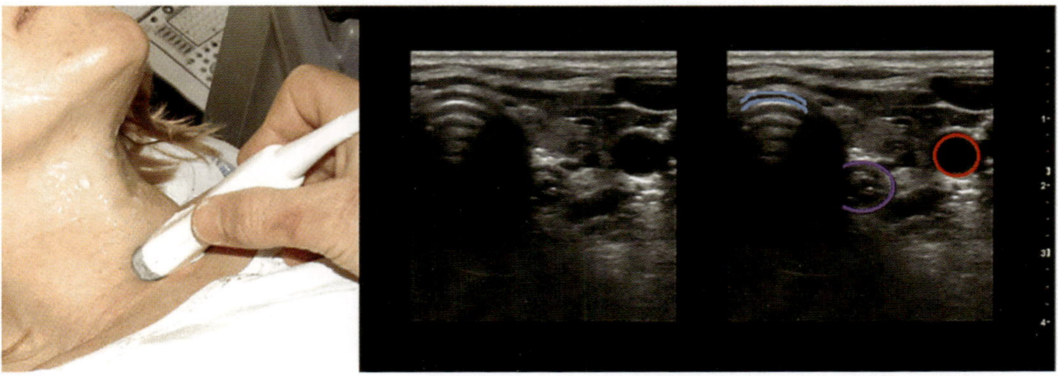

Fig. 34.3: The transverse approach cranial to suprasternal notch and to patient's left side of trachea: (1) Anterior part of tracheal cartilages (light blue), (2) esophagus (purple), (3) carotid artery (red)[54]

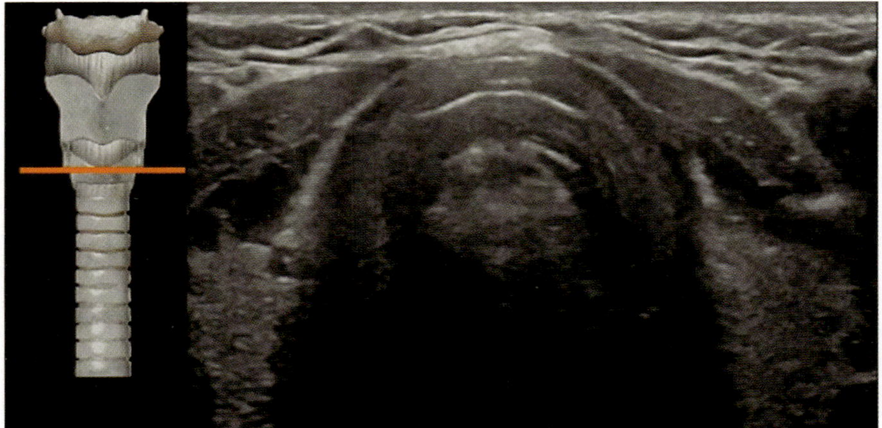

Fig. 34.4: The transverse approach at cricoid cartilage level shows an inverted 'U' appearance of cricoid cartilage[54]

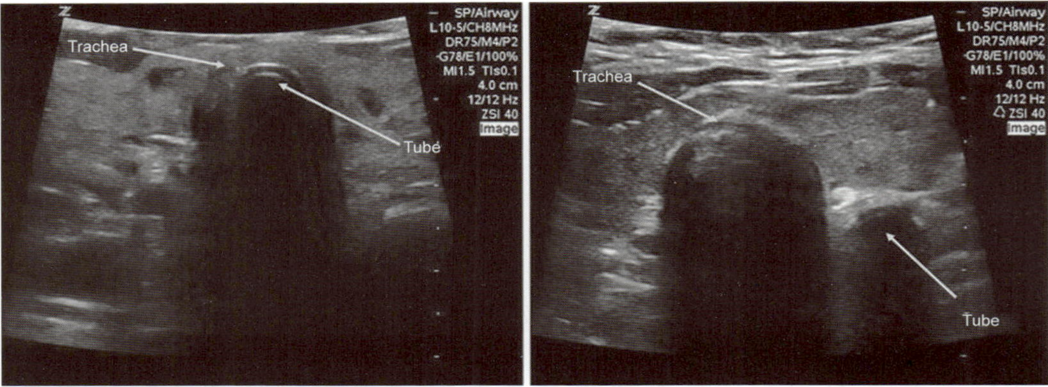

Fig. 34.5: The transverse approach at suprasternal level: On the left: a normal endotracheal intubation is shown with the echogenic semicircular tube visible within the lumen of the trachea. On the right: an esophageal intubation can be identified by the presence of a 'double tract sign' with a second semicircular shadows appearing outside of the trachea[55]

some anecdotal studies. The optimal ETT placement warrants a distance of 2–5 cm between the tip of the ETT and the carina to avoid endobronchial displacement of accidental extubation.[16] And a sufficient distance of 1.5–2.5 cm is required between the upper margin of the cuff to the vocal cords.[17,18] Available literaure suggests that ultrasonographic assessment of a saline-filled ETT cuff at the suprasternal notch is an accurate, objective and rapid way to confirm the optimal ETT insertion depth, thereby to prevent untoward events.[19, 20]

LUNG ULTRASOUND

The advancement of lung ultrasound (LUS) in recent years with better quality and spatial resolution has resulted in greater diagnostic accuracy. Some of the advantages of LUS over chest radiograph and computed tomography include availability, portability, absence of radiation, real-time imaging, documentation, and reproducibility of findings. Hence, in the past two decades, LUS has become a prominent diagnostic tool for assessment and decision-making in care of the ventilated patient. The commonly used modes while performing LUS are the B-mode and M-mode. B-mode, or brightness mode, is the basic mode of ultrasound imaging; it is also known as grayscale or 2-dimensional imaging, which refers to the standard black and white image obtained on the ultrasound monitor. On the other side, M-mode, or motion mode, is used to visualize targets that are physically moving or dynamic, and to assess the movement of structures over time. The LUS examination consists of 12 imaging zones, 6 on each side of thorax. The upper and basal part of each hemithorax is divided into anterior, lateral, and posterior zones, defined by the anterior and posterior axillary lines.[21] It is recommended that to master this LUS imaging technique, one should have a clear understanding of the 7 principles and 10 basic signs of LUS, along with the required skills.

Following are the 7 principles of LUS, as described by Dr Lichtenstein in his work in 2004, with an update on the seventh principle:[22,23]

1. A simple, unsophisticated ultrasound machine is adequate to perform LUS.

2. Artifacts are generated in the thorax because gas and fluids have opposite locations or are mingled by pathologic processes.
3. The lung is the most voluminous organ in the body with an extensive surface area (about 1,500 cm^2). Thus, precise areas need to be defined.
4. All lung signs arise from the pleural line.
5. LUS is largely based on the analysis of artifacts generated, and previously this was addressed as an issue to indicate the infeasibility of LUS.
6. The lung is a vital organ and hence lung signs arising from the pleural line are dynamic.
7. A majority of acute, life-threatening lung disorders abut the pleural line, explaining the potential of LUS. Almost all life-threatening disorders, even those that may be less prominent in other tests, will show an extensive location with LUS, such as a pneumothorax, which can be small but still visible in a reasonably large projection.

The basic 10 signs of LUS are:

1. The baseline normal image obtained during LUS is the pleural line or the bat-wing sign
2. The second sign is the A-line or A-profile, which is a static sign seen in B-mode. These fundamental, hyperechoic, reverberation artifacts of pleural lines are seen normally and are confirmatory for the presence of physiological or free air in thorax
3. Lung sliding is the third sign, and it is normal and dynamic in nature and is seen in B-mode at the same level of pleural line. Lung sliding is synchronized with breathing, as the lungs descend toward the abdomen on inspiration. Lung sliding reflects the normal physiological movement of the lung toward the chest wall.
4. The fourth sign is the quad sign: It is an abnormal static LUS sign seen in B-mode, and it indicates the presence of a pleural effusion and is limited by 4 regular borders
5. The fifth sign is the sinusoid sign, which is an abnormal dynamic LUS sign seen in M-mode, and it indicates the presence of a pleural effusion
6. The sixth sign mentioned is the shred sign, which is an abnormal sign seen in the B-mode. The shred sign represents non-translobar consolidation in most cases. The shred sign is formed when the border between consolidated and aerated lung is irregular, forming the fractal line, which is fully opposed to the lung line. This is a suggestive sign of pneumonia.
7. The seventh sign is the tissue-like sign, an abnormal sign that is observed in B-mode when there is a translobar consolidation. When the lung is excessively filled with fluid, its echogenicity bears a resemblance to the liver, which is also called hepatization of lung.
8. The eighth sign, and one of the most important, is the B-line/lung rocket/comet tail artifacts. B-lines are seen in B-mode, and they are hyperechoic, long, vertical lines that originate from the pleural line and traverse the entire ultrasound screen, down to the bottom of the screen, erasing the normal A-lines. The presence of B-lines is highly suggestive of alevolar-interstitial syndromes, ARDS, and pulmonary edema. B-lines are also known as lung rockets or comet tail artifacts.
9. The ninth sign is the absent lung sliding, which is an abnormal sign observed in the B-mode and is one of the 3 findings to confirm pneumothorax. The presence of air in

the pleural space prevents the visualization of visceral pleura, and lung sliding will not be seen. The typical back and forth movement of the pleural line with breathing will not be seen if there is any pleural involvement such as pneumothorax.

10. The tenth sign is the lung point, which is an abnormal sign seen in the M-mode. Lung point is the point at which the 2 pleural layers re-join one another. Lung point is considered as confirmatory for pneumothorax, provided lung sliding and B-lines are absent.

Since respiratory mechanics is dynamic, LUS requires a structured team effort with standardized reports of detailed examination and scoring, for continuous comparisons and monitoring. Lung aeration loss can be estimated using a validated score called the Lung Ultrasound Score. The LUS score of aeration is calculated for each given region of interest. Points are allocated according to the worst ultrasound pattern observed (**Fig. 34.6**). The lung fields will be scanned by dividing the thorax into 12 zones: 6 on the right (anterior: Upper R1 and lower R2; lateral: Upper R3 and lower R4; posterior: Upper R5 and lower R6) and 6 on the left side (front: upper L1 and lower L2; lateral: Upper L3 and lower L4; rear: Upper L5 and lower L6) (**Fig. 34.7**). For each zone, the scoring criteria assigns 0 points to A lines or <2 separate B lines plus regular sliding; 1 point with lines B ≥ 3 or spaced focal points plus regular sliding; 2 points with coalescing B lines, and 3 points to pulmonary consolidations with a total LUS score ranging from 0 (normal lungs) to 36 (worst scenario).[24] It is also understood that LUS score of aeration changes during a successful spontaneous breathing trial can accurately predict post-extubation distress, i.e. a LUS score of <13 predicts successful extubation, whereas a LUS score of >17 is considered a threshold for post-extubation distress and extubation failure.

Selecting Optimal PEEP

Selection of optimal positive end-expiratory pressure (PEEP) in mechanical ventilation remains debatable in the management of patients with acute respiratory distress syndrome (ARDS). This is because of the varying lung morphology in ARDS patients i.e., in focal ARDS only the dependent areas are usually affected, and in diffuse ARDS where both dependent and nondependent areas are affected. So, it is important to balance re-aeration of collapsed areas to the over distention of non-collapsed areas. LUS being a real-time monitoring tool is found to be useful in this regard. The PEEP titration may be performed as below phases (**Fig. 34.8**).[25]

1. Baseline evaluation of lung morphology with a PEEP of 5 cm H_2O: If normal patterns (A-lines) are observed in the anterior areas of chest wall, this indicates a focal aeration loss on the dependent areas. If well-separated/coalescent B-lines are found in the anterior scan, it represents diffused aeration loss.
2. In case of anterior focal aeration loss, low levels of PEEP (≤ 10 cm H_2O) may be used, however overdistention cannot be identified by LUS. These are candidates for prone ventilation.
3. In case of patients with diffuse loss of aeration, higher level of PEEP (12–16 cm H_2O) can be used. While increasing PEEP, the aeration improvement needs to be monitored by LUS exam of anterior zones. It is suggested to increase the PEEP to 3–4 cm H_2O, until the anterior zones with moderate or severe aeration loss (respectively separated and coalescent B-lines) present normal profile (A-lines).

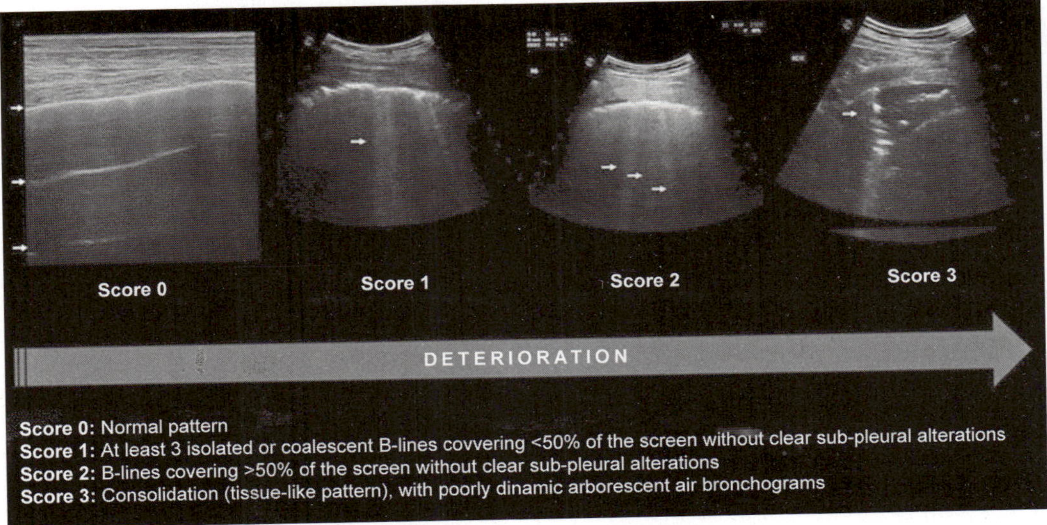

Fig. 34.6: Lung ultrasound severity scoring[56]

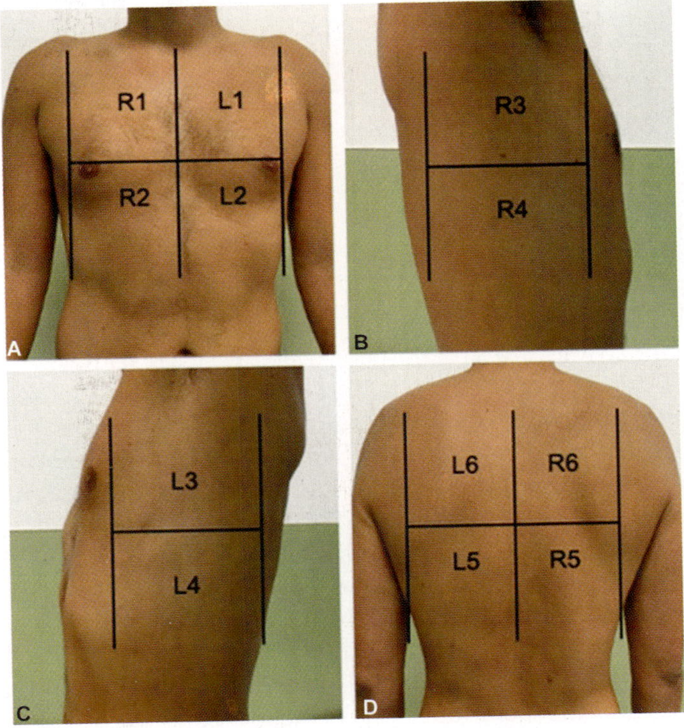

Fig. 34.7: 12 zones of thorax for LUS screening[57]

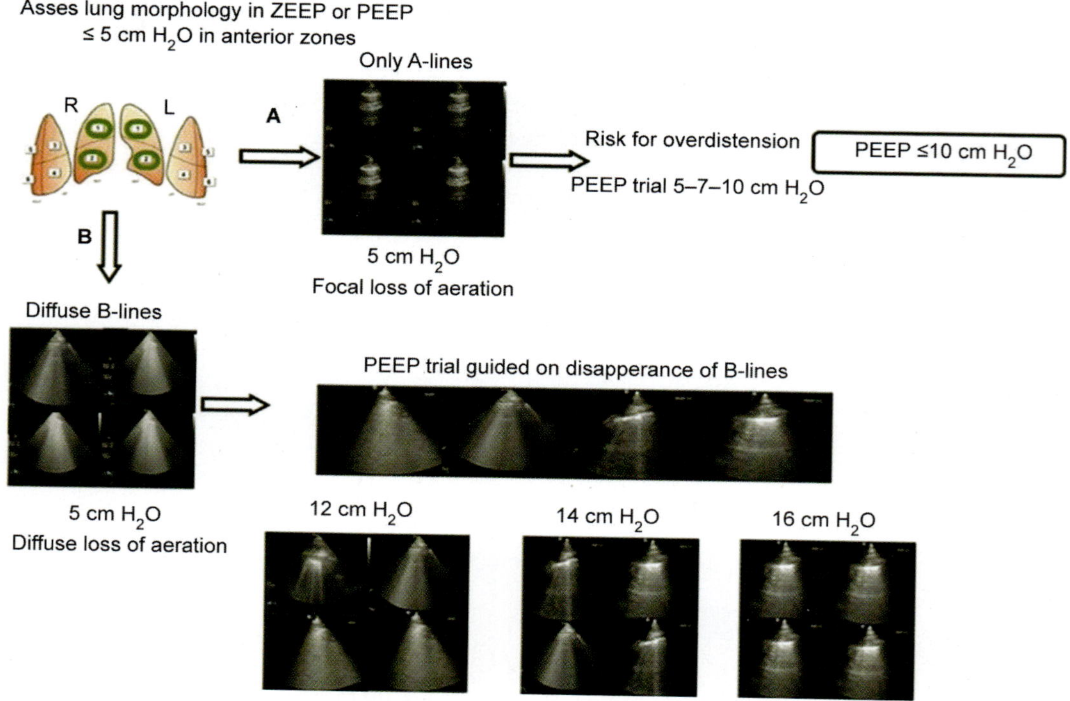

Fig. 34.8: Lung ultrasound to titrate PEEP in ARDS patients[25]

4. The clinician needs to be cautious of over distending the recruited anterior zones, while attempting an increase in PEEP to clear the B-lines in the lateral and posterior zones.

Recruitment Manoeuvres

Recruitment manoeuvres are ventilatory strategies used to open-up the atelectatic lung zones by brief and controlled increment in airway pressures. However, the quantification of optimal pressures for recruitment is still debatable. Unsolved question is how to assess such RM at the bedside. There are literaure support for utilizing LUS as an effective real-time tool to perform and customize recruitment manoeuvres at the bedside.[26] Recruitment manoeuvres mainly benefits anterior and lateral parts of the lung zones, whereas marginal benefits for dorsal dependent lung zones. The effectiveness of recruitment manoeuvres can be visualized as real-time improvement in the aeration lung regions with the disappearance of B lines. Re-aeration will be seen as a sequential pattern, where consolidated pattern to multiple B lines to one or two B lines to normal lung images with A lines. The probe then is placed on the contralateral lung in the same position to confirm normal aeration. This is considered as the opening pressure. After the recruitment manoeuvres a step-wise decrement in PEEP is done to identify the lung's closing pressure. During this process the probe is kept in the same position on the affected lung. The aerated lung zones will transform with decremental PEEP with the presence of B-lines and later with the consolidated pattern, which will define the closing pressure **(Fig. 34.9)**. Identifying the closing pressure will help the clinician to set the optimal PEEP as 2 cm H_2O above the closing pressure.[27,28] If required, the recruitment manoeuvres may be repeated with the targetted opening and closing pressures.

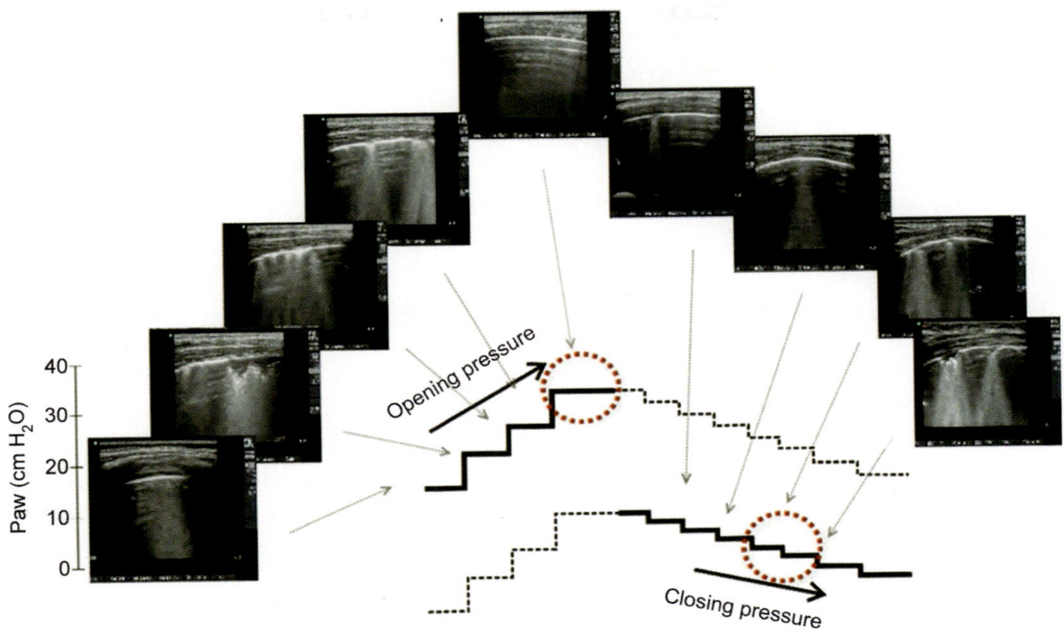

Fig. 34.9: Utility of LUS in recruitment manoeuvres[26]

Prone Ventilation

Prone positioning is widely practiced as one of the important therapeutic approaches for acute respiratory distress syndrome (ARDS). Diseases lungs with diffused patchy loss of aeration usually respond well to recruitment manoeuvres whereas lungs with predominant focal involvement (posteroinferior consolidations) respond better to prone position. However, until the evolution of ultrasound practices in the ICU, there were no effective tools to assess the aeration improvement at the bedside while the patient is on prone position. Literature states that patients with focal loss of aeration on the dorsal dependant lung region, compared to diffuse involvement showed a greater improvement of aeration in prone position.[29] Another study focussed LUS examination on prone ventilation, examined the patients scan zones with the paravertebral line, scapular line, and posterior axillary line, dividing the dorsum of the one side into 3 regions, then every region was divided into 3 equal areas to get 9 examination areas. The aeration of these areas significantly improved after 3 hours of prone positioning in responders. It is also understood that a significant re-aeration of dorsal regions during the first cycle of pronation identified the "long-term" responders to prone position, i.e., a PaO_2/FiO_2 ratio >300 mmHg after 7 days of 6-hour prone position twice daily.[30]

Identifying the Complications

Pneumothorax and ventilator-associated pneumonia (VAP) are the common complications seen in ventilated patients. Accurate diagnosis and timely intervention have been shown to improve the outcome of such presentations. Clinical examinations and imaging methods such as chest X-ray or computed tomography are used for conventional assessment of pneumothorax and VAP; however these imaging techniques are not possible during the real-time assessment of these critical patients. Hence, bedside LUS has been increasingly in recommendation for the continuous monitoring of ventilated patients.

Pneumothorax

Of all the ventilator associated complications, pneumothorax was found to be an independent predictor of mortality during mechanical ventilation and was also associated with significant increase in morbidities such as increased length of ICU and hospital stay.[1] LUS is found to be 78–90% sensitive and >98% sensitive in the detection of pneumothorax.[31] The ultrasonic findings of pneumothorax include abolished lung sliding, absence of B lines, absence of the lung pulse, and presence of the lung point.[32] The sequential assessment of pneumothorax starts with looking for the presence of lung sliding on the highest point of the anterior chest that excludes pneumothorax within seconds. If lung sliding is absent, then the presence of B-lines is checked, to rule out pneumothorax. If there is no sliding and no B lines, then the 'lung point' should be sought, which confirms the presence of pneumothorax.

M-mode is also used to confirm absent lung sliding. Presence of lung sliding will appear as a linear and grainy image, i.e. "seashore sign" (**Fig. 34.10**). And the M-mode image in a pneumothorax will only display one pattern of parallel horizontal lines above and below the pleural line, demonstrating the lack of movement. This pattern bears a resemblance to a 'barcode' and is often termed as 'barcode sign' or 'stratosphere sign' (**Fig. 34.11**).[1]

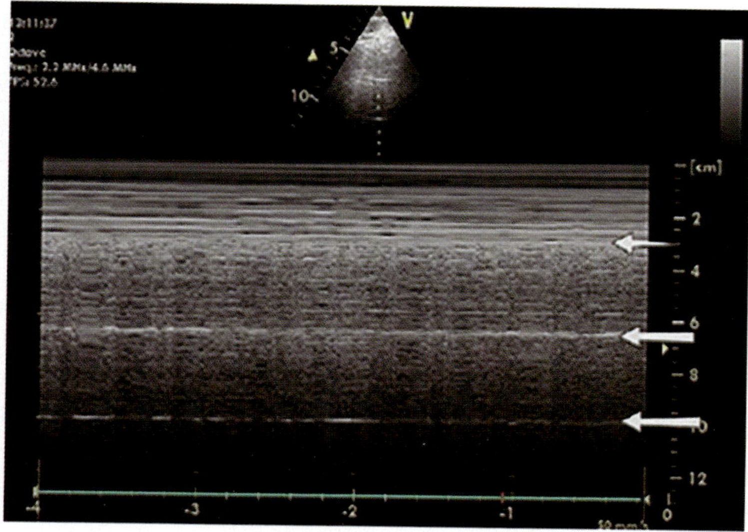

Fig. 34.10: 'Seashore sign' (normal) as seen in M-mode[1]

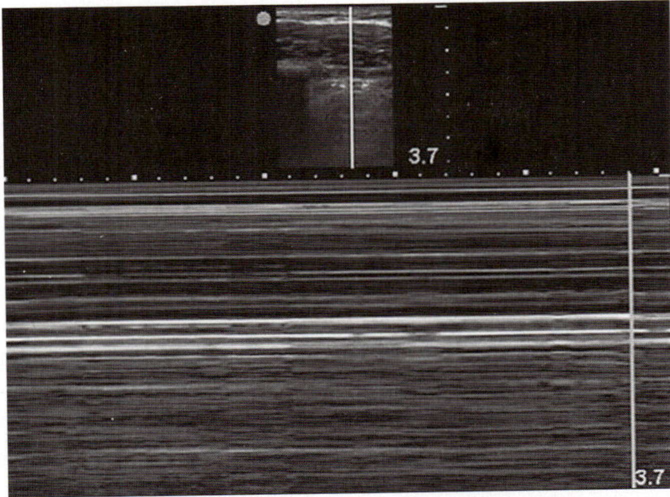

Fig. 34.11: 'Stratosphere/ Barcode sign' (pneumothorax) as seen in M-mode[1]

Ventilator-Associated Pneumonia

VAP remains as one of the major complications in intubated critical patients resulting in hypoxemia and other infectious cascades. LUS, being a bedside tool has the potential for early VAP diagnosis.

The diagnosis of VAP mainly relies on the positive culture of secretion samples; but it takes 24–48 hours for the microbiological results. LUS identifies patients at high risk for VAP, while awaiting the microbiology results.[33]

Conventionally, VAP is suspected when the chest X-ray shows a new infiltrate with fever/hypothermia, leukocytosis/leukopenia, purulent tracheal secretions, and impaired oxygenation. A combination of these clinical findings named as Clinical Pulmonary Infection Score (CPIS) is widely in use for VAP diagnosis, with a score of; 0 to 6 points: Less likely pneumonia; and 7–12: More likely pneumonia.

A new score: The VAP lung ultrasound score (VPLUS) **(Table 34.1)** integrating the lab findings and quantitative analysis of endotracheal aspirate with the LUS findings (two or more focal subpleural consolidations or one or more dynamic air bronchograms) was found to be superior to the CPIS alone in diagnosing VAP.[34] A VPLUS of ≥2 is suggestive of VAP with 71% sensitivity and 69% specificity, with increasing score with confirmed diagnosis **(Table 34.1)**.

Table 34.1: Ventilator-associated pneumonia lung ultrasound score (VPLUS)

Parameter	VPLUS
Two or more areas with subpleural consolidations	1
One or more area with dynamic arborescent/linear air bronchograms	2
Purulent ET aspirate	1
Endotracheal aspirate (EA) + quantitative/qualitative culture	1

HEART LUNG INTERACTION

The main function of the right heart is to maintain adequate pulmonary perfusion pressure to deliver desaturated mixed venous blood to the alveolar level, and low systemic venous pressure to prevent organ congestion. Hypoxia induced by ARDS will result in pulmonary vasoconstriction. Pulmonary vasoconstriction is not only by hypoxia but also by the deranged pulmonary capillary coagulation, resulting in microvascular obstruction in the lung. Lung protective mechanical ventilation with low tidal volume may also result in hypercapnia in ARDS patients, worsening the pulmonary vasoconstriction, thereby increasing pulmonary vascular resistance.[35] Furthermore, microvascular obstruction and inflammation in ARDS contributes to increased afterload of right ventricle resulting in right heart failure.[36] Since the right heart failure contributes to impaired pulmonary circulation, the left heart will also be affected with low cardiac output, decreased systemic hypotension, resulting in impaired global perfusion. Hence mechanical ventilation has a contributing role in acute cor pulmonale and right ventricular failure, as the right of right heart relies on the intrapleural pressure, gas exchange, and the balance between lung recruitment and overdistension.[37] Due to its easy availability and early application, ultrasound has become an important tool in the management of ventilated patients while evaluating their cardiac function due to the complex heart-lung interaction.[38]

Acute cor pulmonale is the acute increased right ventricular afterload, which results in right ventricular dilatation and may compromise the left ventricular filling. Right ventricular volume overload is defined as dilatation of the right ventricle that can be easily identified by echocardiography, while right ventricular pressure overload is defined as dyskinetic movement of the septum during end-systole. Right ventricular volume and right ventricular pressure could interact with each other.[39,40]

There are many echocardiographic manifestations of acute cor pulmonale. One of the simplest criteria to identify acute cor pulmonale in a ventilated patient includes (i) a severe dilatation of the right ventricle and (ii) a paradoxical septal motion with the "D-shape" of the restricted left ventricle, compromising left ventricular diastolic phase. Such a presentation reflects right ventricular failure due to systolic overload (sudden increase in the right ventricular afterload)[38] **(Fig. 34.12)**. A simplified conceptual representation is shown in **Fig. 34.13**.

A statement from the Heart Failure Association and the Working Group on Pulmonary Circulation and Right Ventricular Function of the European Society of Cardiology highlighted on 12 echocardiographic parameters to assess the right ventricular failure, which were (i) pericardial fluid >5 mm in diastole; (ii) RV wall thickness >5 mm; (iii) inferior vena cava diameter >21 mm, inspiration collapse <50% suggests high RA pressure; (iv) tricuspid regurgitation peak systolic velocity of TR > 2.8 m/s; (v) tricuspid annular plane systolic excursion TAPSE <17 mm; (vi) right ventricle dilation RVEDD/LVEDD > 1.0, right ventricle basal diameter >41 mm; (vii) right ventricle fractional area change, FAC <35%; (viii) ventricular interdependence: septal shift, D-shaped left ventricle; (ix) systolic S′ velocity of tricuspid annulus <9.5 cm/s by Doppler Tissue Imaging; (x) longitudinal strain of right ventricle free wall <20%; (xi) right ventricular index of myocardial performance, RIMP >0.54 by Doppler Tissue Imaging; and (xii) 3D right ventricular ejection fraction <45%.[41]

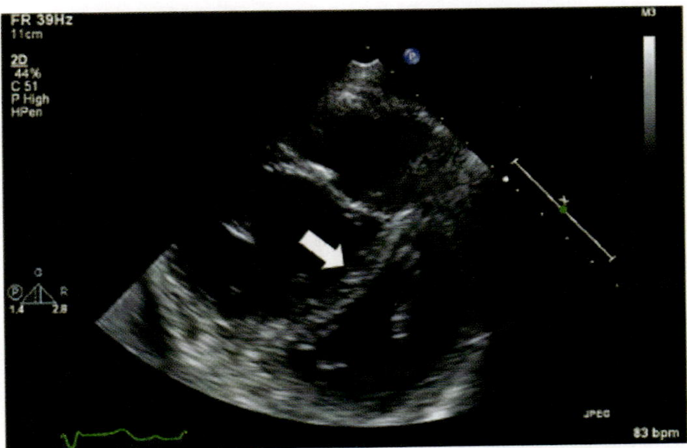

Fig. 34.12: Echocardiographic short-axis view showing the enlarged right ventricle pushing the interventricular septum toward the left ventricle, resulting in the shape of the left ventricle from its normal circular cross-section to a "D" shape.

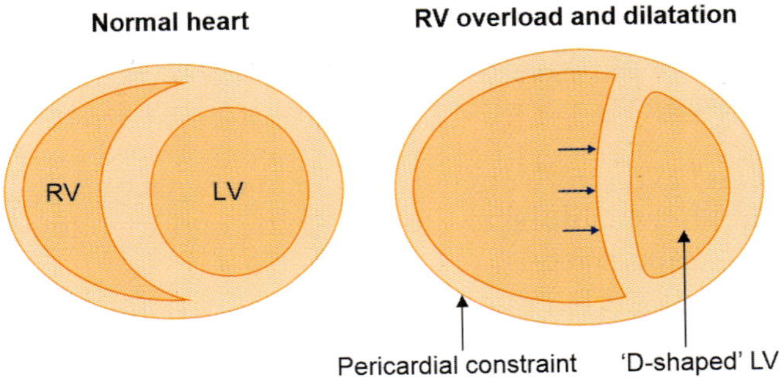

Fig. 34.13: Diagrammatic representation of normal right and left ventricles, compared with the dilated right ventricle and 'D' shaped ventricle following acute cor pulmonale

DIAPHRAGMATIC ULTRASOUND

Over the last two decades, diaphragmatic ultrasound evolved as an important tool to assess the indices such as diaphragmatic excursion, thickness, and thickness fraction. These indices are found to be useful to identify the diaphragmatic size and movement over time, to diagnose diaphragmatic dysfunction and to predict the likelihood of successful weaning.

Diaphragm excursion is usually assessed by a curvilinear array probe, with the probe positioned in the subcostal margin in the mid-clavicular line, to scan the posterior third of the diaphragm (**Fig. 34.14**). B-mode is used to optimize a better position of the probe to yield a good visualization of each hemi-diaphragmatic movement. To record the movement of right hemidiaphragm, the liver is used as a window, and for the left hemidiaphragm, spleen window is used. After obtaining a good window of each hemidiaphragm by B-mode, the machine is switched to M-mode to display the motion of the diaphragm along the selected line.

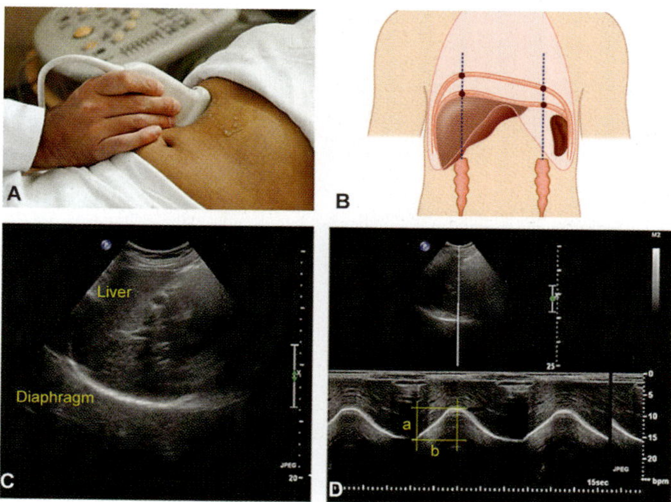

Fig. 34.14: (A) Transducer placement for the anterior subcostal view, with the transducer positioned below the costal margin in the mid-clavicular line; (B) Pathway of ultrasound beam image the diaphragm; (C) B-mode view of the diaphragm with the anterior subcostal approach; (D) M-mode view of diaphragm motion with an anterior subcostal view. "a" represents the amplitude of excursion during deep breathing and "b" represents the time taken for diaphragm contraction, which is used to calculate velocity of movement[44]

The inspiratory and expiratory craniocaudal movements of both hemidiaphragms, (appears as a bright line), resulting in the shortening and a lengthening of the probe-diaphragm distance, respectively.

M-modes are preferable to examine diaphragmatic excursion, due to its real time imaging and precise measurement of diaphragmatic displacement during a respiratory cycle. Excursion is known to positively correlate with inspiratory lung volumes and is higher during forced inspiration. The normal excursion from the resting expiratory position to full inspiration in adults has been reported in the range of 10 to 25 mm, with higher values reported in deep breathing or sniff. However, diaphragmatic excursion of the ventilated patients is affected by the pressure support provided and the active and passive displacement cannot be distinguished. Instead, the active contractility of the diaphragm can be assessed by an increase in diaphragmatic thickness during respiratory efforts, and by the diaphragmatic thickening ratio.

Diaphragmatic thickness is measured in the zone of apposition, using the curvilinear probe or linear array probe (**Fig. 34.15**). The diaphragm is viewed as a three-layered structure, sandwiched between the two echogenic layers of the pleura and the peritoneum. The thickness can be measured by both the B- and M-modes. Diaphragmatic thickness is correlated with the strength of the diaphragm,[42] but not with the endurance.[43] The thickness can be measured at end expiration or end inspiration, and in both tidal and maximal inspiration.

The average thickness of the diaphragm is 0.22–0.28 cm in healthy people and 0.13–0.19 cm in patients with paralyzed diaphragm. A diaphragm thickness less than 0.2 cm, measured at the end of expiration, has been proposed as the cut-off to define diaphragm

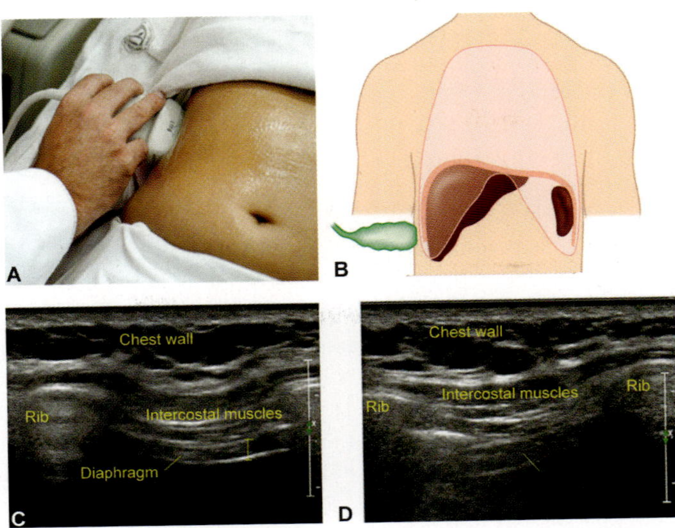

Fig. 34.15: (A) Intercostal view, with the transducer placed on the 9th intercostal space in the anterior axillary line; (B) Diaphragm visualized at the zone of apposition using this approach; (C) B-mode ultrasonography image of the diaphragm; (D) 'Peeling away' of the diaphragm from the chest wall with inspiration with the downward displacement of the lung[44]

atrophy.[44] Diaphragmatic thickness ratio is an indicator of work of breathing.[45] This is used to compare the expiratory and inspiratory thickness, which is obtained from the formula [(End Inspiratory Thickness – End Expiratory Thickness)/End Expiratory Thickness].[46]

Diaphragmatic ultrasound is useful in predicting the weaning outcome. During spontaneous breathing trials, diaphragmatic excursion cut-off values of $<$14 mm[47,48] and $<$11 mm.[49] have both been found to be predictive of weaning failure. The diaphragmatic thickness ratios of $<$20%,[50] $<$30%,[51] and $<$36%[52] are also found to be useful in predicting weaning failure. It is reported that a thickening fraction less than 20% or a diaphragmatic excursion $<$10 mm is an indicator of diaphragmatic dysfunction.[5] It is also documented that a diaphragmatic excursion of 11–14 mm and the thickness ratio of 30–36%, can predict successful extubation with low risk of reintubation in the first hours.[53]

Conclusion

Airway, lung, and diaphragmatic ultrasound provide vital information to enhance the assessment and management of the ventilated patients. Respiratory application of ultrasound also appears to be a promising tool that offers a better diagnostic accuracy in resource and time limited settings.

References

1. Karthika M, Wong D, Nair SG, Pillai LV, Mathew CS. Lung Ultrasound: The Emerging Role of Respiratory Therapists. Respir Care. 2019 Feb;64(2):217–29.
2. Matamis D, Soilemezi E, Tsagourias M, Akoumianaki E, Dimassi S, Boroli F, *et al*. Sonographic evaluation of the diaphragm in critically ill patients. Technique and clinical applications. Intensive Care Med. 2013; 39:801–10.

3. Haji K, Haji D, Canty DJ, The impact of heart, lung and diaphragmatic ultrasound on prediction of failed extubation from mechanical ventilation in critically ill patients: A prospective observational pilot study: Crit Ultrasound J, 2018; 10; 13.
4. Mongodi S, Via G, Bouhemad B, Usefulness of combined bedside lung ultrasound and echocardiography to assess weaning failure from mechanical ventilation: A suggestive case: Crit Care Med, 2013; 41; e182-5
5. DiNino E, Gartman EJ, Sethi JM, McCool FD, Diaphragm ultrasound as a predictor of successful extubation from mechanical ventilation: Thorax, 2014; 69; 423–27.
6. Hangiandreou NJ. AAPM/RSNA physics tutorial for residents. Topics in US: B-mode US: basic concepts and new technology. Radiographics 2003;23(4):1019–33.
7. Aldrich JE. Basic physics of ultrasound imaging. Crit Care Med 2007;35(5 Suppl):S131–S137.
8. Szabo TL, Lewin PA. Ultrasound transducer selection in clinical imaging practice. J Ultrasound Med. 2013;32(4):573–82.
9. Anantham D, Ernst A. Ultrasonography. In: Mason RJ, Broaddus VC, Murray JF, Nadel JA, editors. Murray and Nadel's textbook of respiratory medicine. Philadelphia: Saunders-Elsevier; 2010:445–60.
10. Bakhru RN, Schweickert WD. Intensive care ultrasound: I. Physics, equipment, and image quality. Ann Am Thorac Soc 2013;10(5): 540–48.
11. Abhishek C, Munta K, Rao SM, Chandrasekhar CN. End-tidal capnography and upper airway ultrasonography in the rapid confirmation of endotracheal tube placement in patients requiring intubation for general anaesthesia. Indian J Anaesth. 2017 Jun;61(6):486–89.
12. Osman A, Sum KM. Role of upper airway ultrasound in airway management. J Intensive Care. 2016 Aug 15;4:52.
13. Singh M, Chin KJ, Chan VW, Wong DT, Prasad GA, Yu E. Use of sonography for airway assessment: An observational study. J Ultrasound Med. 2010; 29:79–85
14. Chou HC, Tseng WP, Wang CH, Ma MH, Wang HP, Huang PC, Sim SS, Liao YC, Chen SY, Hsu CY, Yen ZS, Chang WT, Huang CH, Lien WC, Chen SC. Tracheal rapid ultrasound exam (T.R.U.E.) for confirming endotracheal tube placement during emergency intubation. Resuscitation. 2011 Oct;82(10):1279–84.
15. Raphael DT, Conard FU 3rd. Ultrasound confirmation of endotracheal tube placement. J Clin Ultrasound. 1987 Sep;15(7):459–62.
16. Mehta S. Intubation guide marks for correct tube placement. A clinical study. Anaesthesia 1991; 46:306–08.
17. Cavo JW. True vocal cord paralysis following intubation. Laryngoscope 1985; 95:1352–59.
18. Conrardy PA, Goodman LR, Lainge F, *et al*. Alteration of endotracheal tube position. Flexion and extension of the neck. Crit Care Med 1976; 4:8–12.
19. Tessaro MO, Salant EP, Arroyo AC, Haines LE, Dickman E. Tracheal rapid ultrasound saline test (T.R.U.S.T.) for confirming correct endotracheal tube depth in children. Resuscitation. 2015; 89:8–12.
20. Chen X, Zhai W, Yu Z, Geng J, Li M. Determining correct tracheal tube insertion depth by measuring distance between endotracheal tube cuff and vocal cords by ultrasound in Chinese adults: a prospective case-control study. BMJ Open. 2018 Dec 6;8(12): e023374
21. Doerschug KC, Schmidt GA. Intensive care ultrasound: III. Lung and pleural ultrasound for the intensivist. Ann Am Thorac Soc 2013;10(6):708–12.
22. Lichtenstein D. Lung ultrasound in the critically ill. In JL Vincent, editor. Yearbook of intensive care and emergency medicine. Heidelberg: Springer; 2004:625–44.
23. Lichtenstein D. Novel approaches to ultrasonography of the lung and pleural space: where are we now? Breathe 2017;13(2):100–11.

24. Mojoli F, Bouhemad B, Mongodi S, Lichtenstein D. Lung Ultrasound for Critically Ill Patients. Am J Respir Crit Care Med. 2019 Mar 15;199(6):701–14.
25. Bouhemad B, Mongodi S, Via G, Rouquette I. Ultrasound for "lung monitoring" of ventilated patients. Anesthesiology. 2015 Feb;122(2):437–47.
26. Tusman G, Acosta CM, Costantini M. Ultrasonography for the assessment of lung recruitment maneuvers. Crit Ultrasound J. 2016 Dec;8(1):8.
27. Tusman G, Bohm SH, Suarez-Sipmann F (2013) Alveolar recruitment during mechanical ventilation—where are we in 2013? Trends Anaesth Crit Care 3:238–45.
28. Tusman G, Bohm SH (2010) Prevention and reversal of lung collapse during the intra-operative period. Best Pract Clin Res Anaesth 24:183–97.
29. Pierrakos C, Smit MR, Pisani L, Paulus F, Schultz MJ, Constantin JM, Chiumello D, Mojoli F, Mongodi S, Bos LDJ. Lung Ultrasound Assessment of Focal and Non-focal Lung Morphology in Patients With Acute Respiratory Distress Syndrome. Front Physiol. 2021 Sep 14; 12:730857.1
30. Wang XT, Ding X, Zhang HM, Chen H, Su LX, Liu DW; Chinese Critical Ultrasound Study Group (CCUSG). Lung ultrasound can be used to predict the potential of prone positioning and assess prognosis in patients with acute respiratory distress syndrome. Crit Care. 2016 Nov 30;20(1):385.
31. Ding W, Shen Y, Yang J, He X, Zhang M. Diagnosis of pneumothorax by radiography and ultrasonography: a meta-analysis. Chest. 2011; 140:859–66.
32. Volpicelli G. Sonographic diagnosis of pneumothorax. Intensive Care Med 2011;37(2):224–32.
33. Bouhemad B, Liu ZH, Arbelot C, Zhang M, Ferrari F, Le-Guen M, *et al*. Ultrasound assessment of antibiotic-induced pulmonary reaeration in ventilator-associated pneumonia. Crit Care Med. 2010; 38:84–92
34. Mongodi S, Via G, Girard M, Rouquette I, Misset B, Braschi A, Mojoli F, Bouhemad B. Lung Ultrasound for Early Diagnosis of Ventilator-Associated Pneumonia. Chest. 2016 Apr;149(4):969–80.
35. Mekontso Dessap A, Charron C, Devaquet J, *et al*. Impact of acute hypercapnia and augmented positive end-expiratory pressure on right ventricle function in severe acute respiratory distress syndrome. Intensive Care Medicine. 2009;35(11):1850–58.
36. Jardin F, Vieillard-Baron A. Is there a safe plateau pressure in ARDS? The right heart only knows. Intensive Care Medicine. 2007;33(3):444–47.
37. Boissier F, Katsahian S, Razazi K, *et al*. Prevalence and prognosis of cor pulmonale during protective ventilation for acute respiratory distress syndrome. Intensive Care Medicine. 2013;39(10):1725–33.
38. Vieillard-Baron A, Prin S, Chergui K, *et al*. Echo-Doppler demonstration of acute cor pulmonale at the bedside in the medical intensive care unit. American Journal of Respiratory and Critical Care Medicine. 2002;166(10):1310–19.
39. Stanko LK, Jacobsohn E, Tam JW, *et al*. Transthoracic echocardiography: Impact on diagnosis and management in tertiary care intensive care units. Anaesthesia and Intensive Care. 2005;33(4):492–96.
40. Ryan T, Petrovic O, Dillon JC, *et al*. An echocardiographic index for separation of right ventricular volume and pressure overload. Journal of the American College of Cardiology. 1985;5(4):918-27.
41. Harjola VP, Mebazaa A, Čelutkienė J, *et al*. Contemporary management of acute right ventricular failure: A statement from the heart failure association and the working group on pulmonary circulation and right ventricular function of the European Society of Cardiology. European Journal of Heart Failure. 2016;18(3):226–41.

42. Cardenas LZ, Santana PV, Caruso P, Ribeiro de Carvalho CR, Pereira de Albuquerque AL. Diaphragmatic ultrasound correlates with inspiratory muscle strength and pulmonary function in healthy subjects. Ultrasound Med Biol. 2018; 44:786–93.
43. Holtzhausen S, Unger M, Lupton-Smith A, Hanekom S. An investigation into the use of ultrasound as a surrogate measure of diaphragm function. Heart Lung. 2018; 47:418–24.
44. Sarwal A, Walker FO, Cartwright MS. Neuromuscular ultrasound for evaluation of the diaphragm. Muscle Nerve. 2013 Mar;47(3):319–29.
45. Vivier E, Dessap AM, Dimassi S, Vargas F, Lyazidid A, Thille AW, *et al*. Diaphragm ultrasonography to estimate the work of breathing during non-invasive ventilation. Intensive Care Med. 2012; 38:796–803.
46. Vivier E, Roche-Campo F, Brochard L, Mekontso Dessap A. Determinants of diaphragm thickening fraction during mechanical ventilation: an ancillary study of a randomised trial. Eur Respir J. 2017; 50:1700783.
47. Jiang JR, Tsai TH, Jerng JS, Yu CJ, Wu HD, Yang PC. Ultrasonographic evaluation of liver/spleen movements and extubation outcome. Chest. 2004;126(1):179–85.
48. Spadaro S, Grasso S, Mauri T, Dalla Corte F, Alvisi V, Ragazzi R. Can diaphragmatic ultrasonography performed during the T-tube trial predict weaning failure The role of diaphragmatic rapid shallow breathing index. Crit Care. 2016;20(1):305–05.
49. Kim WY, Suh HJ, Hong SB, Koh Y, Lim CM. Diaphragm dysfunction assessed by ultrasonography influence on weaning from mechanical ventilation. Crit Care Med. 2011;39(12):2627–30.
50. Jung B, Moury PH, Mahul M, de Jong A, Galia F, Prades A. Diaphragmatic dysfunction in patients with ICU-acquired weakness and its impact on extubation failure. Intensive Care Med. 2016;42(5):853–61.
51. DiNino E, Gartman EJ, Sethi JM, McCool FD. Diaphragm ultrasound as a predictor of successful extubation from mechanical ventilation. Thorax. 2014;69(5):423–27.
52. Ferrari G, De Filippi G, Elia F, Panero F, Volpicelli G, Aprà F. Diaphragm ultrasound as a new index of discontinuation from mechanical ventilation. Crit Ultrasound J. 2014;6(1):8–8
53. Zedan, A.; Prada Mancilla, W. A..; Rey, P. Diaphragmatic Excursion in Healthy Adults: Normal Values. Analytical Prevalence Study. Rev. colomb. radiol. 2020, 31, 5374–78.
54. https://litfl.com/ultrasound-library/airway/ Accessed November 22, 2022.
55. Chenkin J, McCartney CJ, Jelic T, Romano M, Heslop C, Bandiera G. Defining the learning curve of point-of-care ultrasound for confirming endotracheal tube placement by emergency physicians. Crit Ultrasound J. 2015;7(1):14.
56. Wangüemert Pérez AL, Figueira Gonçalves JM, Hernández Pérez JM, Ramallo Fariña Y, Del Castillo Rodriguez JC. Prognostic value of lung ultrasound and its link with inflammatory biomarkers in patients with SARS-CoV-2 infection. Respir Med Res. 2021; 79:100809.
57. Dell'Aquila P, Raimondo P, Racanelli V, De Luca P, De Matteis S, Pistone A, Melodia R, Crudele L, Lomazzo D, Solimando AG, Moschetta A, Vacca A, Grasso S, Procacci V, Orso D, Vetrugno L. Integrated lung ultrasound score for early clinical decision-making in patients with COVID-19: results and implications. Ultrasound J. 2022;14(1):21.

CHAPTER 35

Basics of Neonatal Ventilation

❑ Tisha Ann Skariah

ABSTRACT

Mechanical ventilation is a lifesaving intervention in preterm and term neonates who are critically ill. A fundamental grasp of respiratory physiology and the underlying disease-induced changes in respiratory function is essential for employing mechanical ventilation. Possessing a thorough understanding of these concepts and fundamental principles of traditional ventilation is crucial for any healthcare professional, whether in medicine or allied fields, engaged in the management of respiratory care for neonates. This chapter aims at novice practitioners to describe the respiratory physiology and initial settings of invasive ventilation in some of the commonest neonatal respiratory conditions.

INTRODUCTION

The approach to respiratory support in newborns differs from that in older children and adults for two reasons. Firstly, the 'normal' respiratory system is in a developing state, with both the neurological control and the respiratory tract at different stages of anatomic and physiologic maturity, depending on gestational age. The second difference relates to the impact of the different neonatal diseases on neonatal respiratory physiology and how the latter influences unique choices in the mode of respiratory support and settings. The objective of mechanical ventilation is to achieve oxygenation and carbon dioxide removal while concurrently striving to minimize potential lung damage. Neonatal mechanical ventilation is no different from adult or pediatric mechanical ventilation but it requires a deeper understanding of the developing lungs as the same disease can present differently at different stages of development.

RESPIRATORY PHYSIOLOGY FOR VENTILATING THE NEWBORN

Newborns are not merely small children or smaller adults. The challenge is to be aware of the many unique aspects of the newborn's respiratory physiology and control of breathing and deliver optimum ventilation and oxygenation. The pattern of breathing in premature newborns is profoundly affected which makes the breathing highly irregular, with frequent pauses or apneas. The heightened activity of peripheral chemoreceptors and the proximity of eupneic and threshold partial pressure of carbon dioxide (PCO_2) contribute to a significant susceptibility to respiratory instability within this population.[1] For better understanding, we will discuss lung mechanics briefly in relation to the respiratory conditions discussed in this chapter.

Lung Mechanics

Compliance

Respiration fundamentally involves a mechanical mechanism wherein the muscles of the thorax and abdomen collaboratively operate under the control of the brain to generate the necessary pressures for lung expansion. The elastic property of the respiratory system is represented as compliance, which is the change in volume resulting from the change in pressure ($\Delta V/\Delta P$). It can be practically calculated by the formula: Tidal volume (V_T)/ pressure change (PIP-PEEP). This would mean that the less compliant lung will need more pressure to displace some volumes in it.[2] In the case of diseases like respiratory distress syndrome (RDS), the compliance is low due to the insufficient pool of surfactant leading to atelectasis and low lung volumes while in the case of meconium aspiration syndrome (MAS) due to partial or complete airway obstruction, there is air trapping leading to high compliance.

Resistance and Time Constant

The other property is the resistance of the respiratory system which has contributing factors from the tissues (viscous resistance) and from the movement of the air in the airways. It can be computed by the formula—change in pressure/flow.[3] In newborns, heightened viscous resistance arises due to the presence of immature small lungs, which have relatively fewer terminal air spaces, increased tissue density, and elevated interstitial fluid, particularly in the initial transition period after birth. Airway resistance refers to the impediment occurring between the movement of gas molecules within the stream and along the respiratory system's walls. Airway resistance is also relatively high in newborns because of the small diameter of the airways in the newborn lung. Resistance is usually lower during inspiration, as lung distending forces (negative intrathoracic pressure during spontaneous breathing or positive airway pressure during mechanical ventilation) increase the diameter of the tracheobronchial system during inspiration. In the case of ventilated neonates there is added resistance to gas flow in the artificial airway, and breathing circuit. The clinical relevance is that in the case of high viscous resistance lungs such as RDS, a higher inspiratory transpulmonary pressure is needed; and in the case of high airway resistance lungs as in MAS, a longer inspiratory and expiratory time to inflate and deflate.[3] This is reflected as the time constant of a respiratory system which is the product of compliance and resistance. One time constant means 63% of pressure equilibration occurs and by 3 times constants 95% of equilibration is reached. The time constant is applicable for both the inspiratory and expiratory phases. The inspiratory time and indirect expiratory time are dependent on time constants.[4] This is the guiding factor for deciding the inspiratory and expiratory time during any pressure controlled/targeted modes.

Choosing the Ventilator Mode: How to set it up?

The fundamental aim of mechanical ventilation is to recover lung function while mitigating the risk of ventilator-induced lung injury (VILI), a significant factor for the onset of bronchopulmonary dysplasia (BPD) in preterm and extremely preterm neonates. Consequently, implementing a lung-protective ventilation approach during invasive mechanical ventilation poses a crucial challenge in neonatal intensive care units (NICU). Ideally, this strategy should steer clear of high tidal volume (V_T) usage, address atelectasis, maintain stability in lung units throughout both inhalation and exhalation, and avoid elevated concentrations of oxygen.[5] The common classification of modes of respiratory support are pressure control (PC) and volume control (VC). As the names imply, in PC, the clinician predetermines how much pressure the ventilator delivers while in VC, the user sets the desired tidal volume. Newer technologies such as microprocessors and flow sensors based on the hot wire anemometer principle or pneumotachograph, allow the measurement of small gas volumes very close to the patient. The ability to reliably measure the volume of gases delivered to even the smallest of preterm neonates has seen PC ventilation rapidly fall out of use. Hybrid modes integrate features of both pressure and volume control.

There is a growing body of evidence to avoid invasive mechanical ventilation via the endotracheal tube whenever feasible for this population particularly. Intubation and invasive mechanical ventilation are warranted in cases of severe respiratory failure, characterized by significantly compromised oxygenation and alveolar ventilation, diminished respiratory effort, and, in specific situations, circulatory failure.[6] Upon the decision to initiate invasive mechanical ventilation, precautions to minimize ventilator-induced lung injury (VILI) should be taken, involving the selection of the suitable ventilation mode and corresponding settings.[7] The following are the basic parameters that need to be set up for any ventilator for the neonate.

a. Positive end expiratory pressure (PEEP)
b. Peak inspiratory time (PIP)
c. Inspiratory time (Ti)
d. Respiratory rate
e. Flowrate
f. Fraction of inspired oxygen (FiO_2)
g. Tidal volume (V_T)
h. Trigger sensitivity

The following section we will discuss the rational of theses settings

Positive end Expiratory Pressure (PEEP)

There is no universal PEEP setting ideal for all lung diseases, or even for one disease, or even for one individual through their disease. The purpose of all ventilation should be to keep the lung volume at functional residual capacity (FRC). At this volume, the pulmonary vascular pressures are minimal. Hyperinflated lung would impede the venous return and may result in reduced preload and shock. With increasing lung volumes—small alveolar vessel resistance decreases but large extra alveolar vessel resistance increases. The exact opposite occurs with reducing lung volume. The pulmonary vascular resistance (PVR) is lowest at FRC. Over-expanded or under-expanded lungs raise the PVR (**Fig. 35.1**).[8] The normal range of this pressure is 3–5 cmH_2O. We decide on this setting depending on the lung volume status. For example, in severe RDS, PEEP of 5 cmH_2O could be set, whereas in the case of severe MAS with over-distension, we may choose a value of 3–4 cmH_2O. In cases of pulmonary hemorrhage, we could consider giving a slightly higher PEEP of 5.5–6 cmH_2O, to reduce bleeding. These values are arbitrary and vary according to the case and the protocol practiced. We can look for clinical lung expansion which is assessed by Chest X-ray. The normal expansion is 8 spaces posterior and 6 spaces anteriorly.

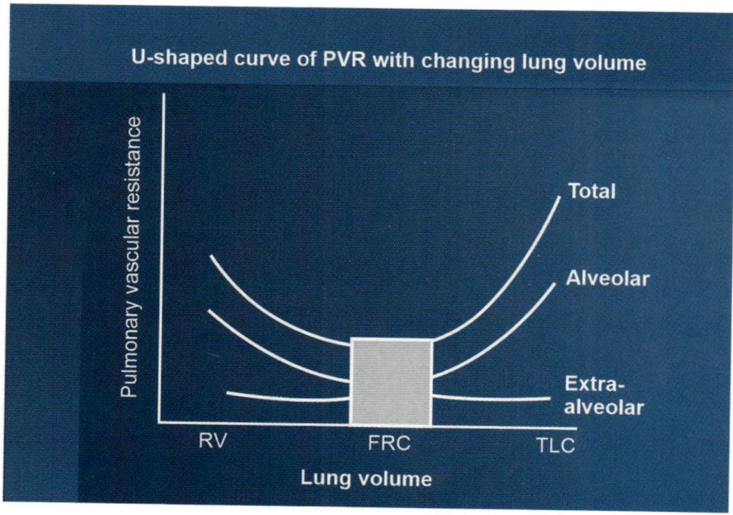

Fig. 35.1: Effect of changing lung volume on PVR.[9] PVR—pulmonary vascular resistance; RV—residual volume; FRC—functional residual capacity; TLC—total lung capacity.

Peak Inspiratory Pressure (PIP)

The pressure required to overcome respiratory system recoil, is estimated by the normal intrathoracic pressure (about –1 to –7 cm H_2O) and about –1 to –7 cmH_2O and that is required to drive gases through the ventilator circuit (in most neonatal ventilators this is 6 cmH_2O). Thus, a PIP of approximately 12 cmH_2O may be sufficient for normal lungs. The former varies according to the respiratory system compliance influenced by the underlying lung condition and the severity thereof. Visually, the adequacy of PIP can be estimated from the chest rise and the presence of retractions. The measured tidal volume is a guide for setting the appropriate pressure for ventilation.[12] PIP in excess of 25–27 cmH_2O is associated with lung injury and, with other indicators such as the oxygenation index or blood gas parameters, signals the need for additional therapies such as high-frequency ventilation (HFV) and treatment for persistent pulmonary hypertension of the newborn (PPHN).

Inspiratory Time (Ti)

As previously discussed in this chapter, the respiratory time constants, which dictate how quickly lung volume re-establishes equilibrium after a pressure change, are influenced by the compliance and resistance of the respiratory system.[4] Neonates facing reduced lung compliance due to respiratory distress syndrome (RDS) exhibit extremely short time constants, necessitating a very brief inspiratory time (Ti) for equilibrium (as short as 0.15 s). However, this brevity may not provide sufficient time for tidal recruitment during the inspiratory phase. Therefore, setting Ti in diseased lungs involves finding a balance between minimizing the duration of plateau pressure at peak inflation and ensuring ample time for the recruiting effect of the plateau pressure. Clinical trials comparing long Ti (0.66–1.0 s) with short Ti (0.33–0.5 s) have subsequently demonstrated advantages in the shorter Ti group, including a slight reduction in mortality and a significant decrease in the risk of air leak, particularly in newborns with RDS.[10,11] Inappropriately long or short set Ti may lead to desynchrony, with the neonate exhaling against the ventilator inflation pressure, or end up having an interruption of expiration with an inspiratory effort. Precise adjustments of Ti can be made based on the flow waveform. Recommended ranges for within which to set Ti in the ventilated neonate are 0.25–0.4s in preterm neonates and 0.4–0.6s in those at full term.[8] For example, in MAS the resistance of the airway is elevated to a greater extent than the reduction of compliance of the lung. So, the overall effect is increased time constants, so slightly higher Ti is used. However, the expiratory time constant is also important, and care should be taken that adequate expiratory time (Te) is also given for expiration.

Respiratory Rate

The rates are determined by the underlying disease condition and the work of breathing (WOB). For example, the case of a severe RDS in the acute stage may require a rate of 50–60 bpm whereas in the case of a neonate intubated due to apnea of prematurity (AOP) may require only 20–25 bpm.

Flow Rate

Generally, the flow rate for all neonatal ventilation is set between 4–8 L/min. Some devices have fixed flow while in others the flow is adjustable. The calculation of flow is based on minute ventilation, which is the product of tidal volume and respiratory rate. The minimum flow required for effective ventilation is 3–5 times the minute ventilation. Inadequate flow setting will cause desynchrony thus leading to increased work of breathing from the neonate. A high flow rate setting would cause a faster flow to the neonate leading to inadequate distribution of the volumes whereas a low flow setting will eventually end up with air trapping.

Fraction of Inspired Oxygen (FiO_2)

To prevent oxygen tissue injury, the general strategy is to start with a lower concentration of 40–50% and titrate according to the target oxygen saturations, with simultaneous appropriate pressures. In some disease states such as MAS with PPHN and CDH with PPHN, the high normal PaO_2 of 80–90 mmHg should be targeted, beyond this there is no extrapulmonary vasodilation expected.

Tidal Volume (V_T)

As mentioned previously, the measurement of small tidal volumes was a big breakthrough in neonatal ventilation. Providing adequate tidal volume for optimum gas exchange and maintaining lung recruitment is the aim of the normal or diseased lung. This becomes more challenging with the background of immaturity, but the latest generation of ventilators helps us achieve this. Tidal volumes are measured during pressure-controlled ventilation and the new hybrid modes enable us to set the target and deliver it with adjusting pressures. It is suggested that the range of neonatal tidal volume in a healthy lung is probably 4-6 ml/kg with minute ventilation of approximately 0.2–0.3 L/min/kg. A lower tidal volume may result in lung collapse and VILI by atelectotrauma whereas larger tidal volumes would increase VILI risk by overdistension.[12–16]

Trigger Sensitivity

The triggering process aims to align the neonate's initiation of breath with the onset of ventilator inflation, delivering the predetermined pressure or volume.[17–19] Ideally, the trigger should be appropriately and optimally configured to accommodate newborns of varying weights. The trigger threshold should surpass artifacts produced by factors like condensation and secretions. If the neonate triggers at a high rate, adjusting the trigger sensitivity is one potential mechanism to address it. However, this adjustment may increase the work of breathing (WOB), which might not be the desired outcome. Therefore, it is essential to investigate auto-triggering caused by moisture condensation in the circuit and the neonate's movements leading to inappropriate triggering before making any adjustments to the settings.

Disease-Specific Ventilation Strategies

Mastering the skill of ventilation in newborns demands a particularly nuanced comprehension of the specific context in which it is employed, possibly more so than for any other age group. The diverse range of scenarios in which ventilation is administered to newborns is exceptionally vast, and each pathophysiological condition necessitates a tailored approach to ensure optimal support. In the gross classification of respiratory disorders that affect the newborn, we can classify it to the conditions that affect the lung parenchymal (diffuse and localized), airway disorders, lung hypoplasia with or without congenital diaphragmatic hernia and the non-respiratory causes in which the lungs would be near normal. In this chapter, we will take you through the initial ventilatory settings based on the understanding of lung mechanics.[13,21–23] provides the common conditions in which conventional ventilation is used in the newborn and it includes the recommendations of initial settings for each condition. Further elaboration of the physiological rationale and available evidence for ventilator settings is explained hereunder.

Lung Parenchymal Diseases

Diffuse or homogenous lung parenchymal diseases

Common diseases that affect the lungs of the newborn in a homogenous pattern are RDS, pulmonary edema, and transient tachypnea of the newborn (TTNB). Surfactant insufficiency and or inadequate surfactant circulation along with the immaturity of the developing parenchymal cause alveolar collapse leading to low compliance with usually no effect on the resistance and thus a short time constant. To expand the lungs with reduced compliance, it is crucial to deliver a sufficient volume of air/oxygen, typically propelled by appropriate flow and pressure with an adequate inspiratory time. A short time constant implies a rapid emptying and collapse of the lung during expiration, and this is mitigated by counteraction with adequate positive end-expiratory pressure (PEEP). Employing a higher ventilator rate can be beneficial, as it may prevent atelectasis during the expiratory phase and constrain peak inspiratory pressure (PIP) by keeping the inspiratory time brief. It is recommended to start with PC-Assist control (AC) ventilation with volume guarantee (VG).[7] Other settings are discussed in **Table 35.1**.

Table 35.1: Common neonatal respiratory disease-specific initial ventilator settings

Conditions	Lung mechanics alterations	Mode of preference	PEEP (cmH_2O)	Ti (s)	PIP* (cmH_2O)	Targeted VT (ml/kg)	RR (bpm)	Considerations
Lung parenchymal disease								
Diffuse lung parenchymal pathology								
✦ RDS	Preterm neonates with low lung volumes, surfactant deficiency leading to micro atelectasis—compliant chest wall, low FRC with low compliance and normal resistance.	PC-AC/ SIPPV or SIMV with VG	5–8	0.3–0.35	Mild 14–16 Moderate 18–20 Severe 20–23	4–6	30–60	Judicious use of PEEP with fixed volume targets are the lung protective strategies to be considered for optimizing the lung volumes with minimal VILI. Guarded use of PIP with close monitoring of the volumes achieved is key for preventing further injury.
✦ Pneumonia edema ✦ TTNB ✦ Pulmonary hemorrhage	Surfactant inactivation, atelectasis – low FRC, compliance and resistance could increase depending on secretions.		5.5–6 (initial) 8–10 (acute phase of hemorrhage)	0.3–0.4	15–17		40–50	
Heterogenous lung pathology								
✦ Atelectatic	Term neonates with aspiration syndromes (MAS), and air leak syndromes will present with airway obstruction, areas of collapse, and or areas of overdistension-increased FRC with high resistance and low compliance.	PC-AC/ SIPPV or SIMV with VG	4–5	0.40	16–18	5–6	30–40	Partial or complete obstruction may result in air trapping. Relatively normal lung units may overdistend. The use of a lower rate should be considered. In the case of surfactant dysfunction, it should be treated as RDS.
✦ Hyperinflated			3–4	0.35	14–16			
Airway disorders	Airway obstruction which could lead to air trapping along with alveolar	PC-SIMV or AC/ SIPPV	3–5	0.3–0.35	12–14	4–6	30–40	Settings are influenced by whether the obstruction can be relieved by the pos

Contd.

Table 35.1: Common neonatal respiratory disease-specific initial ventilator settings (Contd.)

Conditions	Lung mechanics alterations	Mode of preference	PEEP (cmH_2O)	Ti (s)	PIP* (cmH_2O)	Targeted VT (ml/kg)	RR (bpm)	Considerations
	hypoventilation – normal lung compliance with high resistance requiring longer expiratory time.							itioning of the endotracheal tube tip beyond the point of maximal narrowing. Splinting of the airway by titrating PEEP. Slower rates with longer Ti and Te should be considered due to high resistance.
Lung hypoplasia	Low lung compliance related to small total lung volume with normal resistance. The hypoplastic lung is vulnerable to overdistension, stretch injury, and high PVR.	PC-AC/ SIPPV or SIMV with VG	4–6	0.25–0.4	<25	3–5	40–60	Overinflation of the lungs and the use of high VT/ PIP should be avoided. HFV is considered if PIP shoots above 25 cm H_2O, or if there is refractory hypoxic respiratory failure.
Extrapulmonary conditions	Poor respiratory drive, physiological consequences of episodic apnea (bradycardia and desaturation), and postoperative cases with healthy lungs —normal compliance and resistance with normal FRC.	PC-SIMV or AC/ SIPPV with VG	4–5	0.35–0.4	12–14	3–4	20–25	Minimal ventilatory support as the lungs in this condition is often relatively with normal lung mechanics. VILI should be avoided by the use of incongruous settings.

FRC: functional residual capacity, PVR: pulmonary vascular resistance, RDS: respiratory distress syndrome, TTNB: transient tachypnea of the newborn, MAS: meconium aspiration syndrome, PEEP: positive end-expiratory pressure, PIP: peak inspiratory pressure, VT: tidal volume, PC: pressure control, SIMV: synchronized intermittent mandatory ventilation, SIPPV: synchronized intermittent positive pressure ventilation, AC: assist/control, VG- volume guarantee, HFV: high-frequency ventilation, Ti: inspiratory time, Te: expiratory time, PSV: pressure support ventilation, VILI: Ventilator-induced lung injury, s: seconds, bpm: breaths per minute.

*PIP is subjective to sufficient chest rise, severity of pathology and the targeted tidal volume of the neonate.

Heterogenous Lung Diseases

Conditions that affect the lungs in a non-uniform pattern include MAS, pneumonia, aspiration pneumonia, and pneumothorax. In the case of MAS, pathophysiology depends on the distribution of meconium within the lung causing partial and/or complete obstruction of the airways. It has a heterogeneous alveolar lung disease pattern with areas of inflammation and obstruction of airways with areas of atelectasis next to overinflated areas.[12] The overinflated areas are often seen to have a low to normal compliance and high resistance resulting in a longer time constant. Hence, the ventilation strategy of ventilation is adequate PEEP without overdistension, and lower respiratory rates allowing time for exhalation to occur.

Airway Disorders

Conditions that cause supra-glottic, glottic, or sub-glottic airway obstruction like severe Pierre Robin sequence, congenital tracheomalacia, and even esophageal atresia can cause airway compromise that requires an endotracheal tube for airway patency.[12] In most situations, the lungs would be healthy and may only require supportive ventilation.

Lung Hypoplasia with or without Congenital Diaphragmatic Hernia

Congenital hypoplastic lungs with or without congenital diaphragmatic hernia (CDH) are conditions in which the lungs are not developed, or the functionality is compromised. Ventilating these conditions has not only the aim to provide adequate oxygenation but also to avoid the occurrence of PPHN as they are highly susceptible for the latter to develop. With the functioning part of the limited lung, we must adhere to aggressive ventilation strategies. The guiding principle is to ventilate with adequate PEEP and the lowest possible PIP (i.e. a smaller than usual tidal volume).[7]

Extrapulmonary Conditions

These conditions would have healthy lungs where the lung mechanics are not compromised as in the case of apnea, asphyxia, and shock. The ventilatory settings in these conditions are just minimal to provide adequate oxygenation and ventilation. However, these settings are subjective to the worsening of the respiratory system and require close monitoring of the respiratory mechanisms.

Chronic Lung Disease (CLD)/Bronchopulmonary Dysplasia (BPD)

It is a sequel to the injury of the extreme preterm r preterm lungs due to ventilation strategies which results in overdistended, highly compliant lungs along with damage to airway morphology resulting in high resistance. As the name suggests, it is a chronic condition and does not come under the umbrella of initial care. The objective is to continue supportive care and optimize oxygenation and ventilation.

Proportionality of Settings

The various parameters of ventilation should be proportionally moving in the same direction. This is a fundamental principle, e.g. ventilation with FiO_2 of 80% with PIP of 12 cmH_2O and PEEP of 3 cmH_2O is inappropriate. Likewise, if the settings read rate of 50 bpm, PIP of 12 cmH_2O with PEEP of 4 cmH_2O, it is again incongruous whereas FiO_2 of 30% with PIP of 16 cmH_2O, PEEP of 5 cmH_2O and rate of 40 bpm it is proportional.

A Note on Non-invasive Ventilation (NIV) in Neonates

Ventilation of the newborn without the mention of NIV would be incomplete. NIV is one of the most popular approaches of respiratory support in the NICU. It has found its way to the delivery room too, and we use it as early as possible in neonates with respiratory distress to avoid intubation. The use of non-invasive respiratory support in the labor room and NICU has been shown to decrease the need for invasive ventilation in extremely preterm neonates without increasing major morbidities.[24] Some of the commonest modes of NIV include nasal continuous positive airway pressure (NCPAP) and nasal intermittent positive pressure ventilation (NIPPV). As the name suggests NCPAP is providing a continuous pressure that helps in splitting the airway and helping in maintaining adequate FRC, whereas NIPPV has an addition of one more pressure. This bi-level mode provides a higher mean airway pressure (MAP) that would improve gas exchange compared with NCPAP.[25] Over the past thirty years, NCPAP/NIPPV has progressively become the primary preference for respiratory support in preterm and extremely preterm neonates. The key factors contributing to the success of non-invasive ventilation (NIV) include prompt initiation, the proper and assertive administration of surfactant/caffeine, optimal humidification, suitable nasal interface, and attentive nursing care.[26]

Conclusion

In conclusion, a comprehensive comprehension of neonatal lung physiology is essential for effective respiratory support. It is important to recognize that the majority of neonates experiencing respiratory distress are at various stages of lung development and may be particularly vulnerable to ventilator-induced lung injury (VILI). Therefore, adopting a physiology-centric approach appears rational in clinical practice. Each NICU should establish specific protocols grounded in consensus and the best clinical evidence to mitigate the variability in approaches commonly adopted by individual clinicians. The primary goal should be to furnish safe and efficient ventilator management for unwell neonates necessitating invasive mechanical ventilation.

References

1. Alvaro R, Rigatto H. Control of breathing in newborns. Neonatology: A Practical Approach to Neonatal Diseases. 2012:415–22.
2. Keszler M, Abubakar K. Physiologic principles. Assisted ventilation of the neonate: evidence-based approach to newborn respiratory care. 6th ed. Philadelphia, PA: Elsevier Health Sciences Division. 2016 Sep 2:8–30.
3. Pillow JJ, Stocks J, Sly PD, Hantos Z. Partitioning of airway and parenchymal mechanics in unsedated newborn infants. Pediatric research. 2005 Dec;58(6):1210–5.
4. Bancalari E. Inadvertent positive end-expiratory pressure during mechanical ventilation. The Journal of Pediatrics. 1986;108(4):567–9.
5. Van Kaam A. Lung-protective ventilation in neonatology. Neonatology. 2011;99(4):338–41.
6. Carlo WA, Martin RJ. Principles of neonatal assisted ventilation. Pediatric Clinics of North America. 1986 Feb 1;33(1):221–37.
7. Chakkarapani AA, Adappa R, Ali SK, Gupta S, Soni NB, Chicoine L, Hummler HD. "Current concepts in assisted mechanical ventilation in the neonate"-Part 2: Understanding various modes of mechanical ventilation and recommendations for individualized disease-based

approach in neonates. International Journal of Pediatrics and Adolescent Medicine. 2020 Dec 1;7(4):201–8.

8. Chakkarapani AA, Adappa R, Ali SK, Gupta S, Soni NB, Chicoine L, Hummler HD. "Current concepts of mechanical ventilation in neonates"–Part 1: Basics. International Journal of Pediatrics and Adolescent Medicine. 2020 Mar 1;7(1):15-20.
9. Shekerdemian L, Bohn D. Cardiovascular effects of mechanical ventilation. Archives of disease in childhood. 1999 May 1;80(5):475–80.
10. Tarnowmordi W. Multicenter randomized controlled trial of high against low-frequency positive pressure ventilation. Archives of Disease in Childhood-Fetal and Neonatal Edition. 1991 Jul 1;66(7):770-5.
11. Kamlin CO, Davis PG. Long versus short inspiratory times in neonates receiving mechanical ventilation. Cochrane Database of Systematic Reviews. 2003(4).
12. Dargaville PA, Keszler M. Setting the ventilator in the NICU. Pediatric and Neonatal Mechanical Ventilation: From Basics to Clinical Practice. 2015:1101-25.
13. Yoder BA, Goldsmith JP, Karotkin EH, Keszler M, Suresh GK. Mechanical ventilation: disease-specific strategies. Assisted Ventilation of the Neonate, 6th ed. Philadelphia, PA: Elsevier. 2017.
14. Wheeler K, Klingenberg C, McCallion N, Morley CJ, Davis PG. Volume-targeted versus pressure-limited ventilation in the neonate. Cochrane Database Syst Rev 2010.
15. Keszler M, Abubakar KM. Volume guarantee ventilation. Clinics in perinatology. 2007 Mar 1;34(1):107-16.
16. Klingenberg C, Wheeler KI, McCallion N, Morley CJ, Davis PG. Volume-targeted versus pressure-limited ventilation in neonates. Cochrane Database of Systematic Reviews. 2017(10).
17. Keszler M. Volume-targeted ventilation. Early human development. 2006 Dec 1;82(12):811–8.
18. Cleary JP, Bernstein G, Mannino FL, Heldt GP. Improved oxygenation during synchronized intermittent mandatory ventilation in neonates with respiratory distress syndrome: a randomized, crossover study. The Journal of Pediatrics. 1995 Mar 1;126(3):407–11.
19. Bernstein G, Mannino FL, Heldt GP, Callahan JD, Bull DH, Sola A, Ariagno RL, Hoffman GL, Frantz III ID, Troche BI, Roberts JL. Randomized multicenter trial comparing synchronized and conventional intermittent mandatory ventilation in neonates. The Journal of Pediatrics. 1996 Apr 1;128(4):453–63.
20. Chen Jy, Ling Up, Chen JH. Comparison of synchronized and conventional intermittent mandatory ventilation in neonates. Pediatrics International. 1997 Oct;39(5):578–83.
21. Sweet DG, Carnielli V, Greisen G, Hallman M, Ozek E, Plavka R, Saugstad OD, Simeoni U, Speer CP, Vento M, Visser GH. European consensus guidelines on the management of respiratory distress syndrome-2016 update. Neonatology. 2017;111(2):107–25.
22. Chettri S, Bhat BV, Adhisivam B. Current concepts in the management of meconium aspiration syndrome. The Indian Journal of Pediatrics. 2016 Oct;83:1125–30.
23. Logan JW, Cotten CM, Goldberg RN, Clark RH. Mechanical ventilation strategies in the management of congenital diaphragmatic hernia. InSeminars in pediatric surgery 2007 May 1 (Vol. 16, No. 2, pp. 115–125). WB Saunders.
24. Govindaswami B, Nudelman M, Narasimhan SR, Huang A, Misra S, Urquidez G, Kifle A, Stemmle M, Angell C, Patel R, Anderson C. Eliminating risk of intubation in very preterm infants with noninvasive cardiorespiratory support in the delivery room and neonatal intensive care unit. BioMed Research International. 2019 Oct;2019.
25. Claure N, Bancalari E. Non-invasive ventilation in premature infants. Archives of Disease in Childhood-Fetal and Neonatal Edition. 2015 Jan 1;100(1):F2-3.
26. Anne RP, Murki S. Noninvasive respiratory support in neonates: a review of current evidence and practices. Indian Journal of Pediatrics. 2021 Jul;88(7):670–8.

Index

D

E

F

N

O

P

Q

R

S